GW00776121

Hand-Rearing Birds

Hand-Rearing Birds

Laurie J. Gage, DVM
Rebecca S. Duerr, DVM

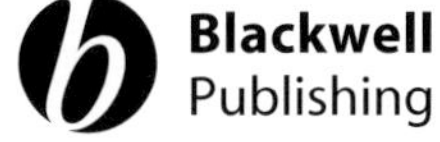

Laurie J. Gage, DVM, served as the Director of Veterinary Services for Six Flags Marine World in Vallejo, California, for 23 years, and then took a veterinary position at the Los Angeles Zoo, where she worked with a large variety of mammals and birds. She is presently the Big Cat Specialist for the United States Department of Agriculture, and also serves as a marine mammal advisor to that agency. She edited *Hand-Rearing Wild and Domestic Mammals* (Blackwell Publishers 2002).

Rebecca S. Duerr, DVM, received her BS in Marine Biology from San Francisco State University and her DVM from the University of California Davis, where she will complete an MPVM degree on oiled seabird care at the UCD Wildlife Health Center in 2007. Since 1988, she has served as staff at several California wildlife organizations including the Marine Mammal Center in Sausalito and Wildlife Rescue, Inc. in Palo Alto. She currently works as an avian and exotic animal veterinarian in Northern California. She serves on the Board of Directors and as wildlife shelter veterinarian for the Wildlife Care Association of Sacramento. She teaches baby bird care and avian trauma and fracture management at various wildlife rehabilitation centers.

©2007 Blackwell Publishing
All rights reserved

Blackwell Publishing Professional
2121 State Avenue, Ames, Iowa 50014, USA

Orders: 1-800-862-6657
Office: 1-515-292-0140
Fax: 1-515-292-3348
Web site: www.blackwellprofessional.com

Blackwell Publishing Ltd
9600 Garsington Road, Oxford OX4 2DQ, UK
Tel.: +44 (0)1865 776868

Blackwell Publishing Asia
550 Swanston Street, Carlton, Victoria 3053, Australia
Tel.: +61 (0)3 8359 1011

Authorization to photocopy items for internal or personal use, or the internal or personal use of specific clients, is granted by Blackwell Publishing, provided that the base fee is paid directly to the Copyright Clearance Center, 222 Rosewood Drive, Danvers, MA 01923. For those organizations that have been granted a photocopy license by CCC, a separate system of payments has been arranged. The fee codes for users of the Transactional Reporting Service is ISBN-13: 978-0-8138-0666-2/2007.

First edition, 2007

Library of Congress Cataloging-in-Publication Data
Gage, Laurie J.
Hand-rearing birds / Laurie J. Gage, Rebecca Duerr.
p. cm.
Includes bibliographical references and index.
ISBN 978-0-8138-0666-2 (alk. paper)
1. Cage birds. 2. Captive wild birds.
I. Duerr, Rebecca. II. Title.
SF461.G33 2007
636.6′8–dc22
2007006837

Cover photo captions: Upper left: Three 42-day-old Toco toucans (photo by Martin Vince, Riverbanks Zoo); Upper center: three 3–5-day-old Northern Mockingbirds (photo by Rebecca Duerr), note yellow color inside mouths and grey down on heads and backs; Upper right: three House Finch nestlings (photo by Rebecca Duerr), note red color inside mouths and four rows of down on heads; Lower right: California Condor chick, 1-1/2 days old, feeding with a condor puppet, (photo by Mike Wallace, Los Angeles Zoo); Lower left: Syringe-feeding a 33-day-old Blue and Gold Macaw (photo © Joanne Abramson).

Disclaimer
The contents of this work are intended to further general scientific research, understanding, and discussion only and are not intended and should not be relied upon as recommending or promoting a specific method, diagnosis, or treatment by practitioners for any particular patient. The publisher and the author make no representations or warranties with respect to the accuracy or completeness of the contents of this work and specifically disclaim all warranties, including without limitation any implied warranties of fitness for a particular purpose. In view of ongoing research, equipment modifications, changes in governmental regulations, and the constant flow of information relating to the use of medicines, equipment, and devices, the reader is urged to review and evaluate the information provided in the package insert or instructions for each medicine, equipment, or device for, among other things, any changes in the instructions or indication of usage and for added warnings and precautions. Readers should consult with a specialist where appropriate. The fact that an organization or Website is referred to in this work as a citation and/or a potential source of further information does not mean that the author or the publisher endorses the information the organization or Website may provide or recommendations it may make. Further, readers should be aware that Internet Websites listed in this work may have changed or disappeared between when this work was written and when it is read. No warranty may be created or extended by any promotional statements for this work. Neither the publisher nor the author shall be liable for any damages arising herefrom.

The last digit is the print number: 9 8 7 6 5 4 3 2 1

Table of Contents

Contributors

Robyn Arnold has been the Bird Department Supervisor at Six Flags Marine World for the past 10 years. During the 14 years employed in the bird department, she has raised over 30 Rainbow and 10 Perfect Lorikeet chicks. She has been working with birds for over 18 years. Her bird experience includes handling and training a variety of species, including parrots, raptors, penguins, and many others.

Veronica Bowers has been a wildlife rehabilitator for 9 years and works exclusively with wild native passerines. She is currently the Director of Avian Care for Sonoma County Wildlife Rescue and is co-leader of insectivore care for WildCare of Marin County, CA.

Kateri J. Davis lives with her husband and daughter near Eugene, Oregon, and together they run the Davis Lund Aviaries. They have specialized in raising and breeding softbill birds for over 15 years.

Rebecca S. Duerr, DVM, received her BS in Marine Biology from San Francisco State University and her DVM from the University of California Davis, where she will complete an MPVM degree on oiled seabird care at the UCD Wildlife Health Center in 2007. Since 1988, she has served as staff at several California wildlife organizations, including the Marine Mammal Center in Sausalito and Wildlife Rescue, Inc. in Palo Alto. She currently works as an avian and exotic animal veterinarian in Northern California. She serves on the Board of Directors and as wildlife shelter veterinarian for the Wildlife Care Association of Sacramento. She teaches baby bird care and avian trauma and fracture management at various wildlife rehabilitation centers. Her favorite baby birds are hatchling American Robins, but House Finches hold a close second place.

Nancy Eilertsen has been a wildlife rehabilitator since 1988. She is the founder and director of East Valley Wildlife based in Phoenix, Arizona, and is state and federally licensed. She is a coauthor of *A Flying Chance* passerine rehabilitation manual and is at work on a second edition focusing on identification of juveniles.

Sandie Elliott, combining a BS in Avian Science with 10 years as an Emergency Medical Technician, has devoted 28 years to the rescue and rehabilitation of wildlife in California. Although her passion lies with avian species, as Founder/Director of Spirit-Wild, a wildlife rescue rehabilitation organization in Lake County California, Sandie works with all species of birds and mammals.

Penny Elliston, one of the founders of Wildlife Rescue of New Mexico, has been working with hummingbirds and other avian species since 1980. She has authored and coauthored a number of papers on hummingbird growth, care, and behavior.

Meryl Faulkner has been a full-time home care volunteer with Project Wildlife, a rehabilitation group in San Diego County, for 20 years. She has raised and rehabilitated various avian species, and also skunks, but specializes in sea and shorebirds. She captive-rears and rehabilitates California Least Terns and Western Snowy Plovers (sometimes hatched from salvaged eggs) for local, state, and federal agencies.

Lisa Fosco is a wildlife biologist and a licensed veterinary technician. She has been involved in wildlife rehabilitation for over 20 years and has been an instructor for the International Wildlife Rehabilitation Council for the last 10 years. Lisa has published several papers on owls and has also participated in several radiotelemetry studies documenting the dispersal and survivability of captive-reared owls. She is presently the Director of Animal Care at the Ohio Wildlife Center.

Wendy Fox is a wildlife rehabilitator and Executive Director of Pelican Harbor Seabird Station in Florida. She has been rehabilitating Brown Pelicans and other species for 15 years. She currently sits on the Boards of Directors for the National Wildlife Rehabilitator's Association and the Florida Wildlife Rehabilitation Association.

Elaine J. Friedman is Director and Owner of Corvid Connection, a nonprofit wildlife education organization that uses permanently injured wildlife in programs for all age groups. A former pharmaceutical chemist for the Food and Drug Administration, Elaine currently does rehabilitation of ravens, crows, magpies, and jays for Lindsay Wildlife Museum, Wildcare and Sulphur Creek Nature Center, all located in the San Francisco Bay Area. She is also a consultant at Wildcare dealing with the handling and care of educational wild animals. Elaine has been involved in wildlife education and rehabilitation for over 20 years and has focused on corvid species for 13 years, publishing a number of papers on corvid care. Previously, she was a supervisor in the educational animal department of Lindsay Wildlife Museum and Corvid Species Manager in the Lindsay wildlife rehabilitation department, and she has worked as a keeper, raptor handler, teacher, and enrichment consultant at a number of wildlife facilities.

Laurie J. Gage, DVM, served as the Director of Veterinary Services for Six Flags Marine World in Vallejo, California, for 23 years, and then took a veterinary position at the Los Angeles Zoo, where she worked with a large variety of mammals and birds. She is presently the Big Cat Specialist for the United States Department of Agriculture, and she also serves as a marine mammal advisor to that agency. She edited *Hand-Rearing Wild and Domestic Mammals* (Blackwell Publishers 2002).

Marge Gibson is Founder and Executive Director of Raptor Education Group, Inc. (REGI), a wildlife rehabilitation, education, and research facility, located in Antigo, Wisconsin (www.raptoreducationgroup.org). A former president of International Wildlife Rehabilitation Council (IWRC), she teaches wildlife rehabilitation classes internationally and maintains an active schedule consulting with wildlife professionals worldwide about avian species. Marge has been active with avian field research and wildlife rehabilitation for over 40 years and has cared for thousands of avian patients from Bald Eagles and Trumpeter Swans to and through warblers and hummingbirds.

Janet Howard has been rehabilitating wildlife for 6 years, specializing in birds for 4 years. She runs a small home-based avian rehabilitation center and works as a photographer outside Atlanta, Georgia.

Linda Hufford is an avian wildlife rehabilitator permitted in the state of Texas and through U.S. Fish and Wildlife. Her area of avian interest includes aerial insectivores. She has been a volunteer with Texas Wildlife Rehabilitation Coalition since 1992 and an independent rehabilitator since 1995.

Sally Cutler Huntington's affinity for animals resulted from time spent as a child working in her father's veterinary clinic in Minneapolis. She now has over 300 finches and softbills in her modern San Diego aviaries. Her daily avian efforts are interrupted somewhat by her full-time private practice as a psychotherapist.

Susie Kasielke started her career as an Animal Keeper at the Los Angeles Zoo in 1977 and has been Curator of Birds there since 2001. She earned a BS degree in Avian Sciences at the University of California Davis. Through her involvement with the California Condor Recovery Program, she worked with the staff at Los Angeles to develop and refine propagation, incubation, and rearing methods for condors and other vultures. She teaches workshops on avian egg incubation for zoo groups in North America. She has also taught aviculture at Pierce College and is a guest lecturer at Moorpark College, UCLA, and UC Davis.

Martha Kudlacik has been a volunteer with Wildlife Rescue, Inc. (WRI) in Palo Alto, California, since 1994, using her degrees in nutrition and medicine to raise birds both in the clinic and in home care for return to the wild. She has also served WRI in several administrative and governance capacities over the years.

Georgean Z. Kyle and **Paul D. Kyle** began rehabilitating avian insectivores in 1984. Over 20 years, they have hand-reared and released more than 1,200 Chimney Swifts. Through banding and an aggressive postrelease study they were able to verify that swifts that they cared for survived, migrated, and successfully bred in the wild. They are the recipients of a Partners in Flight award for public awareness in Chimney Swift conservation, are the founders of the North American Chimney Swift Nest Site Research Project and have written two books about Chimney Swifts as part of the Lindsey Merrick Natural Environmental Series for the Texas A & M University Press.

Nancy Anne Lang, PhD is Director and Owner of Safari West. Previous to that, she was Curator at the San Francisco Zoo where she spent over 15 years propagating birds of prey for reintroduction. Target species included Bald Eagles, Bay-winged Hawks, and Peregrine Falcons. Dr. Lang currently teaches Zoo Biology at Santa Rosa Junior College where she is developing a 2-year degree program for those interested in management of captive exotic wildlife.

David Oehler is Curator of Birds at the Cincinnati Zoo & Botanical Garden. He also founded and operates Feather Link Inc., a nonprofit organization that connects people and birds through education and conservation. David first became involved with alcids while working with these birds in Alaska, in 1992. He has since developed protocols for the captive husbandry of auklet taxa and continued in situ conservation/research programs involving the alcid colonies on the Baby Islands and St. Lawrence Island, Alaska. He has since written several articles and book chapters on these activities with alcids.

Libby Osnes-Erie has been involved with wildlife rehabilitation since 1993. She has worked extensively with terrestrial and marine wildlife in the California central coast region. She was a participant in the California Department of Fish and Game Oiled Wildlife Care Network from 1995–2004 and a California Council for Wildlife Rehabilitators board member from 2000–2006. Libby is a California registered veterinary technician and has a Master's degree in Marine Science, specializing in marine mammals and birds.

Nora Pihkala, DVM, raised and bred chickens in the 4-H youth program in Southern California. She earned her BS in Avian Sciences and her DVM from the University of California Davis. Her professional interests lie in poultry production medicine, small animal practice, and veterinary public health. Her favorite breeds remain Silver Spangled Hamburgs and bantam Barred Plymouth Rocks.

Megan Shaw Prelinger is a wildlife rehabilitator specializing in aquatic birds and oil spill response with International Bird Rescue Research Center. She has presented widely on aquatic bird rehabilitation. She is also an independent scholar and cofounder of the Prelinger Library, a private research library in San Francisco.

Guthrum Purdin has been a lifelong bird enthusiast, and has held staff and volunteer positions at several California wildlife rehabilitation facilities over the past 19 years. He received a BS in Marine Biology from San Francisco State University and is currently attending the School of Veterinary Medicine at University of California, Davis where he intends to become an avian and wildlife veterinarian. He has a particular facility for managing the chaos of overcrowded wild passerine nurseries.

Peter Shannon graduated from Michigan State University with a degree in Zoology in 1977. He later became the Curator of Birds at Audubon Park Zoo in New Orleans where he developed particular interests in flamingos, hornbills, and storks. He spent 3 years in Hawaii running the State's propagation facility for endangered Hawaiian birds and assisting in research and restoration of the state's native species, and then spent several years at the Bronx Zoo's breeding facility on St. Catherine's Island in Georgia. This led to 5-1/2 years as Bird and Primate Curator at the San Francisco Zoo. Significant accomplishments with birds have included the first captive reproduction of three Asian hornbill species, the second institution to breed toucan barbets and plate-billed mountain toucans, the first jabiru stork eggs laid in captivity, and the first year of multiple hatches of Hawaiian crows. Shannon is currently the Curator of birds at the Albuquerque Biological Park.

Louise Shimmel has been a state and federally permitted wildlife rehabilitator since 1985, working for 5 years with all species, and then specializing in raptors. In 1990, she founded Cascades Raptor

Center, a nature center and wildlife hospital in Eugene, Oregon, in order to focus on environmental education, as well as the rehabilitation of individual birds. She served for 7 years on the board, including 2 years as president, of the International Wildlife Rehabilitation Council. She was an IWRC Skills Seminar instructor for 5 years, has been an assistant or associate editor for the IWRC *Journal of Wildlife Rehabilitation* since 1989, authored an article in *Seminars in Avian and Exotic Pet Medicine*, and contributed a number of articles to the IWRC *Journal.*

Dale Smith, DVM, DVSc, is a Professor in the Department of Pathobiology at the Ontario Veterinary College, University of Guelph. Her teaching encompasses various aspects of the veterinary care of nondomestic and nontraditional species to veterinary and graduate students. Dr. Smith first became involved with ratites while working in Africa in the 1980s. She has since lectured and written several articles and book chapters on their veterinary care.

Brian Speer received his DVM degree from the University of California at Davis in 1983. Board specialty status was earned through the American Board of Veterinary Practitioners in 1995, and certification in the European College of Avian Medicine and Surgery (ECAMS) in May, 1999. Brian is the recipient of the Lafeber Practitioner Award, 2003. Brian has served as chair of the Aviculture Committee for the Association of Avian Veterinarians and is the 1999–2000 past president. He currently serves as a consultant for the Veterinary Information Network, and chairs the AAV aviculture committee. Brian is well published in numerous veterinary conference proceedings nationally and internationally, has served as guest editor for a number of veterinary journals and texts, and has authored a number of peer-reviewed journal articles. He is a coauthor of *The Large Macaws* and coauthor of *Birds for Dummies.*

Kappy Sprenger began working in wildlife rehabilitation in Los Gatos, California in 1985, caring for both mammals and birds. In 2002, she moved to Maine where she has continued as a rehabilitator, accepting all avian species but specializing in the fish-eating birds (particularly loons) and all precocial species.

Jane Tollini was the Magellenic Penguin keeper for 19 years at the San Francisco Zoo where she successfully fledged 166 chicks. During that time she held the Magellenic Penguin Studbook for 8 years. She has papers published on the topics of penguin malaria, husbandry, and hand-rearing. Jane was featured on, and told the story of the "Mock Migration," of penguins which received worldwide media coverage.

Martin Vince is the Curator of Birds at the Riverbanks Zoo and Botanical Garden. Vince was co-owner of a 30 acre zoo in England before moving to the Sedgwick Country Zoo, Wichita, Kansas, in 1992, where he worked for 4 years in the tropical jungle exhibit. While at the Sedgwick Country Zoo, Vince wrote *Softbills: Care, Breeding and Conservation* before moving to the Riverbanks Zoo in 1992 as the Assistant Curator of Birds. Vince was promoted to Curator in 2006 and has been the Chair of the AZA's Passerine Taxon Advisory Group since 2000. In addition, Vince oversees the AZA's Population Management Plans for the Toco Toucan and Golden-breasted Starling. Along with Bob Seibels, Riverbanks Curator of Birds Emeritus, Martin Vince coauthored the AZA's *Toucan Husbandry Manual,* which is based on 30 years of toucan breeding at the Riverbanks Zoo and Botanical Garden.

Patricia Wakenell, DVM, PhD, has been a professor of poultry medicine at the University of California Davis since 1990. She received her BS and DVM from Michigan State University. Patricia received a PhD in pathology from MSU and the USDA Avian Disease and Oncology Laboratory in 1985, and is board certified in veterinary clinical pathology. Patricia is a past president of the Western Poultry Disease Conference and is currently president-elect for the American Association of Avian Pathologists.

Patricia Witman is the Avian Care Manager for the Zoological Society of San Diego at the San Diego Zoo's Avian Propagation Center. Her responsibilities include creating protocols for any of the avian species from which eggs or chicks are removed from the parents for hand-rearing. Pat first became involved with hand-rearing hornbills in 1987. Her department has continued to have a very high success rate with other related species, including the Micronesian Kingfisher.

Preface

This book was several years in the making, and is the result of hours of conversations among many colleagues at zoos, wildlife rehabilitation centers, universities and veterinary facilities, as well as with private bird enthusiasts. But ultimately, the idea was hatched with Dr. Gage being heard to utter shortly after she finished writing *Hand-Rearing Wild and Domestic Mammals*, "Hey Becky, we should do a book about raising birds!" Perhaps Dr. Duerr's hearing was a little too good on that day. Nonetheless, with the help of our talented friends and colleagues we were able to create another resource, this time to help feathered creatures find their way in this world.

With over 9,600 species of birds currently recognized, we realized that covering the topic of hand-rearing birds could easily fill a set of encyclopedias. Even if we limited the scope to North American species, it still would not allow for great detail on even those most commonly raised. Although there are several books that discuss hand-rearing specific species, and Dr. Fowler's *Zoo and Wild Animal Medicine* covers medical care of various taxa of birds, there is no single text that gives basic information about hand-rearing the more common species of birds. We finally settled on the following organization: general care of unidentified baby birds in Chapter 1, an identification guide to common North American orphans in Chapter 2, a chapter on general incubation of eggs in Chapter 3, and then 35 chapters dedicated to highlighting species from most of the currently recognized avian orders.

The chapter authors span the breadth of people who hand-rear baby birds, from private breeders to zoo aviculturists, avian veterinarians to wildlife rehabilitators. It has been fascinating for us to see how authors from these diverse backgrounds encounter and surmount the challenges of raising baby birds.

Hand-rearing most species of birds is probably more of an art than it is science. The methods presented in each chapter do not necessarily represent the only way of raising a particular species; indeed, the authors sometimes provide conflicting information or different ways of looking at similar problems or interpreting the same information. Techniques may vary depending on whether one is raising a single chick from an endangered species or several hundred wild orphans simultaneously, or whether a chick is destined to become a pet versus one that needs to learn to survive in the wild. Hand-rearing birds may be frustrating and at times overwhelming, but the expert authors provide proven diets and helpful tips that will improve the chances of having one's hard work pay off by raising strong, healthy, beautiful birds.

Laurie J. Gage, DVM
Rebecca S. Duerr, DVM

Acknowledgments

Many heartfelt thanks to all of our wonderful authors for sharing their vast knowledge and experiences. In particular, Linda Hufford, Penny Elliston, Nancy Eilertsen, Martha Kudlacik, Pat Witman, Susie Kasielke, and Louise Shimmel all went above and beyond to make this book happen. Thanks to Susannah Corona for agreeing to help us in the eleventh hour, and for finding David Oehler, whom we also thank for pulling together his chapter in such short order. Thanks to Marie Travers for providing a last minute brief piece on coots and rails. Thanks from Becky to Susie Brain, Juanita Heinemann, Courtenay Dawson-Roberts, and the rest of the Wildlife Rescue, Inc. Palo Alto, California crews, past and present, for their enthusiasm in teaching her that wild bird care can be done well in a shelter environment. Thanks to Becky's father, Dr. Frederick Duerr, for his assistance with the appendixes; to Ruth Duerr, Jennifer Duerr-Jenkins, Debbie Daniels, and Roger Parker for editorial help; and to Drs. Heather Harris and Anne Dueppen for their support during the long process of getting this book created. Thanks to Laurie's father, James Gage, for his constant moral (and morale) support. And special thanks to our husbands, Guthrum Purdin and Kenji Ruymaker, for all of their help and support this past year.

Laurie J. Gage, DVM
Rebecca S. Duerr, DVM

Hand-Rearing Birds

1
General Care

Rebecca Duerr

NATURAL HISTORY

There are over 9,600 recognized species of birds in the world, with approximately 810 species found in North America north of Mexico (Sibley 2000). Most chicks found as strays in need of care in the U.S.A. or Canada belong to one of these 810 species. There are many other species kept as pets or in zoological institutions, but these chicks typically are identified, and the reader should consult the appropriate chapter for care information.

This chapter provides information on the initial care of unidentified chicks. After reading this chapter, the reader should proceed to Chapter 2, "Chick Identification," for guidance on deciphering the identity of mystery chicks to the level of order or species in some cases. Later chapters in this book cover subsequent care.

Several hundred thousand injured and orphaned wild birds are presented for care annually in the United States (Borgia 2004). Most of these birds are found by Good Samaritans who eventually manage to find the right person or organization in their area to care for the bird. Some are presented to veterinary clinics and are relinquished to the local veterinarian. Others end up in animal control facilities. Many veterinary clinics and animal control agencies have preexisting relationships with local wildlife rehabilitators for transfer of animals. Unfortunately, some finders attempt to give care but are ignorant of the needs of baby birds. These chicks often acquire additional problems before transfer to appropriate care facilities.

Some species of young wild birds may be dangerous to novice handlers. Heron relatives may forcefully stab with their bill, even through the holes in a pet carrier; young raptors have very strong talons with which to pierce; juvenile pelicans may strike at faces with their very powerful bill. Protective goggles and thick leather gloves may be needed with some species. Good hygienic practices are always warranted when handling animals of any kind. Personal protective gear such as a face mask and gloves may be useful to reduce exposure to zoonotic disease as well. If latex gloves are used, wash off the powder before handling birds.

Legal Considerations

There are laws and regulations that protect migratory birds within the United States. Both the general public and veterinarians are prohibited from keeping migratory birds without valid permits from the U.S. Fish and Wildlife Service and applicable state authorities. The vast majority of orphans found are protected by this ruling. As Good Samaritans helping a wild bird in need of care, the public is required to transfer the bird to a permitted wildlife rehabilitator immediately. Wild birds requiring medical treatment may only be kept by veterinarians who do not possess these permits for 24 hours after the bird's condition has been stabilized, after which time it must be transferred to a permitted wildlife rehabilitator (50 CFR 21.12). If a veterinarian is unable to locate a permitted migratory bird rehabilitator, the Regional Migratory Bird Permit Office must be contacted for assistance (see Appendix 1). At press time, the most complete online resources for locating a wildlife rehabilitator in North America are http://www.tc.umn.edu/~devo0028/contact.htm, http://www.nwrawildlife.org, or http://www.iwrc-online.org/emergency/emergency.html. Many states maintain lists of currently permitted rehabilitators within websites of state Fish and Game, Parks and Wildlife, or Division of Natural Resources Departments. For example, Texas Parks and Wildlife lists all permitted Texas rehabilitators by county at http://www.tpwd.state.tx.us/huntwild/wild/rehab/list/.

The chapters in this book make the assumption that any reader applying the knowledge contained herein to protected species possesses the appropriate permits. See Appendix 1 for a listing of state, provincial, or federal wildlife permit offices, and regional wildlife rehabilitation associations.

There are a few nonnative species found throughout the United States that are commonly encountered as orphans, such as feral pigeons (*Columba livia*), European Starlings (*Sturnus vulgaris*), and House Sparrows (*Passer domesticus*). Their care and possession is not regulated in some states, but may be illegal in others. Starlings, in particular, make excellent pet birds and can even learn to speak words. However, identification must be verified because native wild chicks may appear quite similar. Release of nonnative species into the wild is discouraged by most wildlife biologists and natural resource managers, because many nonnative species have deleterious effects on native bird populations.

Altricial versus Precocial

There are two main divisions into which baby birds are divided, *altricial* and *precocial,* although there are numerous gradations between these extremes. Altricial chicks are blind, more-or-less naked, and helpless at hatching. Parents care for altricial chicks in the nest until they are old enough to venture into the outside world, usually at several weeks of age. Altricial chicks include all songbirds, raptors, herons, and many others. Precocial chicks have their eyes open, a full coat of warm downy feathers, and the ability to leave the nest as soon as they have dried off after hatching. Parents of precocial chicks typically provide warmth at night and protection from predators, and—although chicks are able to eat on their own—the parent shows them what to eat, how and where to find it, and what to avoid. Precocial chicks include most waterbirds, such as ducklings and shorebirds, plus chickens, quail, pheasants, and other galliformes.

CRITERIA FOR INTERVENTION

Chicks found in the mouth of a pet, alone in an inappropriate location such as the middle of a parking lot or prone on a baking hot sidewalk, or that are cold, injured, covered with parasites or ants, entangled in a foreign material, or otherwise in obvious trouble, are indeed in need of rescue. Alert, active, mobile chicks that are found without evidence of trauma or distress in the environment in which their parents nested, whether that is a backyard or natural area, should be left alone. If the parents are providing care and the chick is uninjured, the risk of "cats in the neighborhood" is not sufficient reason to bring a found chick into captivity. This risk is faced by every single wild bird in North America.

Precocial chicks are often found alone, apparently parentless. Precocial chicks in obviously bad locations such as running in the street should be immediately rescued or shepherded out of traffic to rejoin their family. Ducks will sometimes nest in fountain planters and when chicks hatch they leap into the water, cannot get out, and eventually drown. Placing a ramp on which the chicks can exit the water is often all that is needed. Once precocial chicks hatch, the family group usually leaves the nest area; it may be consequently very difficult to reunite separated chicks with their parents, although some species will foster extra chicks if an appropriate family group with chicks the same age can be located. Each species varies in the total number of chicks usually accepted.

Many species normally have periods of time when chicks are old enough to begin exploring their environment, but not yet able to fly away from danger. These older chicks are still cared for by the parents, but no longer require moment-to-moment attention. Many fledgling songbirds have a period of approximately 1 week in which chicks are able to perch and move about but the feathers have not yet finished emerging to allow full flight. Chicks of this age group are at the highest risk for capture by domestic pet predators. Persons with chicks of this description in their yards should keep dogs and cats inside for the few days it will take the birds to become fully independent. The parents will usually visit the chick frequently for feedings. The chick will quickly finish growing its feathers and soon be able to follow the parent in flight while learning to be proficient at foraging and other skills.

Parents of certain species may "dive bomb" humans or pets in an effort to save their young from perceived or real predation. The best thing to do in this circumstance is to allow the birds privacy to finish raising their young, which should be over within a few weeks. It may be seen as a hardship to vacate one's backyard for a short period of time, but bear in mind that our backyards may be the only habitat the birds have. They cannot move and finish raising their chicks elsewhere. In addition, it is against federal and state laws to remove migratory bird nests when they are in use.

If a person observing from a distance has not seen a parent visit a suspected orphaned chick within an hour or more of continuous observation, the chick may be in need of care. Parents may not return if the observer is too close. If the parents are known to have been killed or injured, the chicks should be rescued, because they will starve without parental support.

Younger uninjured chicks may be replaced in the nest if its location is known. Always check to make sure that the chicks in the nest are of the same species as the chick being replaced, although some chicks may be days older or younger. It is a myth that humans having handled a chick will cause a parent bird to reject it or abandon its nest.

If a nest has fallen and the chicks appear uninjured, the nest can be replaced by placing it in a larger wicker basket or other container with drainage holes that is wired to the tree as close as possible to the former location. Choose the location such that the nest is high enough to be safe from predators and not in direct sunlight. Nests that have been replaced should be monitored from a distance to ensure that the parents return to feed the chicks. Chicks should always feel warm to the touch. If the chicks are cold, provide supplemental heat while the nest replacement is being arranged. A wet wash cloth inside a ziplock bag or hot water bottle warmed in a microwave oven provides a rapid source of heat. Hot water bottles tend to cool rapidly, so they must be rewarmed frequently. Take care that steam from a heated, moist surface will not reach the chick and scald it. Chemical hand-warmer packs are also an option. Always have cloth or tissues between chicks and any heat source to prevent excessive heating, and check the chicks frequently. If it is near dark and the parents have little daylight in which to find the new nest, bring the chicks inside and provide warmth overnight before re-nesting them in the morning.

Older, healthy, fully feathered chicks may be placed into shrubbery near where found initially and monitored from a distance to watch for parental attention. There are many excellent websites that offer advice, particularly those of wildlife rehabilitation organizations such as Project Wildlife in San Diego at http://www.projectwildlife.org. The International Wildlife Rehabilitation Council (IWRC) maintains a website that provides answers to frequently asked questions about orphaned chicks and other wildlife issues at http://www.iwrc-online.org/emergency/emergency.html.

RECORD KEEPING

Wildlife regulatory agencies have minimum standards for record keeping that require tracking individual animals undergoing rehabilitation. Check with regulating agencies for further information. As a minimum, the following information should be kept: species, age, location and date found, reason brought into captivity, medical problems, final disposition, release location, and release date. Detailed information on the location where the chick was found will serve as a guide for suitable habitat for release and will place the bird back with relatives that may still recognize it.

A detailed medical record should be kept on each individual, with results of the initial examination recorded, and any updated information added as it happens. This should include daily body weights, progress of treatments, and pertinent notes on behavior. For an example of such a record, see Figure 1.1. It is helpful when large numbers of diverse species are being raised en masse, with different volunteer caregivers, to have a "Feeding Instructions" sheet that tells the next caregiver when to feed, what to feed, how much to feed, and any tips for food delivery.

INITIAL CARE AND STABILIZATION

The main rule of initial baby bird care is warmth, rehydration, and feeding, in that order. Warm chicks before giving fluids, and then hydrate them until they start passing droppings. Only then is it safe to commence feedings. Feeding a cold or dehydrated baby bird before it is warm and hydrated may kill it, even if it is begging. Most chicks found in need of care will be cold, significantly dehydrated, and very stressed. Provide a visual barrier against people and other animals. Do not place birds next to barking dogs, noisy children, or other disturbances.

If the bird has come into care at night, remember that most of the commonly encountered species are primarily diurnal (day-active) animals, and require 9–10 hours of uninterrupted sleep. Hence, if a bird is brought into an emergency clinic at night, it is recommended that any life-threatening conditions be treated and rehydration therapy initiated, and then the bird should be allowed to remain warm, dark,

Wildlife Care Association — Giving wildlife a second chance

Species: ______

Date Admitted ______ Time ______ am/pm

Band #or mark:

Bird: ☐ Hatchling ☐ Nestling ☐ Fledgling ☐ Adult

Mammal: ☐ Newborn ☐ Infant ☐ Juvenile ☐ Adult

Other: ☐ Reptile ☐ Amphibian

Sex: ☐ M ☐ F ☐ U

Intaken at: ☐ Nursery ☐ Rehabber

DISPOSITION
Date: ______
Released ☐
Transfer (to other org) ☐
DOA ☐
Expired ☐
EOA ☐
Euthanized ☐
Release site/zip code: ______
Group transferred to: ______

Patient Record

Please promptly return completed forms to: WCA, POBox 60982, Sacramento, CA 95860

Initial Information:Examiner(s) Date:

Mobility: ☐ Normal ☐ Favoring ☐ Unbalanced ☐ Hock sitting ☐ Head Tilt ☐ Prone

Respiration: ☐ Normal ☐ limbFast/Panting ☐ Slow ☐ Gasping ☐ Clicking/Crackling ☐ Open mouth breathing

Stress/fear level: ☐ Low/Calm ☐ Moderate ☐ High

Dehydration status: ☐ None/Mild (0-5%) ☐ Moderate (6-9%) ☐ Severe (>9%)

Attitude: ☐ Bright/Alert ☐ Somewhat alert ☐ Depressed ☐ Unresponsive

Temp ☐ Hot ☐ Warm ☐ Cool ☐ Cold

Color: ☐ normal ☐ pale mouth ☐ pale flesh

Weight (g): ______

Physical exam:Examiner(s): **Date:** ***Check areas with problems, detail below.***

☐ Head ☐ Tracking ☐ Mouth ☐ Bill/Teeth ☐ Tongue ☐ EyesL / R ☐ Nares/NostrilsL / R

☐ EarsL / R ☐ Neck ☐ Throat ☐ Crop: ☐ full ☐ empty ☐ Wings/ForelegsL / R ☐ Legs/HindlegsL / R ☐ FeetL / R

☐ Grip ☐ Back ☐ Chest ☐ Abdomen ☐ Vent/Anus/Genitals ☐ Tail ☐ Ectoparasites: ☐ mites ☐ fleas ☐ lice ☐ fly-eggs ☐ flat flies

☐ Stool ☐ Fur/feathers: ☐ stress marks ☐ bald area(s) ☐ Fracture: ______ ☐ Wounds: ______ Nutritional State: ☐ Normal ☐ Thin ☐ Emaciated

Date	Exam/Progress notes	Initials
	Rehydration: ______ml fluids given SQ or Orally at ______am/pm	
	Over ➡	

Drug/Procedure/Treatment:	Dose:	Dates:	Procedure/Treatment:	Dose:	Dates:
☐ Frontline					to
		to			to
		to			to
		to			to
		to			to

Date:																		
Wt (g):																		

Please fill out the box below with information about the animal.

Date found ______ **Time found:** ______

Reason rescued: ☐ Cat contact ☐ Hit by car ☐ Hit window ☐ Fell from nest ☐ Orphaned ☐ Appears sick or injured:

Other: ______

Describe any care given: ______

Street address or cross streets or city where found: ______

Area found (in road, lawn etc.):

Name ______

Address ______

Zip ______

Email ______

Phone (   ) ______

Would you like to make a donation today? $______

Your donation will help us continue to care for the animals.

All donations are tax deductible and much appreciated!

Figure 1.1. Example of rehabilitation animal record. Use of check-off boxes is handy for data entry into databases, and when admitting large numbers of animals.

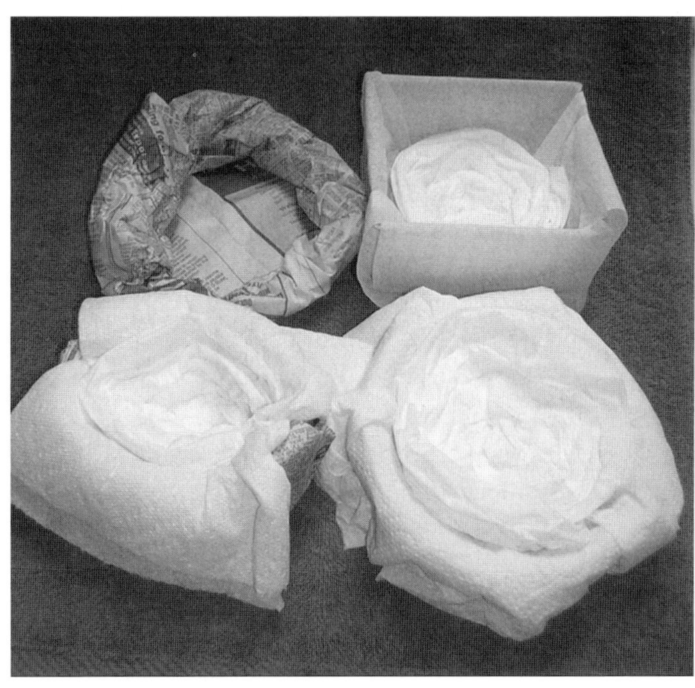

Figure 1.2. Nest substitute examples clockwise from upper left: rolled newspaper nest frame, berry basket nest, ceramic dish nest, rolled newspaper nest with tissue bedding.

and quiet until transferred to an experienced caretaker in the morning. It is not advisable to keep the bird awake all night to be fed because most birds do not feed their young at night and the chick may die of exhaustion if not allowed to rest. However, if the bird is extremely young, a feeding or two once it is warm and rehydrated may be beneficial before bedding it down for the night. Freshly hatched chicks have the benefit of a yolk sac that may continue to provide nutrition for 12–24 hours after hatching.

If the bird is not able to stand, whether due to age, weakness, or injury, it should be placed in a soft support structure such as a rolled cloth "donut" or tissue-lined nest (see Figure 1.2) appropriate for its body size. Do not allow a chick to lie on its side or in other abnormal positions, or on flat surfaces. Chicks should be placed in an appropriately sized nest to support their body with the head slightly elevated and the legs folded beneath the body. Chicks in poorly shaped nests may seem restless and continually try to get out of the nest. Reevaluate the nest replacement if this occurs. Some chicks may be more content with a soft tissue or light piece of cloth draped over the top of the nest. Cavity nesting species may be more comfortable in dim lighting. Some waterbird chicks such as grebes and loons are physiologically unable to stand due to the placement of their legs and need to be placed on ample soft bedding to prevent pressure sores on their legs or keels.

Both altricial and precocial chicks should be placed in a climate-controlled incubator if available, or other high-temperature, moderate-humidity enclosure (see Figures 1.3–1.5, also see Chapter 10, Figures 10.1–10.3, for images of an *aquabrooder*). Heat lamps may be used but are less desirable since it is easy for chicks to overheat under these. Typically, the smaller the body size and less feathered the chick, the higher the temperature required. Older chicks of any body size require less thermal support once stabilized. Start with a very warm 90–100°F (32–38°C) 40–50% humidity environment to normalize the bird's body temperature. Chicks 5–10 g or less may require even higher environmental temperatures (100–104°F, 38–40°C). Larger-bodied chicks such as waterbirds do well in well-padded cardboard pet carriers with one half placed on a heating pad set on "low". Be aware that chicks able to stand may also be proficient at running and jumping. Do not handle the chick more than necessary. Be judicious in application of heat to chicks with head injuries, because high temperatures may exacerbate brain swelling.

Monitor the chick frequently for signs of discomfort. Normal avian body temperature is approximately 104–108°F (40–42°C), but this varies by species and the stress of handling and restraint. It is not practical to measure the temperature of small-bodied birds, but each chick should always feel warm to a warmed human hand. Cold chicks are often lethargic and poorly responsive. Nestbound chicks that are too hot may hang their heads over the edge of nests, lay with their necks stretched out, hold their wings away from their body, or hold their mouths open although not gaping or begging. Hot chicks that are able to stand and ambulate will attempt to move away from the heat source or may pant. Overheated birds are likely to become lethargic and dehydrated, and may cease producing droppings. Dehydrated chicks may feel hot or too firm to the touch; a normally hydrated chick's body feels fleshy and soft. Dehydrated chicks may have wrinkled skin over the abdomen, reduced skin elasticity, sunken eyes, slow eyelid responsiveness, stringy saliva, and dry mucous membranes.

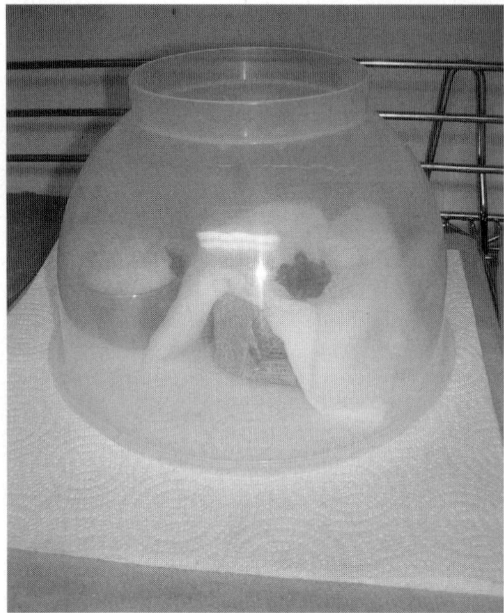

Figure 1.3. Ad hoc incubator: plastic dome on paper toweling on hot pad on "low," with dish of wet paper toweling for humidity. Dome has several vent holes drilled in top.

When the bird is warm and calm, it may be hydrated orally and/or subcutaneously (SQ). Gaping (begging) altricial chicks should be orally hydrated until they produce droppings. Give a few drops of warm oral fluids every 15–20 minutes with a small syringe or eye dropper (see Figure 1.6) and allow the bird to swallow completely before giving more. Once comfortable with the amount the chick is able to swallow, the amount may be raised to 2.5–5% of body weight (25–50 ml/kg) given in several mouthfuls. Human infant electrolyte solutions (unflavored) are excellent for oral rehydration of baby birds, as is lactated Ringer's solution or 2.5% dextrose in

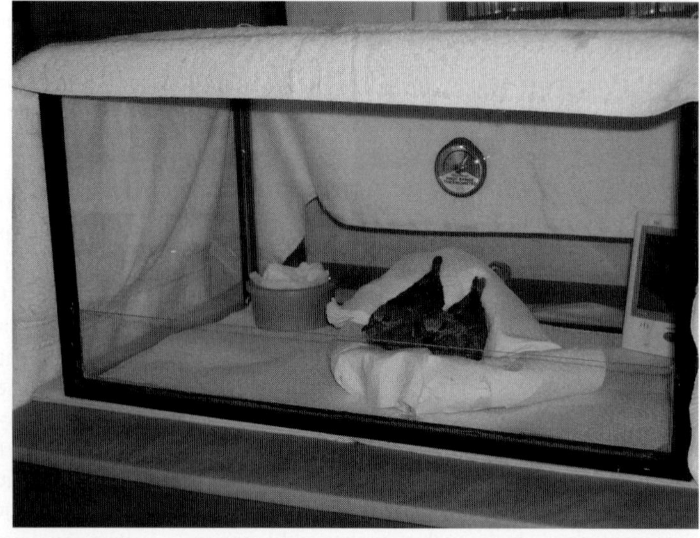

Figure 1.4. Modified glass aquarium incubator, turned sideways to hold heat better. Front has Plexiglas guard high enough to prevent escapes (attached with silicone aquarium cement), dish of soaked paper toweling to add humidity, thermometer, two hot pads underneath with two more possible on top as needed. Cloth flap folds down over opening between feedings.

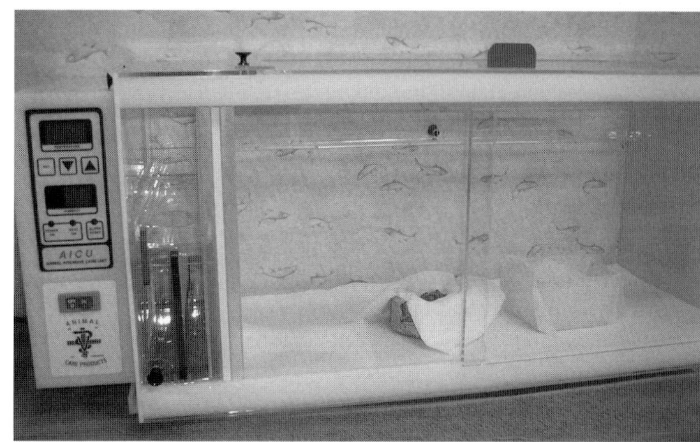

Figure 1.5. Lyon Technologies Animal Intensive Care Unit provides excellent environmental control for chicks requiring high temperatures.

0.45% sodium chloride. Use the smallest gauge needle possible when giving subcutaneous fluids; 25–30 gauge works well for small chicks, 23–25 for larger-bodied chicks. Tiny altricial hatchlings less than 5 g may bruise regardless of how small a needle is used; hence, hydrate these chicks orally whenever possible. Again, ensure that the bird is warm before administering warmed fluids and that the bird is both warm and well-hydrated before receiving food.

Oral fluids may be administered to larger altricial chicks such as herons or raptors by gavage tube (see Figure 1.6). Initial amounts should again be small, 1–2.5% body weight (10–25 ml/kg), until the bird is strong and alert. Herons of any age are generally capable of drinking on their own when fully hydrated; administering fluids by gavage tube is stressful and may cause regurgitation. Subcutaneous fluids are preferred for dehydrated heron chicks to avoid this problem. If SQ fluids are not an option, hold the heron's head upright with the neck stretched up for about 30 seconds after tubing, and then leave the chick alone immediately after to reduce regurgitation.

Precocial chicks such as ducklings may drink and eat on their own once they are warm and feel safe. Provide water in shallow dishes with rocks or other space-occupying masses to prevent the birds falling into the water and drowning or becoming cold and wet. Smaller precocial chicks such as killdeer or other shorebirds are often extremely stressed when brought into captivity. These chicks require hand hydration one drop at a time with a wet cotton swab moved along the bill until a swallowing motion is observed (see Chapter 9, "Shorebirds"). These chicks are very stressed by being alone and may be comforted by the addition of a clean undyed feather duster and small mirror to simulate companionship. However, avoid allowing the chick to spend all its time gazing into the mirror, rather than eating and drinking. Remove the mirror if it is preventing normal activities.

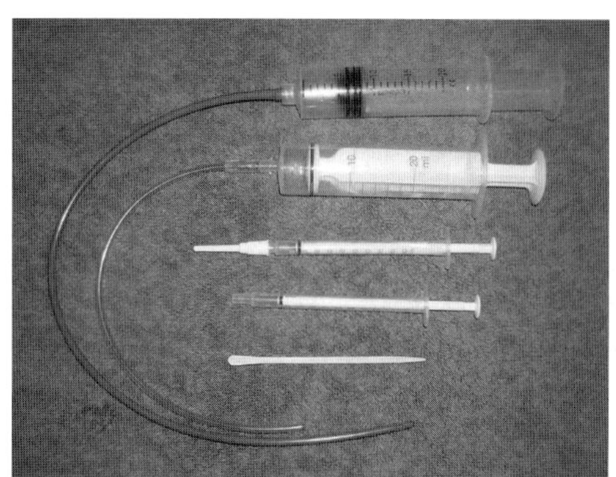

Figure 1.6. Feeding implements from top: 20 ml syringe with red rubber catheter feeding tube, 20 ml O-ring syringe with cut section of IV extension set tubing (note cut end has been burned to round sharp edges), 1 ml O-ring syringe with plastic cannula tip, 1 ml O-ring syringe, wooden feeding pick to use as tiny spoon for small gaping species.

If a chick is depressed or not swallowing well, oral rehydration must be done very carefully because there is a substantial risk of aspiration of fluids into the respiratory system. It may be better in this circumstance to wait for the animal to absorb SQ fluids, rather than giving oral fluids too quickly. If SQ fluids are not an option, give tiny amounts of oral fluids deep into the mouth and ensure that the bird swallows everything before giving more.

Start altricial birds on a hand-feeding diet after they begin passing droppings (see Chapter 34, "Passerines: Hand-Feeding Diets"). If an altricial chick does not begin passing droppings within 1 hour of giving rehydration fluids, begin feeding a hand-feeding diet, but keep the diet dilute and the meal size small until droppings are seen. See Chapter 2, "Chick Identification," for assistance identifying the chick, and then proceed to the most appropriate chapter for further instructions and information on what to feed.

PHYSICAL EXAMINATION

Each chick should receive a complete physical examination. This should be performed in a habitual, systematic manner to avoid missing subtle problems possibly missed if distracted by glaringly obvious abnormalities. With practice, a complete physical should only take a few minutes. However, before the physical examination takes place, it is important to get as complete a history on the bird as possible. Ask the finder whether he or she can provide any clues as to what happened. Did the bird fall into a pool? Did a cat catch it? Was it lying on the side of the road? Had it fallen below a window? Has the yard or property been recently treated for rats or mice or termites? Has the yard been sprayed with pesticides? Were other fallen birds found in the same location?

A visual exam should include the container in which the chick arrived. Any droppings, blood, parasites, or food should be noted. Assess the chick's general posture and attitude: Is it alert or depressed, standing or prone, showing normal movements or convulsing, open-mouth breathing or regurgitating? Is the head drooping or held tilted or straight? Are the wings symmetrical? Is the bird limping or does it have an obvious fracture? Are there visible areas of swelling? Are there signs of bleeding or disturbed areas of feathering? Are there any unusual odors? What is the species and age? Is the chick covered with food? If so, what kind?

Restrain the chick carefully for a full physical examination. Be as gentle as possible and do not allow the chick to become chilled again. The exam can occur in numerous short periods spread out over several hours if necessary. If the chick shows any open-mouth breathing during handling, stop and allow the chick to rest and become calm before further handling. If a major injury is found immediately, stop active bleeding and then complete the rest of the physical examination, evaluating the major injury last. Prognosis for recovery from a single severe injury may be good; multiple serious problems hold a much graver prognosis. In the author's experience, emaciated or malnourished chicks with major injuries do not do well, but well-fleshed chicks may recover fully from surprisingly severe injuries.

Fractured limbs must be considered life-threatening injuries in wild chicks because they need to have fully functional limbs in order to qualify for release. Permanent placement for disabled wildlife is usually not available. If a wild chick is likely to be disabled to the point of not being able to function in the wild, euthanasia should be considered. With a small amount of handling or thrashing in a cage (or restraint for radiographs), a formerly fixable fracture may quickly become a limb that requires amputation, which is usually a death sentence. Hence, it is very important to keep the chick from flapping or kicking a fractured limb while finishing the rest of the exam. As soon as the bird is stable enough to tolerate the handling, the fracture should be at least temporarily immobilized. Fracture stabilization is described in Stocker (2005) and in many avian medicine texts.

Is the chick old enough to expect the eyes to be open? If so, are they open? Are they caked with food? Wild chicks that have been fed by the general public often have food in their eyes that requires flushing with ophthalmic saline solution. Are the eyes symmetrical? Is the bird tending to hold one eye closed? Check pupil size and response to light, although this may be difficult to interpret in young birds. Are the pupils dilated or constricted? Look for lacerations and scratches, hemorrhage, conjunctivitis, discharge, or swelling of the eyelids. Are there any cloudy or opaque areas to the lens or cornea? Is there blood visible inside the eye? Is the third eyelid functioning? Is its movement normal or slow? Is the iris normally positioned within the globe? If warranted, use fluorescein stain to examine for corneal ulcers and examine the retina with an ophthalmoscope.

Check the color of the oral mucous membranes. Bird species vary widely in normal oral mucous membrane color from yellow to purple to pink to black. The conjunctiva may be a better gauge of perfusion than the mouth in some species. Look for parasites or blood within the mouth. The presence and state of gape flanges will help determine how old the bird is. These flanges are sometimes torn in injured chicks. Stringy saliva suggests significant dehydration. Check the nares and bill for discharge, patency, symmetry, dried food, masses, or parasites. Fly eggs or freshly hatched maggots are clear and easily overlooked, but are frequently found in the nares. Beak fractures and dislocations are sometimes seen. Examine the beak for cracks, bruises, and proper occlusion. In all wild species in North America with the exception of crossbills, the top and bottom beak tips should be well aligned.

Check the throat for difficulty in swallowing, breath odor, foreign bodies, and lacerations. A paper clip inserted flat between the upper and lower bill then twisted will generally open the mouth without harm. Look for plaques, swellings, discharges, and abscesses. Some species such as roadrunners and cuckoos have normal markings within the mouth that must not be mistaken for lesions. *Trichmonas gallinae* affects many species and may result in malodorous whitish plaques and masses within the mouth, throat, or crop. Similar lesions can be seen with vitamin deficiencies or viral, yeast, and bacterial infections. Perform a wet mount of a throat swab to differentiate potential pathogens if suspicious lesions are present.

Are there any signs of parasites, blood, or infection in the ears? Are there any lacerations, discharge, or swelling?

Is there evidence of swelling, bruising, or lacerations on the skull? Gently palpate the skull for indentations, scabbed areas, or crepitus. The skulls of chicks are not fully calcified and normally feel soft. If a chick appears to have a skull puncture, clean the wound carefully and use the chick's neurologic status as a guide for prognosis. Scalp lacerations exposing the skull should be closed or dressed as any other wound. Old, dry, skull-exposing lacerations heal well when dressed to keep moist and clean.

Palpate the crop for contents if the species has a crop. Is it empty or full? Does it feel like normal food or is it mushy or hard? Is it leaking contents from a laceration? Crop tears are quite common in young doves and pigeons or birds caught by predators. Impactions are common for chilled, dehydrated birds with food in the crop due to lack of gut motility.

Assess body condition by palpating the muscle mass of the breast and over the hips. Look and feel for areas of scabbing, bruising, and feather loss or damage. In most passerines, one can blow air to part the feathers, allowing a view of the skin between the feather tracts. This works well to spot punctures, lacerations, bruising, and subcutaneous emphysema (air under the skin).

Gently palpate the abdomen. It should feel soft. Many altricial hatchlings have abdominal organs that may be easily visualized through the skin. Markedly dehydrated chicks may have firm or hard-feeling abdominal organs and wrinkled skin over the abdomen, both of which may resolve with fluid therapy. Hatchlings that have fallen onto hard surfaces may have blood visible inside their abdomen or even herniated viscera. Hatchlings with intraabdominal bleeding do not do well. However, older chicks may recover, depending on the severity. Use the chick's attitude as a guide for prognosis. Check the vent for lesions, diarrhea, patency, crusted droppings, and normal sphincter tone. Gently wash the vent with warm water if necessary, without soaking or chilling the chick.

If the chick is unfeathered, what is the color of its skin and flesh? Although skin color varies, most altricial chicks should be pinkish. Although some doves and roadrunners may have black skin, white and grey are not often normal colors for the flesh of young birds. With a modicum of experience one can spot a bird that is pale.

Inspect the limbs and joints. Gently palpate, flex, and extend all limbs and each joint separately. Note the presence of pain, heat, swelling, deformities, and asymmetries, limitation of motion, crepitus, dislocation, or fractures. Midshaft tibiotarsus fractures are the most common, with many times more leg fractures than wing fractures seen in chicks. Check for lacerations, other lesions, and missing nails and toes. Lacerations are especially common around the knees and thighs of small birds, especially if caught by cats. Evaluate muscle tone of the tail as limpness may indicate a spinal injury.

Is the chick abnormally unsteady when walking or trying to perch if it is old enough to do so? Is it dragging any limbs? Limping? Do the feet grip? Does the animal exhibit normal and symmetrical responses to manipulation of its limbs?

Evaluate feather condition. Malnourished chicks often exhibit poor feather condition with ragged or broken feathers, adhered feather sheaths, and stress marks. Abnormally whitish feathers are sometimes seen in malnourished crows, jays, house sparrows and others. Missing or broken feathers may also provide evidence of predator attack. If there is soft tissue damage to the area of the primary or secondary feather follicles on the wings, be conservative in debriding damaged tissue and avoid plucking these important feathers unless actively bleeding. It is best to allow the follicles to heal with a feather inside, and then later remove the feather if necessary once the soft tissue has healed. Ectoparasites such as mites and feather lice are common.

Normal droppings vary widely by species, but in most small-bodied altricial chicks, feces are enclosed in a mucus envelope. When these species have diarrhea, encapsulation is lost and the droppings are wet, messy, sometimes malodorous, and often soil the chick. If the droppings look or smell odd or the bird has diarrhea, a fecal examination should be performed to look for parasites. Emaciated animals should always have fecal smears and flotations done because a heavy parasite load may be a primary problem. This may need to wait until the bird passes significant feces. Routine fecal examination of all wild birds admitted for care is prudent. Bacterial infection is another common cause of diarrhea in chicks. Gram stains of feces may be informative.

COMMON MEDICAL PROBLEMS AND SOLUTIONS

In the author's experience, the most common problems encountered in wild chicks presented for care include one or more of the following: hypothermia; dehydration; lacerations from attack by cats (approximately 1/3 of all chicks seen); fractures and soft-tissue trauma from falls from nest or cat attack; emaciation secondary to either parasite load, parental separation, or poor care by finder; malnutrition with poor feather condition, with or without accompanying metabolic bone disease; and parasite infestations.

Lacerations from predators should be cleaned, debrided, and closed primarily, whenever possible, to speed healing and reduce development of stress bars on growing feathers. All debris should be removed from wounds and the feathers carefully plucked within 3–5 mm of the margin, with the exception of flight feathers. Take care to avoid tearing skin by gently plucking in the direction of feather growth or toward the wound edge, if close to margins. Never cut or shave feathers. Be very conservative in removing any feathers from seabirds: Use tape to hold feathers back during wound closure instead. For very young chicks or for wounds that do not have much tension, surgical glue such as Nexaband (Abbott) may provide adequate closure. Semipermeable self-adhesive dressings such as Biodres (DVM Pharmaceuticals) or Tegaderm (3M) may be used for wounds that are unable to be sutured or glued. The author's preference is to suture, glue, or dress all open wounds, especially in crowded wild-bird nursery situations. Whenever possible, facilitate the fastest possible wound healing, in order to lead to rapid progress through rehabilitation and an expeditious release. The longer the bird must stay in captivity, the more likely it is to develop secondary problems.

There are many other wound care products that are appropriate for use in young birds; however, merely dabbing some cream onto a wound does not foster optimal wound healing. Silver sulfadiazine cream is often used to treat exposed wounds if secondary intention healing is necessary, because it has both antifungal and antibacterial properties, and it is water-soluble. Collasate (PRN Pharmacal) is a product that is gaining popularity for its ability to foster granulation tissue, and it may be used underneath Tegaderm or Biodres. Avoid the use of petroleum-based products, such as ointments, due to their inevitable undesirable contamination of feathers.

Subcutaneous emphysema (air under the skin) is a common result of a cat attack or severe impact, in which one or more air sacs have been ruptured and leak air into subcutaneous spaces. This often resolves without treatment, but it may be helpful to remove the pressure if it is interfering with mobility or if it is causing the bird to become depressed. If necessary, puncture the bubble with a sterile needle, avoiding any visible skin blood vessels. Many cases will reinflate quickly and may require repeat punctures several times over the course of a few days. This problem may manifest 24–48 hours after presentation.

All chicks with wounds including subcutaneous emphysema should be placed on a course of broad spectrum antibiotics that are likely to cover *Pasteurella multocida* such as amoxicillin with clavulanic acid (Clavamox, Pfizer) at 125 mg/kg orally twice daily or cephalexin at 100 mg/kg orally twice daily until the problem resolves (Carpenter 2005). Be sure antibiotics are not discontinued until the wound has completely healed. Some wildlife veterinarians continue antibiotics for several days after external wounds have healed to reduce the likelihood of complications, especially in cases of body cavity punctures.

Wild birds may become depressed if encumbered by heavy or confining splints, and wraps may damage growing feathers. Hence, minimally restrictive wraps and light weight splints are recommended. The author uses Micropore paper tape (3M) on feathers because it comes off fairly easily without pulling out feathers and does not leave a residue behind.

Chicks with metabolic bone disease (MBD) may show rubbery long bones on physical examination and perhaps one or more fractures. Mild cases may present with subtle fractures of the proximal tarsometatarsus. In some species, the tough scaly skin of this segment of leg will provide some stability for fractures, and fractures here may not be noticed until a small callus or mild angular deformity forms at the fracture site. On small-bodied chicks, these fractures heal well with a light stabilizing external splint that does not immobilize the intertarsal (hock) joint. Surgical fixation is often futile because the extant bone lacks enough density to hold fixators and pins.

Sometimes MBD is seen in the smallest chick in a clutch if the parents were not able to adequately provision all chicks, or if the female was nutritionally depleted at the end of egg laying. If the chick does not have conformational deformities or joint abnormalities, it may recover with nest rest and application of lightweight external splints as necessary. Once placed on a balanced diet, many birds will quickly calcify their long bones, especially if supplemented with calcium glubionate orally at 150 mg/kg twice daily. If there are marked skeletal deformities, euthanasia should be considered.

External parasites can cause severe debilitation due to anemia in nestbound chicks and may spread many blood-borne diseases. They can also cause allergic reactions in sensitive humans, warranting treatment to safeguard caregivers. Treatment is also necessary to prevent spread to other birds, as well as provide relief for the affected bird. Mites are often treated with Ivermectin at 200 µg/kg once orally (Carpenter 2005) or a single application of Fipronil (Frontline spray, Merial) at 20 mg/kg topically onto skin. Both of these products take many hours to have an effect; hence, many rehabilitators and wildlife veterinarians lightly dust the bird with Sevin Dust (GardenTech) in severe cases, and it works very quickly. The Environmental Protection Agency has a fact sheet on this class of chemicals available online at http://www.epa.gov/oppsrrd1/REDs/factsheets/carbaryl_factsheet.pdf. As mentioned in Ritchie, Harrison, and Harrison (1999), "lightly salting" with pyrethrin or carbaryl powder is often sufficient. Paper sprinkled with Sevin Dust may be placed underneath the container holding the affected bird to reduce mite contamination of adjacent birds. Kelthane (Dow Agrosciences) is also used by some as a miticide. Gloves are recommended when applying chemical pesticides. See each chemical's Material Safety Data Sheet (MSDS) before handling. Investigation is ongoing at several wildlife rehabilitation centers into whether Nitenpyram (Capstar, Novartis) has an effective safe dose for avian mites. Bathing the chick is another option to reduce mite numbers if the bird is strong enough to tolerate the stress; do not allow the chick to become chilled during the washing or drying process.

As previously discussed, internal parasites should be diagnosed by fecal examination and treated accordingly. However, not all endoparasites can be diagnosed by fecal examination. Either the parasites are not being shed at the time of examination, or they are not shed in feces. For example, herons and egrets commonly have nematode worm infestations with migrating worms in the subcutaneous tissues and coelomic cavity that can significantly impact these chicks, but will have no ova visible on fecal examination. Multiple diagnostics may be necessary.

TEMPORARY CARE DIETS

Caregivers should make every effort to avoid covering chicks in food. Sloppy feeding techniques will create more problems for already compromised birds, including poor feather development, follicle damage, eye infections, and other problems.

Commercial diets intended for baby parrots are for the most part not appropriate for wild songbird, seabird, shorebird, or raptor chicks, all of which have much higher protein requirements. However, Kaytee Exact Hand Feeding Formula is adequate as a temporary tube-feeding diet for chickens, pheasants, doves, and pigeons.

Dog food is not an appropriate food for growing birds; milk and bread, hamburger, condensed milk, uncooked rice, or monkey biscuits also are not appropriate. To provide a decent short-term food for songbird chicks of any age, soak a high-quality kitten chow in water until fully saturated and feed as soft nuggets or blend to make slurry and feed by syringe (J. Perlman, pers. comm.). Canned Hills A/D is another acceptable option found in most veterinary clinics. Neither of these foods have enough calcium for growing birds; hence, if the bird must stay in a clinic for more than a few hours, oral supplementation with calcium glubionate is recommended at up to 150 mg/kg twice daily (Carpenter 2005). Commercially available crickets are another option for temporary food for those species with high protein requirements.

Metabolic bone disease may be quickly induced in raptor chicks by feeding meat products that have not been supplemented with adequate calcium. Bone meal is not appropriate as a calcium supplement because it cannot be used to change the ratio of calcium to phosphorus; it already contains both in a fixed ratio. Calcium carbonate powder is the most commonly used oral calcium supplement.

Most partially or fully feathered songbird chicks should be fed approximately 5% of body weight (1 ml per 20 g body weight) in food every 30–45 minutes, with hatchlings fed every 20–30 minutes for 12–14 hours per day. Droppings should be formed and moist for most species, and should be produced with nearly every feeding. Some species stop begging when they are full and some species do not.

Hummingbird chicks must be kept warm and fed every 20–30 minutes while awaiting transfer to experienced care. Giving oral 5% dextrose or dilute hummingbird nectar (6 parts water to 1 part table sugar) for hydration will keep the bird hydrated and alive for a brief period but is nutritionally deficient and is inappropriate for more than very short-term emergency support.

It is essential to not allow sugar water to spill and dry on feathers. This will result in permanent damage, which is life threatening for a hummingbird. If a bird is old enough it can be persuaded to drink from a syringe or dropper by inserting the tip of the bill into the end of the tube until rapid swallowing motions are observed.

ACKNOWLEDGMENTS

Many thanks to Penny Elliston, Daphne Bremer, Martha Kudlacik, Marianne Brick, and Linda Hufford for reviewing this chapter, and thanks to all the avian wildlife veterinarians who have graciously allowed me to pick their brains over the years: Greg Massey, Vicki Joseph, Nancy Anderson, Marianne Brick, Mira Sanchez, Mike Ziccardi, and Tina Peak.

SOURCES FOR PRODUCTS MENTIONED

BioDres: DVM Pharmaceuticals, Subsidiary of IVAX Corporation, 4400 Biscayne Blvd, Miami, FL 33137, (305) 575-6000.

Capstar (Nitenpyram): Novartis Animal Health, (800) 637-0281.

Collasate (PRN Pharmacal) 8809 Ely Road, Pensacola, FL 32514, (800) 874-9764.

Frontline spray (Fipronil): Merial, (888) Merial-1.

Kaytee products: 521 Clay St, PO Box 230, Chilton, WI 53014, (800) KAYTEE-1.

Kelthane miticide: Dow AgroSciences LLC, 9330 Zionsville Road, Indianapolis, IN 46268, (317) 337-3000.

Nexaband: Abbott Animal Health, North Chicago, IL 60064, (888) 299-7416.

Sevin Dust: GardenTech, PO Box 24830, Lexington, KY 40524-4830, (800) 969-7200.

Tegaderm: 3M Corporate Headquarters, 3M Center, St. Paul, MN 55144-1000, (888) 364-3577.

REFERENCES

Borgia, L. 2004. NWRA membership survey 2003: Results and comparisons. Wildlife Rehabilitation Bulletin 22(1):37–42.

Carpenter, J.W., ed. 2005. Exotic Animal Formulary, 3rd Edition. Elsevier Saunders, Philadelphia, pp 135–344.

Code of Federal Regulations. 2006. Title 50: Wildlife and Fisheries, Sub Part B General Requirements and Exceptions, §21.12 (d) General Exceptions to Permit Requirements. U.S. Government Printing Office.

Ritchie, B.W., Harrison, G.J., and Harrison, L.R. 1999. Avian Medicine: Principles and Applications. HBD International, Inc. Delray Beach, Florida, pp 1196.

Sibley, D.A. 2000. The Sibley Guide to Birds. Alfred A. Knopf, Inc., New York. 544 pp.

Stocker, L. 2005. Practical Wildlife Care. Blackwell Publishing Ltd. Oxford, UK, 335 pp.

2
Chick Identification

Guthrum Purdin

INTRODUCTION TO THE TABLES

The purpose of this chapter is to provide clues as to the identity of unidentified chicks, at least to the level of order or family, through attention to a few physical characteristics. There are nearly 1,000 species of wild birds breeding in North America, and currently there is no extant comprehensive identification guide available. A complicating factor to identification is the rapid growth rate of chicks; the appearance of many changes daily. Hence, an ID guide covering chicks would need to be even more sizable than the many excellent volumes covering adults. Many species are secretive during breeding and there are still great gaps in our knowledge about the chicks of some species.

When an unidentified chick is presented for care it is imperative that its species becomes known. Although there are many common themes to the needs of any baby bird, many species have special requirements for diet, housing, or behavioral enrichment. Species may be rare or endangered as well and there may be legal ramifications to their care.

Despite superficial similarities among bird families, physiological and metabolic needs are markedly different. For example, altricial parrot chicks need much lower levels of protein in their diets (about 20%) than altricial passerine chicks (50% or more). Even this generalization is highly variable between species. Parrots also have much larger crops relative to their body size than passerines; feeding regimens must be tailored accordingly to avoid over- or underfeeding. Other chicks, such as cranes, are likely to imprint on human caregivers, rendering them incapable of reproducing once released into the wild if they are not reared with techniques to avoid this problem.

Casual identification of chicks is often misguided. Even if a finder feels absolutely confident about the species of the chick, caregivers must evaluate chicks with a critical eye. Finders may never have looked very closely at adult birds and may be unlikely to have seen a baby before. Identification may have been made based on personal expectations rather than observation. Some species are brood parasites of other species; hence, even being from the nest of an identified species does not guarantee correct identification of the chick.

People frequently identify large chicks or even adult birds of other species as infant raptors. Grounded adult Caprimulgiformes such as Common Poorwills are often thought to be baby owls; nestling Rock Pigeons are not uncommonly thought to be baby hawks or even eagles. Most people are not aware of how quickly chicks gain weight. Obviously undeveloped nestlings may be as large as adults and may even be heavier than their parents, as is the case with cliff swallows and some raptors. In many species, the chick reaches adult body size well in advance of feather development.

Most young birds do not look like miniature versions of their parents; however, as soon as the first tips of feathers emerge from the sheaths, some species show a suggestion of adult plumage to come. Dark-eyed Junco chicks show the adult form's white outer tail feathers. Black Phoebe chicks show the white belly of the adult. Cliff Swallow chicks have a distinctive orange-brown patch of feathers on the top of their rump. The tail of wren nestlings tends to stick up at a sharp angle like the adult's with the tightly spaced transverse stripes becoming quickly apparent.

When presented with a chick of unknown identity, attention to particular features helps guide the caregiver to at least a tentative identification. Is the chick precocial or altricial? Precocial chicks are born with their eyes open and a warm coat of downy feathers. Altricial birds are born in an almost fetal state with eyes closed, nearly or completely naked, with some covered sparsely in natal down. Chickens are an example of precocial chicks familiar to most people. Once their down has dried after hatching, they are out of the nest following after the hen and able to start pecking at food. An internalized yolk remnant allows them a day or two to develop feeding skills. Their ability to thermoregulate is generally limited, and the parent typically uses its body heat to maintain the brood. Duck dams may shelter their precocial hatchlings under their wings, and parents of semiprecocial grebes carry chicks on their backs. Altricial chicks are dependent on parents for thermoregulation and must be closely monitored in captivity. Hatchlings are poorly aware of their surroundings, often responding by gaping to any disturbance of the nest. They are nestbound and entirely dependent on parental care. Semiprecocial birds represent an intermediate developmental style. Like precocials, they hatch with eyes open but have variable amounts of down and thus variable needs for thermal support from parents. Some species may be able to leave the nest for short excursions, but more remain until fledging and require feeding by the parents.

The next most helpful trait in determining identity is the arrangement of the toes. Birds have several foot types. *Anisodactyl,* the foot morphology most frequently associated with birds, has three toes forward and one pointed back. Raptor feet are basically anisodactyl but are characterized by heavy hooked talons. Owls have the same large talons but are *zygodactyl,* with two toes forward and two toes back, although sometimes owl feet may appear like the toes are at 90 degrees to each other or may vary from an *X* shape to a + shape. Ducks are *palmate:* The forward three digits are fully webbed and the rear toe, the hallux, is small and above the plane of the standing foot. *Semipalmate* birds are anisodactyl, but have only partial webs between the front toes that do not extend very far up the digits. The hallux on these birds is often greatly reduced or may be absent. Many sandpipers and some breeds of chicken have this morphology. Grebes have yet another variation on the anisodactyl foot: the *lobate* toes have webbing but do not attach to each other. When swimming, on the upstroke, these webs fold closed. On the downstroke, they spread open and propel the bird forward. American coot feet appear similar but have separate lobes on each joint of the toes; thus, they are termed *semilobate.*

Pelicans, cormorants, and their kin are *totipalmate.* Webbing connects all the toes, and the hallux is pulled medially. Swifts are *pamprodactyl,* with the ability to rotate the hallux fully forward so all four toes are anteriorly directed. Combined with strong sharp claws, this allows them to cling to sheer rock faces; even hatchlings can cling vertically 24 hours posthatch. Chimney Swifts are more likely to hold toes anisodactyl, and White-throated Swifts more habitually have all toes on the foot facing forward.

As an example, suppose a hatchling has been presented for care. First note whether the chick is altricial or precocial and what type of feet it has. Then look for other clues: color, beak, weight, color of gape, color and distribution of down, and so forth. This chick is completely naked, eyes are closed, it is a translucent pink color overall, and it has a flat midsized wedge-type beak. This could describe a number of species' altricial hatchlings. However, the feet are zygodactyl. Two toes point forward and two back. With this information it may be determined that it is a woodpecker, and Chapter 31, "Woodpeckers," can be consulted for further information. Were the legs black or grey, it could be a roadrunner or a cuckoo. Were the beak heavy and hooked, it would be a psittacine chick. Geography also plays a role in identification: Trogons have similar hatchlings, but since their range barely extends into Arizona from Mexico, chances of a trogon baby are slim in northern North America.

Table 2.1 presents a sampling of characteristics from a few commonly seen species from most major taxonomic groups. Tables 2.2 and 2.3 reprint highly useful information comparing the attributes of commonly encountered passerine chicks. These latter two tables were developed at Wildlife Rescue, Inc. in Palo Alto, California, and have since been used extensively by numerous wildlife shelters. Although many of the species covered in these latter two tables are oriented toward the West Coast, the tables can be quite valuable in identifying similar-appearing, closely related species. Closely related species' chicks often have similar needs even if adults diverge in lifestyle. All passerine chicks are altricial with anisodactyl feet, so these characteristics are not mentioned in the songbird tables.

Table 2.1. Chick identification based on developmental characteristics and morphology for selected species from most avian orders.

Hatching Status	Foot Topography	Weight	Integument	Mouth	Vocalizations	Species	Order
ALTRICIAL.	ANISODACTYL. Legs very tiny.	3 days: 0.9 g. Some hummingbird species as little as 250 mg at hatch.	Skin black. Natal down a "smoky fuzz" in 2 lines (11 pairs) running along dorsum. Significant pinfeathers after 1 week.	Yellow mouth, short and squat. Very different from long thin adult bill.	Begging call: high thin *seet.*	Anna's Hummingbird (*Calypte anna*) (BNA-226)	Apodiformes Chapter 27
ALTRICIAL. Cannot stand or lift head at hatch. If disturbed after first week, regurgitates. Iris grey.	ANISODACTYL. Legs/feet dark grey. May appear dirty white from feces.	Hatch: 60 g.	Naked, black face, throat, crop. Otherwise, short dense white down on head, long fluffy on body. By day 25, down dirty white and thicker.	Bill dark, short, and hooked. Nares large and perforate.	No syrinx. Hatch: weak hissing. After first week, uses various loud hissing sounds when threatened (wheezing snore, snake rattle, roaring wind, etc.). Lasts 3–7 sec.	Turkey Vulture (*Cathartes aura*) (BNA-339)	Ciconiiformes Chapter 14
ALTRICIAL. 5 cm length.	ANISODACTYL. Feet pink to slate.	Hatch: 15.2 g. Gains 4–8 g /day.	Long, silky, bright yellow natal down on head and body. Skin pink, visible under down; may be darker on head.	Bill leathery and pinkish to dark, light at distal tip. Lumpy around nares. Texture smooth.	Peeping call becomes persistent by 1 week. Nestlings will "dance" in circles while begging.	Rock Pigeon (*Columba livia*) (BNA-13)	Columbiformes Chapter 20
ALTRICIAL.	ANISODACTYL. Legs and feet dark, bare.	Hatch: 5 g. Day 10: 60 g. Fledge: 80 g.	Off-white natal down on head and body with dark, blackish grey skin visible.	Bill leathery and dark. Lumpy around nares. Texture smooth. Sharp egg teeth on maxilla and mandible.	Weak peeping becomes stronger as squabs develop.	Mourning Dove (*Zenaida macroura*) (BNA-117)	Columbiformes Chapter 20
ALTRICIAL.	ANISODACTYL, raptorial.	Hatch: 17.4 g. Gains 12 g/day first month.	Natal down light tan to yellowish. May be grey by week 1.	Hooked raptorial bill.	No information on hatchlings. By 2 weeks, will raise wings and gape if threatened but remain silent.	White-tailed Kite (*Elanus leucurus*) (BNA-178)	Falconiformes Chapter 14

Table 2.1. *Continued*

Hatching Status	Foot Topography	Weight	Integument	Mouth	Vocalizations	Species	Order
ALTRICIAL. Very weak on first day, more active after 24 hrs.	ANISODACTYL, raptorial. Femur bare.	Hatch: 57.6 g.	Hatch: white, short down. White occipital spot. White to pale gray after 1 week. By day 9, head is lighter.	Hooked raptorial bill.	Soft peeping (*pipsee*).	Red-tailed Hawk (*Buteo jamaicensis*) (BNA-52)	Falconiformes Chapter 14
ALTRICIAL. Weak. Dark eyes open first or second day. Crawls well by day 3.	ANISODACTYL, raptorial. Legs yellowish. Talons whitish pink.	Hatch: varies by region. About 8–10 g.	Skin pink. Down white, sparse. Distended abdomen largely bare. After 1 week, wing skin bluish.	Bill is not hooked, but has distinct "falcon tooth." The actual egg tooth is 1–2 mm. Bill and cere white-pink.	Hatch: peeping. Day 3: peep supplanted by *klee*.	American Kestrel (*Falco sparverius*) (BNA-602)	Falconiformes Chapter 14
ALTRICIAL, but with ears open and eyes partially open. Can move about, weakly. Cannot perceive movement.	ANISODACTYL, raptorial. Legs/feet pale pinkish. Talons pinkish to white.	Hatch: 110.6 g (105– 115 g)	Hatch: covering of short natal down, white. grayish	Hooked raptorial bill. Black. Prominent egg tooth.	Chirping starts well before hatch. Later adds cheeping and high-pitch chitters.	Golden Eagle (*Aquila chrysaetos*) (BNA-684)	Falconiformes Chapter 14
ALTRICIAL. Iris brown.	ANISODACTYL.	Hatch: 6.61 g.	Skin: pale salmon. Sparse down on dorsum, head, limbs long, grey.	Gape red.	A weak *peep* at hatch. Faint, high *peeping* if nest disturbed. Begging call louder, hoarser. Fledglings make a harsh squealing if captured.	Great-tailed Grackle (*Quiscalus mexicanus*) (BNA-576)	Passeriformes Chapter 36 most relevant for chick care. Check additional sources for wild diet for weaning.
ALTRICIAL. Doesn't move unless parent's arrival stimulates gaping.	ANISODACTYL.	Hatch: 3.5 g. Day 2: 6.3 g. 1 week: 23.1 g.	Naked. Feather tracts have sparse, fine grey down (6–11 mm). Skin orange.	Hatchling gape reddish orange, edged in yellow. Nestling grey to black. Gape flanges cream.	By fifth day, begging call loud.	Northern Cardinal (*Cardinalis cardinalis*) (BNA-440)	Passeriformes Chapter 36 most relevant for chick care. Check additional sources for wild diet for weaning.

ALTRICIAL. Maintains a vertical posture. Swallows without closing mouth.	ANISODACTYL. Legs/feet apricot orange. Pinkish beige by fifth day.	Hatch: 3 g. Day 3: 6 g. Day 4: 10 g.	Naked, apricot orange skin. Sparse 1 cm white down along feather tracts. None on ventrum.	Bill apricot orange. Gape reddish apricot with ivory white edging. Gape flanges yellow.	Quiet, high *peeps*. Nestlings have continuous *wheeur* that builds to loud begging when parent arrives.	Black-headed Grosbeak (*Pheuticus melanocephalus*) (BNA-143)	Passeriformes Chapter 36 most relevant for chick care. Check additional sources for wild diet for weaning.
ALTRICIAL. Eyes closed until about fourth day.	ANISODACTYL. Legs/feet orange-red.	Unknown.	Naked with some tufted grayish down Skin orange-red. By third day, dark lines on back, wings, and spot on head indicate emerging feathers.	Bill orange-red at hatch. Gape red with yellow edging from bill/gape flanges.	Fledglings start calling, *zee-zee-zee*, about a day before departure from nest.	Magnolia Warbler (*Dendroica coronata*) (BNA-136)	Passeriformes Chapter 37 most relevant for chick care. Check additional sources for wild diet for weaning.
ALTRICIAL. Once eyes open, iris is vibrant blue, becoming grey as bird fledges out. Adult iris dark brown.	ANISODACTYL. Legs/feet pinkish at hatch, becoming grayish black in nestling.	Hatch: 15.6 g.	Appears naked, but sparse grayish down wings, head, dorsum. Older chicks dark-skinned. Skin pink, by fourth day "drab rose" and pinkish slate after 1 week.	Bill pink at hatch, later grey-black. Gape blood-red. Darkening to grey-black as bird ages. Medium wedge shape.	At first weak, but gradually louder with age. A variety of *churrs*, *chee-aps*, *wa-eeks*, and squeaks among other sounds. Nestlings make a distinctive wet *yumyumyum* noise during hand-feeding.	American Crow (*Corvus brachyrhynchos*) (BNA-647)	Passeriformes Chapter 33
ALTRICIAL. Weak, quiet. Can barely lift head for first few days. Eyes remain closed first week.	ANISODACTYL. Unable to grip until about fifth day. Doesn't perch well until about day 10.	Hatch: 3.1 g.	Skin pink. Completely naked. By third day, rectrices barely appearing.	Gape bright red, edged with yellow of bill.	By fifth day, faint buzzing or chirping. Begging call a long excited trill using several *chip* syllables.	Cedar Waxwing (*Bombycilla cedrorum*) (BNA-309)	Passeriformes Chapter 36
ALTRICIAL. Can cling vertically day after hatch.	PAMPRODACTYL. Hallux rotates from ANISODACTYL to all forward. Claws greyish.	Hatch: 1.0–1.5 g. Day 10: 14.5– 21.0 g.	Naked. Pink.	Egg tooth on maxilla with matching hardened cap on mandible. Bill greyish. No gape flanges. Inside mouth drab.	Hatch: weak squeaking. Day 3: a stronger, repeating "*cheh-cheh-cheh*." Day 5: loud, ratcheting "*chuh-chuh-chuh*."	Chimney Swift (*Chaetura pelagica*) (BNA-646)	Apodiformes Chapter 28

Table 2.1. *Continued*

Hatching Status	Foot Topography	Weight	Integument	Mouth	Vocalizations	Species	Order
ALTRICIAL. Chicks huddle together, wings and necks intertwined.	SYNDACTYL.	Hatch: 9–13 g.	Naked. Bright pink. No down.	Upper bill shorter than lower. Egg tooth on both. No gape flanges. Inside of mouth pink. Color blackish.	Continuous chattering in nestlings. After day 1: warbling call. By 1 week, a "harsh, mechanical" rattle call similar ro adult.	Belted Kingfisher (*Ceryl alcyon*) (BNA-84)	Coraciiformes Chapter 30
ALTRICIAL. Weak and feeble. Stiff limb movement.	TOTIPALMATE.	Hatch: 27.6–34.7 g.	Naked. Skin a translucent, shiny brown. Develops thick, woollike, black down by week 2.	Culmen avg. length: 9 mm. Egg tooth present.	Chirps when begging or overheated. Hisses if threatened.	Double-crested Cormorant (*Phalocrocorax auritus*) (BNA-441)	Pelicaniformes Chapters 7 and 11 most relevant
ALTRICIAL. Unable to lift head, frequent vocalization. Eyes open at hatch, but with nonfunctioning nictitating membrane.	TOTIPALMATE.	Hatch: 73.5 g (54.9–87.0 g).	Hatch: naked with some natal down along posterior manus. Purpley-pink skin. Purple by end of week 1. Ectothermic at hatch. Grade into endothermy as white down grows (starting on rump), mass increases, and gullar fluttering develops by 3 weeks.	Initially, bill wedge-shaped and much, much shorter than adults. Growth is fast and linear from day 4–5 through to fledging. Full adult length not achieved until after fledge. Tip slightly hooked.	Begins "squawking" a day or two before hatch. Makes "shrill, rasping squawk" frequently after hatch.	Brown Pelican (*Pelecanus occidentalis*) (BNA-609)	Pelicaniformes Chapter 7
ALTRICIAL. Active and alert minutes after hatch. The sound of leaves rustling induces gaping.	ZYGODACTYL. Legs and feet light slate grey.	Hatch: 7.4 g. 24 hrs: 8.5 g.	Skin shiny black. Grey, hairlike natal down along feather tracts.	Bill a light slate grey. Gape red with elaborate pattern of large, flat, creamy-white, disk-shaped papillae on tongue and palate.	Insectile buzzing.	Black-billed Cuckoo (*Coccyzus erythropthalmus*) (BNA-587)	Cuculiformes Chapter 23 most relevant

ALTRICIAL, but strong and active. Touch induces gaping.	ZYGODACTYL. Legs black.	Hatch: 14 g. 24 hrs: 20 g. 3 days: 34 g.	Skin black, appears oily. White natal down along feather tracts.	Mandibles black. Commissure dull pink. Tongue tip black. Hard palate white. Buccal cavity red with 4 white markings. Rictus red. Beak wide, triangular at hatch. Narrows by fledging.	Whining, growling sounds.	Greater Roadrunner (*Geococcyx californianus*) (BNA-244)	Cuculiformes Chapter 23
ALTRICIAL. Chicks face toward center of nest with necks intertwined.	ZYGODACTYL. Legs pale, pink/white. Heel callouses large. Tiny white nails.	Hatch: 3.3 g.	Skin bright, translucent pink. Completely naked.	Bill pink/white. Maxilla is narrower at its base and sits in large white gape flanges, turning upward from mandible. Maxilla shorter than mandible with white egg tooth.	"Strident, rasping squeek" when begging. Otherwise silent.	Red-Cockaded Woodpecker (*Picoides borealis*) (BNA-85)	Piciformes Chapter 15
ALTRICIAL. The shadow of parent entering nest elicits gaping, even before eyes open.	ZYGODACTYL. Legs pink. Callous pads on heels.	Hatch: 1.67 g (1.55–1.77 g).	Skin "translucent pink." Completely naked. Tiny feather tips at rectrices and ventral tract barely visible.	Maxilla has shiny white covering tipped with egg tooth. Mandible pink/white and protrudes ~1 mm past upper beak. Oral flanges light pink. Tongue tip white and shiny.	Low, rhythmic *pip*. A rasping call when begging.	Downy Woodpecker (*Picoides pubescens*) (BNA-613)	Piciformes Chapter 31

Table 2.1. *Continued*

Hatching Status	Foot Topography	Weight	Integument	Mouth	Vocalizations	Species	Order
ALTRICIAL. Weak lifting of head to feed. Chicks huddle at bottom of nest.	ZYGODACTYL. Legs/feet beige to pink.	Hatch: 5.5 g.	Completely naked. Pink.	Bill pink. White, fleshy fold at commissure.	Buzzing starts shortly after hatch.	Northern Flicker (*Colaptes auratus*) (BNA-166)	Piciformes Chapter 31
ALTRICIAL. Unable to move around or raise head at hatch, but do gape.	ZYGODACTYL.	Hatch: 4.07–5.45 g.	Largely naked. Yellow down distributed sparsely over body.	Hooked, parrot-type bill.	Silent for first 2 days. A complex food-begging call used after day 10. A similar feeding call when eating (shorter note, longer interval).	Monk Parakeet (*Myopsitta monachus*) (BNA-322)	Psittaciformes Chapter 21 most relevant
ALTRICIAL. Low mobility. Especially sensitive to hypothermia.	ZYGODACTYL.	Hatch: 11.5–13.5 g.	Sparse whitish down over otherwise naked body.	Heavy hooked bill. Beige.	A rackety begging call.	Red-crowned Parrot (*Amazona viridigenalis*) (BNA-292)	Psittaciformes Chapter 21 most relevant
ALTRICIAL. Largely immobile after hatch. Egg tooth and yolk sack vestiges for 4–6 days, possibly longer.	ZYGODACTYL. Feet pink.	Hatch: 34.7 g. Gains about 33.3 g/day for first month.	Naked, pink. White down ventrally.	Hooked raptorial bill	Begins snapping bill at 1 week. Food call and whimper in response to adult hooting after a couple of days. After 2 weeks, hisses and clatters bill when threatened.	Great Horned Owl (*Bubo virginianus*) (BNA-372)	Strigiformes Chapter 24
ALTRICIAL. At first unable to rise. Weak crawling on day 1, improves until good walking on about day 14.	ZYGODACTYL. White down on front of legs and on digits.	Hatch weight varies a bit by subspecies. Average: 15.08 g.	Pink, bare areas on sides of neck, abdomen, and midback. White natal down elsewhere. By weeks 3–4, very fluffy, white, may be more greyish. Developing facial disk evident.	Bill color ivory. Hooked, raptorial.	Early on: a twittering call to get attention or show irritation. Food call a "raspy snoring." Loud hissing when disturbed.	Barn Owl (*Tyto alba*) (BNA-1)	Strigiformes Chapter 24

SEMIALTRICIAL. Light grey iris.	ANISODACTYL. Leg color varies "yellow to grayish to black." Digits lighter than legs. Long legs relative to body.	Hatch: 20 g.	Hatch: except for wings, covered in white down. Long hairy down on crown. Skin greyish. Bare areas at eye have pinkish and greenish tint, dark blue around eye. Pinfeathers visible by week 1.	Pale pink grey darkens distally to black tip. Has a yellowish or dark grey base to upper bill. All black by 1 week. Culmen day 1: 11.9 mm. Day 4: 15.9 mm. Inside mouth pale pink. Long spearlike bill.	"Soft buzzing calls" in nest. Begging call 2–3 syllables.	Snowy Egret (*Egretta thula*) (BNA-489)	Ciconiiformes Chapter 16
SEMIALTRICIAL. Eyes open at hatch. Iris grey-olive at hatch, light yellow by third day. Unresponsive at first. Sitting upright by next day.	ANISODACTYL. Legs drab, may be bluish. Digits lighter drab on top and yellowish ventral. Pink-ivory nails. Long legs relative to body.	Hatch: 24.2 g.	Skin pink. Gray down on dorsum, neck, head. White crown filaments. White femoral down. Lighter grey ventral.	Upper bill light drab, grayish tip. Becomes yellowish between 1 and 2 weeks. Black with yellowish sides around 2 months. Egg tooth (persists into second month). Pink interior. Long, spearlike.	Begging call *pip pip pip* begins day after hatch. Downy chick uses *yip yip yip* "like two stones being hit together." Later uses a *chuck chuck-a-chuck chuck* call. When threatened, uses a very loud "ghastly, sharply accented *Sque-e-e-e-e-e-ak.*"	Black-crowned Night-Heron (*Nycticorax nycticorax*) (BNA-74)	Ciconiiformes Chapter 16
PRECOCIAL, nidifugous. Will become motionless if approached. Iris dark.	ANISODACTYL (not webbed) and lacking hallux. Legs pink-buff. Nails black.	Hatch: 9.6–10.1 g on average.	Downy. From above: mottled buff, brown, black. Ventrum, throat, forehead white. A black stripe runs back from the eye. Wreathlike stripe around crown. Broader black band collars neck. Black middorsal stripe (normally broken). Bare eye ring: yellow grey.	Bill a glossy black. Gape pink (maybe grayish pink). Short, blunt wedge.	Begins peeping before hatch. Distress call: short piping notes.	Killdeer (*Charadrius vociferus*) (BNA-517)	Charadriiformes Chapter 9

Table 2.1. *Continued*

Hatching Status	Foot Topography	Weight	Integument	Mouth	Vocalizations	Species	Order
PRECOCIAL. Leaves nest right after hatch with parent, begins foraging, pecking. Iris brown, dark, but lighter than adult.	ANISODACTYL. Legs/feet dark grey. Hallux short.	Day 2: 6.1 g. Gains 2 g/day first 90 days.	Covered in down. Buff white, rusty on back and white underneath. Dark spot at ears. Large dark brown patch back of head with buff border. A pair of black stripes on dorsum.	Bill grey. Like chicken chick, but very short.	Chick call: trill (shortly posthatch). Juvenile call: peeping. Distress call: *pseu-pseu.*	California Quail (*Callipepla californica*) (BNA-473)	Galliformes Chapter 18
PRECOCIAL. Leaves nest soon after hatch. Self-feeding. About 7.6 cm tall by week 1. Iris dark brown.	ANISODACTYL. Legs/feet pink-white. Becomes browner with age. Hallux short.	Hatch: avg. 18.5 g. One month: 135 g.	Covered in down. Pale tawny to yellow buff. Dark stripes on flanks and dorsum. Black spots over ears, black patches on wings. Sides of crown and brow cinnamon.	Bill pink horn-colored with black at base of upper beak. Egg tooth not retained very long. Short, like chicken chick.	Contentment call: *ter-it* or *ter-wit.* Caution call: *terreep* or *turreep,* is "louder . . . more bubbling." Flock call: *tee-erp* or *pre-erp* when distressed.	Ring-necked Pheasant (*Phasianus colchicus*) (BNA-572)	Galliformes Chapter 18
PRECOCIAL, nidifugous. Fed by hen first few days.	ANISODACTYL. Yellowish.	Males: 48 g. Females: 46 g.	Natal down-covered. Throat white. Cinnamon head, back. Breast, sides lighter. Dark brown spotting extensive on crown, upper body. Sides of head, ventral body light pinkish buff to yellow.	Like chicken chick, but somewhat heavier.	A soft purr call is common. Especially noticeable when held. Three types of peep call (single, double, and multiple notes).	Wild Turkey (*Meleagris gallopavo*) (BNA-22)	Galliformes Chapter 18

PRECOCIAL, nidifugous. Hocksitting by 2–3 hours posthatch and can stand weakly. Can leave nest next day and start active feeding. Eyes dark umber.	ANISODACTYL. Legs/feet yellowish. Hallux short and above plane of other digits; doesn't reach ground. Long legs relative to body.	Hatch: 114.2 g. By week 1: 315 g (variable by subspecies).	Covered in thick, rusty brown down. Unlike adult, crown is feathered.	Bill beige-pink. Darkens distally. Length: 22.7 mm. Narrow.	Soft, continuous purring maintains contact with parent. Starting a day prehatch to about 9–10 months, uses several peeping and trilled whistle calls.	Sandhill Crane (*Grus canadensis*) (BNA-31)	Gruiformes Chapter 19
PRECOCIAL. Iris brown to grey-brown. Skin around eyes brown-grey. Cavity nest departure may involve prodigious falls.	PALMATE. Legs/digits brown, yellow highlights. Webs black.	Hatch: 23.7 g (19–28 g).	Covered in down. Dark brown dorsum and crown with stripe at eye. Buff yellow otherwise. Light yellow spots on shoulders and rump, wing patch. Tail very dark.	Maxilla grey brown, edge light yellow. Mandible yellow-pink. Nail reddish, paling distally. Egg teeth ivory, with lower bilobed.	Click call: 2–3 days prehatch. Alarm call: high pitched *peep*. Also shriek call and hiss if threatened.	Wood Duck (*Aix sponsa*) (BNA-169)	Anseriformes Chapter 12
PRECOCIAL. Iris brown. Leaves nest with hen day after hatch. Self-feeding.	PALMATE. Legs/feet orange with some grey-brown patterning.	Avg. hatch weight in North America: 31.8 g (27.2–40.6 g).	Fully covered in down. Face/body yellow base with brown-eye stripe, ear-spot, forehead. Also brown patches on dorsum (4) and wings.	Duck bill. Pink-beige with black spotting, black tip. Egg tooth.	Contentment call: quiet *pipi*. Distress call: loud *peep*. After week 1, air-alarm call: a shrill *pii*.	Mallard (*Anas platyrhynchos*) (BNA-658)	Anseriformes Chapter 12
PRECOCIAL. Departs nest 24–48 hrs. May rest on hen's back. Iris greyish brown.	PALMATE. Legs olive brown.	Hatch: 46.2 g.	Down-covered. Head dark brown to black, white eye-stripe, white cheeks. Rufous patch on neck, tawny brown patch over eye. Dark streaks bill to below eye. White ventral surface. Flanks, dorsum dark brown. White patches on rump and wings.	Grey bill. Slender. Relatively shorter than adult, not "ducklike." Sharply serrated in adults.	NA	Common Merganser (*Mergus merganser*) (BNA-442)	Anseriformes Chapter 12

Table 2.1. *Continued*

Hatching Status	Foot Topography	Weight	Integument	Mouth	Vocalizations	Species	Order
PRECOCIAL. Hardy. Self-feeding. Iris blue-grey. Shades to dark brown in adults. Long necks.	PALMATE. Leg/foot color varies: greyish yellow-green, olive grey, blackish grey, to black.	Varies by subspecies. 68–103 g.	Covered in down. Round dark crown. Body color varies bright yellow to greenish yellow. Fades to dirty grey as gosling develops.	Blue-grey to black. Egg tooth lighter than bill. Ducklike.	Calls either single strong peeps or warbling trills reflecting a range of social contexts.	Canada Goose (*Branta canadensis*) (BNA-682)	Anseriformes Chapter 12
PRECOCIAL. Ambulatory a few hours posthatch. Iris dark brown. Very long necks.	PALMATE. Legs/digits light pink. Light grey blue at distal toe joints and edges of tarsi/digits.	One day: 179 g (170.5–189.5 g).	Down light grey, darker dorsally, more whitish ventrally.	Bill light pink. Greyish blue along tomia and edge of nail. Nail bluish pink. Maxillary egg tooth ivory to yellow-green. Scalelike mandibular egg tooth translucent white. Ducklike.	Call: *kuk kuk*. A "squawking *aw*" when stressed.	Tundra Swan (*Cygnus columbianus*) (BNA-89)	Anseriformes Chapter 12
PRECOCIAL. Quickly self-feeds and begs from adults. Iris red. Prominent pollex with 1 mm claw.	SEMILOBATE. Lateral lobes indented at each toe joint. Legs/feet very large. Greenish grey scaled skin. Compare grebe foot in Fig. 6.1 to American Coot in Fig. 12a.1.	Hatch: 19–22 g.	Covered in thick down. Predominantly black, but grayish ventrally. Down has long red to orange waxy tips on neck and head. Yellow tips on wing down.	Bill orange at nares, shades to black distally. Proximal bill and frontal shield of face blood-red. Egg tooth.	Four calls. Twitter is most common, a contentment call. *Witou*: contact call, mild distress call. Squawk: distress call. *Yeow*: severe distress, as when held.	American Coot (*Fulica americana*) (BNA-697)	Gruiformes Chapter 12 most relevant

PRECOCIAL. Walks/swims to follow parents. Awkward for first 24 hrs. On hearing parent's alarm call, may stand and look around or crouch down. By week 3, may just run.	SEMIPALMATE. Legs/feet greyish blue. Legs long. Webs more developed between digits 3 and 4. Hallux is extremely small, clawed. Nails brownish. Edges of webs may be orangey.	Day 1: 20.2 g Day 7: 44.0 g Day 14: 90.8 g.	Covered in down. Cream to white underneath. Viewed from above, drab with cinnamon tone. Dorsum and crown spotted/ mottled with black. Grey on nape. Thin black line through eye may be solid, broken, or indistinct. A black line separates upper and lower tail from let to tip. Dark lines start at shoulders, meet as a single line midback, and become spotty caudally.	Bill short and jet black. Egg teeth on upper bill (larger) and lower lost in 24 hrs. Nestling bill nearly straight, without adult's pronounced upward curve.	Begins to *peep* and click prehatch, continuing into posthatch. When caught: *chip-chip-chip*.	American Avocet (*Recurvirostra americana*) (BNA-275)	Charadriiformes Chapter 9
PRECOCIAL, nidifugous. Can walk and jab at food at hatch.	SEMIPALMATE. Legs/feet long, blue-grey. Smallish hallux.	Hatch 37 g.	Covered in down. From above: pale buffy brown with darker dapples. From below: pinkish buff. Light brown wings. Dark crown patch and temporal spots. Stripe from lores doesn't reach eye. Diamond mark lower back meets central stripe. Another dark stripe leg to tail.	Bill 12.9 mm, feathers to tip (adult is 80–135 mm). Egg teeth upper and lower (last 1–2 days).	Unknown	Marbled Godwit (*Limosa fedora*) (BNA-517)	Charadriiformes Chapter 9

Table 2.1. *Continued*

Hatching Status	Foot Topography	Weight	Integument	Mouth	Vocalizations	Species	Order
SEMIPRECOCIAL. Eyes open, black. Ectothermic at hatch. Begins to move outside nest after day 2. Endothermy by 3 weeks.	ANISODACTYL. Legs small for body. Leg/foot grey-brown.	Weight N/A. Length at hatch: 65 mm when stretched. Adult: 19–21 cm, 31–58 g.	Natal down buff colored, ventrally paler. Sparse at hatch.	Black bill. Tubular nares. Bill small, but gape very large.	Peeping during hatch. First note vocalized about day 25. Full adult *poor-will* call day 65.	Common Poorwill (*Phalaenoptilus Nuttallii*) (BNA-32)	Caprimulgiformes Chapter 25
SEMIPRECOCIAL. Eyes open. Can locomote day after hatch.	ANISODACTYL. Small weak legs.	Hatch: 5.8–6.1 g. Length: 48–55 mm.	Sparse soft down. Dark grey above, pale to cream ventrally. Malar stripe and chin patch nearly black. Bare areas of dark skin midback and lateral lumbar regions.	Mouth appears much smaller closed than open. Bill small.	Largely silent. Soft peeping if disturbed.	Common Nighthawk (*Chordeiles minor*) (BNA-213)	Caprimulgiformes Chapter 25
SEMIPRECOCIAL. Climbs onto parent's back while still wet from hatch.	LOBATE. Legs and digits grayish black. Legs placed posteriorly, making walking and standing difficult. Compare grebe foot in Fig.6.1 to American Coot in Fig. 12a.1.	Hatch: 14.9 g (13.3–16.2 g).	Down-covered. Black on back and flanks. Longitudinal white striping. Two v-shaped stripes on crown. Black marks on sides of head and neck. Black spots reach to white chest. Cinnamon bar on nape, spot on crown. Lores bare, pink.	Proximal bill pink, black in middle, white egg tooth upper and lower bill (larger on maxilla). 5.1 mm, nare to tip, 4.6 mm top to bottom.	Weak begging call ("*ee-ee-ee-ee-ii-ii-iah*") during first few days. Remains soft until week 3, and then volume rises. Single *peep* every few seconds if distressed.	Pied-billed Grebe (*Podilymbus podiceps*) (BNA-410)	Podicipediformes Chapter 6

SEMIPRECOCIAL. Climbs onto parent's back while still wet from hatch. Iris black to grey, becomes adult red after day 80.	LOBATE. Legs and feet slate, almost black, lobed webs greenish. Legs placed posteriorly, making walking and standing difficult. Compare grebe foot in Fig.6.1 to American Coot in Fig.12a.1.	Within 1 day posthatch: 21.7– 36.0 g.	Featherless, "straw yellow" patch on crown, becomes red if begging or isolated from parent. Head has thick, velvet down black-grey with white strands (upper) and white (lower). Large white eye ring and bare white lores. Very light striping on sides of head. Body a velvety grey.	Black. The white egg tooth on maxilla tip has matched white spot on mandible (retained until about 156 g). Length about 11.5 mm. Between day 40–80, assumes nearly adult color of yellow-green.	Loud peeping before hatch. Continues after hatch, frequent and loud. Responds to foraging parent's "clucking" by emerging from brooding parent's back and begging.	Western Grebe (*Aechmophorus occcidentalis*) (BNA-26)	Podicipediformes Chapter 6
SEMIPRECOCIAL. Eyes open. Iris dark. Hatch in burrow.	PALMATE, but lacking a hallux. Leg/digits dark grey. Webbing pinkish grey.	Hatch: 61.4–70.3 g.	Covered in long down: 25–30 mm on dorsum, shorter elsewhere. May be black or brownish black. Some may be dark grey ventrally. A small percentage will have white ventrally. Cere is dark brown.	Maxilla dark grey, mandible pinkish grey. Egg tooth on upper bill may be lost early or maintained 2–3 weeks. Stumpy wedge.	Begging is a repetitious *peep peep peep.* Otherwise, *uiiiep uiiiep uiiiep.*	Tufted Puffin (*Fratercula cirrhata*) (BNA-708)	Charadriiformes Chapter 11
SEMIPRECOCIAL. Upright on tarsi within 24 hrs. Iris dark.	PALMATE, but lacking hallux. Feet/legs very large relative to body. Dark grey feet with black nails.	Hatch: 75.8 g.	Covered in down of medium grey color. 11 mm on body, head 8 mm. Paler ventrally. Down of head/neck has silver tips. After 2 weeks, white throat and side of head. Mask of dark grey. Dark line separating white patches extending from mask.	Mouth pale pink beige to purplish. Bill blue-grey. A conical wedge shape, tapering to point.	Early call a *peep.* More complex calls develop after first week.	Common Murre (*Uria aalge*) (BNA-666)	Charadriiformes Chapter 11

Table 2.1. *Continued*

Hatching Status	Foot Topography	Weight	Integument	Mouth	Vocalizations	Species	Order
SEMIPRECOCIAL, nidifugous. Eyes open, iris dark. Leaves nest soon after hatch.	PALMATE. Legs/feet: grey-pink at hatch, darkens with age.	Hatch: 60–75 g. Day 5: 100–150 g.	Body covered in thick, pale grey down. Dark spotting head/body/thighs. Mottled spots on back may look like lines. Fine grey-black spots on head: stellate to oblong. Paler ventral surfaces generally unmarked.	Bill black, sometimes horn-colored. Distal third pink buff. Base may be pinkish. Pinkish egg tooth lasts 2–3 days. A wedge shape.	Begins peeping once egg is pipped. Peeping persists as begging call. A "shrill waver" produced if threatened.	Herring Gull (*Larus argentatus*) (BNA-124)	Charadriiformes Chapter 10
SEMIPRECOCIAL, nidifugous. Eyes open, iris dark brown. Can stand/walk.	PALMATE. Legs/feet pink. May become somewhat more orange in first 2 weeks.	Hatch: 15 g. Day 3: 25 g. Day 14: 100 g.	Covered in thick down. Wings, flanks, dorsum: cinnamon brown to grey brown. Black spots or streaks, indistinct lines dorsally. Throat, neck-sides, lores are fuscous to brown black. Ventrum white. Rare individuals have spots only on head with cinnamon buff upper bodies.	Bill pink, tip black. Base may become somewhat more orange in first 2 weeks. A gracile wedge shape.	Begins soft *peep* at pipping and uses same while pecking parent's bill. Becomes a "squeaky cheeping" after a few days. Begging call an insistent *Kri-kri-kri-kri-kri*. Distress call: penetrating *zeee*.	Common Tern (*Sterna hirundo*) (BNA-618)	Charadriiformes Chapter 10

Table 2.2. Guide to identification of hatchling and nestling songbirds.*

Pink to Red Mouth Birds

SPECIES	*MOUTH COLOR*	*GAPE FLANGES*	*BEAK CONTOUR*	*DOWN*	*LEGS/ FEET*	*APPROX. WEIGHT in grams*			*FEEDING CALL*	*FEATHERS*	*SPECIAL FEATURES*
						Hatchling	*Nestling*	*Adult (F)*			
HOUSE SPARROW	pink	med. yellow, prominent	short, cone-shaped	none	short, chunky	2–13	14–20	27	melodic, single chirp	smooth, gray-white chest	
RUFOUS SIDED TOWHEE	pink	pale yellow	conical and pointed	dark gray	long legs, big feet	3–18	20–29	39		dark back, white spots on wings and tail	
CALIFORNIA TOWHEE	pink to red	pale yellow not prominent	conical and pointed	long, brown-gray on head, back and wings	long legs, big feet	4–20	25–39	52	high-pitched repeated, like crickets. changes to single peep	brown	

Table 2.2. *Continued*

Pink to Red Mouth Birds

SPECIES	*MOUTH COLOR*	*GAPE FLANGES*	*BEAK CONTOUR*	*DOWN*	*LEGS/ FEET*	*APPROX. WEIGHT in grams*			*FEEDING CALL*	*FEATHERS*	*SPECIAL FEATURES*
						Hatchling	*Nestling*	*Adult (F)*			
BROWN-HEADED COWBIRD	deep pink	white to cream not prominent	heavy, to a point narrower than a towhee's	long, snow-white	long legs, big feet, blk. tipped nails	2–20	25–30	39	continuous, high-pitched vibrating sound	breast yellowish when coming in	bald face, parasitic, often found in nests of towhees
NORTHERN ORIOLE	deep pink	pale yellow	long, pointed, narrow	long, white-lt. gray on back, wings. 2 rows on head	long, slate-gray legs	2.5–18	20–25	33	high, staccato, repeated notes, similar to blackbird	yellow breast, gray back, white wing bars	insect eater
LESSER GOLDFINCH	red	pale yellow	similar to finch	grayish	short, pink, stubby	1–6	7–8	10		green to rust back, yellow abdomen	red dot at corner of gape flanges
RED-WINGED BLACKBIRD	red	yellow, not prominent	long, pointed	scant, white on back, lower wings, and thighs	long legs	3–15	20–30	42			bald face, similar to cowbirds

BREWER'S BLACKBIRD	red	white, not prominent	long, pointed	blackish gray, fairly plentiful	long legs, white toenails	3–15	20–30	42	raucous, repeated call, sounds like a rusty hinge	black	
SCRUB JAY	red	while, not prominent	long and wide	none	long legs, grabby feet, white toenails	6–30	35–70	87	hatchling—short repeated peeping, later a single squawk	furry gray head, blue wings and tail	ruddy skin
HOUSE FINCH	red	white to yellowish	short, conical	white, long and plentiful. 4 rows on head	short, stocky	1.5–8	10–15	21	none when newly hatched, then high-pitched peeping	stripey, gray/white chest	
CROW	red	white	very long, large, heavy	sparse, gray-brown on head, underparts	long, heavy	18– 70	70–328	438		black	ruddy skin

PINK TO RED MOUTH SONGBIRDS INCLUDE: Blackbirds, Cowbirds, Crows, Finches, Goldfinches, Grosbeaks, Jays, Orioles, Sparrows, Tanagers, Towhees, and Waxwings

**Source:* Marty Johnson, Wildlife Rescue, Inc., Palo Alto, CA 94303, 1995. *By Permission:* International Wildlife Rehabilitation Council. *Journal of Wildlife Rehabilitation* Vol.18, No. 3.

Table 2.3. Guide to identification of hatchling and nestling songbirds.*

Yellow to Orange Mouth Birds

SPECIES	*MOUTH COLOR*	*GAPE FLANGES*	*BEAK CONTOUR*	*DOWN*	*LEGS/ FEET*	*APPROX. WEIGHT in grams*			*FEEDING CALL*	*FEATHERS*	*SPECIAL FEATURES*
						Hatchling	*Nestling*	*Adult (F)*			
STARLING	bright yellow	bright yellow, very prominent, lower larger than upper	very wide	grayish white, long and plentiful on head, back, and wings	long legs	5.5–30	40–60	80	hatchling —single squeaky note	gray-black	
MOCKINGBIRD	yellow	yellow	wide	dark gray, plentiful	long legs	5–18	20–32	43	hatchling —single, clear, piping note; then throaty bark	gray and white striped wings and tail	gray, irides., crescent markings on roof of mouth
ROBIN	yellow to yellow-orange	pale yellow	wide	sparse, cream on head, back, legs	long legs	5–35	40–60	77	hatchling —staccato trill	rust-tipped speckled y chest	skin often yellowish

BLACK PHOEBE	bright yellow-orange	bright yellow	wide, flat, tapering to a point	gray and sparse	long, thin legs	2–5	7–15	18	peep-peep	brown-tipped black feathers	insect eater
PACIFIC SLOPE FLYCATCHER	bright yellow-orange	yellow	flat, wide, pointy tip, "arrowhead" look	white on head, back and wings in a "star" cluster	long, thin, delicate, dark blue-gray, white toenails	2–6	7–8	11	insistent crow-like squawk, frog-like when older	buff abdomen, buff and white striped wings	insect eater
CLIFF SWALLOW	orange-yellow	flesh	very wide, flat, pointy beak	light gray head and back	short legs, small chubby feet	2–13	13–15	22	barking type chirp	nestlings—light tan on back by tail, otherwise adult	insect eater, cavity nest
VIOLET-GREEN SWALLOW	orange-yellow	cream	very wide, pointy beak	cream on head, shoulders, and back	short legs	1.5–8	8–10	14		white eyebrows	insect eater, cavity nest
CALIFORNIA THRASHER	orange-yellow	cream	curves down as nestling grows	dark gray on head, back, wings, thighs, plentiful	long legs	6–35	40–60	84		medium gray	

Table 2.3. *Continued.*

Yellow to Orange Mouth Birds

SPECIES	*MOUTH COLOR*	*GAPE FLANGES*	*BEAK CONTOUR*	*DOWN*	*LEGS/ FEET*	*APPROX. WEIGHT in grams*			*FEEDING CALL*	*FEATHERS*	*SPECIAL FEATURES*
						Hatchling	*Nestling*	*Adult (F)*			
CHESTNUT-BACKED CHICKADEE	orange-yellow	very yellow, prominent	flat, wide	gray on head and back	long, pale bluish purple	1–4	6–8	10	squeaky cheep	buff abdomen, black head, buff-white circles on side of head	insect eater
BEWICK'S WREN	orange	yellow	flat, wide, pointy	long, gray on head only	long, delicate	1–4	6–8	10			
BUSHTIT	deep orange-yellow	yellow	short	none	long, delicate	1–3	3.5–4	5	3 syllable "locator" call, "mohawk" look	gray, first feathers on crown of head	females have blue eyes, cavity nesters
WRENTIT	deep orange	yellow	pointy	none		1.5–6	7–11	14		gray-brown	yellow irides.

YELLOW TO ORANGE MOUTH SONGBIRDS INCLUDE: Bushtits, Chickadees, Creepers, Dippers, Flycatchers, Mockingbirds, Robins, Shrikes, Starlings, Swallows, Thrashers, Thrushes, Titmice, Wrens, and Vireos

**Source:* Marty Johnson, Wildlife Rescue, Inc., Palo Alto, CA 94303, 1995. *By Permission:* International Wildlife Rehabilitation Council. *Journal of Wildlife Rehabilitation* Vol.18, No. 3.

It is advisable to develop a library of field guides that targets the avifauna one expects to see but includes other types that may be present unexpectedly. The *Sibley Guide to Birds* (Sibley 2000) has excellent reference paintings and the sister volume *The Sibley Guide to Bird Life and Behavior* (Elphick et al. 2001) goes into greater detail on how birds conduct themselves. The most complete commercially available book on chicks is Baicich and Harrison's *Nests, Eggs and Nestlings of North American Birds* (2005).

Most of the information in Table 2.1 was derived from the Birds of North America Online, an amazingly comprehensive and continually updated compendium of information about America's birdlife. Reasonably priced online subscriptions are available to the public at http://bna.birds.cornell.edu/BNA/. Other pieces of information were gleaned from the chapters themselves.

It cannot be overemphasized that not all birds are alike. Neonates must be treated according to the individual needs of their family and species. However, making that vital first identification can be daunting, in many ways not so much a science but rather an art developed with practice and research. With diligence, caregivers can build a unique body of knowledge. It is necessary to make use of all available clues to target the correct rearing techniques to the right species. The reward is a healthy and vibrant living bird.

ACKNOWLEDGMENTS

Many thanks to Marty Johnson for creating the songbird tables and the International Wildlife Rehabilitation Council for allowing their use.

REFERENCES

Baicich, P.J. and Harrison, C.J.O. 2005. Nests, Eggs, and Nestlings of North American Birds, Second Edition. Princeton University Press, Princeton, NJ, 347 pp.

Elphick, C., Dunning Jr., J.B., and Sibley, D.A. 2001. The Sibley Guide to Bird Life and Behavior. Alfred A. Knopf, Inc., New York, 588 pp.

Poole, A., ed. The Birds of North America Online. Cornell Laboratory of Ornithology, Ithaca; retrieved from The Birds of North American Online database: http://bna.birds.cornell.edu/BNA/; AUG 2005. [Individual species papers are indicated by BNA number under each species in Table 2.1.]

Sibley, D.A. 2000. The Sibley Guide to Birds. Alfred A. Knopf, Inc., New York, 544 pp.

3
Incubation of Eggs

Susie Kasielke

INTRODUCTION

Artificial incubation of bird eggs, like everything we do to care for animals, requires both art and science. A large body of scientific work on avian embryonic development has been done to optimize production in the commercial poultry industry. Fortunately for those working with nondomestic birds, the process of development and hatching avian embryos is highly conserved across all species, so most of the knowledge derived from domestic species may be directly applied to other taxa. Variation among species is seen in incubation periods (terms), temperature and humidity requirements, and, to some extent, the hatching process. This is where the art, our collective avicultural expertise, refines science-based techniques to achieve optimal hatchability.

Artificial incubation may be used as a tool to increase production in rare and endangered species, because many birds will lay replacement eggs if the first clutch of eggs is removed. In this case, timing of removal of eggs may be carefully planned. Most often, however, artificially incubated eggs have been rescued due to parental abandonment or other emergency. In some cases, a combination of natural and artificial incubation may give the best results. Certain species, such as raptors, have better hatchability if eggs are naturally incubated, either by actual or foster parents, for one-quarter to one-third of the incubation term before placing under artificial incubation. With a new or contentious pair of birds who may squabble over incubation duties with freshly laid eggs, replacing them with artificial or "dummy" eggs during most of the term will protect valuable eggs from breakage. Once parents have settled in and proven themselves with dummy eggs, the real eggs may be carefully returned to them, usually at internal pip, to allow parental hatching and rearing.

In order to manage the process of artificial incubation, and to some extent natural incubation, it is important to first have a thorough understanding of the structure of the egg, the functions of its components, the development of the embryo and its extraembryonic membranes, and the hatching process. This chapter provides a cursory review of these. The reader is strongly encouraged to take advantage of more detailed references on the subject (Anderson-Brown 1979; Hamburger and Hamilton 1951; Romanoff and Romanoff 1949, 1972) and to practice incubation techniques with chicken eggs or other domestic species.

When the egg is laid, the embryo is positioned over the least dense area of yolk and so rises to the uppermost position regardless of the position of the egg. The yolk is surrounded by layers of albumen, including the chalazae, which keep the yolk suspended in the egg and prevent the embryo from sticking to the shell. In addition to serving as a source of water and protein for the embryo, the albumen contains antimicrobial proteins that are a barrier to infection. Surrounding the albumen are two nonliving membranes, the inner and outer shell membranes. The air cell forms between these two membranes, at the blunt end of the egg in most species, initially as the egg contents cool and contract after laying and then during incubation through evaporation of water through the pores of the shell. The shell provides not only physical protection but also the primary source of calcium and other minerals for the developing embryo. The shell is covered by the cuticle layer, which ranges from glossy to chalky to barely visible in various species. This coating helps regulate water loss and, along with the shell and shell membranes, provides a mechanical barrier to infection. The embryo begins to develop before the egg is laid and does so initially in a flat plane, with the four extraembryonic membranes extending outward from the body wall.

The yolk sac is the first of these living membranes to develop. It is a highly vascular structure, initially forming a roughly circular pattern as it begins to envelop the yolk. Before other membranes have formed and because, along with the embryo, it is in contact with the inner surface of the shell membranes at the high point of the egg, it serves as the first respiratory organ for the embryo, providing a limited amount of gas exchange. As it grows, it becomes thicker and develops folds lined with villi to increase surface area for the uptake of nutrients much like the mature intestinal wall. The yolk is the primary nutrient source for the embryo, and for the chick even after hatch for a few days, and contains maternal antibodies providing some passive immunity to the embryo, which has no active immune function.

The amnion is the next membrane to develop, also extending outward from the body wall. This nearly transparent membrane is minimally vascular. It grows up and over the embryo, eventually closing and filling with fluid that will cushion the embryo during development. The amnion also contains fine muscle fibers that contract rhythmically to prevent the embryo from sticking to it until embryonic muscles are developed enough to perform this function.

The chorion is formed by the extension of the amnion folding back on itself from the seam where it sealed over the embryo. It extends out to line the entire inner shell membrane, fusing with it and with the allantois, which is the last membrane to form.

The allantois is highly vascular. It emerges balloonlike from the hind gut of the embryo, continuing to expand and coming in *contact* with the chorion, with which it fuses, forming the chorioallantoic membrane or chorioallantois. The fluid that expands and is contained by the allantois is urinary waste, with uric acid crystals held in suspension until shortly before hatching, when they precipitate out of suspension into strands of opaque, white urates. The chorioallantois is the primary respiratory organ for the embryo throughout most of incubation, allowing transpiration of oxygen, carbon dioxide, and water vapor from its dense vascular network across the shell. It also forms the albumen sac, which ruptures its contents into the amniotic fluid just after the middle of incubation, allowing the embryo to consume the albumen protein that facilitates its final growth stage. Lastly, the chorioallantois transports calcium and trace minerals, etched from the shell, to the developing embryo.

HATCHERY FACILITIES AND EQUIPMENT

Before the first egg arrives, the hatchery must be well organized and equipped. Although few facilities have the resources to build and equip an ideal hatchery, most of the following principles can be achieved in any facility with some creativity and attention to detail.

Because eggs and chicks are vulnerable to infection and disturbance, the hatchery should in effect be treated as a quarantine facility with access restricted to only essential personnel. The design should allow the primary functional areas to be separated and a one-way traffic flow, from cleanest to dirtiest, should be maintained. The incubation room, with only intact eggs, has the least contamination. Before they are externally pipped, eggs should be moved to the hatching room because the shell waste and feather dander of hatched chicks might provide substrates for microbial growth. Once hatched and rested, chicks should be moved to the chick rearing room where food, feces, and more feather dander create the greatest source of contamination. Tools and equipment should also follow this one-way path, being thoroughly disinfected before returning to previous areas.

The rooms should be constructed with materials that allow all surfaces to be washable, including floors, walls, and ceilings. Only equipment and supplies in current use should be kept in the room, and clutter should not be allowed to accumulate. Historic paper records and reference materials are invariably dusty and should be stored elsewhere. Rooms should have adequate ventilation with frequent air changes and, ideally, a separate system for each functional area. The environment should be kept at 65–70°F (18–21°C) and must be as dry as possible to minimize microbial growth and optimize incubator function.

In developing the hatchery design, consideration should also be given to every aspect of its function. An efficient design facilitates easy servicing of incubators, routine weighing and candling of eggs, frequent cleaning, and maintaining and moving equipment.

Although the skill of the person operating an incubator is far more important than the machine itself, investment in high-quality equipment invariably pays off. There is no one incubator that is best, and in fact all have potential quirks. The number and type acquired will depend on each facility's species, number of eggs, and budget. Talking over the options with those in established hatcheries is very helpful in making these decisions. For many operations, a good strategy is to have at least three incubators, all set at the same temperature but each at a different humidity so that eggs may be moved among them as needed rather than making risky adjustments during incubation.

Most incubators currently available for avicultural incubation are tabletop models, making it possible to have several in a relatively small room. Popular brands available in the United States include Grumbach (Lyon Electric), Alpha Genesis (China Prairie), Lyon Roll-X (Lyon Electric), Georgia Quail Farm (GQF Manufacturing), and Brinsea (Brinsea Products). A.B. Newlife incubators (A.B. Incubators) are sold only in the United Kingdom, but have been used in some U. S. facilities with good results. Brinsea has recently begun marketing a "contact" incubator, which is intended to more closely simulate natural incubation. The air above a flexible plastic membrane is heated by a forced-air system. This membrane is then in contact with the tops of the eggs in the tray underneath, creating a temperature gradient from the top to bottom through each egg, which is somewhat similar to a still-air system. Inexpensive incubators made primarily for classroom use with chicken eggs are usually not reliable enough for avicultural incubation. The Humidaire Incubator Company is now out of business, but its popular table-top Models 20 and 21, as well as its older freestanding Model 50, Ostrich and Gooser incubators, may be worth purchasing used although replacement parts may be difficult to find. The Petersime Company has also discontinued making its excellent freestanding incubator models 1 and 4.

Nearly all current models have electronic temperature controls that are accurate and dependable. Older incubators may employ mercury contact thermometers or ether wafers to control temperature. Contact thermometers are also accurate but have a fatal flaw: When they fail, the heating element stays on rather than shutting off and eggs are rapidly overheated. Ether wafers are still used as a backup temperature control system in some incubators. They are less accurate than electronic controllers but are useful in a secondary system. They deteriorate over time and should be replaced annually.

Humidity may be provided by an automatic humidifier with either an evaporative pad or fine mist, or by simple evaporation from open water reservoirs. Automatic humidifiers are usually quite accurate and effective but are nearly impossible to clean and disinfect, particularly during use. Unless mounted into the machine, most open reservoirs are easily changed out for cleaning. If not, using simple water pans in lieu of the humidifier built into the machine may make things easier. Humidity is controlled by increasing or decreasing the surface area of water, usually by adding or removing pans. To ensure consistent humidity, pans should be straight-sided, made of nonreactive material such as stainless steel or plastic and kept full (distilled water only) at all times. With multiples of the same-sized pans, both changing humidity and changing pans is easily done.

Turning mechanisms fall into three types: trays that are rotated, rollers on which eggs rest, and grids (or bars) that push eggs along a substrate. Rotating trays are usually safe because eggs do not actually move, but many do not rotate through an adequate radius of 90°. Used properly, rollers provide sufficient turning radius for most eggs, although small eggs receive more turning and large eggs receive less. If rollers are improperly spaced, eggs may "ride" the rollers and receive little or no turning. Eggs with a conical shape tend to "walk" toward one end of the rollers. Placing eggs point-to-point will minimize this. Grids or bars that push eggs have a greater chance of breaking eggs.

Incubators may also be used as hatchers, but these functions should be done in separate machines to prevent contamination of incubating eggs and to accommodate changes in temperature and humidity during the hatching process. Machines designed specifically for hatching are also available. In addition to the models listed above, both Brinsea and A.B. Newlife make hatchers. Spare parts for both incubators and hatchers should be kept on hand to quickly repair mechanical problems during incubation.

Thermometers are often frustrating monitoring equipment because it is almost impossible to get two of them to agree when placed side by side. Nonetheless, it is important to invest in high-quality thermometers. Better mercury, digital, and bimetal dial thermometers with a range bracketing that of incubation and readable increments of 0.1°C or F should be used. All should be calibrated annually. A laboratory-grade ASTM-certified mercury thermometer, model 18F, (VWR Scientific catalog #61127-006 or

Fisher Scientific catalog #15-059-438) is useful for this and can be used directly in some incubators. The VWR or Fisher Humidity/Temperature Pen with Memory (VWR catalog #35519-049, Fisher catalog #11-661-14) is one of the most accurate for use in incubation and has the advantage of being able to stay on continuously, allowing accurate readings without opening the incubator door. Similar-looking models are available from some incubator vendors but have not performed as well and do not stay on continuously. Alcohol or "spirit" thermometers are not accurate enough for egg incubation.

Humidity in egg incubators has traditionally been measured using wet-bulb thermometers, otherwise known as *sling psychrometers*. One end of a cotton wick is placed over the bulb of a secondary thermometer and the other end in a small water reservoir, usually a glass tube. Often only the reading of this wet bulb is used to record humidity, but true relative humidity is actually calculated from the differential between the dry- and wet-bulb temperatures. The same wet-bulb temperature will indicate different humidities at different dry temperatures. If the wick is not rinsed daily and changed at frequent intervals, increasingly inaccurate readings will result and it may become a source of contamination in the incubator. Dial hygrometers give direct relative humidity readings but must be calibrated for the humidity range in which they are used. Digital hygrometers are both accurate and reliable, but it is important to buy a high-quality model (VWR catalog #35519-049, Fisher catalog #11-661-14) rather than those made for monitoring rooms, because these are more variable.

Precise scales are essential for effective egg weight loss management. Digital scales are more affordable than in the past. Scales should be laboratory quality if possible. The range of egg sizes seen in the hatchery will determine the capacity and weighing increments needed for effective egg weight loss management. For eggs weighing less than 30 g at lay, the scale should weigh in increments of and have an accuracy of 1/100th g. For eggs greater than 30 g but less than 500 grams, increments and accuracy of at least 1/10th g are needed. If the only eggs incubated are from ratites and weigh over 500 g, whole gram increments and accuracy are sufficient.

In most hatcheries, it is important to have an egg candler with the greatest light intensity available. The Lyon High-Intensity Zoo Model Candler (Lyon Electric) is currently the brightest available. An old-fashioned slide projector, adapted to focus the beam and prevent light leaks, works nearly as well. For facilities incubating only small, white eggs, such as parrots, less powerful candlers are fine. The Probe Light Candler (Lyon Electric), an inexpensive, battery-powered, fiberoptic candler is ideal for checking small eggs in the nestbox. Prototype models of infrared and ultraviolet light candlers may be useful for imaging with eggs that are difficult to candle with incandescent light but are not commercially available.

A room dehumidifier is essential in humid climates and with species whose eggs have difficulty losing sufficient weight, such as condors and ostrich. An emergency backup generator is indispensable, even if it produces only enough power to run one machine. A portable incubator may be useful, especially if eggs must be transported long distances between facilities or from the field, or in freezing weather. Dean's Animal Supply's The Brooder Mini is small enough for use on an airplane (contact the airline well in advance for security assistance) and may be run on 110 V household current, a car cigarette lighter outlet, or portable batteries.

HATCHERY SANITATION

A rigorous sanitation protocol will minimize egg and chick mortality due to infection. Access to the hatchery should be restricted to essential personnel, and only the equipment and supplies in immediate use should be stored in the rooms.

Before the onset of the breeding season each year, the hatchery and all its equipment should be thoroughly cleaned and sanitized. A strong disinfectant such as Synphenol-3 (Veterinary Products Laboratories), a synthetic phenol product, is recommended. The interiors of incubators and hatchers are now more frequently sanitized with such a product between uses, but great care must be taken to rinse and air all parts and ensure that sensitive electronics are not damaged because the solution is somewhat corrosive. In the past, formaldehyde fumigation was the preferred method, but due to serious human health hazards this is now strictly regulated or prohibited by state laws. All machines should have any necessary annual maintenance performed, and then operated for testing and stabilization before eggs are likely to arrive.

Once the hatchery is operational, routine cleaning of the rooms should be done at least weekly. This should include wiping down all working surfaces, washing the floor, and cleaning water reservoirs in the incubators. Iodine-based, chlorhexidine, and quaternary ammonium disinfectants are good choices for this. Chlorine bleach is inexpensive but creates noxious fumes and is corrosive to equipment. Water pans and wet-bulb wicks should be replaced with freshly sterilized (autoclaved) or disinfected pans and wicks. Water reservoirs that cannot be removed for cleaning should be drained and flushed periodically during the season. A disinfectant footbath placed outside the door will reduce contaminants that may be tracked into the rooms. The trash receptacle may also be kept just outside to minimize the potential for contamination in the room.

Staff working in the hatchery should organize daily work to minimize the potential for contaminants to enter the hatchery. It is essential to service the hatchery first, before entering any other bird area. Some facilities choose to use protective clothing, such as lab coats or coveralls, over work clothes in the hatchery but this may also serve as a reservoir of contaminants in the rooms. Clean dedicated clothing for the hatchery is preferred. Hands should be washed thoroughly with antibacterial scrub before servicing incubators and aseptic technique should be observed. When handling eggs, the use of exam gloves in addition to hand-washing is strongly recommended.

EGG HANDLING AND STORAGE

Many factors affect hatchability even before the egg is laid. These include genetics, nutrition, and exposure to toxins, as well as physiological factors, such as age and disease, and behavioral influences, such as stress or physical trauma that may affect egg formation. Much research has been done on all of these and many other publications are available for reference (Kuehler 1983; Landauer 1967; Romanoff and Romanoff 1972).

Additional factors influence hatchability once the egg is laid but before incubation starts. Infection of the incubating egg is one of the main causes of reduced hatchability. Microbial contamination of the shell may come from feces, nest material, or human hands. Physical trauma such as cracking or breaking of eggs is an obvious cause of egg mortality, but any jarring, shaking, or vibration may disrupt the loosely adhered cells of the blastoderm, much like a sand painting, and cause abnormal twinning, duplications, or complete failure of the embryo. Allowing an egg to roll or turn over and over in the same direction may cause the chalazae to wind up like rubber bands and break, causing the embryo to stick to the inner shell membrane.

Environmental conditions prior to incubation affect hatchability. At a temperature of 70°F (21°C) or higher, embryonic development will initiate, but different tissues will form at abnormal rates, resulting in embryonic mortality. Eggs will also lose too much weight through water evaporation if held at ambient humidity.

Many taxa, such as waterfowl, do not begin incubating until the clutch of eggs is complete. Eggs of these species tolerate short periods of storage better than those of single-egg clutches, such as flamingos, or multiple-egg clutches of species that begin incubation with the first egg, such as parrots. When incubating a lot of eggs of certain precocial species, such as ostrich or pheasant, it is desirable to synchronize hatching by storing eggs and then setting a group at once. Such eggs may be stored up to 7 days without significant decrease in hatchability. Ideal parameters for egg storage are 55–60°F (13–15°C) and 70–80% relative humidity (RH). Refrigerators designed for wine storage may be set to the appropriate temperature, and humidity can be provided the same ways as in an incubator. Ventilation, although not crucial, is important to prevent condensation moisture from forming on the eggs. Eggs may be stored in cardboard egg flats or clean sand and should be rotated through at least a 90° angle once daily. Stored eggs should be allowed to warm gradually, usually overnight, to room temperature before being set in the incubator.

INITIAL CARE OF EGGS

Eggs that have been partially incubated prior to transfer to the hatchery must be placed in the incubator as soon as possible, especially if they have already become chilled. More time may be taken with unincubated eggs. In either case, eggs should be handled with exam gloves or paper towels and should be transported to the hatchery with great care taken to avoid rough handling or jarring. Many types of transport containers have been used, from cardboard boxes to buckets to small ice chests, which are filled or lined with cushioning materials such as clean paper or cloth toweling, waterfowl down, or small seed such as millet. Hot water bottles or chemical warming packs may be used if transport time or outdoor temperature puts eggs at risk of prolonged cooling. Caution must be used to ensure that these do not come in direct contact with the eggs and that the eggs are maintained below incubation temperature, because even slight overheating would damage developing embryos. For longer trips, portable electronic incubators or brooders made for chicks (Dean's Animal Supply) are useful, with the option of using wall outlets, car cigarette lighter jacks, or rechargeable batteries for power. Whatever the container, it should be handheld during transport if possible to reduce the risk of shaking and jarring.

Once at the hatchery, the egg should be carefully examined both directly and with the candler. Cracks and flaws may not be obvious until the egg is candled. These should be carefully marked with a blunt pencil during candling to ensure that potential openings for infectious agents will be completely sealed. An identification number may also be written on the shell in pencil. A fine black marker may be necessary for heavily pigmented eggs. Embryonic and membrane development, if initiated, should be described along with any anomalies in or on the egg.

Soiled eggs should have loose, dry material such as down, nest substrate, or feces gently brushed off with a dry paper towel, gauze sponge, or swab, depending on the size of the egg. Large deposits of dried fecal material may be mostly removed by carefully sanding with a clean, fine sanding block or emery board, taking great care not to disrupt the cuticle or shell. This will leave a visible stain or thin coating, which should be left undisturbed.

Eggs should never be spot-cleaned with liquid. Even using an antiseptic or disinfectant solution fluid on the shell may facilitate the movement of infectious microbes through the pores of the shell and into the egg. In commercial production of domestic species, unincubated eggs may be dipped in a disinfectant solution to reduce contamination. This is done with products designed specifically for this purpose and using strict protocols of concentration, temperature, agitation, and immersion time. The temperature of the solution must be sufficiently higher than the egg contents but not so high as to kill the embryo. If the solution is too cool, the egg contents will shrink, drawing surface contaminants rapidly into the egg. Dipping is generally contraindicated for nondomestic bird eggs, especially those with more delicate or thin-shelled eggs. Eggs that may have received any incubation should not be dipped. Fumigation with formaldehyde gas has also been used commercially to sanitize eggs, but it is more strictly regulated and less often used these days as the fumes are highly toxic to humans. Formaldehyde gas has been shown to cause lethal embryonic defects in the eggs of nondomestic species. Other methods of sanitizing eggs, such as exposure to ultraviolet light, have not been shown to be effective. The best way to prevent soiling of eggs and resulting infections is to ensure a clean nest environment whenever possible.

Cracked, flawed, punctured, or dented eggs are often hatchable if carefully repaired. If not repaired, they are vulnerable to infection and excessive weight loss. Even if there is a slight leakage of albumen or blood, repairs may usually be made. Eggs leaking yolk material, however, are not repairable. Various materials have been used to repair eggs, with some more suitable than others. Tape and wound dressing products do not make an adequate seal over an opening in an egg. Similarly, surgical tissue glue or other cyanoacrylate glues are often too fluid and do not fill in fine cracks or punctures. In a laboratory setting, where a large number of eggs is undergoing invasive procedures, high–melting-point paraffin is typically used but is less practical in a small hatchery. Clear nail polish is quick-drying and has been used successfully, especially with small eggs, but it contains volatile solvents that have the potential to be toxic to the embryo. White glue, such as Elmer's Glue All® or Wilhold (not school glue), although slow-drying, is an excellent, nontoxic material for repair that also provides some structural support.

White glue should be applied with a sterile swab and using aseptic technique, thoroughly sealing the entire crack or puncture but only covering the affected area so as not to interfere with chorioallantoic respiration. For large dents or cracks that compromise the structural integrity of the egg, thin, sturdy paper toweling (or tissue paper for tiny eggs) may be used to create a papier maché patch. The patch should be torn (not cut) just larger than the area to be supported and carefully pressed onto a layer of glue, eliminating air bubbles, and sealed over with another layer of glue. Because white glue will become more fluid at incubation temperature and may run down the side of the egg, the egg should be placed in a paper-towel–lined dish on the bottom of the incubator or on a leveled tray until the glue is thoroughly dried. If necessary, slight hand-turning can substitute for machine turning during this time. It is better to take this precaution, even with a small repair, than to come back later to find an egg glued to the tray.

Eggs compromised by cracks or excessive soil that are too valuable to discard should be incubated in a separate machine from sound eggs if possible or, if this is not an option, at least in a separate tray.

INCUBATION PARAMETERS

Natural incubation conditions create a temperature gradient from the top to the bottom of the egg, humidity varies within the nest microclimate, and turning occurs with varying timing and radius. Artificial incubation does not strictly mimic the natural process, but it should strive to achieve the same outcome. Eggs should hatch in the same incubation term for the species as is seen under parental incubation. The chicks should be able to hatch without assistance and be vigorous after hatching. And as with any scientific effort, these results should be consistently repeatable.

Temperature

Incubating machines may be either still-air or forced-air. Although still-air incubators, those with a radiant heat sources that circulate air by convection rather than fans, create a temperature gradient, the temperature is difficult to control, ventilation is poor, and capacity is limited due to the necessity of setting eggs in a single layer. Temperature in a still-air incubator is usually, but not always, measured at the top of the egg. When using parameters developed by others, it is important to verify how and where temperatures are taken. Nearly all incubators in current use have a forced-air design, with air circulated by a fan that creates a uniform temperature throughout the cabinet. Only forced-air incubation parameters will be discussed here.

Domestic poultry species are normally incubated at 99.5°F (37.5°C) and this temperature works well for many nondomestic species. Particularly large eggs with longer incubation terms typically require lower temperature. For example, 96.5°F (35.8°C) is typically used for penguins, 98.0°F (36.7°C) for condors, 98.5°F (36.9°C) for waterfowl and 99.0–99.2°F (37.2–37.3°C) for psittacines. The smallest eggs, such as small passerines and others with shorter incubation terms may hatch best at temperatures of 100.0–100.5°F (37.8–38.1°C).

If the temperature is a little too high, embryonic development will be slightly accelerated but at different rates in different tissues. If chicks hatch, they are likely to be reduced in size, have rough umbilical seals, and be thin and noisy. During hot weather, power failures affecting air conditioning may cause overheating in incubators despite the power loss to the machines. Once incubation starts, embryos usually survive temporary drops in temperature, but do not tolerate increases in temperature. An increase of even 1.0°F (0.5°C) is often fatal in a few hours or less. If eggs must be moved in an emergency, such as during a machine or power failure, they should always be moved to a machine with the same or lower temperature.

If the temperature is too low, embryonic development will be retarded, with different rates in different tissues if this is extreme or prolonged. It is not usually lethal unless to an excessive degree or duration, but chicks are often large, sluggish, and sticky with incomplete yolk sac retraction or partially open umbilical seals. Power failures causing cooling for more than a few hours will prolong development. Although embryos may survive the initial insult, detrimental effects are usually not seen until the hatching process is initiated and some late mortality may occur.

During the hatching process for commercial poultry, the incubation temperature is dropped by 0.5–1.0°F (0.3–0.5°C), which has been shown to improve hatchability. This seems to work well for nondomestic species as well, although it has not been scientifically tested.

Humidity

Avian eggs lose weight during incubation, usually 15% ± 3%, by water evaporation through the pores of the eggshell. Because this is a physical process, not a metabolic process, it is not influenced by the stage of embryonic development and follows a linear pattern throughout incubation. Under artificial incubation conditions, this weight loss is managed by controlling the humidity in the incubator.

Domestic poultry are normally incubated at 55–60% relative humidity. This is a good starting point for most nondomestic species. Eggs of species such as ostrich that are from exceptionally dry climates, however, are incubated without supplemental water in the incubator and may require a room dehumidifier. Similarly, eggs from wet-climate species will require high humidity from the start.

Eggs should be weighed as soon after they are laid as possible and weight loss tracked throughout incubation to ensure successful hatching. If the humidity is too high, weight loss will be insufficient and embryos are likely to be edematous and/or malpositioned or have residual albumen or fluids, potentially resulting in drowning. Chicks that do hatch may have unretracted yolk sacs and/or open umbilical seals and will be lethargic. Humidity that is too low will result in excessive egg weight loss. This causes poor bone mineralization due to impaired calcium transport and weak, dehydrated (red) chicks with rough/bloody umbilical seals. Ambient humidity is naturally low at high altitudes and even parent-incubated eggs may lose too much weight. In this situation, good strategy is to remove eggs for artificial incubation at an appropriate humidity and give the parents dummy eggs, returning their own eggs just before hatching.

For artificially hatched eggs, the humidity in the hatcher should be increased as soon as eggs are externally pipped in order to limit the drying of shell membranes, which can restrict the embryos' movement. The amount of humidity needed varies by species, but those eggs with longer pip-to-hatch intervals are at greatest risk of having dry membranes.

Turning the Eggs

Eggs must be turned at regular, frequent intervals during incubation to facilitate normal membrane development and nutrient uptake and to prevent the embryo from sticking to the inside of the shell. Chickens turn their eggs every 35 minutes on average; most incubators with automatic turning mechanisms turn eggs hourly. Some machines can be set to turn at greater or lesser intervals, but hourly turning is generally sufficient for nondomestic species. Although commercial poultry eggs are set with their air cells uppermost and rotated around the short axis in order to maximize the number of eggs that will fit in the incubator, nondomestic species are not adapted to hatch well in this position. They should be set on their sides and rotated around the long axis. Eggs must be turned in opposite directions each time to prevent rupture of the chalazae and should turn through a radius of at least 90°. Supplemental hand-turning, usually two to three times daily through ~180° in opposite directions, may improve hatchability, particularly in large eggs. In machines that do not turn through at least 90°, additional hand-turning is essential to ensure completion of the chorioallantoic membrane. When automatic turning is not available and eggs are hand-turned, they must be turned a minimum of five times daily, preferably more, but always an odd number of times to prevent eggs from being in the same position overnight every night.

Ventilation

Because embryos are respiring throughout incubation, they are sensitive to abnormal levels of oxygen and carbon dioxide in the incubator. In most avicultural settings, only a few eggs are incubated at a time, so ambient outdoor oxygen and carbon dioxide concentrations are naturally maintained in the incubator as long as the hatchery is adequately ventilated. The exception to this is at high altitude where the oxygen concentration in the air is lower. In that case, testing and supplementing oxygen levels in the incubator may increase hatchability. Commercial incubation facilities, however, must always work to ensure adequate ventilation, especially late in incubation when eggs are generating high levels of carbon dioxide. During a power failure with incubators containing large numbers of eggs, opening the incubator for ventilation within an hour becomes more important than keeping it closed to conserve heat.

CANDLING

Candling is the primary method for monitoring embryonic development. Excellent photos of candled eggs, healthy and not, at all stages of development are available on the internet (Delaney, et al. 1998; Ernst, et al. 1999) and in published materials (Jordan 1989). Many eggs have pigmented shells that make candling difficult or even of little value later in incubation. It is important to have a room that can be completely darkened and to use a candler with the strongest light available. The brighter the candler, the hotter the light, so great caution must be used to avoid damaging eggs. Eggs should not be held against the light for more than a few seconds at a time and their surfaces should be felt to ensure they do not overheat.

Before eggs are placed in the incubator, they should be candled to evaluate shell quality, check for cracks and flaws, note yolk quality and mobility, and determine air cell formation and position. During incubation, development of the embryo and its extraembryonic membranes should be monitored to the extent possible, based on visibility. The progression of the air cell may be tracked by tracing its margin on the shell with a blunt pencil at regular intervals, usually every 4–7 days.

The first observable evidence of development is often the shadow of the blastoderm, appearing as a faint crescent along one edge of the yolk, although this is not visible in all fertile eggs. The yolk will also begin to increase in size and appear more fluid as water from the albumen moves into the yolk material. By 1/7th of the incubation term (3 days of 21 for the chicken) the embryo and yolk sac vessels should be clearly visible in even the smallest eggs. Practiced eyes may discern this even in the most heavily pigmented eggs, although candling will quickly become impossible as vessels line the shell in such eggs. Note that while it is possible to confirm fertility by candling once the embryo has reached the stage of blood development, it is not possible to confirm infertility by candling alone. In eggs that remain "clear" on candling, fertility may be determined only by breaking them open and carefully examining the contents.

It is useful to record landmarks of development, such as heartbeat, eye pigment, membrane progression and embryonic movement, and other detailed comments on candling observations, including sketches. Review of past records may help determine whether eggs are progressing normally, but only if notes are written in sufficient detail.

Initially, the yolk sac will appear as a roughly circular red "spider" shape with the embryo in the center. As this membrane surrounds the yolk and becomes more complex, it will appear less distinct, an effect that is soon compounded by the vessels of the chorioallantoic membrane (CAM) as they line the inside of the shell. This "streaky" stage is often incorrectly interpreted to be the breakdown of vessels. Eggs at this stage have even been removed from incubation by those who were convinced they were dead or dying. The vasculature of the CAM eventually becomes more distinct and heavy. It should completely line the inside of the shell soon after the middle of the incubation period, usually forming a visible "seam" along the back side of the egg. Insufficient turning radius and setting eggs with the air cells uppermost will prevent the CAM from completing. This is easily checked by candling the egg from the small end.

The first indication that the hatching process has begun is the apparent sudden enlargement of the air cell, termed *drawdown*. This is caused by the slight separation of the inner and outer shell membranes rather than a true increase in air cell size. The inner shell membrane that has been taut above the embryo during incubation is now loosely draped like a blanket, allowing the embryo more flexibility of movement. Prior to internal pip, the shadow of the embryo's beak may be seen pushing against the membrane. The hatching contractions will appear irregular and jerky. Once the embryo has internally pipped, or pierced into the air cell, regular, rhythmic respiration is observed. After external pip, candling can verify whether the outer shell membrane has been pierced, ensuring the embryo's access to outside air. As the hatching process progresses, candling at the small end and sides may be used to monitor the regression and shutdown of the CAM vessels, at least in light-shelled eggs. This is especially useful in deciding if and when hatching assistance may be safely initiated.

EGG WEIGHT LOSS MANAGEMENT

Eggs must lose the appropriate amount of weight during incubation in order to hatch successfully. Generally this is about 15% of the initial egg weight at laying, or fresh weight, for most species. Because this is not a metabolic function but occurs by the physical process of water evaporation through the pores of the eggshell, it is linear and can be manipulated by increasing or decreasing the humidity during incubation. Carefully monitoring and controlling egg weight loss is key to hatching success.

Eggs should be weighed as soon after laying as possible. Using a starting weight taken after eggs have started incubation will result in inaccurate weight loss calculations that may affect hatchability. If a true fresh weight cannot be obtained, it can be approximated by the following formula:

$$\begin{array}{l}\textit{Fresh}\\ \textit{Weight}\\ \textit{Estimate}\end{array} = \frac{\begin{array}{c}\textit{Current}\\ \textit{Weight}\end{array}}{1-\left(\dfrac{\begin{array}{c}\textit{Days Incubated From}\\ \textit{Setting to Current}\end{array}}{\begin{array}{c}\textit{Total Days of}\\ \textit{Expected Incubation}\end{array}}\times(0.15)\right)}$$

This equation assumes that the egg has had a weight loss trend of 15% under the incubating parents, as represented by the term "0.15" in the equation. This number may be adjusted as indicated by individual circumstances.

Once the fresh weight is known or estimated, the expected weight loss may be calculated and the actual weight loss tracked graphically (see Figure 3.1). This may be done using computer software

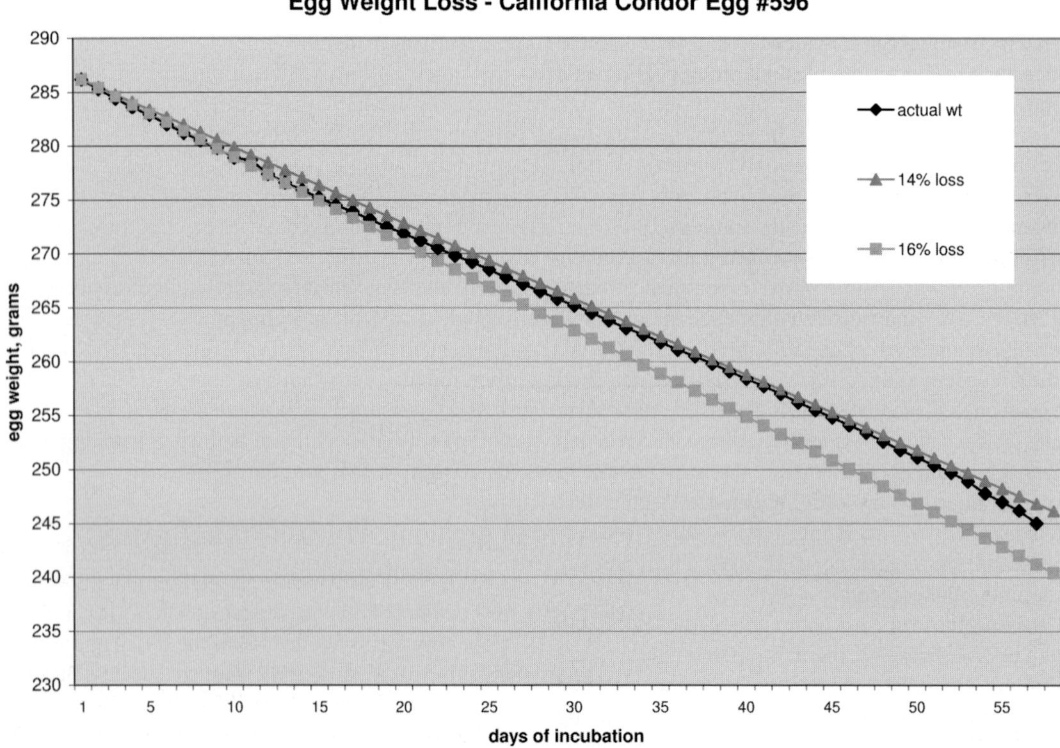

Figure 3.1. Graph of California condor egg weight loss.

designed especially for hatchery management, such as AIMS (Brinsea), a generic spreadsheet application, or simply graph paper and pencil. Egg weight is plotted on the Y-axis, with a scale range from fresh weight to fresh weight less 20% (approximately). Days of incubation are plotted on the X-axis, with the lay date as day 0 and continuing a few days beyond the expected incubation term. If the expected weight loss is 15%, lines that bracket this, e.g. 14% and 16%, should be plotted on the graph. Then, as actual egg weights are plotted, it will be easy to see whether the weight loss is staying within the expected range and whether the slope of the line projects the appropriate trend.

If the date the egg was laid or incubation started is unknown and cannot be estimated, it is more difficult to manage weight loss. Such eggs should be set with parameters used successfully for the same or similar species and the progression of the air cell closely tracked. If there are records for eggs of very similar size, the expected daily weight loss for the current egg(s) may be estimated.

Weigh eggs daily at the same time each day. This is particularly important during the early part of incubation because it becomes increasingly difficult to change an established weight loss trend later in incubation. When incubating large numbers of eggs, weight loss may be recorded and managed for the average of all eggs or for a representative subset.

RECORD KEEPING

Consistent, detailed record keeping is essential to successful hatching of eggs and to analyses and ongoing refinement of techniques of artificial incubation. The following basic data should be collected on each egg and/or clutch:

- Species
- Individual egg identification number
- Dam's and sire's identification, age, and reproductive history

- Lay date
- Set date (the date either natural or artificial incubation commenced)
- Expected term
- Expected egg weight loss
- Fresh weight (egg weight on lay date, actual or estimated)
- Incubator and hatcher (identify individual machines)
- Temperature and humidity settings prescribed

Each time the egg is handled for weighing, candling, or moving to a different machine, the following data should be recorded:

- Day of incubation (lay date = day 0)
- Date and time
- Actual temperature and humidity
- Current egg weight
- Candling observations, changes to the incubation environment, and other comments
- Initials of the person recording data

These data may be recorded directly into a spreadsheet or egg management software program for egg management during incubation, including monitoring of egg weight loss, and later analysis of overall hatchery results.

In addition to egg incubation records, data on individual incubators and hatchers should be recorded. Subtle problems with individual machines may become obvious only through poor hatchability. Records will help identify specific problems, such as excessive temperature fluctuation or failed turning mechanisms, and indicate needed repairs or adjustments. The following information should be recorded about each machine:

- Make, model, serial number, and local identification
- Date, time, temperature, humidity, and egg tray position at least twice daily and whenever the machine is opened
- Type of event, including routine monitoring or servicing the machine, such as adding water or cleaning reservoirs
- Adjustments to parameters, weighing, candling, or movement of eggs, and seasonal cleaning or repair
- Initials of the person recording data

Similarly, monitoring room temperature and humidity on an ongoing basis will aid in management of the hatchery.

THE HATCHING PROCESS

As the time of hatching nears, the embryo approaches its maximum size, occupying nearly the space within the egg except for the air cell. The gas exchange capacity of chorioallontois becomes insufficient causing the onset of hypoxia (low O_2 in blood) and hypercapnia (high CO_2 in blood). The embryo consumes remaining fluids while positioning for hatching. The spine is aligned with the long axis of the egg, with the dorsal side corresponding to the "highest" edge of the air cell; the head is between the thighs in the small end of the egg. The head gradually moves up alongside the body to under the right wing, positioning the egg tooth under the air cell (inner shell membrane) (see Figure 3.2). The hatching muscle along the back of the neck engorges with lymph. At this stage, the entire head may be edematous despite normal egg weight loss, but pulmonary respiration will normally dissipate this edema. Correct positioning is correlated with adequate egg weight loss, incubation position (on the side versus air cell up) and adequate ventilation (excess CO_2 often causes upside-down embryos).

The first indication that the hatching process has begun is air cell drawdown seen on candling as the inner and outer shell membranes begin to separate. The inner membrane is then draped over the embryo rather than being taut, and the air cell margin appears irregular. Internal pip occurs as contraction of the hatching muscle causes the egg tooth to pierce the inner membrane. Pulmonary respiration is then initi-

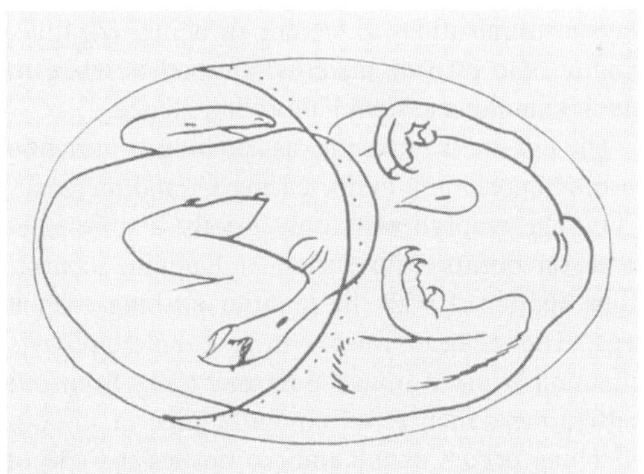

Figure 3.2. California condor embryo in correct hatching position with the head under the right wing (drawing credit: Mike Clark, Los Angeles Zoo).

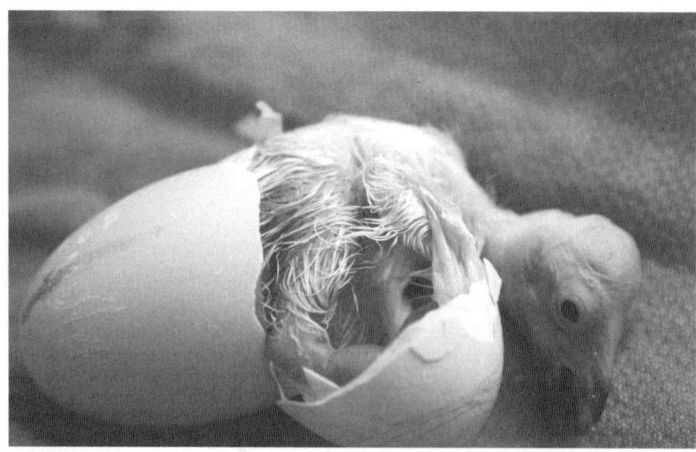

Figure 3.3. California condor chick hatching (photo credit: Mike Wallace, Courtesy of the Los Angeles Zoo).

ated. This may be audible, including vocalization in response to stimulation by the parent or surrogate. The contractions subside as gas exchange improves and the embryo rests. With exposure to air and the rubbing movements of the embryo, the chorioallantoic vasculature begins to recede, initially around the air cell, finally at the umbilical seal just prior to hatch. External pip occurs as hatching contractions resume in response to decreasing O_2 and increasing CO_2 and the egg tooth pierces the shell. The contractions again subside as gas exchange improves and the embryo rests.

The yolk sac is gradually drawn into the abdomen, facilitated by embryonic movement. By hatching, the yolk sac is fully internalized behind a tight umbilical seal. The remaining yolk continues to be a food and water source for the chick for up to 3 days as it transitions to feeding or being fed. It also continues to provide maternal antibodies while the chick's immune system gains competence.

The pip site is broken up as hatching contractions resume in response to decreasing O_2 and increasing CO_2. The embryo rests only briefly at this stage. Rotation occurs with sustained hatching contractions combined with the embryo pushing with its legs. The embryo rotates in a counterclockwise direction (viewed from the air cell end), from one-half to more than a full circumference of the egg. Hatching occurs as the embryo pushes the cap off and frees itself from the shell (see Figure 3.3). The chick then rests and dries off. Residual chorioallantoic vessels protrude from the seal but normally dry quickly. It may remain on its side for some time, even continuing to push as if still hatching. Healthy, artificially hatched chicks are usually ready to move from the hatcher to the brooder when they can maintain sternal posture, will give a feeding response, and have defecated. They should be weighed and have their umbilical seals swabbed with a tamed iodine solution such as Betadine.

HATCHING ASSISTANCE

Even under ideal conditions, a proportion of embryos will fail to hatch, often due to malpositioning. Because of this, the imperfect nature of artificial incubation and the likelihood that eggs are in the hatchery because they were already compromised, it is sometimes appropriate to assist the hatching process. There is no simple formula for all species, or even individual species, to determine when this is necessary. Careful observation of many healthy eggs, particularly during the hatching process, will make it more obvious when something goes wrong.

Failure of the embryo to make expected progress during the hatching process warrants more frequent observation and possible assistance. When malpositioning is suspected, eggs may be radiographed, using film and/or screens that give very fine detail. A piece of thin surgical wire may be loosely taped along the surface of the egg as a marker to correspond with a pencil line drawn on the shell. In order to determine which structures are in front of others, four views will be useful: presumed V-D (ventral-to-dorsal), and then rotated 45° counterclockwise (viewed from the air cell end) around the long axis three times so that the last view is presumed to be left lateral/dorsal oblique. Interpreting the images takes considerable time and patience because the bones are poorly calcified and overlay one another.

If the embryo has internally pipped but failed to make progress within the expected time, providing an air hole may be helpful at this stage. A small hole, ~2 mm, may be drilled at the apex of the air cell, well away from the embryo, using a Dremel tool with a clean abrasive bit. A 16 or 18 gauge hypodermic needle may also be used as a drill, but extreme caution must be used to avoid slipping and injuring the embryo. Some embryos require no further assistance and go on to hatch on their own, making us wonder whether the assistance was necessary in the first place.

If the embryo has failed to internally pip and is either losing strength or becoming frantic, it may be necessary to manually provide an internal pip. A larger hole may be made in the shell nearer the tip of the beak and a hole made through the membranes over the beak and nares, using blunt dissection technique to minimize bleeding. The location blood flow to the chorioallantoic membrane and location of large vessels may be checked by moistening a sterile swab with sterile water (or normal saline or lactated Ringer's solution) and gently pressing or rubbing the area. If necessary, repeating this process will eventually reduce the refill rate of the vessels, making it safer to break the membranes.

Once this is done, it is most often necessary to fully assist the embryo from the shell when it is ready. Both the retraction of the yolk sac and shutdown of chorioallantoic vessels take time. It is important to try to make sure that both these have occurred before the shell is completely removed. Candling all areas of the egg is helpful in monitoring vessels. It is difficult and sometimes impossible to see whether the yolk sac is exposed, but removing too much shell will allow the embryo to push out prematurely. In the meantime, the hole in the shell should be covered with cellophane tape or dressing material such as Tegaderm that is perforated or loose around the edges to allow air exchange while retaining moisture. Membranes usually become too dry during a lengthy assisted hatch and can even shrink, compressing the embryo. Application of sterile water or isotonic solutions seems to aggravate this drying, but oil-based artificial tears or ophthalmic ointment, used sparingly, can be helpful. Care must also be taken to ensure that the tip of the beak and the nares remain clear.

There also is a risk of infection at this stage because both the membranes and yolk sac are exposed to the air and microbes in the environment. Using sterile, or at least aseptic, technique will minimize the risk. Because California condors have a protracted hatching period (an average of 72 hours from external pip to hatch in self-hatching eggs at the Los Angeles Zoo), it is routine to treat them prophylactically with antibiotics when the egg must be opened for assistance. An antibiotic least likely to cause kidney damage, such as Rocephin (Roche Pharmaceuticals), is dripped onto the inner surface of the chorioallantoic membrane.

Malpositioned embryos with the beak not near the air cell are more difficult to assist. Radiographs can determine the position of the beak and an air hole made directly in over the beak. This is certain to result in some bleeding but usually not enough to be life threatening. Because it has not pipped into the air cell, the embryo will not have that additional space to allow movement and yolk sac retraction. An additional small hole should be drilled at the apex of the air cell and the egg positioned such that the weight of the embryo will gradually push out the air at that end, gaining more room to move. This is also a good technique for embryos that externally pip on their own away from the air cell. These may even hatch without further assistance, although they warrant frequent checks.

Most chicks, even those requiring hatching assistance, will have fully retracted their yolk sacs and tightly closed their umbilical seals. A few, however, may have partially or fully unretracted yolk sacs. If there is a small amount exposed and the seal is slightly open, it may be possible to ease the yolk sac into the body cavity and suture the seal closed. If the seal has tightened around a small knob of yolk, the chick may be kept especially clean until the material dries and eventually sloughs off. If there is a large part or all of the yolk exposed, it is usually surgically amputated. Great care must be taken when tying it off because there is normally a loop of intestine external to the body cavity until the yolk sac is retracted. Chicks that have had their yolk sacs amputated will require supportive care, including feeding frequent small amounts as early as possible, as well as a course of antibiotics.

EGG NECROPSY AND ANALYSIS OF HATCHING FAILURES

Thorough analysis of hatching failures is crucial to future hatching success. This chapter will provide a simple outline for this process. The reader is strongly encouraged to take advantage of more detailed references on the subject (Ernst, et al. 1999; Joyner and Abbott 1991; Kuehler 1983; Langenberg 1989).

The two main statistics that are most useful are fertility and hatchability, expressed as percentages. Fertility is the ratio of the number of fertile eggs to the total number of eggs received. For commercial poultry, this is usually 90% or more. Similar fertility should be seen in aviculture as well with mature, healthy, compatible birds. Hatchability is the ratio of the number of hatched eggs to the number of fertile eggs set (*not* the total number of eggs—infertile eggs are incapable of hatching). This is typically 87–93% in commercial poultry hatcheries but tends to be lower in aviculture even under good conditions for a variety of reasons.

This expected or normal mortality falls into specific developmental periods. One-third, or about 2–5% of all expected mortality occurs during the first few days of incubation and is primarily due to chromosomal anomalies when the gametes form. The remaining two-thirds, about 5–9%, occur during the last few days of incubation and are usually associated with the hatching process, including malpositions. There should be little or no mortality during the middle of incubation.

It is important to break out and examine all unhatched eggs, including those that are "clear" on candling. If all clear eggs are assumed to be infertile, efforts will likely be made to solve a fertility problem when in fact there may be a hatchability problem with a vastly different cause.

The first step in a thorough egg necropsy is a review of the parental history and the incubation record. The egg should be candled to locate the embryo, air cell, and any unusual characteristics. It may be desirable to take microbial culture samples from the shell surface and/or egg contents, particularly the yolk contents, but the embryo will likely have been dead for more than a day, resulting in a high number of decay organisms and masking infectious ones. It is sometimes very difficult to determine whether an embryo is still viable and usually wise to risk leaving the egg under incubation a few days longer.

Clear eggs and those with younger embryos are best opened in water. The shell can be cracked (much like for cooking), and the egg held submerged in a bowl of water while the shell halves are eased apart. Broken yolk is likely to obscure everything else, so it may be necessary to carefully strain and rinse the egg contents to find membrane tissue or a tiny embryo. Eggs with older embryos may be opened with forceps, beginning with a hole over the air cell and carefully noting the condition of the extraembryonic membranes and fluids and the position of the embryo as the shell and shell membranes are removed. Using a standard system of characterizing embryos by developmental stage (Hamburger and Hamilton, 1951), breakout results should be characterized as follows.

"Clear" on Candling:

- I = infertile—blastodisc centrally dense white, not "donut-shaped" as in fertile egg
- PD = positive development—no discrete embryo but white membranous tissue covering a watery yolk
- FND = fertile, no development—rare case of development ceasing at lay due to genetic defect or thermostabilized blastoderm

"Blood Ring" on Candling:

- BWE = blastoderm without embryo—membranes and blood only
- ED = early dead embryo (see below)

Obvious Dead Embryo on Candling:

- ED = early dead embryo—H&H stage 1–19 (≤3 days in chick embryo)
- MD = mid-dead embryo—H&H stage 20–39 (3–14 days in chick embryo)
- LD = late dead embryo—H&H stage 40–45 (≥14 days in chick embryo)

All embryos should be examined to determine whether they are normal for their developmental stage and whether that stage is consistent with the number of days of incubation.

Hatching failures due to obvious causes such as insufficient egg weight loss are easy to diagnose with individual eggs, and to prevent in the future. Most causes of poor hatchability will be more subtle and difficult to detect, so careful analysis of data over time will prove invaluable. For example, if there is a high incidence of mortality during mid-incubation, it may be traced back to a nutritional problem with the breeding birds or to a source of infection of the eggs. The problem may be as simple as a malfunctioning turning mechanism on a particular incubator. Diligent and detailed record keeping followed by objective data analysis is the best way to ensure optimum hatchability.

SOURCES FOR PRODUCTS MENTIONED

A.B. Incubators, Unit 1, Church Farm, Chelmondiston, Ipswich, Suffolk, IP9 1HS, UK, +44(0)1473-780-050, http://www.abincubators.co.uk.

Brinsea Products, Inc., 704 North Dixie Avenue, Titusville, FL 32786, (321) 267-7009, (888) 667-7009, http://www.brinsea.com/default.html.

China Prairie Company, P.O. Box 2000, 121 Briceland Road, Redway, CA 95560, (888) 373-7401, http://www.chinaprairie.com.

Dean's Animal Supply, Inc., P.O. Box 701172, Saint Cloud, FL 34770, (407) 891-8030, http://www.thebrooder.com.

Fisher Scientific Worldwide, One Liberty Lane, Hampton, NH 03842, (603) 929-2410, http://www.fisherscientific.com/index.cfm?fuseaction=order.map.

G.Q.F. Manufacturing Company, P.O. Box 1552, Savannah, GA 31402-1552, (912) 236-0651, http://www.gqfmfg.com.

Lyon Technologies, Inc., 1690 Brandywine Ave, Chula Vista, CA 91911, (888) 596-6872, http://www.lyonelectric.com.

Roche Pharmaceuticals, Hoffman-La Roche, Inc., 340 Kingsland Street, Nutley, NJ 07110, (973) 235-5000, http://www.rocheusa.com/products/rocephin/pi.pdf.

Veterinary Products Laboratories, P.O. Box 34820, Phoenix, AZ 85067,(602) 285-1660, (888) 241-9545, http://www.vpl.com.

VWR Scientific, 1310 Goshen Parkway, West Chester, PA 19380, (610) 431-1700, (800) 932-5000, http://www.vwr.com.

REFERENCES

Abbott, U.K. 1992. Cockatiel Embryonic Development. poster. publication #21504. University of California, Division of Agricultural and Natural Resources. http://anrcatalog.ucdavis.edu/InOrder/Shop/ItemDetails.asp?ItemNo=21504.

Abbott, U.K., Brice, A.T., Cutler, B.A., and Millam, J.R. Embryonic Development of Cockatiel. 1992. University of California, Davis. http://animalscience.ucdavis.edu/research/parrot/c/c.htm.

Anderson-Brown, A.F. 1979. The Incubation Book. Spur Publications Co./Saiga Publishing, Surrey.

Burnham, W. 1983. Artificial incubation of falcon eggs. Journal of Wildlife Management 47(l): 158–168.

Delany, M.E., Tell, L.A., Millam, J.R., and Preisler, D.M. 1998. Orange-winged Amazon Parrot Incubation Series. University of California, Davis. http://animalscience.ucdavis.edu/research/parrot/d/d.htm.

Ernst, R.A., Bradley, F.A., Abbott, U.K., and Craig, R.M. 1999. Poultry Fact Sheet No. 32: Egg Candling and Break Out Analysis for Hatchery Quality Assurance and Analysis of Poor Hatches. Animal Science Department, University of California, Davis. http://animalscience.ucdavis.edu/Avian/pfs33.htm.

Gilbert, S.F. 2003. Chick Embryo Staging. Swarthmore College. http://www.swarthmore.edu/NatSci/sgilber1/DB_lab/Chick/chick_stage.html.

Hamburger, V. and Hamilton, H.L. 1951. A series of normal stages in the development of the chick embryo. Journal of Morphology 88: 49–89.

———. 1951. A series of normal stages in the development of the chick embryo. Reprinted in Developmental Dynamics 195: 231–272 (1992).

———. 1951. A series of normal stages in the development of the chick embryo. poster. John Wiley and Sons, Inc., New York. http://www.wiley.com/legacy/products/subject/life/anatomy/hamburger.pdf.

Hamilton, H.L. 1952. Lillie's Development of the Chick. Holt, Reinhart & Winston, New York.

Harvey, R. 1990. Practical Incubation. Birdwood Holt Pound, Surrey.

Jordan, R. 1989. Parrot Incubation Procedures. Silvio Mattacchione & Co, Ontario.

Joyner, K.L. and Abbott, U.K. 1991. Egg necropsy techniques. AAV Proceedings 146–152.

Kuehler, C. 1983. Causes of embryonic malformations and mortality. AAZV Proceedings 157–170.

Kuehler, C.M. and Good, J. 1990. Artificial incubation of bird eggs at the Zoological Society of San Diego. International Zoo Yearbook 29: 118–136.

Landauer, W. 1967. The Hatchability of Chicken Eggs as Influenced by Environment and Heredity, Monograph I (Revised). University of Connecticut, Storrs, Connecticut.

Langenberg, J. 1989. Pathological evaluation of the avian egg. AAZV Proceedings 78–82.
Patten, B.M. 1971. Early Embryology of the Chick. McGraw-Hill, New York.
Rahn, H., Ar, A., and Paganelli, C.V. 1975, How bird eggs breathe. Scientific American 46–55.
Romanoff, A.L. and Romanoff, A.J. 1949. The Avian Egg. John Wiley & Sons, New York.
———. 1972. Pathogenesis of the Avian Embryo. John Wiley & Sons, New York.

4
Ratites

Dale A. Smith

NATURAL HISTORY

Ratites are flightless birds in five families of the order *Struthioniformes*: ostriches, emus, cassowaries, rheas, and kiwis. (Folch 1992a–e) The term *ratite* comes from the Latin *ratis* meaning raft and refers to the flat smooth sternum that is characteristic of these birds. Ostriches, emus, and rheas are raised commercially for meat, leather, feathers, and oil. Cassowaries and kiwis are handled more as specimens in zoological or display collections, or—for the kiwi—as part of conservation and rehabilitation projects. All species have lived for 30 years or more in captivity.

The ostrich (*Struthio camelus*, Order Struthioniformes, Suborder Struthiones, Family Struthionidae) was originally found throughout Africa and extending into the Middle East. Wild birds are currently found in greatly reduced numbers in geographically limited pockets. Four subspecies have survived: the North African Ostrich (*Struthio c. camelus*), the Somali Ostrich (*S. c. molybdophanes*), the Masai (East African) Ostrich (*S. c. massaicus*), and the South African Ostrich (*S. c. australis*) (Folch 1992e). In the 1800's, North African and South African Ostriches were interbred in South Africa to produce the domesticated South African or Cape Black Ostrich (*Struthio camelus domesticus*). Because of the color of the skin on the legs and necks of males during the breeding season, North and east African birds are commonly known as *Red-neck,* and Somali and South African birds as *Blue-neck*. Ostriches are the largest living birds; males commonly stand 2–3 meters in height (6.5–9.8 ft) and may weigh up to 180 kg (400 lb). Females are smaller with weights up to 150 kg (330 lb). Male birds have black and white plumage; females and juveniles are brownish grey. Ostriches have relatively large wings and two unequally sized toes pointing forward.

The emu (*Dromaius novaehollandiae*, Order Struthioniformes, Suborder Casuarii, Family Dromaiidae) is found in a variety of open and semiarid habitats through most parts of Australia. (Folch 1992b). Birds stand up to 1.8 meters (6 ft) in height and weigh up to 50 kg (110 lb); females are slightly taller and heavier than males. Both sexes have brown and black feathering. Emus have vestigial wings and three forward-facing toes.

The rhea is native to South America (Order Struthioniformes, Suborder Rheae, Family Rheidae). There are two species, the Greater or Common Rhea (*Rhea americana*) and the Lesser or Darwin's Rhea (*Pterocnemia pennata*) (Folch). Rheas are the smallest of the three commercially raised ratites. Common Rheas may stand up to 1.5 meters (5 ft) in height and weigh 20 to 25 kg (44–55 lb); the Lesser Rhea is approximately half this size. Rheas have grey-brown plumage and are not sexually dimorphic, although males are slightly larger and darker. Rheas have moderately sized wings and three forward facing toes.

Cassowaries (Order Struthioniformes, Suborder Casuarii, Family Casuariidae) are found within tropical rainforests in Australia, Papua New Guinea, and Indonesia (Folch 1992c). There are three species, the Southern or Double-wattled Cassowary (*Casuarius casuarius*), the Northern or Single-wattled Cassowary (*Casuarius unappendiculatus*), and the Dwarf Cassowary (*Casuarius bennetti*). The Southern Cassowary, the species most commonly held in captivity, measures 1.3–1.7 m in height (4.3–5.6 ft), with weights of 29–34 kg (64–75 lb) for males, and up to 58 kg (125 lb) for females. Northern and Southern Cassowaries are similar in size; Dwarf Cassowaries are smaller. Cassowaries have glossy black hairlike feathers and brightly colored featherless facial and neck skin, with colored wattles hanging from the sides or front of the neck. Cassowary wings are vestigial and end in a claw. Cassowaries have three forward-facing toes ending in strong and sometimes very long nails.

Kiwis (Order Struthioniformes, Suborder Apteryges, Family Apterygidae) live in forested zones in New Zealand. Three species of kiwi exist: the Brown (Apteryx australis), Little Spotted (Apteryx owenii), and Great Spotted (Apteryx haasti) (Folch 1992a). These small birds, the larger females weighing up to 3.5 kg (7.7 lb), are nocturnal, spending their days in burrows. Kiwis have long decurved beaks with nostrils at their tips; they rely more on scent and hearing than they do vision. Kiwis have three cranial-facing and one rear-facing toe.

The information contained in this chapter refers primarily to the species held most commonly in captivity, the ostrich, emu, and rhea, unless otherwise noted.

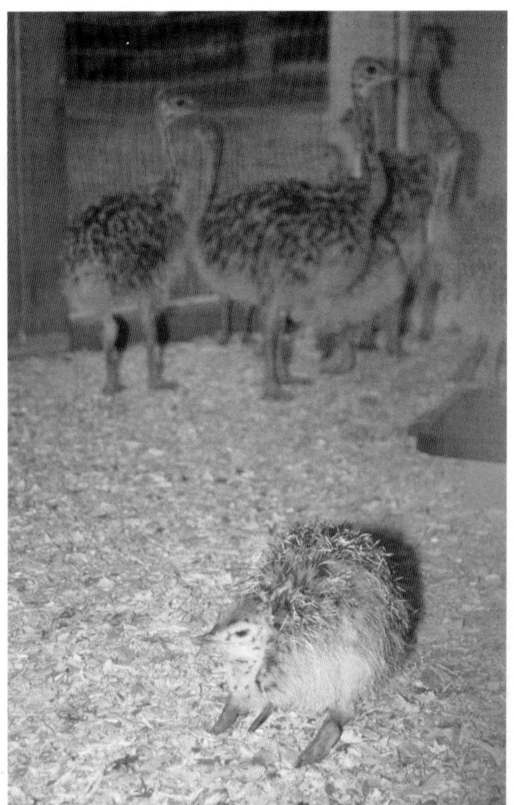

Figure 4.1. Depressed young ostrich separating from other chicks.

CRITERIA FOR INTERVENTION

In captivity, natural incubation and parental raising of ratite chicks is unusual. In commercial settings ostrich, emu, and rhea eggs are collected, artificially incubated, and most commonly raised apart from adults, although they may occasionally be fostered back to breeding pairs. Ratite chicks are precocial but would normally stay with their parents for a period of months. Chicks may be recognized as requiring intervention at the time of hatching, or might be removed from their groups of conspecifics for reasons including obvious illness (e.g., anorexia, dehydration, depression, inactivity), injury, and significantly delayed growth (see Figure 4.1).

Ratite chicks are normally alert, social, and inquisitive and, especially ostriches, are highly stressed by changes in management and by being isolated from their companions. Extensive picking at nonfood items may indicate stress and be a predictor for poor-doing ostrich chicks, with anorexia, gastric stasis, and death resulting (Deeming and Bubier 1999).

RECORD KEEPING

Commercial ratite farms keep extensive records on breeding, egg laying, incubation parameters, egg weight loss during incubation, hatch times, and chick growth and development (Minaar 1998). Although recommended parameters are listed in many texts and references (Doneley 2006, Huchzermeyer 1998, Jensen et al. 1992, Minaar 1998, Tulley and Shane 1996), considerable variation can result from farm and location-related factors such as type of incubator, number of eggs being hatched, and ambient temperature and humidity. General incubation and hatching guidelines are presented in Table 4.1.

The days of incubation and percentage of weight loss during incubation follow normal distribution curves; hence, a spread of values within a hatch is to be expected. Specifically designed and commercially available computer programs and computerized incubation systems are also available. Careful record keeping and frequent assessment of incubation parameters and growth of chicks is essential to maximize production and for early

Table 4.1. Incubation and hatching parameters for ratites.

Species	Egg Weight (g)	Temperature	Relative Humidity	Days of Incubation	Weight Loss over Incubation	Approx. Chick Weight at Hatching (g)
ostrich	1300–1700	36.0–36.5°C 96.8–97.7°F	20–40%	42	15%	860–1100
emu	550–600	36.1–36.4°C 97.0–97.5°F	25–40%	50–52	10–15%	360–400
rhea	500–800	36.4°C 97.5°F	30–60%	36–40	15%	330–530
cassowary	500–800	35.5–36.7°C 95.9–98.1°F	40–60%	47–54	12–15%	330–530
kiwi	400–450	35.5–36.5°C 95.9–97.7°F	60–65%	70–90		280

identification of management errors and impending health problems.

INCUBATION OF EGGS

Ratites are seasonal breeders, with egg production linked to increasing daylight in ostrich, rhea, and kiwi; decreasing daylight in emu; and availability of food sources in cassowary (Anonymous 2006, Folch 1992a–e). Eggs are laid in depressions in the ground; hence, environmental cleanliness is important to reduce egg contamination and maximize hatching success. Eggs should be collected and given a specific identity as soon as possible after lay. Eggs are often stored after collection to synchronize incubation of groups of eggs. Hatchability generally decreases with increased storage time, i.e., after 7–10 days for ostrich eggs. Ostrich eggs are stored at 50–68°F (10–20°C) with twice-daily turning during this period. Emu eggs are stored at temperatures of 40–60°F (4–15.5°C) and may be more tolerant of longer storage periods (Minaar 1998). Hatching rates of ratite eggs, especially ostrich, are considerably less than those for commercial poultry.

The environmental quality inside the incubator is of paramount importance to embryo development and growth. Eggs should be examined and weighed at weekly intervals to ensure that weight loss and embryo development are progressing appropriately. As in other avian species, abnormal embryo development and embryonic mortality may be associated with elevated or depressed temperature or humidity, with inadequate or inappropriate egg-turning, or with bacterial or fungal contamination. Adequate air flow through the incubator is particularly important with ratites to provide adequate oxygen for the large embryos and to ensure that incubator temperature does not rise excessively. Specific incubators are manufactured for ostriches and emus in order to provide the appropriate frequency and mechanics of egg rotation. Ostrich eggs are set air cell up, and are rotated over a 90° arc, 45° each side of vertical. Emu eggs are more generally laid on their sides and are rotated back and forth around the long axis with a series of roller bars. Visual assessment of embryonic development (i.e., candling eggs) requires strong light sources to pass through the thick shells of ostrich and rhea eggs. An infrared candler may be used for dark-shelled emu eggs (see Figure 4.2).

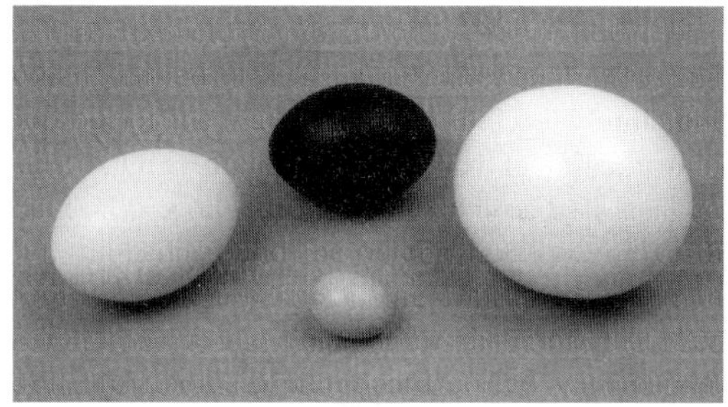

Figure 4.2. Rhea, emu, and ostrich eggs (left to right), with chicken egg in foreground for scale.

Specific references should be consulted for details regarding the incubation and hatching of kiwi eggs (Doneley 2006).

HATCHING, INITIAL CARE, AND STABILIZATION

Ratite eggs are moved to a hatcher 1–4 days before the end of incubation to provide higher humidity, slip-free flooring, and reduce contamination in the incubator. Chicks may take 1–3 days from internal pipping (entry into the air cell) to external pipping (opening of the shell). It may take several hours to days for the chick to fully emerge from the egg. Ratite chicks open their shells with a combination of pushing with their legs and head. Hatching problems are almost always a result of weak chicks due to incubation difficulties, inadequate nutrient stores provided by the hen, or embryonic developmental anomalies. It is a quite common practice to assist hatch in ostrich chicks by chipping away some of the egg shell once external pipping begins; however, prematurely forcing the hatch may result in bacterial contamination of the yolk sac. After hatching, chicks are inspected to ensure that the yolk sac is completely internalized and the navel closed; if not, the navel is treated with a topical disinfectant e.g., Betadine solution (Purdue Frederick) and covered with a bandage or other temporary protection. A visible identification tag is placed to allow accurate record keeping. Microchips are sometimes placed in the large pipping muscle at the back of the neck at this time. Chicks are left in the hatcher for a few hours up to a few days, depending on their strength and activity (see Figure 4.3).

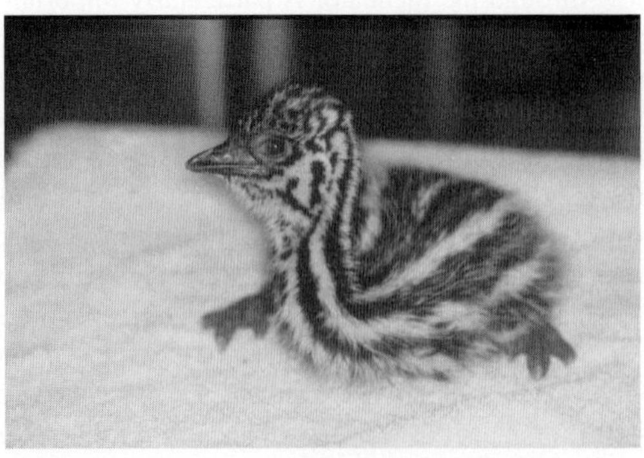

Figure 4.3. Emu chick shortly after removal from hatcher.

The navel should be closed before the chick is removed from the hatcher. It is important that the flooring in the hatcher be nonslippery to prevent leg injuries as the chicks move around and attempt to stand. It is common practice to place tape hobbles on all chicks for first few days to prevent splaying.

Chicks of several days to several months of age may be sexed by direct cloacal observation. The bird is restrained on its back and the cloaca gently everted to reveal the male phallus or female clitoris. Experience is required for accuracy, and caution should be taken in guaranteeing the sex of young birds.

COMMON MEDICAL PROBLEMS AND SOLUTIONS

Ratites are susceptible to a variety of infectious and noninfectious disease conditions. Evaluation of incubation and hatching records should be the first step in the clinical evaluation of poor-doing or ill ratite chicks. Problems seen within the first week of life often reflect the quality of the egg (and hence the nutrition of the hen) and incubation and egg handling procedures. Congenital abnormalities can occur. Mortality rates are generally highest for the first 3 months of life; beyond 6 to 8 months ratite juveniles are generally hardy, as are adult birds. Ostrich chicks appear to be more easily stressed and more prone to infectious diseases than the other species of ratites. Noninfectious conditions, particularly those predisposed to by management factors, are the primary causes of losses on many farms. Major outbreaks of infectious disease are less common.

Chicks should be observed at rest before restraint and handling in order to assess mental alertness and demeanor, and the respiratory, nervous, and musculoskeletal systems. Ratites are normally extremely curious. Birds should be assessed for conformation, stance, and gait because leg deformities are a significant problem. Scoliosis and other spinal deviations occur and may be the result of genetics or problems during incubation. Stunted growth and poor feathering are evidence of chronic disease.

Supportive care, including provision of supplementary heat and fluid and nutritional support, is critical regardless of the primary concern. Because there are no medications licensed for use in ratites in the majority of countries of the world, veterinarians must prescribe and use drugs in an "off-label" manner as governed by their veterinary associations. Medications may be administered orally via stomach tube, or birds may be manually pilled. Many will even preferentially peck at and consume tablets or capsules because of their unusual appearance. Placing medication in the food or water may be appropriate in some circumstances. Esophagostomy tubes have been used for long-term nutritional supplementation. Ratites do not have a crop in which to store food. Injections can be made subcutaneously, into the muscle masses of the legs or lumbar area, or intravenously via the medial metatarsal vein. In larger juveniles, the jugular—or in the ostrich, the brachial vein—are also used. In older birds intended for the slaughter market, intramuscular injections can result in condemnation or trimming of meat.

Young ratites are easily caught and handled. Small chicks may be supported under the body with the legs folded or left to hang. The birds may also be laid upside down in one's lap to examine the abdomen or legs. As chicks grow, their running speed increases exponentially and it is important not to cause injury by panicking the birds or by rough handling of the legs during catching. The use of corrals or chutes, or boards used for herding, can aid in isolating and capturing individual birds in need of attention. Juvenile birds may be lifted off the ground from behind, leaving their legs dangling free. After a short period of kicking most birds relax and may be carried without a struggle. Older juvenile birds should be treated like adults, which are large and strong and may seriously injure the handler.

Common medical problems in ratite chicks include yolk sac retention and infection, nutritional deficiencies, limb deformity, gastric impaction, enteritis, respiratory disease, and fading ostrich syndrome. For a more detailed description of these and other diseases of ratites the reader should consult the veterinary literature (Anonymous 2006, Boardman 1998, Doneley 2006, Jensen et al. 1992, Huchzermeyer 1998, Smith 2003, Tulley and Shane 1996, Tulley and Shane 1998, Verwoerd 1998).

Yolk Sac Problems

Yolk sac retention and infection are generally identified in birds under 2 weeks of age, but may result in more chronic ill-thrift. Chicks with yolk sac problems are often reluctant to feed and fail to gain weight and grow at the same rate as their clutchmates. The yolk sac should be completely retracted into the body at the time of hatch, the navel closed before removal from the hatcher, and the yolk sac completely resorbed by 2–3 weeks after hatch. The abdomen in chicks with persistent and infected yolk sacs is more full than normal, and the normal intestinal tract and its contents cannot be palpated. Ultrasound examination can help confirm the diagnosis. Improper incubation and hatching parameters resulting in delayed umbilical closure, prematurely assisted hatching, and inadequate hygiene leading to umbilical infection are the common predisposing factors for these conditions. If only a small portion of the sac remains external at hatch it may sometimes be replaced in the abdomen, and the navel sutured or bandaged closed. Large or abnormal portions of the sac should be removed surgically and the yolk sac stalk ligated and umbilicus closed; however, these chicks are often weak and reluctant to eat. In older chicks, surgical removal of the sac and systemic antibiotic therapy are required, along with supportive care.

Nutritional Deficiencies

A wide range of nutritional deficiencies have been suggested to occur in ratite chicks; however, these are often based on clinical signs that might be seen in domestic poultry rather than actual knowledge of the conditions as they occur in ratites. Classic and phosphorus-deficient (in rhea) rickets, vitamin E/selenium–responsive myopathy, and suspect vitamin B deficiency syndromes including dermatitis and curled toes have been identified in ratites. Some ostrich chick management protocols include injection with a vitamin E/selenium product shortly after hatch. Recently hatched emu chicks with twisted necks or that "tumble" and roll may respond to vitamin B supplementation.

Leg Deformities

Long-bone deformity is probably the most widespread problem in young chicks. A number of interrelated factors are likely involved in the development of this condition. These include overfeeding (excessive calorie intake) or excess dietary protein leading to too rapid growth, nutritional deficiencies and imbalances (e.g., calcium, phosphorus, vitamin D, vitamin E, selenium, methionine, choline, manganese, zinc), damage to the leg during hatching or within the hatcher, inadequate exercise, and genetic predisposition. The extremely rapid growth rate of ratite chicks exacerbates any nutritional imbalances that may be present. The most successful methods for prevention appear to be providing large pens to encourage exercise, reducing the protein level of the chick diet to under 20% within approximately 2 weeks of hatching, and reducing the total amount fed.

Leg deviations may be rotational—that is, around the axis of the bone—or to the side. The resulting turnout of the lower leg and foot can be severe enough to completely prevent the bird from standing or walking. The tibiotarsal bone is most frequently affected, but not all cases are alike. Because of the rapid growth rates, problems may appear overnight and can progress rapidly. Lateral displacement of the gastrocnemius and other tendons can occur either at the same time, or secondarily. A variety of splinting and surgical procedures have been attempted, with almost uniformly poor results unless the leg is splinted correctly within a few hours of the onset of the problem.

A separate problem seen in ostrich chicks is rotation of the large toe. This problem usually responds well if corrective splints are immediately applied. Again, a variety of causes have been suggested, including genetic predisposition and riboflavin deficiency.

Gastric Impaction

Ratite chicks will eat and possibly impact on various foreign objects and almost any substrate: sand, gravel, straw, long grass, or plastic turf materials (Astroturf). Emus seem slightly less prone to this than ostriches or rheas. Ingested foreign bodies may also perforate the proventriculus or gizzard causing septic peritonitis, similar to *hardware disease* in cattle. Management activities that may predispose to impaction include irregular feeding routines, rapid changes in diet, lack of grit, movement of birds onto a substrate that is novel to them, and any change in routine that stresses the birds. Clinical signs may be acute and resemble colic as seen in other species, or they may be chronic and include listlessness, reduced appetite and fecal output, decreased size and increased dryness of fecal pellets, and stunted growth. The impacted proventriculus or ventriculus may be palpable in the abdomen, but often plain or barium contrast radiographs are necessary. If the condition is identified quickly, laxatives may assist in passage of the proventricular and ventricular contents, but in most cases surgical removal is required. The prognosis depends very much on the condition of the bird at the time of surgery; the survival rate is poor for weakened birds.

Proventricular and ventricular function may also be disrupted by localized infections by fungi, including *Candida* and *Aspergillus* spp., and by megabacteriosis (*Macrorhabdos ornithogaster*). These are often secondary to immunosuppression or another insult.

Enteritis

Enteritis may be an important problem in chicks less than 6 months of age. Inadequate sanitation, combined with the propensity of chicks to be coprophagic, may result in outbreaks of disease. The establishment of a normal intestinal flora within the first days of life is considered important in preventing enteric infections. A variety of pathogens have been implicated, including gram-negative bacteria such as *E. coli, Campylobacter jejuni, Pseudomonas,* and *Salmonella* spp; *Clostridium* spp, spirochete organisms in rhea, and paramyxo-, reo-, corona-, adeno-, and herpes viruses. Systemic infection frequently follows bacterial enteritis. Cloacal prolapse may occur secondary to diarrhea and straining and has also been associated with cryptosporidial infection in ostrich chicks. Appropriate antibacterial therapy should be provided along with fluids and supportive care. Investigation into underlying sanitation and management protocols is essential to prevent and control outbreaks of enteritis.

Parasitic Disease

A variety of intestinal and external parasites have been identified in ratites. The most clinically significant of these is *Libyostrongylus douglassi*, the proventricular worm of ostriches. Clinical signs in affected chicks include anorexia, weight loss, depression, and death. Regular fecal evaluation and deworming programs are essential for parasite control.

Respiratory Disease

Respiratory disease may be significant in chicks under 6 months of age. Clinical signs include conjunctivitis, rhinitis or sinusitis, and respiratory distress. A variety of bacterial, fungal, mycoplasmal, and viral agents have been implicated, including *Pasteurella hemolytica, Bordetella avium, Pseudomonas aeruginosa, Hemophilus* spp., and *Neisseria* sp. Aspergillosis is a disease of particular concern to ratite farmers. Infection occurs by exposure to overwhelming numbers of fungal spores in situations with poor husbandry (in the brooder or later), or after reduction in a bird's immune function due to concurrent disease or other stress. Poor ventilation leading to high levels of ammonia in the barn may predispose to outbreaks of respiratory disease. Aspergillosis may be seen as explosive outbreaks in flocks of young chicks. Smoldering infections in individual older birds may become clinically apparent under stressful conditions—for example, after transport to a new farm. Birds may show nonspecific clinical signs even when severely affected. Treatment is rarely effective, but a variety of systemic and aerosolized antifungal medications have been recommended.

Fading Ostrich Syndrome

The cause of this syndrome, which may cause anorexia, gastric stasis, and extremely high mortality in ostrich chicks less than 6 months of age, has not been determined. A combination of management-induced stress and immunosuppression and one or more infectious agents is likely responsible. Careful attention to management, hygiene, and biosecurity appear to be the best prevention at present.

Other Conditions

Other husbandry-related diseases include trauma, predation, exertional myopathy, hypothermia, heat stroke, intestinal accidents, and plant, heavy metal or chemical poisoning.

DIET AND FEEDING PROCEDURES

Ratites, with the exception of kiwis, are primarily herbivores; however, their digestive systems and natural diets differ (Cillers and Angel 1999, Perron 1992, Sales 2006). Ostrich, emu, and rhea graze on a variety of low energy vegetation in semiarid environments. Gastrointestinal transit time is more rapid in the emu (5–6 hours) than in the ostrich (36–39 hours for immature birds) or rhea, species that rely more heavily on hindgut and cecal fermentation. Commercial feeds are formulated specifically for ostrich, emu, and rhea, and for birds of different ages and are sold by a variety of feed companies and co-ops (Mazuri, Blue Mountain Feeds, Floradale Feed Mill). Cassowaries feed on a variety of fruits of the tropical forest, but in captivity are fed a mixture of fruit, pellets, and sometimes small amounts of animal matter (e.g., chicks, rats, meat) (Anonymous 2006, Folch 1992c, Perron 1992). Kiwis are insectivorous, feeding primarily on earthworms and a variety of soil invertebrates (Folch 1992a).

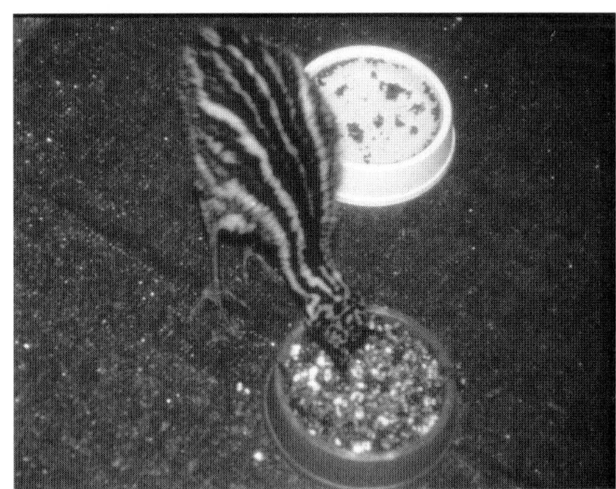

Figure 4.4. Emu chick eating from feed top, dressed with fresh greens to encourage foraging behavior.

Although ratite chicks rely on the yolk sac for nutrients and fluid for up to a week after hatching, a pelleted or crumbled starter ration should be offered soon after hatching to encourage development of normal feeding behavior and early weight gain (Deeming and Bubier 1999). Without older birds to act as role models, newly hatched chicks may need assistance to identify food and water. White dishes with patterns on the bottom, or freshly chopped greens or brightly colored vegetable matter floating in the water or placed on dried feed may encourage interest (see Figure 4.4).

Chicks may feed more readily from the ground than from dishes or pans. For biosecurity reasons, species such as domestic chickens should not be placed with the chicks to encourage eating. It is a matter of debate whether grit is necessary for birds fed a pelleted diet; however, the following general recommendations have been made for grit size: starter (3 mm; 2/16 in) at hatch to 3 weeks, grower (2 mm × 5–6 mm; 2/16 in × 3–4/16 in) at 4 to 7 weeks, developer (6 mm × 9–13 mm; 4/16 in × 6–8/16 in) at 8 to 16 weeks, and turkey (9 mm × 16–22 mm; 6/16 in × 10/16–14/16 in) after 16 weeks (Mazuri/PMI Nutrition International 2004).

There is no universal program for chick nutrition (Minaar 1998, Minaar and Minaar 1992, Sales 2006). Most chicks are initially fed a ratite crumble or starter with at least 20% protein free choice. If specific ratite diets are not available, a pelleted feed with approximately 15–20% protein could be substituted (Sales 2006). Dietary utilization of nutrients is poor initially as the digestive and absorptive capabilities of the gastrointestinal tract mature over the first few weeks of life. The establishment of normal GI flora is felt to occur within the first week of life. Some producers place fresh feces from healthy adult or juvenile birds in the pen with chicks in order to transfer the appropriate bacterial and protozoal organisms. This practice has also led to severe disease outbreaks. Some farmers feel that probiotics assist in development of balanced flora, but this has not been substantiated scientifically. Fresh water should be provided at all times; automatic livestock waterers are useful as birds age. Birds will cease eating if water is not available.

At approximately 2–3 months of age, the protein level of the feed is progressively decreased to reach 13–15% by the time birds are 6–10 months of age (Cilliers and Angel 1999, Mazuri/PMI Nutrition International 2004, O'Malley 1996). Feeding frequency should also be decreased to limit growth rates. Chicks placed in outdoor paddocks will supplement their food intake by grazing. Maintenance and breeder rations are used for birds over a year of age, as appropriate.

EXPECTED WEIGHT GAIN

Commercial species of ratites grow rapidly. Ostrich chicks may increase in height by 30 cm per month and can reach 4 kg in weight by 1 month of age, 9–14 kg by 2 months, 20–30 kg by 3 months, and 40–50 kg by 4 months (Huchzermeyer 1998). Ostrich chicks develop their juvenile plumage at approximately 3 months of age, and gain adult plumage and weight by the second year of life. Emu chicks gain juvenile plumage at approximately 2 months of age; full adult plumage and full height are reached at approximately 1 year of age. Emu chicks should achieve hatch weight by day 6–7, will weigh approximately 1.5 kg at 1 month, 6 kg by 10 wks, 16 kg by 20 wks, and continue to grow steadily until reaching adult weight (O'Malley 1996).

HOUSING

A number of references describe the management of young ratites (Jensen et al. 1992, Huchzermeyer 1998, Minaar 1998, Minaar and Minaar 1992, Tulley and Shane 1996, Verwoerd et al. 1999). Chicks are moved from the hatcher into a brooder pen—a confined area with supplementary heating to compensate for the young birds' poor thermoregulation—and then into larger pen or paddock areas, preferably with access to the outdoors if climate conditions permit (see Figure 4.5).

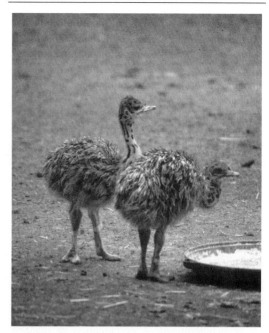

Figure 4.5. Ostrich chicks in outdoor pen (photo courtesy of Brian Beck.)

Pen size is dependent on the size and number of animals in the group, but should be sufficient to allow the birds to move about freely and to exercise as they grow. A rough guide for brooder pen size is 2.4 m^2 (8 ft^2) with 0.6 m (2 ft) sides (Jensen et al. 1992). The temperature is gradually dropped from an initial high of 90°F (32°C) to approximately 79°F (26°C). Chicks are kept in groups so they can socialize and huddle together for comfort and warmth at night. Similar-sized chicks should be kept together to prevent bullying and crowding at feeders. As birds grow, they are given access to larger pens and, depending on ambient temperature, may be confined to or simply provided with heated areas at night. Localized heat may be provided by under-floor and radiant heaters (see Figure 4.6).

Runs must be well drained with good footing, and should be practical to clean and sanitize. All in–all out systems and leaving pens fallow after a group of chicks has been in them helps reduce pathogen load.

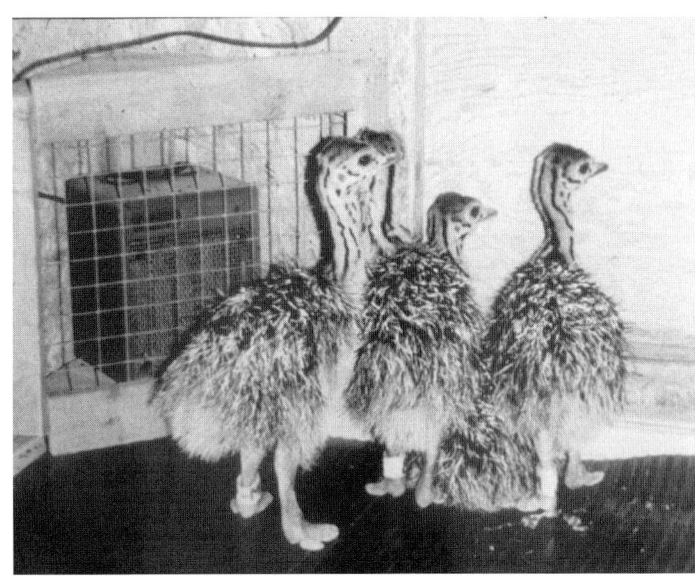

Figure 4.6. Ostrich chicks near supplementary heat source in a brooder pen.

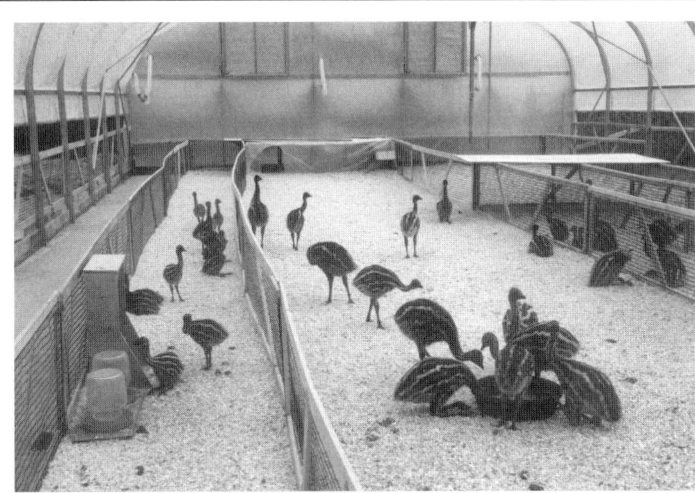

Figure 4.7. Emu chick pens in a large plastic greenhouse.

Chicks respond poorly to changes in their environment; therefore, it is recommended to keep groups of birds together during the growing period, and whenever possible to maintain them in the same physical location until they are well established. Chicks are housed indoors with supplementary heat during cold seasons.

It is essential that even the youngest chicks be given sufficient room to allow adequate exercise. In the wild, young birds of all species follow their parent(s) for many kilometers each day. Lack of exercise is felt to be one of the main predisposing factors for the variety of leg deformities seen in growing birds. Minimum pen area is approximately 3.7 m^2 (40 ft^2) for birds less than 2 months of age, or less than 9 kg (20 lb) in weight, and 21–23 m^2 (225–250 ft^2) for older or heavier birds (Raines 1998). Pens should be rectangular with lengths of 30–60 m (100–200 ft) and a minimum width of approximately 3 m (10 ft) (Jensen et al. 1992, Minnar 1998, Raines 1998). Width and total pen size will depend on the number of chicks in the group. In colder climates, the use of large greenhouse structures is effective in providing chicks hatched in winter months—for example, emus—with exercise as well as exposure to sunlight and natural light cycles (see Figure 4.7).

Older birds are kept outdoors in fenced paddocks or pens. To prevent injuries, fences should be 6 ft (1.8 m), have a smooth and solid top rail, and be easily visible. Shade should be provided in the summer, and in temperate climates protection must be given from the coldest weather and wind. Adult ratites of commercially raised species are able to tolerate full winter temperatures if appropriate shelters are present; however, icy or slippery footing may be dangerous for the birds. Barns are rarely heated unless they also contain young birds.

It is critical that ratites are exposed early to the types of bedding used on the farm. The rate of proventricular impaction in ostrich and rhea chicks is extremely high, and is often associated with changes in management that include alterations in bedding substrates. Chicks that will be put out on grass should be watched carefully for early signs of impaction if they have not had access to the outdoors as young birds.

WEANING

Ratites are precocial and do not require weaning.

PREPARATION FOR SOCIALIZATION OR INTRODUCTION TO CAPTIVE FLOCK

Ratites are sociable and become easily accustomed to human contact. Caution should be taken working with birds as they gain adult sizes, particularly as they reach sexual maturity and in breeding season. Cassowaries and male ostriches can be extremely dangerous.

In general, young birds are not aggressive toward each other; however some caution must be undertaken when chicks or juveniles are reintroduced to similarly aged conspecifics. Smaller birds may be at a disadvantage getting to food and water sources. Rabbits and pygmy goats have been used as "company" and role models for young chicks that are raised on their own.

ACKNOWLEDGMENTS

I would like to thank Sharon Patterson for assistance with manuscript preparation, and Alison Downie, Dr. Graham Crawshaw, and Dr. Colin Peace for reviewing the manuscript.

SOURCES FOR PRODUCTS MENTIONED

Betadine Solution, Purdue Frederick Co. (manufacturer), Norwalk CT, (203) 853–5667, www.pharma.com.

Blue Mountain Feeds, (303) 678–7343, www.blue-mountain.net. Floradale Feed Mills, Floradale, Ontario, (800) 265-6126, www.ffmltd.com/index.php.

Mazuri, a division of PMI Nutrition International, (800) 277-8941 www.mazuri.com.

REFERENCES

Anonymous. Accessed June 2006. The cassowary workshop. http://www.cassowary.com/workshop.html.

Boardman, W. 1998. Causes of mortality in captive kiwi. Kiwi Workshop Proceedings, Aukland, New Zealand, pp. 61–68.

Deeming, D.C. and Bubier, N.E. 1999. In Deeming, D.C., ed., The Ostrich Biology, Production, and Health. CAB International, New York, pp. 83–104.

Doneley, B. 2006. Management of captive ratites. In Harrison, G.J. and Lightfoot, T.L., Clinical Avian Medicine, Volume 2. Spix Publishing, Palm Beach, Florida, pp. 957–989.

Cilliers, S.C. and Angel, C.R. 1999. In Deeming, D. C., ed., The Ostrich Biology, Production, and Health. CAB International, New York, pp. 105–128.

Folch, A. 1992a. Family Apterygidae (Kiwis). In del Hoyo, J., Elliott, A., and Sargatal, J., eds., Handbook of the Birds of the World, Vol. 1. Lynx Edicions, Barcelona, pp. 104–108.

———. 1992b. Family Dromaiidae (Emu). In del Hoyo, J., Elliott, A., and Sargatal, J., eds., Handbook of the Birds of the World, Vol. 1. Lynx Edicions, Barcelona, pp. 98–102.

———. 1992c. Family Casuaridae (Cassowaries). In del Hoyo, J., Elliott, A., and Sargatal, J., eds., Handbook of the Birds of the World Vol. 1. Lynx Edicions, Barcelona, pp. 90–97.

———. 1992d. Family Rheidae (Rheas). In del Hoyo, J., Elliott, A., and Sargatal, J., eds., Handbook of the Birds of the World Vol. 1. Lynx Edicions, Barcelona, pp. 84–88.

———. 1992e. Family Struthionidae (Ostrich). In del Hoyo, J., Elliott, A., and Sargatal, J., eds., Handbook of the Birds of the World Vol. 1. Lynx Edicions, Barcelona, pp. 76–82.

Huchzermeyer, F.W. 1998. Diseases of Ostriches and Other Ratites. Onderstepoort Agricultural Research Council, Onderstepoort, South Africa.

Jensen, J.M., Johnson, J.H., and Weiner, S.T. 1992. Husbandry and Medical Management of Ostriches, Emus and Rheas. College Station, Texas, Wildlife and Exotic Animal Teleconsultants.

Mazuri/PMI Nutrition International. 2004. Accessed June 2006. Mazuri ratite starter. http://www.mazuri.com.

Minaar, M. 1998. The Emu Farmer's Handbook, Volume 2. Nyoni Publishing Company, Grovetown, Texas.

Minaar, P. and Minaar, M. 1992. The Emu Farmer's Handbook. Induna Company, Grovetown, Texas.

O'Malley, P.J. 1996. An estimate of the nutritional requirements of emu. Proceedings of Improving our Understanding of Ratites in a Farming Environment, pp. 92–108.

Perron, R. 1992. The Cassowary in Captivity. International Zoo News No. 240, Vol 39:7. Online at http://www.species.net/Aves/Cassowary.html.

Raines, A.M. 1998. Restraint and Housing of Ratites. In Tulley, T.N. and Shane, S.M., eds., The Veterinary Clinics of North America—Food Animal Practice (Ratites), WB Saunders, Philadelphia, Pennsylvania, pp. 387–399.

Sales, J. Accessed June 2006. Feeding guidelines for ratites in zoos. http://www.eznc.org/DataRoot/docs/Ratitestandard2.pdf.

Smith, D.A. 2003. Ratites: Tinamiformes (Tinamous) and Struthioniformes, Rheiiformes, Casuariiformes (Ostriches, Emus, Cassowaries, and Kiwis). In Fowler, M.E. and Miller, R.E., eds., Zoo and Wild Animal Medicine, Edition 5. Saunders, St. Louis, Missouri, pp. 94–102.

Tully, T.N. and Shane, S.M., eds. 1996. Ratite Management, Medicine, and Surgery. Krieger Publishing, Malabar, Florida.

———. 1998. The Veterinary Clinics of North America—Food Animal Practice (Ratites), WB Saunders, Philadelphia, Pennsylvania.

Verwoerd, D.J. 1998. Ostrich Diseases. Revue Scientifique et Technique 19(2): 638–661.

Verwoerd, D.J., Deeming, D.C., Angel, C.R., and Perelman, B. 1999. In Deeming, D.C., ed., The Ostrich Biology, Production, and Health. CAB International, New York, pp. 191–216.

5
Penguins

Jane Tollini

NATURAL HISTORY

Penguins are southern hemisphere birds. There are 17 to 18 species distributed between the equator and Antarctica. Their paddlelike wings allow them to "fly" through water and their bones are not hollow. Fish, squid, and a variety of crustaceans make up their diet, the composition of which changes depending upon prey availability. Migration varies within the species. The Magellanic penguin has the longest migration, 2,000 km, breeding in Argentina and wintering off the coast of Brazil; the Galapagos penguins never travel more than a few hundred km from their nest site. They have a longevity of 20 years in the wild and even longer in zoos.

Most species do not start breeding until they are 3–4 years old; some wait until they are 12 or 14 years old before laying their first egg or finding their first mate. Most penguins lay one or two eggs. Emperor and King penguins lay only one egg every 2–3 years. King penguins take up to 18 months to rear their chick; the Galapagos penguins may rear two chicks in just over 3 months and lay eggs up to three times a year.

Most penguins are monogamous but not necessarily faithful, although some individuals in some species stay with the same partner for their reproductive lifetime.

Unlike other species of birds, penguins are adapted to feast or famine. Adults gain weight while at sea and fast on shore while courting, incubating, and guarding their chicks. They regularly fluctuate in weight depending on where they are in their breeding cycle.

In contrast to most birds that molt a few feathers at a time, penguins molt all their feathers at once and fast while they grow new feathers on land. Most penguin species molt once a year with the exception of the Galapagos penguins, which molt twice a year.

CRITERIA FOR INTERVENTION

Common criteria for intervention include abandonment of the nest, egg, or chick by the parents, ill parents, and hatching problems. Generally, penguins chicks experience few problems in hatching, however managers should be familiar with the normal hatch sequence (pip-to-hatch interval, appearance of a newly hatched chick, etc.), which will help in determining when a problem arises. If the vocalizations of a hatching chick become weak or stop, especially when no discernible progress with the pip hole is observed, intervention is necessary.

General indicators of improper hatching, either in the incubator or observed under the parent are as follows:

- Chicks have made an internal pip but have failed to progress for over 12–15 hours.
- Chicks have not pipped and are well over the expected incubation period.
- Chicks have chipped through the shell but have not progressed for 12–15 hours.
- Chicks have rotated within the egg after pipping and the beak is no longer visible at the pip hole.
- In Aptenodytes and Pygoscelis, parental behavior can be indicative of a problem with hatching progress because these birds will lift the brood pouch and bow more frequently.

The most common hatching difficulty for penguin chicks is malpositioning of the chick inside the egg. This may or may not be accompanied by unabsorbed yolk and/or residual albumen. Once a chick is determined to be having hatching difficulty, the egg should be removed from the incubator or from the under the parent for assistance. When performing an assisted hatch, hands should be washed and gloved and all instruments cleaned to prevent introducing bacteria to the chick. The pip should be examined and an evaluation should be made before assisting the chick to hatch. The egg should be candled to assess vascularization, which is a robust growth of blood vessels surrounding the embryo inside the egg, indicating that the chick is then ready to hatch. The pip location should be assessed to determine whether it is above or below the air cell, and a small flashlight may be used to look inside the pip hole for unabsorbed yolk, residual albumen, or other problems. Once these steps are completed, carefully peel away small portions of the shell from the pip site with forceps.

After the pip area has been further exposed, the membrane should be moistened with sterile saline on a swab to check for active vessels. If no vessels are present, the membrane may be peeled back to expose the chick. Be sure the membrane does not stick to the nares and occlude breathing. Efforts should be made to expose the head first. In extreme cases, it may be necessary to manipulate the head out from under the wing.

If the chick is to be parent-reared, it should be returned to the nest as soon as possible following a careful examination to rule out other problems. Sticky chicks (those with residual albumen) or chicks with protruding yolk sacs should be considered for hand-rearing.

Nesting problems should be addressed. If the nests become excessively soiled or wet, they may be "freshened" by doing the following:

1. If both parents are in the nest area, carefully remove the parent that is not on the egg and place away from the nest.
2. Carefully remove the parent from the nest and hold the parent until the nest is clean.
3. Remove the egg (this is a good time to do a candling check).
4. If removing a chick, this is a good time to do a health analysis.
5. As quickly as possible, replace soiled nest substrate. If any part of the original nest is salvageable, return it to the nest.
6. Return the egg or chick and very slowly release the parent back into the nest and monitor from a distance.

RECORD KEEPING

Accurate records are essential for long-term management of penguin populations. It is recommended that all institutions participate in the International Species Information System (ISIS) and comply with data requests by species coordinators and/or studbook keepers.

Minimum records should include ISIS Accession number, whether the bird is wild-caught or captive-hatched, parentage, date of birth or capture, capture location if known, individual identification method, studbook data (if applicable), breeding history, molting, and weights. If in-house record keeping systems are used, essential data should also be entered into ARKS (Animal Record Keeping System). Valuable reproductive data include egg weights, chick growth rates, and incubation and brooding information. Other records that may be kept include behavioral observations, environmental parameters, molting data, and food consumption. Thorough accurate medical records should be maintained for all animals in the collection. Medical information should also be recorded and entered into MedARKS if possible.

Record keeping relating to reproductive management should begin at the time of egg laying. Marking the first egg laid is important if the expected incubation dates are to be calculated. Egg logs should be used to record data such as lay date, number of days incubated, sire and dam, sibling identification, and method of rearing. By tracking a pair's reproductive history, trends in success and/or failure may be identified.

Hatch weight and subsequent daily or weekly weights are important in determining the overall growth weight. Many institutions develop records that include first morning weight, weight before and after each feeding, amount of food offered and consumed at each feeding, types of food consumed, behavioral comments, vitamins, and medication. It is useful to record ambient temperature and brooder temperature (if applicable). Chick records should be maintained through fledgling. In the following pages there will be actual charts of egg-laying intervals, incubation, feeding, and growth data. These data apply to hand-reared birds only. During the hand-rearing process it is imperative to fill in daily criteria, *especially* all health comments. Table 5.1 is an example of a feeding record for a 200 g hand-reared chick.

Table 5.1. Feeding record for 200 g penguin.

Date	Time	I.D.	Diet	General/Health Comments
	6:00 a.m.		20 ml formula	
	9:00 a.m.		15 ml formula, 1–2 ml Pedialyte, 3–5 g fish	
	12:00 noon		20 ml formula	
	3:00 p.m.		15 ml formula, 1–2 ml Pedialyte, 3–5 g fish	
	6:00 p.m.		20 ml formula	
	9:00 p.m.		20 ml formula	

ARTIFICIAL INCUBATION AND EGG MANAGEMENT

Removing Eggs

The age of the pair, reproductive experience, environment, and social conditions, as well as the goals of the reproductive program factor into any decision to remove eggs from the nest. Other considerations that might necessitate the removal of the egg include overdue hatching, improper incubation, replacement with dummy egg to avoid recycling, fostering to another pair, transportation to another facility, contraception, and egg damage.

If eggs are to be removed for the purpose of contraception, it is advisable to remove them soon after they are laid to avoid any development. A dummy egg may be placed with the parents to prevent double-clutching, to keep parents in sync with the colony, and to keep the pair ready to be potential foster parents.

Eggs removed for fostering to another pair may be taken at any point during incubation. Options at this time include placing the egg in an incubator until the target foster pair is ready to receive the egg or transferring the egg immediately to the target pair. If this is the case, the target pair should be incubating a dummy egg before replacement with the fostered egg.

Preparation of the Incubator

It is common practice to fumigate with formalin/potassium permanganate to disinfect the incubator. Some institutions combine the use of disinfectant solution to wash the inside of the incubator with fumigation. There are stringent regulations governing the use of potassium permanganate; in California, special training is required and proper personal protective gear must be worn.

Because many penguin eggs become soiled in the nest before being transferred to the incubator, there may be concern regarding cleaning and/or disinfecting eggs. Penguin eggs naturally get soiled in the nests. Use dry gauze to wipe but only if absolutely necessary. The majority of institutions do not fumigate the incubator with eggs present.

Types of Incubators

There are a variety of suitable incubators available for incubating penguin eggs. These include Petersime Models 1 and 4, Humidaire (models 20, 50, and 120), and Grumbach. Considerations in choosing an incubator include the incubator room/ambient conditions, size and number of eggs to be incubated at one time, and turning requirements (see Chapter 3).

Temperature and Humidity

There are two temperatures to monitor for the incubator. The first is the dry-bulb, which should be about 96.5°F (35.8°C). The dry-bulb temperature measures the air temperature inside the incubator. The wet-bulb temperature ranges between 82–83°F (27.7–28.8°C). The wet-bulb thermometer is usually mounted on the inside of the door of the incubator, with the thermometer wick dipped into a water tube. The temperature should be clearly visible from the outside of the incubator. The geographic locale and humidity may dictate more-or-less frequent additions of water to the incubator reservoir. Type of incubator and number of eggs being held at one time will affect overall humidity.

Egg Setting, Egg Turning Technique and Frequency

Eggs should not be set on end, but rather they should be laid flat in the incubator. The majority of institutions that have attempted artificial incubation report that mechanically turning the eggs every 1–2 hours is necessary. In addition to mechanical turning, some institutions also perform a 180° manual turn of the egg. This practice facilitates a more even development of vascularization in the egg. For incubators without an automatic turning capability, manual turning may be done every 2–3 hours, with preferably an odd number of turns in a 24-hour day. It is not clearly known why an odd number of turns is necessary, but experience indicates this is a more valuable technique. Eggs should be turned slowly to avoid rupture of developing blood vessels in the egg.

Candling

Candling may be a useful tool in determining the fertility and development of an egg. Candling techniques require practice, and a person with experience should be consulted before handling the eggs. Some managers are of the opinion that the eggs should not be handled before the tenth day following onset of incubation due to potential damage to the embryo. Care should always be taken to avoid jarring the egg during handling or burning the embryo with the light source. Cooling should be kept to a minimum; however, slight cooling of the egg during candling does not appear to have deleterious effects. During the majority of the incubation period, the air cell will be clearly visible. The shape of the air cell will usually change during the 24–48 hours before internal pip. This is described as *draw-down,* which is when the air cell at the larger end of the egg expands as the embryo develops. The embryo "draws" down more on one side at an angle when it is within days of pip. At this point, turning the egg is discontinued. The chick penetrates through the membrane into the air cell. The drawdown is followed by the external pip or chipping of the shell itself.

Managing the Pip-to-Hatch Interval

Before candling or handling eggs, consider that penguins do not like to be disturbed during nesting. Cautiously weigh the pros and cons of handling the eggs. Eggs may need to be candled more frequently in the week before the expected hatch. Some institutions report daily candling of eggs in the incubator at this time. A penguin egg is ready to move to the hatcher following the external pip. Turning the egg is no longer necessary at this time. At the time of the pip, the humidity should be increased 2–3°F (1–2°C) on the wet-bulb thermometer. This may be accomplished in a hatcher separate from the incubator. Utilizing the hatcher is important for several reasons, including the ability to increase humidity without adversely affecting other earlier-stage eggs and preventing contamination of the incubator by hatching eggs. However, this may not be feasible for those with one incubator. Hatching eggs should be checked four to five times per day, and the area surrounding the pip should be misted with distilled water. Water for misting should be kept at the same temperature as the hatcher, and may be stored there for convenience. Average pip-to-hatch interval is 24–48 hours (see Table 5.2). A normal pip should

Table 5.2. Pip-to-hatch interval.

Species	Egg Lay Interval	Mean Incubation Period	Incubation Period Range	Pip-to-Hatch
Emperor		67 days	64–73 days	48–72 hrs
King		56 days	53–62 days	48–72 hrs
Adelie	3–4 days		34–42 days	24–48 hrs
Chinstrap	3–4 days	37 days	35–39 days	36–48 hrs
Gentoo	3–5 days	38 days	36–41 days	36–48 hrs
Macaroni	4–6 days	36 days	33–39 days	24–48 hrs
Rockhopper	3–5 days	36 days	32–36 days	24–48 hrs
Humboldt	2–4 days	42 days	40–46 days	24–48 hrs
Magellanic	3–4 days	42 days	38–48 days	24–48 hrs
African	3–4 days	38 days	36–42 days	24–48 hrs
Little Blue	2–3 days	35 days	32–35 days	48–56 hrs

occur at the large end of the egg, nearly in alignment of drawdown.

INITIAL CARE AND STABILIZATION

After hatching, chicks are brooded for a period of approximately 15 days. Down color is species-specific, although Adelie penguin chicks may exhibit either a silvery grey or a sooty grey down. In the wild, some chicks are not fed until 3 days of age (Spurr 1975). Food begging by chicks has been observed on the day of hatching but is apparently not essential to initiate feeding. When feeding a hatchling, the parent bends over and places its bill beneath that of the chick. Subsequent begging by the chick then stimulates regurgitation of food by the parent into the chick's open bill.

The normal weight for newly hatched, dry chicks of various genera and species is listed in the growth data charts (Table 5.9). Chicks below the lowest range for hatch weight for their species should be monitored carefully and hand-reared if necessary, especially if there is a sibling in the nest. There is considerable competition between nestmates, and weaker chicks frequently fail to thrive.

Chicks remaining with the parents also should be monitored closely. If a problem is suspected, parent-reared chicks may be carefully removed from the nest, examined, and weighed. The weight gain within the first 5–7 days should be substantial, nearly doubling their weight daily. Upon examination, chicks should be checked for adequate hydration by lightly pinching the skin on the back of the neck and assessing resilience. If the skin stays in the pinched position, the chick is dehydrated. The lungs should be clear, the eyes should be moist and the feet plump. A healthy chick may be heard vocalizing as it solicits food from the parents. It should be noted, however, that at least one institution has reported hearing no vocalizations from some chicks.

24–36 Hours after Hatch

After the egg hatches, wait 24–36 hours to weigh the chick and to check for strength and hydration. If the chick is dehydrated, administer 1–3 ml Pedialyte (Abbott Labs) via gavage. Do not overfill the chick, because this may cause it to cease begging, which is essential to stimulate the parents to feed it. Parents should be observed from a distance to ensure they are feeding the chick. It may be slow or inactive for the first 24–36 hours, after which the parent's heaving motions and chick's preening activities should be noticeable. When the chick starts eating, each parent should be given 500 mg vitamin B-1 daily. In the beginning, parents will not be eating much as they digest their food to feed the chick. They may not feed if they feel they are being watched, so observe at a distance.

36 Hours through 4 Weeks

Chicks should be checked each day without disturbing parents. This should be done from at least 10 ft away and using binoculars if necessary. Chicks should be weighed weekly at the same time and day. It is easier to remove chick for weighing if only one parent is in the burrow; if both are in the nest, remove the parent not on the chick or the least docile one. Do not let the remaining parent leave the nest while the chick is being weighed. Return the chick carefully as the parent will try to bite, wing beat, and protect the nest and the chick could be injured in the process. As the chick begins to grow, feed the parents as much as they will consume, continuing with the 500 mg vitamin B-1 daily. Parents with chicks 3–4 weeks old will require three feedings a day.

Weaning 5–6-Week-Old Chicks with Parents

It is necessary to pull chicks of most species at this age. This will make it easier to teach them to hand-feed from keepers. Pull chicks from parents and try to pull two or more chicks at once. Hand-rearing a single chick by itself is more difficult.

It is imperative to put chick type identification bands on chicks as soon as they are pulled. Because their wings are limp, typical wing-bands do not work. Use a cable tie with different-colored tape placed on the wing of each chick. Check bands daily for tightness, because the chicks will grow quickly. Then place the chick into a holding pen and/or pool with no water. Make sure to cover the floor using a good substrate; dry plastic turf material (Astroturf) is preferred. Place the top of an extra-large flight kennel in the pen so they can use it as a collective burrow and a spot to hide.

When selecting fish to feed the chicks, pick out tiny herring and small smelt, and keep it frozen until

Table 5.3. Feed recipe.

Makes 16–18 oz (480–540 ml)	
330 g	Herring
330 g	Smelt
420 ml	Pedialyte (Abbott)
3	Capsules Vitamin E (400 I.U.)
3	Capsules Cod liver oil*
2	Capsules acidophilus
1	Vitamin package+

*Cod liver oil may be removed if using Mazuri Vita-Zu Bird Vitamin; may be too much vitamin A.
+Vitamin Package Mazuri Vita-Zu bird tablet, 375 mg vitamin B-1, 9 dicalcium phosphate capsules (145 mg Ca/112 mg Phos).

it is ready to be fed. Offer three feedings per day. Weigh chicks once a week until they reach 3,000 g (for the larger species) or until they are able to swim. Feed 10% of body weight at each feeding. It is easier to prepare all of the diets for one day by weighing the total amount of fish calculated for that chick and dividing it into three bags. Keep the fish frozen and thaw just before a feed. They do not need to consume the entire calculated amount per day, and likewise they may be offered a small amount more if they consume all of the diet for the day. It is recommended to adhere to the 10% of body weight rule at each feeding until chicks are more than 3,000 g or able to swim. Note that some species and individuals are smaller and they may not reach 3,000 g (see Table 5.3).

7–12 Weeks Old

Once chicks reach approximately 3,000 g or near maximum weight, their wings have stiffened, and they are swimming, you may remove their temporary identification bands and replace them with adult wing bands. At this point remove the flight kennel lid or they will seek burrows when they return to the colony. The adult birds will peck and chase them off if the chicks try to go into an occupied burrow. Chicks do not need burrows for 1–2 years. At over 3,000 g, the weekly weighing may be discontinued and the chicks may be fed like the adults, which is generally ad libitum twice a day, and may begin the adult vitamin protocol.

SWIMMING

At 5–6 weeks, the chick's wings are limp and awkward, and they are mostly covered in down. When their wings have stiffened and they have lost most of their down, begin introducing them to water. Place the chicks in a shallow pool. They will generally respond negatively and exit the water immediately. Continue putting them into the pool 2–3 times daily. Eventually they will prefer to stay in the pool. At that point, fill up the pool and allow them to swim at will. If they are capable of swimming normally, the depth of the water is not an issue.

COMMON MEDICAL PROBLEMS AND SOLUTIONS

Overheating and underheating may lead to medical problems, but they may be avoided by careful monitoring. Chicks should be observed closely for signs of heat or cold stress. The symptoms most frequently observed in overheated chicks include lethargy, inappetence, panting, and extension of the feet and flippers. Overheating may be problematic for chicks of any age but may quickly become life threatening in very young chicks unless corrective measures are taken. Underheated chicks may be observed shivering and huddled against the side of the brooder, and their feet will be cold to the touch. Chicks in this state will be slow to respond to a feeding stimulus.

Overfeeding may be avoided by careful evaluation of each chick's weight gain. Even when strictly following feeding protocols, problems from overfeeding may arise. It is always best to address each chick's needs individually. What may be an appropriate amount of formula for one chick may be excessive for another. Generally, a substantial weight gain is expected during the first few weeks but will vary between species. Behaviors associated with overfeeding include lethargy, regurgitation, and disinterest in food. Food should be withheld until the chick is hungry. A dark, grainy stool may be an indicator of improper digestion and medical advice should be sought.

Hydration throughout development should be carefully monitored. This is essential when solid fish is introduced into the diet. Symptoms of dehydration include dry appearance of the eyes, shriveled appearance of the skin on the feet, or thick pasty feces. The skin along the back will remain "tented up" after pinching it if the chick is inadequately hydrated. Water feedings of appropriate amounts will improve this condition. Depending on the size of the species, 10–20% of their body weight would be appropriate. Generally 100 to 200 ml of fluids may be given subcutaneously once a day.

Another problem, although not common, is splayed legs (the feet are rotated laterally). This condition may result in serious and long-term complications. Therefore, early detection is important. The brooder or nest substrate should be textured enough to prevent the feet from slipping. Some have experienced good results treating this condition by tying the legs together with a soft material, being careful to maintain a normal spacing between the legs. Another successful treatment method is to place the chick into a bowl approximately the same size as the chick's body so that the legs cannot splay. In very young chicks, this often corrects the problem in 5–7 days.

Eye irritation may develop at any age, and may be caused by a variety of factors such as bacteria, injury, or foreign material in the eye. Keepers should note whether the chick's eyes tear excessively or appear red, swollen, or cloudy. If eye irritation is noticed, the eyes should be examined carefully for foreign materials. Chicks that are actively losing downy feathers also release tiny flecks of skin or dander that may adhere to the surface of the eye and cause damage to the cornea. Irrigating the eyes with saline solution may provide relief. If necessary, ophthalmic drops may be prescribed by the veterinarian.

Other common medical problems are enteritis and respiratory tract infections.

Penguins may be rehydrated with 50 ml/kg subcutaneous fluids, administered 2–3 times daily. Antibiotics that may be used are penicillin derivatives such as Piperacillin, as well as Enrofloxacin. Trimethoprim sulfdiazine may be used after chicks are nearly adult size (3–4 kg). Antifungals such as fluconozole 20–30 mg/kg may be administered once daily as prophylaxis during antibiotic use. In general when chicks do show signs of illness, it will progress quickly. Immediate action, especially with Aspergillosis and malaria will yield the best chance of recovery.

HAND-FEEDING EQUIPMENT

Catheter Tubes

Start with 10 French catheters for neonates (infants), and graduate to 12, 16, and 18 French as the chick grows.

Syringes

Use the following steps with 12 ml, 35 ml, or 60 ml:

1. Cut the feeding tube (do not cut the tip or insertion end) to fit the syringe. Ensure cuts are smooth. Measure tube to go from beak to midabdomen or lower; this avoids tubing into trachea.
2. Lubricate the tube with a small amount of sterile petroleum jelly or KY jelly to allow it to slide easily down the open mouth of chick. Even small chicks can accept a fairly large tube. Using a larger tube will help ensure that you do not introduce the tube into the trachea.
3. "Bleed" all air out of syringe and tube before feeding by pushing formula into the tube.
4. Initially to make the formula pass easily and quickly through tubes, it may need to be strained through a medium mesh plastic colander. As the chicks grow, give them more chunks and bones.
5. All syringes filled with formula must be kept on ice but not frozen until they are used.

Tubes and syringes may be used again, provided they are disinfected and as long as the syringes work easily. To disinfect the syringes and tubes, first wash in detergent immediately after using. Soak in disinfectant Chlorhexidine (Nolvasan) solution (Fort Dodge) for 10–20 minutes. Rinse thoroughly and allow to dry.

When tube-feeding Pedialyte (Abbott) first, do not remove the tube from the chick but follow-up by attaching the formula syringe to the tube and continue the feeding. This reduces retubing, which may cause irritation.

HAND-REARING DIET FORMULA

Preparation of Diet

Blend in a high-powered blender (Vita-Mix) as follows, keeping the formula cold:

1. Add Pedialyte (Abbott) and vitamins first, mix briefly.
2. Fish should be kept frozen until ready to prepare formula, and then remove head, tail, and the larger bones, cut into "steaks" (crosscut pieces), and quarter.
3. Add fish a little at a time to prevent the machine from jamming.

4. Initially strain the formula for smoothness.
5. Label with the date and time prepared. Refrigerate.
6. Discard unused portion after 24 hours.

FEEDING PROCEDURES

Wait at least 12 hours after hatching before offering a penguin chick its first feeding. The first feeding should be only water and/or Pedialyte in order to assess the chick's feeding response and ability to swallow. Chicks with a large, unabsorbed yolk sac should be given water for the first two to three feedings to allow time for yolk absorption. Once feeding begins, check the consistency and color of the stool daily. A black or foul-smelling stool may be indicative of improper digestion.

A feeding response may be initiated from a penguin chick by forming a "V" with the middle and index fingers and then placing the "V" upside down on the top of the chick's bill and wiggling the fingers (see Figure 5.1).

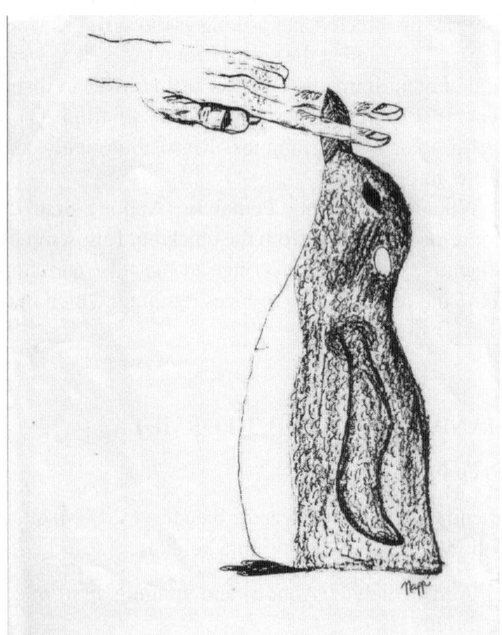

Figure 5.1. A feeding response may be initiated from a penguin chick by forming a "V" with the middle and index fingers, then placing the "V" upside down on the top of the chick's bill and wiggling the fingers.

The chick should respond by pushing up the crook of the fingers. At this time, the formula may be delivered by inserting the tube into the throat at least 5 cm. The fingers should be simultaneously wiggling to stimulate chick response and lifted very slightly to encourage the chick to stretch up its neck. As the formula is delivered, it is important that the feeder watch the back of the throat for formula backup. This may be a signal that the chick is no longer swallowing or that the formula is being delivered too quickly. If the chick tires and stops swallowing, remove the tube and syringe and wait until the chick recovers. This process may be repeated until the feeding is completed. Chicks 1–5 days of age tire easily; therefore, it is important to be prepared to deliver the formula immediately after initiating the feeding responses.

Newly hatched chicks should be fed just 1–2 ml of Pedialyte for the first two to three feedings. This is true of most species with the exception of Emperor and King penguin chicks, in which case you would double the amount of Pedialyte to 2–4 ml in those two species.

After the initial Pedialyte feedings, feedings #3–6 would be 1–2 ml of Pedialyte and 1–2 ml Formula, yielding a formula-to-Pedialyte ratio of 50 : 50.

Weigh each chick at the same time each day, starting at 1 day old, and calculate the diet for the day (24 hours) (see Figure 5.2). Feed about 10% of body weight in volume at each feeding, being careful not to exceed 10%.

Use the sample feed charts (see Tables 5.4–5.7) to determine which formula to feed, based on the

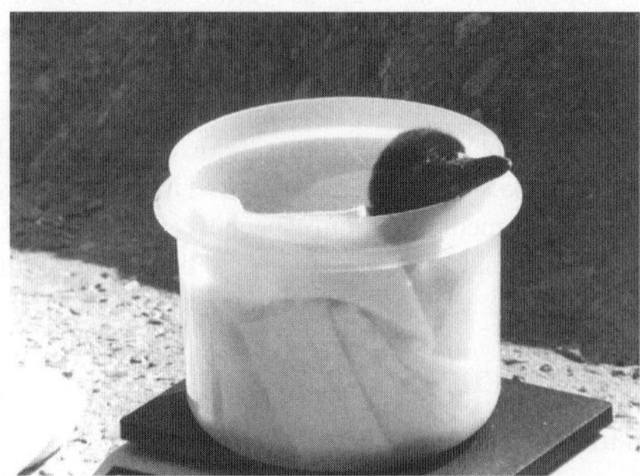

Figure 5.2. A 5-day-old Magellanic Penguin chick being weighed.

Table 5.4. Example of hand-feeding diet procedure for 6 daily feedings for penguin chicks from hatch day to 500 g. For 5 feeds per day, start at 7 a.m. and feed every 3 hours until five feedings have occurred.

	Feeding 1 6 a.m.	Feeding 2 9 a.m.	Feeding 3 12 p.m.	Feeding 4 3 p.m.	Feeding 5 6 p.m.	Feeding 6 9 p.m.
Diet 1 Hatch day	1–2 ml Pedialyte only	1–2 ml Pedialyte only	Formula: Pedialyte ratio (50 : 50) 1–2 ml Pedialyte, 1–2 ml formula	Formula: Pedialyte ratio (50 : 50) 1–2 ml Pedialyte, 1–2 ml formula	Formula: Pedialyte ratio (50 : 50) 1–2 ml Pedialyte, 1–2 ml formula	Formula: Pedialyte ratio (50 : 50) 1–2 ml Pedialyte, 1–2 ml formula
Diet 2 One day old	Formula: Pedialyte ratio (75 : 25)	Formula: Pedialyte ratio (75 : 25)	Formula: Pedialyte ratio (75 : 25)	100% formula	100% formula	100% formula
Diet 3 2–3 days old or when chick is 200 g	100% formula	100% formula	100% formula	100% formula	100% formula	100% formula
Diet 4 Body weight ≥200 g but <250 g	20 ml formula	15 ml formula, 1–2 ml Pedialyte, and then 3–5 g fish	20 ml formula	15 ml formula, 1–2 ml Pedialyte, and then 3–5 g fish	20 ml formula	20 ml formula
Diet 5 Body weight <250 g but <300 g	25 ml formula	20 ml formula, 3 ml Pedialyte, and then 3–5 g fish	25 ml formula	20 ml formula, 3 ml Pedialyte, and then 3–5 g fish	25 ml formula	20 ml formula, 3 ml Pedialyte, and then 3–5 g fish
Diet 6 Body weight ≥300 g but <400 g	20 ml formula, 3 ml Pedialyte, and then 3–5 g fish	20 ml formula, 3 ml Pedialyte, and then 3–5 g fish	20 ml formula, 3 ml Pedialyte, and then 3–5 g fish	20 ml formula, 3 ml Pedialyte, and then 3–5 g fish	20 ml formula, 3 ml Pedialyte, and then 3–5 g fish	20 ml formula, 3 ml Pedialyte, and then 3–5 g fish
Diet 7 Body weight ≥400 g but <500 g	25 ml formula, 5 ml Pedialyte, and then 15 g fish	25 ml formula, 5 ml Pedialyte, and then 15 g fish	25 ml formula, 5 ml Pedialyte, and then 15 g fish	25 ml formula, 5 ml Pedialyte, and then 15 g fish	25 ml formula, 5 ml Pedialyte, and then 15 g fish	25 ml formula, 5 ml Pedialyte, and then 15 g fish

Table 5.5. Feeding chart for chicks 500–600 g.

	Feeding 1 6 a.m.	Feeding 2 10 a.m.	Feeding 3 2 p.m.	Feeding 4 6 p.m.	Feeding 5 9 p.m.
Diet 8 Body weight ≥500 g but <600 g	20 ml formula (adjust formula to equal 10% of body weight for total of formula, Pedialyte, and fish), 5 ml Pedialyte, and then 20 g of fish chunks (fish should not exceed 50% of meal)	20 ml formula 5 ml Pedialyte, 50 mg vitamin B-1, and then 20 g fish chunks	20 ml formula 5 ml Pedialyte, and then 20 g fish chunks	20 ml formula 5 ml Pedialyte, 50 mg vitamin B-1, and then 20 g fish chunks	20 ml formula 5 ml Pedialyte, and then 20 g fish chunks

Table 5.6. Feeding chart for chicks 600–700 g.

	Feeding 1 6 a.m.	Feeding 2 11 a.m.	Feeding 3 4 p.m.	Feeding 4 9 p.m.
Diet 9 Body weight ≥600 g but <700 g	100% formula and then fish chunks	100% formula and then fish chunks, 50 mg vitamin B-1	100% formula and then fish chunks	100% formula and then fish chunks, 50 mg vitamin B-1

Table 5.7. Feeding chart for chicks 700–2500 g.

	Feeding 1 7 a.m.	Feeding 2 1 p.m.	Feeding 3 7 p.m.
Diet 10 Body weight ≥700 g but <900 g	35 ml formula, 10–15 ml Pedialyte, and then 20 g fish chunks (formula and Pedialyte not to exceed 50 ml, rest of volume in fish)	35 ml formula, 10–15 ml Pedialyte, and then 20 g fish chunks (formula and Pedialyte not to exceed 50 ml, rest of volume in fish)	35 ml formula, 10–15 ml Pedialyte, and then 20 g fish chunks (formula and Pedialyte not to exceed 50 ml, rest of volume in fish)
Diet 11 Body weight ≥900 g but <1,000 g	40 ml formula, 15 ml Pedialyte, and then 45 g fish chunks (formula and Pedialyte not to exceed 55 ml, rest of volume in fish) 50 mg vitamin B-1	40 ml formula, 15 ml Pedialyte, and then 45 g fish chunks (formula and Pedialyte not to exceed 55 ml, rest of volume in fish)	40 ml formula, 15 ml Pedialyte, and then 45 g fish chunks (formula and Pedialyte not to exceed 55 ml, rest of volume in fish), 50 mg vitamin B-1
Diet 12 Body weight ≥1,000 g but <2,500 g	40 ml formula, 15 ml Pedialyte, (formula and Pedialyte not to exceed 55 ml, rest of volume in fish) Vitamins: 1 50 I.U. vitamin E, 1/2 tablet of Mazuri Vita-Zu bird, 100 mg vitamin B-1	40 ml formula, 15 ml Pedialyte, (formula and Pedialyte not to exceed 55 ml, rest of volume in fish)	40 ml formula, 15 ml Pedialyte, (formula and Pedialyte not to exceed 55 ml, rest of volume in fish) Vitamins: 1 50 I.U. vitamin E, 1/2 tablet of Mazuri Vita-Zu bird, 100 mg vitamin B-1

weight and the age of the chick. Start with six feedings every 3 hours beginning at 6 a.m. and ending with a 9 p.m. feed. Five feedings every 3 hours starting at 7 a.m. is also acceptable. Record the chick's weight at the same time each day. Calculate diet for about 10% of body weight in volume at each feeding. Do not feed more than 10% of body weight per feed. Note that the number of feedings will change with weight change. When fish is introduced to diet, it is important to feed the fish last. If not, it may cause the chick to regurgitate. If the chick regurgitates at any point, go back a diet step. If the chick is not gaining weight, increase the intake volume slowly.

Begin the fledgling protocol for chicks weighing 2,000–3,000 g at 5–6 weeks. Please note that not all chicks will reach 3,000 g due to difference in species or smaller parent individuals.

Table 5.8. Vitamin chart.

Body Weight	Frequency	Vitamins
500–1,000 g	BID	50 mg vitamin B-1
1,000–3,000 g	SID	100 I.U. vitamin E 1-Mazuri Vita-Zu bird tablet 200 mg vitamin B-1
>3,000 g	SID	100 I.U. vitamin E 1-Mazuri Vita-Zu bird tablet 250 mg vitamin B-1 1 dicalcium phosphate caplet

PARENT AND HAND-RAISED FLEDGLINGS

Expect some weight loss and they may go for a few days without food. Then force-feed based on their weight (10% of body weight per feeding). When one chick understands that you are the source of food, the others soon follow. Once they begin to eat, let them eat as much as they want within reason; this also depends on the species. You can expect them to eat as much or more than the adults; then they will plateau and slow down or stop eating, and then start again. This is normal providing they appear to be fat, active and in good health.

Vitamin Protocol for Chicks Eating Whole Fish

Vitamins are placed in the gills of the fish (see Table 5.8). If the holding area has fresh water, add one 1 g salt tablet to the vitamin protocol. Salt should be introduced gradually to the diet to stimulate the activity of the salt gland. Give 1 g of salt to each penguin twice the first week, three times the second week, and from the third week forward, the chicks should be getting 1 g of salt daily in their diet. Some institutions with penguins housed in freshwater pools prefer to give 1 g salt tablets 3 times a week for the life of an adult penguin. Penguins housed in salt water pools do not require salt supplementation.

EXPECTED WEIGHT GAIN

Table 5.9 lists expected penguin weight gains.

HOUSING

Brooders

Primary concerns when choosing a brooder include the following:

- *Adequate air circulation:* Penguin chicks require a dry rearing environment and should never be reared in an enclosed area where humidity is high. Do not overheat. Heating half of the holding area will allow chicks to select their comfort zone. Increase or decrease heat and cool ratio accordingly.
- *Ease of maintenance and disinfection:* Brooders should be cleaned at least twice daily. If wood is used, it should be sealed; however, ensure that the sealer is compatible with the heat source that will be used to prevent combustion.
- *Size and temperature gradient:* There should be an approximate 10°F (5°C) temperature difference from one side to the other to allow the chick to adjust its behavior to meet its own thermoregulatory needs (after 5–7 days of age). If the brooder is too large, chicks may venture too far from the heat source and suffer serious cooling.
- *Number of chicks to be reared together:* It is recommended that no more than 2–5 chicks be reared in a single brooder. Overcrowding may lead to overheating of the chicks and increase the likelihood of transferring disease.

Typical early brooder dimensions might be 40 cm × 83 cm × 38 cm (16 in × 33 in × 15 in) to accom-

Table 5.9. Growth data.

HAND-REARING GROWTH DATA POST-HATCH
Mean Weights in Grams

Days	1	5	10	15	20	25	30	35	40	45	50	55	60	65	70
Species															
Emperor	190	219	307	459	657	929	1260	1593	1990	2487	3210	4065	4921	6171	7188
King	204	195	247	334	437	564	740	1000	1386	1948	2692	3531	4355	5183	5991
Gentoo	89	124	275	606	1169	1764	2420	3087	3735	4525	5234	5839	6092	6020	6021
Adelie	80	101	192	329	535	825	1172	1599	1901	2290	2656	2701	2596	2551	2500
Chinstrap	69	105	207	423	689	1009	1430	1996	2582	2962	3112	3094	3150	2962	2903
Macaroni	107	165	401	650	959	1356	1741	2237	2669	2998	3214	3232	3211	3104	3004
Rockhopper	68	96	203	392	564	716	882	1088	1345	1490	1561	1565	1517	1453	1255
Humboldt	82	86	144	229	313	445	504	776	974	1197	1487	1847	2145	2362	2625
Magellanic	81	121	313	539	799	1076	1422	1834	2252	2557	2763	2949	3177	3253	3150

Source: Penguin Taxon Advisory Groups Husbandry Manual (2003).

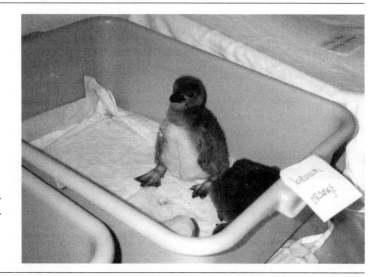

Figure 5.3. A 7-day-old Magellanic Penguin chick in a restaurant-bus brooder, with an absorbent lap pad covering a towel for substrate.

modate one to four chicks of smaller species or one to two chicks of larger species (see Figure 5.3). The most common heat source provided is a forced air heater. Heat lamps, heating pads, and electric heaters were also reported as heat sources used. To prevent burns, heat lamps should not be situated closer than 3 ft of the brooder. Heat sources should be adjusted to maintain 80–90°F (26.6–32.2°C) in the brooder for the first 14 days posthatch. Depending on ambient brooder room conditions, the temperature may need to be lowered as the chick approaches 14 days of age. Severely overheated chicks often lie flat with flippers and feet outstretched and may be panting. Other subtle indicators of overheating are slight dehydration and unexplained inappetence. When setting up brooder or tub, try to create a burrow/cave-like covering over the chicks. Ensure that it is stable and will not collapse on them. The covering will give the chicks a sense of security.

Substrate and Cleaning

Cloth toweling is the most commonly used substrate in the brooder for the first 2 weeks of rearing. Disposable lap pads wrapped around a towel would also be satisfactory (see Figure 5.3). Towels are readily available and may be easily laundered with bleach for adequate cleanliness. Roughly textured or frayed towels should be avoided because of reports of leg injuries resulting from snagged toenails. Other early brooder substrates are matting, paper toweling, and surgical drape material. It is important that the substrate not be so smooth that the chick's feet slide out from under it. Temporary or permanent damage to muscles, tendons, and joints may result from improper footing.

Brooders should be cleaned twice daily. It is advantageous to correspond cleaning with feeding to reduce overall handling of the chick. Use special care when handling chicks that have just been fed, because they may regurgitate. Additionally, toweling may be replaced as needed between scheduled cleanings. Disinfectants should be thoroughly rinsed and brooders allowed to dry before the chick(s) are returned. Betadine sprayed directly on toweling and allowed to dry before adding the chick may reduce fungal spores. The San Francisco Zoo uses diluted Nolvasan as its primary disinfectant.

Older Chick Handling and Brooder Requirements—Day 15 through Fledgling

As chicks grow, larger brooder accommodations will be required. Most institutions utilize an in-house design plywood box. Wood should be painted or sealed with a suitable product. Some designs incorporate a 3/4 cm wire or mesh flooring and are elevated from ground level on legs or casters. Typical dimensions might be 2.4 m × 1.2 m × 0.6 m (7.8 ft × 4 ft × 2 ft) with wooden dividers, which allow partitioning based on chicks requirements. This size can accommodate eight chicks in four sections or four chicks in two sections. Brooders should never house more than four chicks together. As chicks grow older and more timid, it may be useful to supply shelters or a cover. One method is to provide half of a pet airline kennel, or a sheltered area may be built into the brooder design. To expedite habituation to handling and desensitization to external stimuli, the shelter should be removed for portions of the day.

Generally, dependent on the chick's response and ambient temperature conditions, a heat source may not be required at this stage. For high-latitude species, further cooling may be required. For *Spheniscus* penguins, addition of a fan or air conditioner to the brooder area may improve thermoregulatory conditions and air quality. Previously described symptoms of overheating are the best indicator of a chick's thermoregulatory needs. At this stage, the brooder substrate most commonly used is indoor/outdoor carpeting. It is easily hosed for cleaning and may be soaked in a disinfectant and rinsed before drying. Other substrates used are rubberized matting and cloth toweling. Surfaces that are too smooth should be avoided to allow chick proper traction. Brooders may require more frequent cleaning but should be done a minimum of twice daily.

ACKNOWLEDGMENTS

I thank Christa Pu, Dr. Freeland Dunker, Carol Ann Hutchins, and Jan Nicholas for their assistance with the preparation of this chapter. Thanks also to Nancy Lang, Linda Henry, and Dr. Dee Boersma. This chapter is dedicated to penguins around the globe and to those folks who have spent countless hours of selfless dedication in the service of penguins.

SOURCES FOR PRODUCTS MENTIONED

Mazuri Vita-Zu Bird Tablet (5M25), Mazuri, 1050 Progress Drive, Richmond, IN 47374, (800) 227-8941, www.mazuri.com, Product information at http://www.mazuri.com/Home.asp?Products = 2&Opening = 2.

Nolvasan, Fort Dodge, Wyeth, 5 Giralda Farms, Madison, NJ 07940, (800) 533-8536, www.wyeth.com.

Pedialyte Abbott Laboratories, Columbus, OH 43215, www.abbott.com.

REFERENCES

Ainley, D.G., Leresche, R.E., and Sladen, W.J. 1983. Breeding Biology of Adelie Penguins. Berkeley: University of California Press.

Ainley, D.G. and Schlatter, R.P. 1972. Chick-Raising Ability in Adelie Penguins. Auk 89: 559–566.

Boersma, P.D., Stokes, D.L., and Yorio, P.M. 1990. Reproductive Variability and Historical Change of Magellanic Penguins (Spheniscus magellanicus) at Punto Tombo, Argentina. In Penguin Biology, Davis, L.S. and Darby, J.T., eds. Academic Press, San Diego.

Cooper, J. 1980. Breeding Biology of the Jackass Penguin with Special Reference to Its Conservation. Proceedings of the Fourth Pan-African Ornithological Congress, pp. 227–231.

Ellis-Joseph, S. 1990. Patterns of Incubation Behavior in Captive Housed Adelie Penguins: Implications for Long Term Penguin Breeding Programs. American Association of Zoological Parks and Aquariums Regional Conference Proceedings, pp. 115–120.

Gailey-Phipps, J. 1978. A World Survey of Penguins in Captivity. International Zoo Yearbook 18: 7–21.

———. 1978. Breeding Black-Footed Penguins (Spheniscus demerus) at the Baltimore Zoo. International Zoo Yearbook 18: 28–35.

Geraci, J.R. and St. Aubin, D.J. 1980. Nutritional disorders of captive fish-eating animals. In The Comparative Pathology of Zoo Animals, Montali, R.J. and Migaki, G., eds. Smithsonian National Press, Washington, D.C., pp. 41–49.

Henry, L.M. and Twohy, F. 1990. Hand Rearing Guidelines for the Humboldt Penguin (Spheniscus humboldth) with Special Emphasis on Common Hand Rearing Concerns. AAZPA Regional Conference Proceedings.

Kuehler, C.M. and Good, J. 1990. Artificial Incubation of Bird Eggs at the Zoological Society of San Diego. International Zoo Yearbook, 29. Zoological Society of London, London.

Lishman, G.S. 1985. The Food and Feeding Ecology of Adelie Penguins (Pygoscelis Adeliae) and Chinstrap Penguins (P. Antarctica) at Stigny Island, South Orkney Islands. Journal of Zoology, London (A) 205: 245–263.

Miller, K.A. and Searles, S. 1991. The Handrearing of Humboldt Penguins. Proceedings of the 16th Annual Conference, American Association of Zookeepers.

Montague, T.L. 1982. The Food and Feeding Ecology of the Little Penguin Eudyptula minor at Philip Island, Victoria, Australia. Unpubl. M.Sc. thesis, Monash Univ.

Nagy, K.A. and Obst, B.S. 1992. Food and Energy Requirements of Adelie Penguins (Pygoscelis Adelie) on the Antarctic Peninsula. Physiological Zoology 65: 1271–1284.

Osborn, K. and Kuehler, C. 1989. Artificial Incubation: Basic Techniques and Potential Problems. Proceedings of the Annual Meeting of the American Association of Zoo Veterinarians.

Penguin Taxon Advisory Groups Husbandry Manual 2nd Edition. 2003. Tom Schneider, Penguin Tag Chair, Detroit Zoo. Phone: (248) 398-0903; Fax: (248 0 398-0504; email: www.penguintag.org.

Schofield, N.A. 1991. The Effects of Diet and Feeding Regimen on Growth Rate of Magellanic Penguins. Spheniscus Penguin Newsletter 4 (2): 12–17.

Spurr, E.B. 1975. Behavior of the Adelie Penguin Chick. Condo 77: 272–280.

Stevenson, M.F. and Gibbons, M.P. 1993. Bringing new penguins into the collection 90's style. Penguin Conservation 6(2): 2–6.

Von Bocxstele, R. 1978. Breeding and Hand Rearing the Black Footed Penguin (Spheniscus Demersus) at Antwerp Zoo. International Zoo Yearbook 18: 42–4.

Williams, A.J. 1981. The laying interval and incubation period of rockhopper and macaroni penguins. Ostrich 52: 226–229.

6
Grebes

Sandie Elliott

NATURAL HISTORY

There are 19 species of grebes in the suborder Podicipedidae of the order Podicipediformes. Seven species of grebes found in North America include Black-necked (also called Eared), Clark's, Horned, Least, Pied-billed, Red-necked and Western. All species in this order are aquatic, communal, have three individually lobed toes on each foot, build nests of floating vegetation, hatch precocial young, and feed on aquatic invertebrates and fish. These stocky birds are well adapted for diving with lobed toes and legs set far back on the body, but these same aquatic adaptations preclude walking on solid surfaces. Grebes walk and stand poorly at best, and when found on land may be erroneously thought to have two broken legs (see Figure 6.1).

Grebes are best known for their amazing aquatic mating displays, such as the Western grebe's courtship ritual where the male and female run on the surface of the water, dive, and come together with breasts touching to form the shape of a heart with their outstretched necks and long thin beaks. Because they spend their entire lives in the water, other information about these birds is limited.

Grebes spend spring and summer on freshwater lakes and marshes where they mate and nest. Three to ten white to light-blue eggs are laid on a floating nest of aquatic plant material that is anchored to reeds in shallow waters. Incubation takes approximately 21–23 days for smaller species: Pied-billed, Eared, Horned, and Least, and 25–28 days for larger species: Red-necked, Clark's, and Western. Both parents participate in incubation and rearing of the young. Hatch weights of the young range from approximately 15 g in smaller grebes such as the Pied-billed (Muller and Storer 1999) to 30 g in the larger Western Grebe (Storer and Nuechterlein 1992).

The precocial young hatch covered with thick down and eyes open, and are mobile but need parental care for food, warmth, and protection. The first plumage transition from hatchling down to juvenile down takes place over the first 6 weeks of life, and flight feathers appear at about 10 weeks of age for the larger Clark's and Western Grebes. Juvenile grebes reach approximately 75% of their adult size at 6 months of age (see Figure 6.2).

Predators of eggs include crows, ravens, and gulls. Hatchlings are preyed upon by carp, large-mouthed bass and predatory birds. Environmental concerns include mercury and other toxin accumulation in lakes, and human activities and recreation that disturb nesting areas.

Grebes are migratory but not all grebes migrate. Some grebes move to coastal waters in the fall; others of the same species and colony remain on large inland lakes. Grebes are diurnal feeders, but coastal migrants have been observed participating in nocturnal feeding behaviors (Clowater 1996).

CRITERIA FOR INTERVENTION

Hatchling grebes are carried on the backs of the parent birds secured beneath the adults' wings for approximately the first 2–3 weeks of life. The hatchlings slip into the water to defecate, drink, take short swims, and forage on aquatic insects and surface debris throughout the day. Most young grebes brought into captive rearing situations have been separated from their parents by boaters moving through the colonies causing the adult birds to dive, spilling the young off their backs. Larger hatchlings and fledglings commonly present with severe injuries to their legs and feet caused by boat propellers or entanglement in fishing line. Some are simply

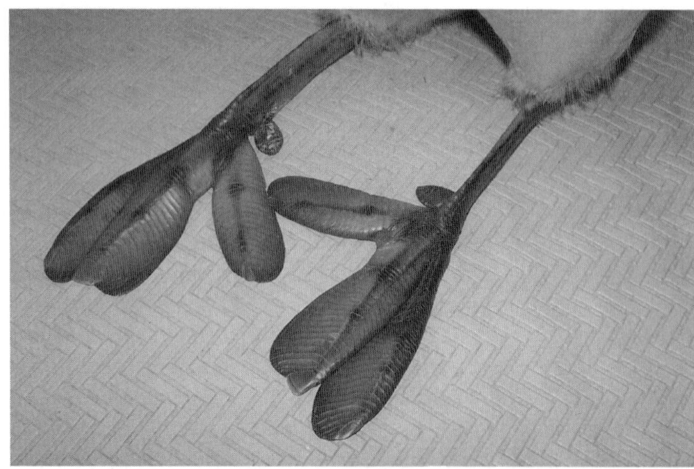

Figure 6.1. Close-up of Western Grebe feet showing the characteristic lobed toes.

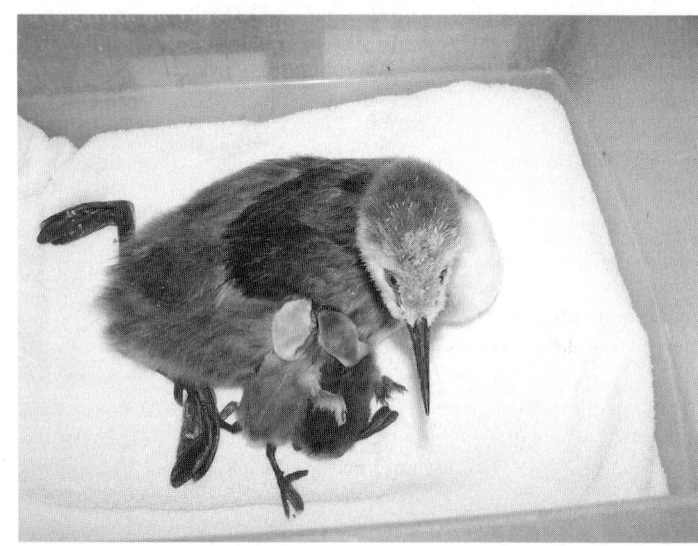

Figure 6.2. Fledgling Western with hatchling Western (right) and Clark's (left) Grebes. Some immature grebes have a tolerance for hatchlings and will allow them to climb on their back and will actually feed them.

high-centered on the shoreline and unable to get back into the water. It is not currently known whether young grebes can be returned to the area of the colony and be accepted by adoptive parents. Some data suggest this may be a possibility but more research is needed. Therefore, any young grebe still covered with down, found alone, injured, or on land warrants intervention.

Undertaking the rearing of these diving birds needs careful consideration because they have special needs including a pool for swimming and diving, excellent water quality, and an ample continuous supply of live food. Transfer to a facility that specializes in diving birds should be a priority consideration.

RECORD KEEPING

Record keeping information listed in Minimum Standards for Wildlife Rehabilitation (Miller 2000) should be adhered to in compliance with state or regional wildlife agency and Federal Fish & Wildlife Service regulations. As a minimum the following information should be kept: species; date admitted;

location found; approximate age; reason admitted for care; medical problems; admission weight; and final disposition, including transfer, death, euthanasia, or release date and location.

A detailed medical record should also be kept with each bird detailing findings of the initial examination, medications administered, daily body weight, progress of treatment, and behavioral notes. A daily feed and care chart should be maintained throughout the birds' stay in captivity.

Each bird should be assigned a patient number. If multiple birds are being cared for, small plastic numbered leg bands available from avian and poultry suppliers should be used (National Band and Tag Company).

INITIAL CARE AND STABILIZATION

Newly arrived orphans are generally cold, exhausted, and hungry. Do a quick preliminary examination to determine the level of hydration and whether there are any obvious injuries that need immediate attention, such as bleeding or breathing difficulties. Address life-threatening situations at once. If there are any injuries that disqualify the bird from continuing rehabilitation efforts, such as fractures at joints or other gross injuries that will render the bird incapable of supporting itself in the wild, rehabilitation should not be undertaken. If the youngster meets the criteria for rehabilitation, warm the bird.

Birds should be warmed by placing them on a padded surface in a climate-controlled incubator (if available) set to 86°F (30°C) with relative humidity of 40–50%. Grebes of any age may be placed on a towel-covered heating pad set to low contained in a plastic tub or cardboard box. The heating pad should take up only one-half of the container so that if the bird gets too warm it can move to a cooler location. Allow the bird to warm and relax for 15–20 minutes before conducting a full examination. Warm birds will become more alert, active, and vocal.

Following an in-depth, head-to-toe examination and if the bird is thoroughly warmed and has control of its neck and head movements, it may be placed in a plastic tub of shallow water warmed to 80–85°F (26–29°C). It will usually drink on its own. If it does not drink immediately, use a finger to gently push its head into the water. Repeat this several times if needed until it begins drinking, being careful not to overexert the bird. If it does not drink following several attempts, or if it is too weak to lift its head, fluids must be delivered bolus via orogastric tube. Due to the thick downy plumage, subcutaneous and intraperitoneal (IP) hydration should be avoided unless the care provider is adept at these methods. Grebes do not exhibit open-mouth begging behavior (gaping), so oral administration of fluids increases the risk of aspiration. Fluids may also be administered intravenously (IV) into the medial metatarsal vein if technical expertise and sterile equipment are available.

The degree of dehydration should be determined to institute a proper care protocol for the youngster. To determine the correct amount of fluids to give, use the Maintenance and Deficit Replacement Method: estimated dehydration (%) × body weight (g) = fluid deficit (ml) with half the deficit amount over the first 12–24 hours and the remainder divided over the next 48 hours (Bailey 2000). This amount is added to the daily maintenance requirement, which is calculated as 50 ml/kg/day for most birds. An alternate method is the Body Weight Percentage Method: fluid replacement in ml = body weight (g) × 2.5%. This amount should be delivered 8–12 times over a 24-hour period. For example, for a 100 g bird the amount of fluids needed is (100 g) (0.025) = 2.5 ml; therefore, 2.5 ml of fluid should be administered 8–12 times over a 24-hour period or until the bird begins to drink on its own.

All birds are assumed to be suffering from mild dehydration upon admission. Healthy birds can be given hydrating fluids calculated at 2.5% of their total body weight once and then be fed. A bird that is moderately dehydrated and exhibits dry mouth and tenting of the skin may need two or three doses of fluids given hourly prior to feeding. A severely dehydrated bird exhibiting ropey saliva, pale oral cavity, sunken eyes, and prolonged tenting of the skin will need a full course of fluids, as previously described, before feeding is initiated. As a general rule, with very young birds the sooner food can be introduced the better, but never before rehydration has at least been initiated.

Lactated Ringer's Solution and Normasol are both excellent isotonic rehydration fluids. If these are not available, human infant oral rehydration solutions comparable to Pedialyte may be substituted. Fluids should be warmed to 100.4–102.2°F (38–39°C) before delivery (Bailey 2000). Once the grebe is warm, hydrated, and has defecated, it may be considered stable.

Grebe chicks will defecate out of water but prefer to be in water. The paddling motion of their legs while swimming stimulates excretion.

These chicks vocalize not only due to hunger but for social reasons as well. Placing a small mirror beside a solitary bird will calm and quiet it between feedings.

COMMON MEDICAL PROBLEMS AND SOLUTIONS

Hatchling grebes often present with signs of hypothermia, dehydration, and starvation. They need heat, fluids, and food. They may also suffer from a form of gastritis commonly called *bloat* or from aspiration pneumonia. Both of these conditions are usually the result of well-intentioned but untrained individuals administering fluids and/or inappropriate foods before presenting the birds for professional help.

Bloat may be caused by an obstruction of the gastrointestinal tract, but more often it is a biological reaction of the intestines to food or bacterial activities. During gastritis (bloat), intestinal gases expand and rapidly fill the body, causing organ failure due to the pressure exerted on the organs. Gastritis is often accompanied by metabolic acidosis. If a grebe presents with gastric distention, decompression must be initiated immediately. Gastric decompression may be accomplished with insertion of an orogastric (esophageal) tube passed from the mouth along the esophagus and into the stomach to allow the gas to escape.

Decompression should be followed by gastric lavage with warm water or normal saline to eliminate any remaining irritants. Hydrating fluids can then be given IP or IV, or via orogastric tube. If the first attempt is unsuccessful or if the care provider is untrained in these procedures, an avian veterinarian should be seen immediately due to the severity of this problem.

Aspiration pneumonia results from food or water being introduced into the lungs or air sacs. A young grebe that has been paddling half submerged and exhausted may inhale lake water. More often it will be human error that causes this complication, such as inappropriate feeding technique. A bird that shows distressed respiratory efforts (open-mouth breathing) often accompanied by wet or congested lung sounds will need a 7–10 day course of antibiotics such as Amoxicillin at 15–25 mg/kg two to three times daily. An avian veterinarian should be consulted for the proper treatment protocol. If oxygen is available, an oxygen-rich environment will be beneficial. Keep the bird warm and well hydrated. It may be prudent to give the bird antifungal agents as well while it's being treated with antibiotics, because many waterbirds are very susceptible to aspergillosis.

It is uncommon for hatchling grebes to arrive with fractures or other injuries. However, fledglings are often admitted with fractures of the legs and toes and other traumatic impact injuries. Due to the anatomy of the legs and physical agility needed by these birds to capture prey, birds with fractures often have a poor prognosis, and splinting or wrapping fractures may be an exercise in futility. However, this may be useful to stabilize a fracture temporarily. An avian veterinarian should be consulted for any fractures.

Traumatic head injuries require that the bird be kept in an unheated container so as to not exacerbate brain swelling, and steroids or nonsteroidal antiinflammatory drugs (NSAIDS) such as Celebrex or Meloxicam may be administered. The utility of corticosteroids, given their impact on the immune system, is highly controversial. The author prefers not to treat with medications, but rather to keep the bird at 70–75°F (21–24°C), dark, quiet, hydrated, and fed via orogastric tube if unable to feed itself.

Grebes are susceptible to avian influenza, bacterial diseases such as Erysipelas or Pasteurella, and toxins including avian botulism and methylmercury poisoning. Nasal leeches are common as well (USDI/USGS 1999).

Parasites are rarely a problem for young grebes. However, fecal flotation and microscopic examination should be done as part of routine care procedures. The most important parasites of these birds are flukes (*Trichobilharzia spp.).* Anthelmintics commonly used to treat waterfowl include Fenbendazole (5–15 mg/kg PO once daily for 5 days), Levamisole (20–50 mg/kg PO once), Mebendazole (5–15 mg/kg PO once daily for 2 days), Praziquantel (for trematodes 5–10 mg/kg PO or SQ once daily for 14 days) and Ivermectin (0.2 mg/kg PO, SQ, or IM once) (Carpenter 2005). An avian veterinarian should be consulted for exact laboratory diagnosis of illness and always before administering any medications.

DIET RECIPES

Precise nutritional requirements for grebes have not been established, but the fact that they are live-insect and fish eaters indicates that this is the diet they need. Nutritional values of live, whole feeder gold-

Table 6.1. Nutrient values of common foods.

Nutrient Value per 100 Grams Edible Portion	Kcal	Calcium mg	Phosphorus mg	Thiamine mg
Chicken breast, raw[a]	110	11	196	0.07
Herring, wild, raw[a]	195	83	228	0.06
Shad wild, raw[a]	197	47	272	0.15
Carp wild, raw[a]	127	41	415	0.12
Trout wild, raw[a]	119	67	271	0.12
Smelt wild, raw[a]	97	60	230	0.01
Crickets, adult[b]	140	41	295	0.04
Mealworms[b]	206	17	285	0.24

[a] USDA Agricultural Research Service. Nutrient Data Library; http://www.ars.usda.gov/ba/bhnrc/nd/.
[b] Finke 2002.

fish, guppies, and minnows are not available but they have long been used in rehabilitation of small aquatic birds and can be fed to hatchling grebes. Live crickets and mealworms are another good source of nutrition and are helpful in stimulating self-feeding behaviors. Water fleas and water beetles may also be fed.

Raw deboned freshwater fish are useful for hand-feeding, force-feeding, or tube-feeding any age grebe for short periods of time. When feeding a diet of dead fish, 25–30 mg thiamine and 100 mg vitamin E must be supplemented per kilogram of fish fed (Carpenter 2005). The calcium-to-phosphorus ratio should be adjusted in all diets to optimum 2:1 calcium-to-phosphorus by weight (see Table 6.1 for nutrient values of some common foods). If nutrient values of the diet are unknown, calcium glubionate may be supplemented orally at 150 mg/kg body weight once or twice daily (Carpenter 2005). Because deboned fish is very high in phosphorus and low in calcium, a large amount of added calcium is needed to bring the calcium and phosphorus back into the correct ratio for a growing bird. If a bird is to remain on deboned fish for very long, add 12.0 g calcium carbonate powder (4800 mg of elemental calcium) to each kilogram of deboned fish. Calcium should be 0.4–0.8% of the diet as fed.

Fledglings may be fed live or dead freshwater trout, fingerling carp, threadfin shad, crayfish, or saltwater fish such as herring or smelt up to approximately 5 in (0.13 m) in length. It is important to remember that these birds swallow their prey whole; hence, if it does not fit in the bird's mouth, the bird cannot eat it. Healthy grebes will regurgitate a cast pellet of undigestible material, including feathers and fish bones.

Insects may also be added to increase the protein diversity and caloric value of this diet. Use a food processor to process the ingredients to a texture that will move smoothly through a feeding syringe and orogastric tube. When using this diet, do not attempt to warm the food prior to feeding, because fish cooks at relatively low temperatures. This diet should be fed at room temperature and the excess refrigerated for use within 24 hours.

Recipes using canine or feline foods, cereals, and eggs should be avoided because they have a tendency to cause bloat. Raw chicken meat may be used as an emergency overnight food source, but carries the risk of bacterial contamination. Use of raw meat products necessitates close adherence to hygienic food handling practices.

FEEDING PROCEDURES

Grebe chicks hatch, spend a few hours drying off, crawl to the edge of the nest, plop into the water and climb onto the adult's back. Their eyes are open and they know they are grebes, so unless the baby was found on the nest, the chance of imprinting is negligible. This is important because baby grebes are very social and close interaction is necessary for successful rearing.

Grebe hatchlings that are 24–48 hours old have been fed by their parents and already know how to take food from the adult's beak. At 72 hours of age, they have been attempting to eat things they find in the water during short swims. Feeding these birds

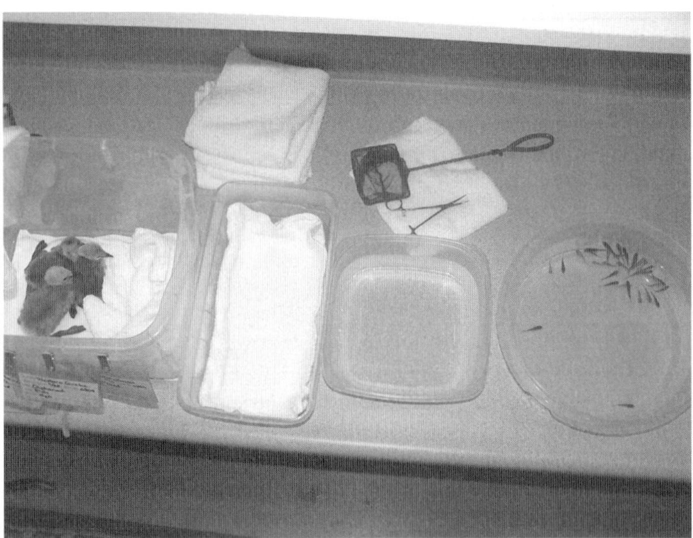

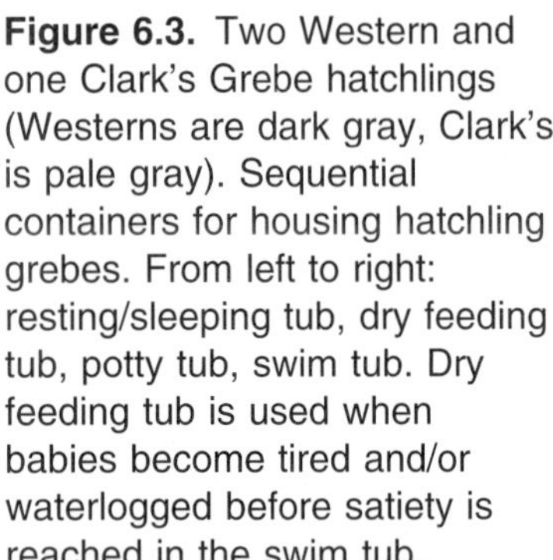

Figure 6.3. Two Western and one Clark's Grebe hatchlings (Westerns are dark gray, Clark's is pale gray). Sequential containers for housing hatchling grebes. From left to right: resting/sleeping tub, dry feeding tub, potty tub, swim tub. Dry feeding tub is used when babies become tired and/or waterlogged before satiety is reached in the swim tub.

combines getting them to focus and waiting for them to improve their beak-to-food coordination skills. Getting them to focus will be the greater challenge.

Let the bird demonstrate its abilities. All grebe chicks should be tested for the ability to self-feed by placing them in a tub of shallow water containing live fish or in a container with live crickets (see Figure 6.3). This may require the care provider to step out of the room for a few minutes to get the bird to focus on the task. All grebe chicks over 200 g are already capable of feeding themselves unless debilitated by illness or injury. Food presentation should be as compatible with their normal feeding behavior as is possible, and food items should be of a size they can easily eat.

Feeder goldfish are the easiest fish to keep alive for self-feeding youngsters and they come in a range of small sizes. A 30 liter (or larger) aquarium with filter system should be set up and stocked with the proper size fish.

A cricket/mealworm feeder box may be constructed simply by placing a deep, bottomless, plastic container on a towel and then placing the bird and the insects in it. Placing a towel in the bottom of a container will not work because the crickets and mealworms will hide beneath the towel.

Birds should be weighed daily and the amount needed to be fed recalculated. The 5% of body weight per feeding rule-of-thumb may be used until the proper amount to feed can be established (see Appendix 2 for tables of kcals/day to support growth in juvenile birds).

There are four basic ways that a grebe of any age can be fed: (1) orogastric tube or (2) force-feeding are recommended for birds that are sick or debilitated; (3) hand-feeding with blunt-tip forceps for very young birds that do not have the strength, stamina, or skill to dive and capture food; and (4) placing live food in the water for birds that are self-feeding.

Hatchlings

Hatchlings that are stable but need to be tube- or force-fed should be placed in a container of water 3–4 in (8–10 cm) deep, approximately 65–75°F (18–24°C) and large enough to allow the bird some movement prior to each feeding. It is prudent to have two water containers set up because some babies will drink and then defecate, and others will defecate immediately upon touching the water. If they defecate before drinking, they should be removed immediately and placed in the second container with clean water for drinking and swimming. Very young chicks usually stay in the water only long enough to defecate and drink. They will then call loudly and demonstrate a need to get out of the water, at which time the care provider should place a hand in the water and allow the bird to climb onto it. Tube and force-fed birds should be fed following a swim time at 1-hour intervals during daylight hours. If the youngster cries between feedings, decrease the intervals or increase the amount being fed.

For tube feedings, soft rubber size 12 or 14 French urogenital catheters or tubing from an intravenous extension set cut to an appropriate length and attached to a luer-lock syringe make excellent feeding apparatuses. Any cut plastic tubing ends must be filed or burned to round sharp edges before use. Determine the length for the tube by holding the bird with its neck extended and measure from the tip of the beak to the caudal end of the rib cage where the stomach is located. Mark this measured distance on the tube. Attach the tube to the syringe and draw up the required amount of fluid or food, making sure there is no air in the tube. To insert the tube, hold the bird with fingers behind the mandibles and extend the neck vertically. Gently open the beak and carefully pass the tube into the oral cavity and along the right side of the neck down the esophagus, avoiding the glottis (tracheal opening at the back and center of the tongue). If the tube is correctly placed it will slide easily and may be observed beneath the skin as it moves down the right side of the neck. Use gentle pressure while inserting and stop when the mark on the tube is at the tip of the beak or when resistance is met. Keep the neck fully extended while delivering the contents of the feeding syringe to avoid reflux and aspiration. A 60 g grebe will tolerate 1.5–2 ml of fluid or 2–3 ml of pureed fish bolus delivery without risk of aspiration. Following feeding, the tube should be withdrawn carefully to prevent reflux. If reflux occurs, the bird should be released immediately and allowed to clear the oral cavity on its own.

To force-feed, use a fingernail inserted between the upper and lower beak close to the face (never at the tip) to open the mouth. Use blunt-nose forceps to place small insects, fish, or slivers of fish to the back and right side of the throat. Watch for the bird to swallow. If the bird does not swallow, gently massage the neck downward to move the food along the esophagus toward the stomach.

Hand-feeding may be done while the bird is in the water if it can swim long enough to eat, or after the swim with the bird back in its nest box. Simply offer the food items with forceps and allow the bird to take the food with its beak. Those birds just learning to eat will shake the food and fling it across the nest box or onto a nearby wall. Keep in mind that force-feeding is still an option but will inhibit the bird's learning. Hand-fed birds need to be fed at 1-hour intervals during the daylight hours.

Healthy hand-fed chicks should be encouraged to self-feed by placing them in a cricket box or adding a few live feeder fish to their water at least once a day until they figure out how to capture prey. Do this prior to feeding using hunger as a motivator. Remember to step out of sight momentarily if the bird will not focus on the food.

For self-feeding youngsters, set up two containers of water 3–4 in (8–10 cm) deep, approximately 65–75°F (18–24°C) and large enough to allow them to swim and dive. Put live feeder fish in one container. Place the bird into the first container until it defecates, and then move the bird into the second container to drink, swim, and feed. Adjust the depth of the water to accommodate the bird's diving ability and allow the bird to eat its fill before returning it to its nest container. Self-feeding birds should be fed at 1–2 hour intervals throughout the daylight hours. The fish should be weighed and counted to keep track of the amount being eaten. Younger birds may tire before eating enough. If this occurs, remove them from the water and offer crickets and mealworms; hand-feed, force-feed, or use an orogastric tube to complete the meal.

Between 200 and 240 g of weight, young Clark's and Western Grebes go through a rapid growth phase that may last from 1–3 days. During this time, they become ravenous and may eat an amount equal to their own body weight or more during a 24-hour period. During this phase, feeding intervals need to be decreased while the amount fed per feeding needs to be increased dramatically.

There is speculation that young grebes are fed feathers to line their stomachs and protect them from fish bones. Whether this is actively practiced for a reason or just a matter of the birds eating floating debris that happens to be feathers is an issue for debate. Feeder goldfish, guppies, and small minnows have no hardened bones that will harm the digestive system of young grebes. However, if small downy feathers are available, offer them to the bird.

Fledglings

Fledglings are birds that are self-sufficient, nearly the size of adults, feathered, waterproof, and learning to fly. They should be fed live fish when possible but will generally accept dead threadfin shad or other small freshwater fish or chunks of deboned large fish dropped into their water tank. The movement of the fish in the water stimulates them to feed. Large dead fish should be deboned to ensure that the sharp ends of cut bones will not injure the bird's gastrointestinal tract.

Healthy self-feeding fledglings should be fed to satiety at 4-hour intervals during daylight hours. Fledgling birds needing orogastric tube or force-feedings should be fed every 2–3 hours during daylight hours.

EXPECTED WEIGHT GAIN

There is no set daily weight gain recorded for grebes, only generalizations that are geographic region- and species-specific. If the bird is active, alert, and appears healthy and normal, it probably is and these birds will vocalize hunger. Each bird should be weighed daily to be certain it is continuously gaining weight. The author's experience is that hatchling Western and Clark's Grebes gain approximately 8–12 g per day while Pied-billed Grebes gain 6–10 g per day during the early growth stages.

HOUSING

Accommodations for grebes must change as they grow and become self-sufficient. It is important that at all ages their feet are protected from abrasion by not being placed on hard or rough surfaces such as wood, gravel, dirt, wire, or screen. Grebes must always be on a padded surface until spending all of their time in the water, and they must be allowed maximum pool time at all ages. Keep in mind that the accommodations must be determined by the bird's ability, not its age and weight. They are social birds so same-size preadult birds may be safely housed together.

Any softly padded incubator, climate controlled nursery unit, or container with heating pad will accommodate young, sick, and/or injured grebes. Incubators or climate-controlled nursery units should be set to 86°F (30°C) with a relative humidity of 40–50%. Toweling or padding materials should be changed a minimum of twice daily. It is imperative that plumage does not become soiled with droppings or food debris. Frequent brief swims in clean water will help reduce fecal contamination of bedding.

Water containers for defecating, feeding, and exercising must be on hand for all age grebes. Allowing the bird to swim for as long as it can before, during, and/or after feedings will greatly improve its muscle tone and diving ability, and keep the gastrointestinal tract motile. Never leave young grebes unattended in the water for extended periods of time until they are fully waterproof.

Water containers should be of a size to allow the bird room to swim and dive (see Figure 6.4). The level of the water should always be several inches below the top of the container so the bird does not propel itself over the side, and never deeper than the bird can dive to retrieve food on the bottom. There are many commercially available plastic or rubber

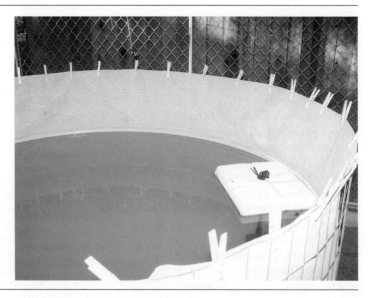

Figure 6.4. Regulation 6 feet diameter by 2 feet deep (1.8 × 0.7 m) pool with nylon net covered foam haul-out. Tank "surround" is wire fencing covered with shade cloth secured with clothespins. It rises one foot (30 cm) above the water surface.

containers of graduated sizes that are acceptable as swim/feed pools for young grebes, are easy to clean and transport, and make transitioning easy and inexpensive. A 50–60 g hatchling may do nicely in a dishpan, but by 200 g will need at least a bathtub-sized swimming pool.

When the bird is completely self-feeding and capable of spending a good deal of time in the water, it may be placed in a small human children's pool or the recommended 6 ft (1.8 m) diameter × 2 ft (0.6 m) deep pool (Miller 2000). Careful observation will dictate the depth of the water necessary to accommodate the bird's diving and food capture capabilities. The pool must have a haul-out area so the bird can get out of the water to rest, preen, and warm itself.

A haul-out for young grebes with little feet can be made by wrapping a piece of closed-cell foam 1 ft wide × 1 ft long × 1–2 in thick (30 cm × 30 cm × 3–5 cm) with tightly stretched 1/4-in (0.6 cm) knotless nylon netting (Nylon Net Company) or similar material. For larger birds use a piece of foam 2 ft wide × 2 ft long × 3 in thick (60 cm × 60 cm × 7 cm) wrapped with 1 in (2.5 cm) knotless nylon netting (Christensen Net Works). Make a hole in the center of the foam pad and run a piece of plastic rope through it. Tie a large bulky knot in the top of the rope that will not slip back through the hole. Measure the lower section of rope equal to the water depth to be used and then tie it to a brick or a rock to act as an anchor for the floating platform. Leave the extra rope intact so the length can be adjusted as the depth of the water is increased during the course of rehabilitation. Portable, custom-made frames with netting stretched across four uprights, hammock style, can also be used. The haul-out must rise out of the water allowing the bird to climb out, dry off, and warm up and must be positioned in a way that the bird can easily climb on and off without injury.

Younger grebes should be supplied with a lamp for heat located overhead of the haul-out anytime the ambient temperature drops significantly below the seasonal normal. The water in the pool should be 65–70°F (18–21°C) or the approximate temperature of lakes in the area for that time of the year. The pool should be placed in a quiet outdoor area where the bird can receive natural light during daylight hours. If the pool is indoors, full-spectrum lighting must be supplied with a normal day/night cycle. Outdoor pools must be in predator-proof enclosures, and a visual barrier is recommended around the pool to provide security and minimize visual contact with humans. This can be easily accomplished with tall potted plants or shade netting hung on the enclosure walls.

At this stage, the youngster may still need to be removed to a safe nest container for the night or when there is no supervision for long periods of time. Careful observation will determine its needs. When raising a lone bird, a mirror placed near the haul-out can be important for its psychological well-being.

Placing the grebe in a larger or deeper body of water will allow the fish an increased opportunity to escape the bird. Fish that are added to the pool for feeding should be weighed and counted before and after feedings to be sure the bird is getting enough to eat.

Following the first plumage transition from hatchling down to juvenile down or when it is waterproof and capable of swimming for extended periods of time, the bird should be permanently placed in a 6 ft (1.8 m) diameter × 2 ft (0.6 m) deep outdoor pool. When startled or attempting to escape, grebes may pop out of the water and over the side, so the pool must have a safety barrier or *surround*. A surround can be constructed of any flexible material that can be wrapped around the outer circumference of the pool to create a barrier rising 1 ft (0.3 m) above the water level in the pool. Some materials that work well are linoleum, cardboard coated with paraffin wax, the thin plastic used for shower stall applications, or even wood or metal stakes driven into the ground with 1.4 in (3.5 cm) wire mesh, netting, or screen attached. Alternatively, a pool 3 ft (0.9 m) or deeper may be used and be filled only to the 2 ft (0.6 m) level. The pool must be in a predator-proof enclosure with a visual barrier and have a haul-out or resting area. No external heat source is needed.

Overflow cleaning of pools is recommended when no filtering system is available and can be easily accomplished by placing a garden hose in the pool and allowing fresh water to run in until the pool overflows for a few minutes. This will reduce the likelihood of droppings or oils from prey items fouling the birds' plumage.

PREPARATION FOR WILD RELEASE

Grebes may be released when they are 10–12 weeks of age (flight feathers present but not necessarily completely grown in), self-feeding on live fish, fully waterproof, and no longer in need of medical treatment. Testing for waterproofing is done by removal of the haul-out for a minimum of 48 hours. If the bird is ready, its waterproofing should not be compromised. The downy underfeathers should be dry with no areas where water penetrates to the skin.

Release should be done when calm weather is expected for three consecutive days, in suitable habitat, and near others of the same species when possible.

ACKNOWLEDGMENTS

Many thanks to David Stoneberg for reviewing the chapter.

SOURCES FOR PRODUCTS MENTIONED

Leg bands: National Band and Tag Company, 721 York St, Newport, KY 41072-0430, (800) 261-TAGS (8247).

Netting: Nylon Net Company, 845 N Main St, Memphis, TN 38107, (800) 238-7529.

Netting: Christensen Net Works, 5510 A Nielsen Ave, Ferndale, WA 98248, (800) 459-2147.

REFERENCES

Bailey, T.A. 2000. Fluid therapy. In Avian Medicine. Samour, J., ed. Mosby, London, pp. 103–104.

Carpenter, J.W., ed. 2005. Exotic Animal Formulary, 3rd Edition. Elsevier Saunders, Philadelphia, pp. 135–344.

Clowater, J.S. 1996. Western Grebe Research: Nocturnal Foraging of Western Grebes. http://webs.ii.ca/clowater/default.htm.

Finke, M.D. 2002. Complete nutrient composition for commercially raised invertebrates used as food for insectivores. Zoo Biology 21: 269–285.

Miller, E.A., ed. 2000. Minimum Standards for Wildlife Rehabilitation, 3rd Edition. National Wildlife Rehabilitation Association, St. Cloud, MN, 77 pp.

Muller, M.J. and Storer, R.W. 1999. Pied-billed Grebe (*Podilymbus podiceps*). In The Birds of North America, No. 410, Poole, A., and Gill, F., eds. The Birds of North America, Inc., Philadelphia, PA.

Stocker, L. 2000. Practical Wildlife Care for Veterinary Nurses, Animal Care Students and Rehabilitators. Blackwell Science Ltd. London, pp. 26–32.

Storer, R.W. and Nuechterlein, G.L. 1992. Western and Clark's Grebe. In The Birds of North America, No. 26, Poole, A., Stettenheim, P., and Gill, F., eds. Philadelphia: The Academy of Natural Sciences; Washington, DC: The American Ornithologists' Union.

U.S. Department of the Interior and U.S. Geological Survey. 1999. Field Manual of Wildlife Diseases: General Field Procedures and Diseases of Birds. Biological Resources Division Information and Technology Report 199-001. National Wildlife Health Center. Madison, WI, 425 pp. Manual available as free download at http://www.nwhc.usgs.gov/publications/field_manual/index.jsp.

7
Pelicans

Wendy Fox

NATURAL HISTORY

In the United States there are three subspecies of the Brown Pelican occidentalis group. *Pelecanus occidentalis occidentalis* is found throughout the Gulf Coast, from Mexico to both coasts of Florida. *P.o. carolinensis* breeds from Maryland, around Florida and through the Gulf Coast to Central America. *P.o. californicus* ranges from British Columbia down the Pacific coast typically breeding from California into Mexico.

Sexual maturity is reached between 3 and 5 years of age. Pelicans nest colonially, on the ground or in trees such as mangroves. The male selects the site and after attracting the female, the male begins gathering sticks, which the female arranges. Ground nesting sites may be no more than a depression in the ground.

A normal clutch size is three eggs laid over a period of several days, normally with a 2-day interval between eggs. Both parents incubate the eggs and the incubation period varies by species and region but appears to be between 30–35 days.

CRITERIA FOR INTERVENTION

Reasons for human intervention are most likely to involve a mass event caused by disruption or devastation to a rookery site, such as an oil spill or hurricane.

Although it is unusual for members of the public to find and bring baby pelicans to a wildlife rehabilitation facility, as humans continue to encroach on coastal areas the chance increases. Pelicans prefer to nest on small coastal islands or on dredge islands in intracoastal waterways, many of which are easily accessible to recreational boaters and fishermen.

It is always in the best interests of the chick to be raised by its own parents or at a wildlife facility where foster parents are available. Not all eventualities can be dealt with in this chapter, and it is cruel and inappropriate (and illegal) for wild birds to be raised incorrectly or by inexperienced individuals and then released into the wild.

RECORD KEEPING

Wildlife rehabilitators and others handling migratory birds must hold state and federal rehabilitation permits requiring an annual report on each bird treated. Information required is as follows: date of admission, species, disposition, and date of disposition.

In addition, it is recommended that the following information be collected to ensure the best continuity of care for the bird: the location the bird was found (because it is hoped that the bird can be returned to the same location), the general condition and weight of the bird on intake, the location of any injuries on intake and follow-up treatment, records of fluids and any medications given, a feeding schedule, and notes pertinent to whether the chick is eating unassisted or whether it needs help. A growth chart may be useful to assist in targeting birds that are not progressing normally.

INITIAL CARE AND STABILIZATION

It is critical that the chicks be warmed first and then hydrated before taking any other action. Place the chick in a warm quiet area in a towel nest. Baby pelicans feed from the nest floor, so it is recommended that paper, especially shredded paper, not be used as a nesting material, because it will be ingested.

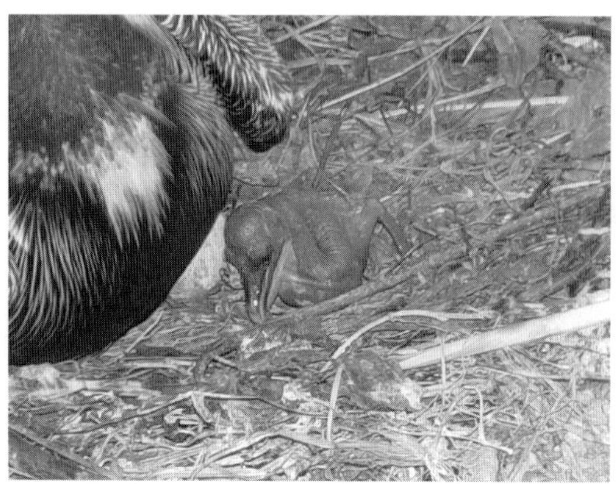

Figure 7.1. Hatchling pelican. Skin color is purplish before down grows in.

For approximately the first 3 weeks of life, until they are covered in down, pelican chicks have trouble thermoregulating and are constantly attended by a parent (see Figure 7.1).

Hydration may be given orally, subcutaneously or by IV bolus. Many different hydration fluids are available, and the choice should be made on your wildlife veterinarian's recommendation. Fluid therapy charts are available for wildlife (see the "References" section at the end of this chapter). Once the chick is warmed and hydrated feeding may begin.

COMMON MEDICAL PROBLEMS AND SOLUTIONS

Minor skin lacerations are not uncommon. Make sure the affected area is kept clean; this type of minor skin nick normally heals quickly.

More serious wounds may occur if a chick is or has been attacked by older siblings in the nest. Another problem can occur during weaning. Juveniles may try to feed from any available adult, becoming quite aggressive in their attempts to force the adult's beak open. The adult will on occasion retaliate by biting the juvenile around the head sometimes resulting in head injuries. Most injuries are superficial and will scab over and heal quickly. At this age the beak is still soft and is damaged easily. Normally, the injuries are closer to the jaw. Scabbing can be quite severe, and the beak may take several weeks to fully heal. Birds with scratches to the eyes and birds exhibiting neurological symptoms should be seen by an experienced wildlife veterinarian. Hematological and biochemical reference values can be found in Zaias et al. (2000).

It is normal for Brown Pelicans to have what appears to be subcutaneous emphysema under the skin. This assists with buoyancy. When palpated, it will feel like bubble wrap and may make a crackling sound. If an air sac is ruptured there will be an obvious, larger outpouching of the skin. If a ruptured air sac is suspected, the bird should be referred to a wildlife veterinarian. The air sac may need draining, and the bird may also require ventilatory assistance.

DIET

In the wild, Brown Pelicans feed by plunge diving and bringing to the surface up to three gallons of fish and water in their pouches. Brown Pelicans will also catch fish while floating on the surface if large, dense schools of small bait fish are available. In captivity, smelt, minnows, and anchovies are useful in small chicks, increasing in size to small threadfin herring, sardines, mullet, menhaden, and other small whole baitfish for juveniles. The nutritional value of fish varies depending on fish type, season, and whether the fish is alive or dead. Fish with a higher fat content will have a higher caloric density. Very oily fish such as mackerel can cause fish oil to adhere around the pelican's beak and will eventually end up on the feathers causing waterproofing problems. Although fish are normally a good source of vitamins, changes can occur in dead or frozen fish. Birds fed dead or frozen fish should receive thiamine and vitamin E supplements and a good general vitamin supplement. Even birds being fed live fish in captivity will benefit from an appropriate good-quality vitamin supplement. Dosage is by weight and will depend on the diet given and combination of supplements used. Choices include Vionate powder (Rich Health Inc.) and SeaTabs, which are formulated for fish-eating birds and mammals (Pacific Research Laboratories).

A general rule would be to use a variety of seasonal, locally available fish if possible, because the best diet should closely resemble what would be available to the birds in the wild during nesting season. Chunks of large fish or fish with large bones, gill plates, or skulls are not appropriate, because the bones are difficult and sometimes impossible for the pelican to digest. Large, sharp bones can perforate the stomach causing peritonitis or become lodged in

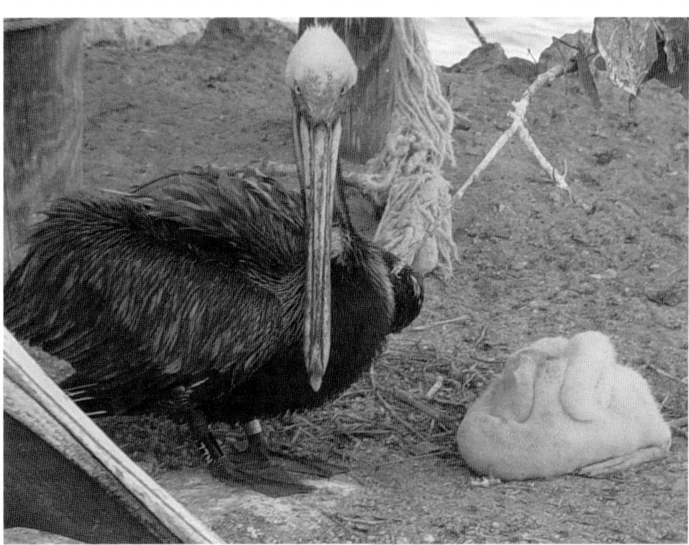

Figure 7.2. Foster parent with sleeping chick.

the esophagus, making it difficult for the bird to swallow.

Caloric/energy requirement charts and calculations are available for wildlife (see "References" and Appendix 2).

FEEDING PROCEDURES

In the wild, feeding begins within hours of hatching. The parent regurgitates partially digested fish into the nest for chicks to pick up. This behavior lasts for approximately 3 weeks. The transition to a different feeding method coincides with the chicks becoming completely down covered. At about 2–3 weeks of age, the chicks begin feeding by reaching into the parent's throat for fish. This behavior lasts until the chick is ready to fledge. Once the chick can fly, the parent limits the number of feedings. Pelican Harbor Seabird Station is located on a flyway in Biscayne Bay near a pelican nesting site. The author frequently sees young pelicans chasing adult birds both on land and water. Normal behavior is for the fledgling to waggle its wings, bob the head, and snap at its own wings to attract the parent's attention. More aggressive behavior includes trying to force the adult's beak open.

For small chicks without down, offer slivers of fish or small whole fish, such as small smelt, on the cage or nest floor. Leave the area, because the chick may become distracted and not eat while humans are present. It is important to count the number of fish placed with the chick so you can monitor eating habits. Introduce the chick to foster parents as soon as possible (see Figure 7.2).

Older down-covered chicks may be more of a challenge as they have become used to eating from the pouch (see Figure 7.3). If they will not pick fish off the floor, try presenting fish on the end of a hemostat or pair of scissors. They will learn quickly. Chicks that are standing well and developing feathers can be introduced to fish in a bowl of shallow water.

If foster parents are not available, it is in the chick's best interests to be transferred to a facility with foster parents and experience in raising pelicans. Foster parents are normally nonreleasable pelicans used for fostering or education purposes. Permits are required. Adults undergoing rehabilitation should not be used as foster parents.

When placing chicks with foster parents, it is normally readily apparent if the chick will be accepted or not. Normal behavior is for the adult to circle the chick, with head swaying and open beak; "hissing" may also occur. The adult will settle over the chick fairly quickly (see Figure 7.4). Pairs or single adults will foster.

Older chicks are best when kept in groups with adult foster parents as role models. The number in each group depends on aviary size. In addition, be aware that young pelicans can become quite

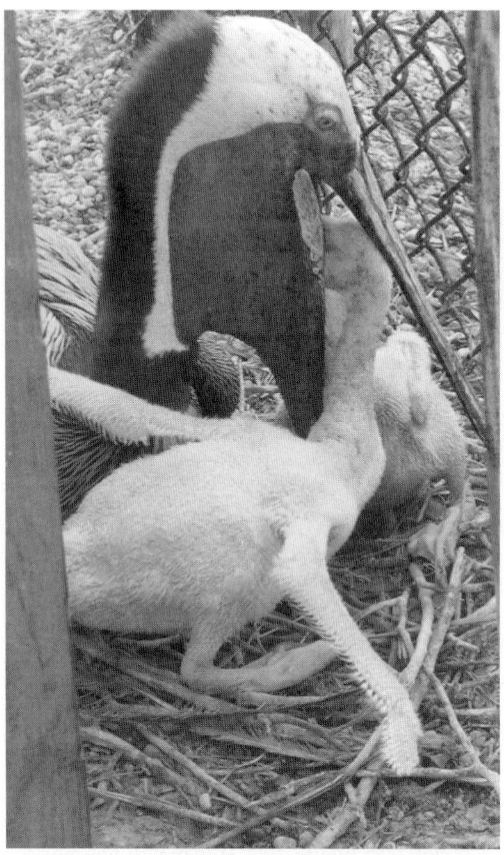

Figure 7.3. Nestling feeding from foster parent's pouch. Note thick woolly white down.

aggressive in their feeding techniques, often overwhelming adults or older juveniles with their anxiety to feed. This is a dangerous situation for both the chicks and adults.

A slow introduction technique through a joint aviary fence needs to be used when introducing large groups of displaced pelican chicks, such as when a rookery island is destroyed after a hurricane. These pelicans tend to be traumatized by rescue and transportation issues and may have been in a large group for at least several days. After Hurricane Dennis in 2004, the author raised 50 6–10-week-old pelican chicks. The chicks were divided into three age-specific groups in aviaries that shared a common fence with foster adults. As night approached at the end of the first day, the chicks settled down to sleep against the common fence and the adults settled down next to the chicks on their side of the fence. By the next day, a calm and successful introduction was possible.

EXPECTED DEVELOPMENT

Weight gain is rapid during the first 3 weeks. After 3 weeks, a steady, but not as rapid, weight gain will occur. Because pelicans vary greatly in size, weight gain should not be the only indicator of successful growth. Daily checks should show an increasingly active chick, well-hydrated with a well-rounded body and plump breast.

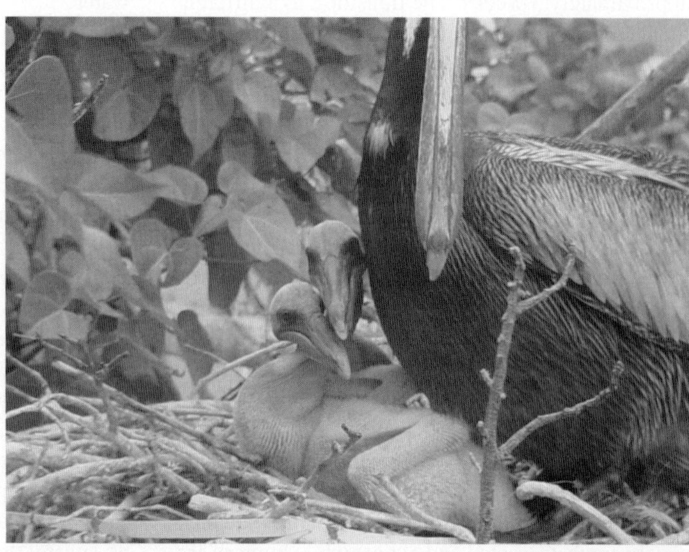

Figure 7.4. Foster parent brooding two chicks.

Chicks are altricial with purplish skin for about 7 days. Then white down begins to appear on the rump area first, and the chick will be completely downy at about 3 weeks. Contour feathers begin to appear at about 4 to 5 weeks, beginning in the scapula area and extending onto the humerus.

Nestlings begin holding their heads up at 2 to 4 days. By 10 to 14 days they are moving in the nest and are able to hold themselves upright. At 3 to 4 weeks they sit or stand for prolonged periods of time, and after that ground-nesting chicks become very mobile. They will leave the nest and begin to explore, closely watched over by their parents, although sometimes from a distance. Chicks in tree nests will move to perches next to the nest. First flight is normally between 12 to 14 weeks.

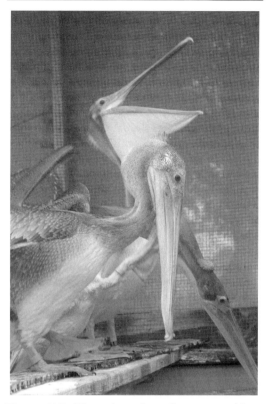

Figure 7.5. Three juvenile pelicans stretching (photo courtesy of Marie Travers IBRRC).

FLIGHT CAGES AND POOLS

Caging standards for rehabilitating wild birds are regulated by the United States Fish and Wildlife Service. In the federal regulations, Miller (2000) is cited as the guideline for caging sizes. Although the guidelines call for an aviary 12 × 30 × 10 ft high (3.6 × 9 × 3 m high), the author believes that pelicans needing flight conditioning or fledglings being prepared for the wild receive better conditioning in a cage approximately 24 × 30 × 14 ft high (7.3 × 9 × 4.3 m high). This allows for turning while in flight. Different height perches should be made available. Pool size is also specified and should be at least 2 ft deep. Saltwater pools are the ideal. It is recommended that all pools have an intake on one side and outlet on the other side. This overflow arrangement allows for good water circulation and in particular keeps the surface of the water free of fish oil, feces, and other contaminants. Before release, water birds' feathers must be waterproof and in top condition. This is essential to their success in the wild.

PREPARATION FOR WILD RELEASE

It is crucial to their success in the wild that pelicans are raised by foster parents or other pelican role models. Pelicans are naturally fairly curious, naturally fairly friendly, and will do just about anything for a fish. Sadly, at Pelican Harbor Seabird Station in Miami, over 90% of the injuries seen are caused by recreational fishing. Pelicans cannot tell the difference between a handout and a fish with a hook in it that is being used as bait. If, as chicks, they learn to associate people with food they will continue this behavior into adulthood making them even more vulnerable to injury and possible death. When raised in the appropriate caging with foster parents or in a group setting with other pelicans, they will have a much better chance of success in the wild. Although it is very difficult to teach plunge diving in a rehabilitation setting, with the appropriate type pool, caging, foster parents, and other pelicans to serve as role models the chicks will quickly learn that fish come out of water. It is important to present them with live fish so that they experience catching live fish in their pouch, draining the water and swallowing the fish without losing it.

A soft release is preferable if possible. It is also recommended that juveniles are released in groups in the vicinity of flocks of adult pelicans and, if possible, near a rookery site. At Pelican Harbor Seabird Station in Miami, rehabilitated and wild pelicans are banded with USGS metal bands and plastic sight bands making identification easy. Juvenile pelicans released from the facility are often seen swimming and flying in the bay with wild adults. They leave with these wild groups of adults for the spring migration north. An avid birder has been active in reporting sightings and sending photographs of a rookery site 200 miles north of Miami. These reports show captive raised and/or rehabilitated juveniles interacting in the wild with adults and other juveniles.

ACKNOWLEDGMENTS

Thanks to Beth Hirschfeld, DVM, for her input.

SOURCES FOR PRODUCTS MENTIONED

SeaTabs, Pacific Research Laboratories, El Cajon, CA.

Vionate powder, Rich Health Inc., Irvine, CA.

REFERENCES

Miller, E.A., ed. 2000. Minimum Standards for Wildlife Rehabilitation, 3rd Edition. National Wildlife Rehabilitation Association, St. Cloud, MN, 77 pp. http://www.nwrawildlife.org/documents/Standards3rdEdition.pdf.

Miller, E.A. and Wolf, L.A. Quick Reference, 2nd edition. National Wildlife Rehabilitators Association, St Cloud, MN.

Shields, M. 2002. Brown Pelicans (*Pelecanus occidentalis*). In The Birds of North America, No. 609, Poole, A. and Gill, F., eds. The Birds of North America Inc. Philadelphia, PA.

Zaias, J., Fox, W., Cray, C., and Altman, N. 2000. Hematologic, plasma protein, and biochemical profiles of Brown Pelicans. American Journal of Veterinary Research 61(7): 771–774.

8
Flamingos

Peter Shannon

NATURAL HISTORY

The six species/subspecies of flamingo share similar natural histories. The Greater Flamingo (*Phoenicopterus ruber roseus*) and the Lesser Flamingo (*Phoeniconais minor*) occur in the Old World; the Caribbean (*Phoenicopterus ruber ruber*), Chilean (*P. chilensis*), Andean (*Phoenicoparrus andinus*), and James' (*Phoenicoparrus jamesi*) are found in the New World. Their habitats range from sea-level tropics for the *P. r. ruber* to high-altitude Andes for the *P. chilensis*, James', Chilean, and Andean.

Typically found in large congregations, their movements are generally dictated by the availability of food resources. Breeding is typically seasonal, but the timing may vary depending on changes in local conditions.

Group displays serve to synchronize breeding condition within the colonies and promote simultaneous egg laying. Nests are typically raised mounds of mud and debris (see Figure 8.1). In some locations this nest structure probably serves to reduce the temperature on the nest by raising the eggs off the surface. Elsewhere, the raised mounds can serve to prevent flooding of the nests during heavy rains or tidal surges.

In the wild, pairs are most likely monogamous during the nesting season but probably have different partners every year. In captivity, pairs can be stable for several years, but promiscuity is common. Captive flocks often have trios, quartets, and same sex pairings, most likely because choices for mates are very limited and most captive flocks are closed communities (Shannon 2000).

Typically, a single egg is laid. If the egg is lost or broken and the colony remains actively nesting, replacement eggs may be produced.

Incubation and chick care responsibilities are shared by the pair. The incubation period for most species ranges from 27 to 30 days. Vocalizations between the parents and the chick in the shell are critical for bonding. Chicks are fed a regurgitated fluid. Flow is stimulated by vocalizations of the chick. Chicks will generally start leaving the nest mound after about 5 days, but they may stay on the nest for as long as 2 weeks.

In the wild, chicks would be fed by the adults up to about the age of fledging when they are capable of flight, at about 2–3 months. During the rearing period, once the chicks stop returning to a nest to be brooded and have finally left the nest, they will congregate in creches while the parents leave to feed. A few adults typically stay with the chicks. Due to the limited size of captive flocks, this behavior is seldom observed or is not as apparent.

CRITERIA FOR INTERVENTION

Intervention during the nesting cycle might be necessary at any point during the stages of incubation, hatching, or posthatching.

Incubation

During incubation, eggs may be rolled out of nests by accident or as a result of aggressive attacks by other birds. Eggs may be replaced in the nests if the adults seem to be capable of properly defending and incubating them. They may also be fostered into other nests. Flamingos do not recognize their own egg prior to hatching, only the nest they are defending. Exchanging eggs for a dummy egg and artificially incubating them until hatching is a strategy for ensuring an egg will survive.

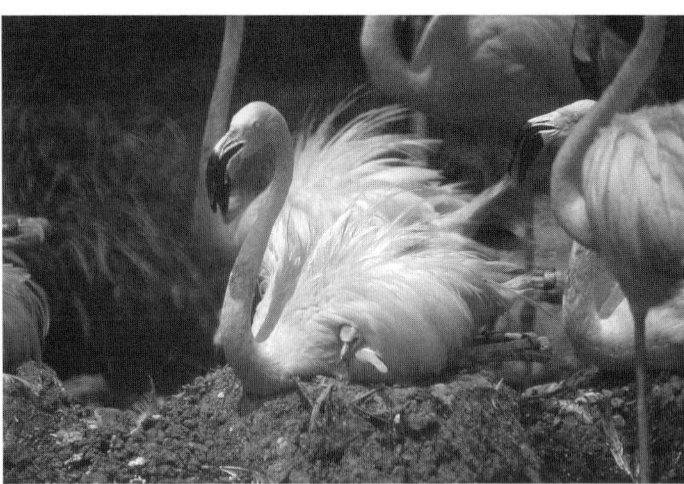

Figure 8.1. Flamingo chick on a mud nest with parent.

If one of the parents dies or is otherwise no longer able to participate in nesting, eggs must be fostered or artificially incubated because a single bird cannot adequately defend a nest on its own.

In the case of disturbance to the colony (predator, flooding, other site-specific issues) or concern about a pair's ability to incubate properly (inexperience, single female without a mate, history of poor incubation), eggs may need to be replaced with dummies or salvaged for artificial incubation. As a management tool, eggs from some birds might be removed to encourage recycling because some females have been known to produce up to four eggs in a season.

In any case, where a fertile egg cannot be returned to a nest, the chick must be hand-reared.

Hatching

Generally, if the bill of a chick enters the air cell, it should have an excellent chance of hatching. Eggs being artificially incubated must be returned to a nest at this stage in order for the chick and parents to learn the others' voice prior to hatching. Chicks hatched in an incubator generally can not be placed in a nest because the incubating adults will not recognize it as theirs and will attack it. Incubator-hatched chicks need to be hand-reared.

Chicks may be injured at the time of hatching due to inexperience of the parents or aggression by other birds. Weak chicks may also be at risk if they are unable to successfully free themselves from the shell or maneuver under the brooding adult within the first 24 hours.

Posthatch

Just as eggs can be rolled from a nest, chicks may accidentally fall off a nest or be pushed off by other birds. Chicks generally begin to leave the nest on their own for short periods of time within 5–7 days of hatching. A chick leaving the nest sooner than this may be unable to return to the nest on its own. The adults remain devoted to the nest site, and although they continue to recognize their young chick, they are unable to assist its return to the nest. Chicks at this age may be returned to the nests, but great care must be taken not to inadvertently cause young chicks to jump out of other nests. Older chicks will be followed by the parents and brooded wherever they may be.

Typically, chicks will continue to return to the natal nest mound to be fed and brooded for several weeks posthatch. As they wander further from the nest site, the parents should be in close proximity at all times. If empty nests are available, the chick may climb onto them and the parents will often brood the chick regardless of its location. If, during these first few weeks, the chick does not appear to be as hardy as other chicks of the same age, assistance may be required. Inexperienced parents sometimes have difficulty coordinating their feeding efforts with the chick, or one parent may abandon the rearing duties leaving a single parent with the chick. As long as the initial vocal bonding has occurred, chicks may be pulled for a day or two at a time for supportive care and returned to the flock without ill effect. Each individual pair is different, as are different colonies, and may respond to disturbance differently, so it is important to know the unique behavioral traits of the birds involved in order to know how conservative or aggressive the intervention care may be.

RECORD KEEPING

Record keeping is invaluable to help track the behavioral idiosyncrasies of the individuals in the flock. Record which birds incubate their eggs well, which might not be able to defend their nests/eggs/chicks from other more aggressive birds, and which have and which have not successfully reared chicks in the past. The best way to achieve this flock history is to have the birds visually identifiable from a distance and to keep detailed records of pairings, nesting, and chick rearing. Color leg bands with engraved numbers (Ogilvie 1972) can be made in a variety of styles and are the easiest system of distant identification. Colored-coded leg bands or those with large numbers are the preferred methods of identification. Tracking the incubation history of the chick, the weight gains, and the amounts of formula fed, and noting any behavioral or medical abnormalities are useful parameters to record.

INCUBATION OF EGGS

Standard incubation parameters apply to flamingo eggs (see Chapter 3). Dirty eggs should be cleaned as much as possible. The chalky surface of flamingo eggs facilitates removal of mud/dirt. Eggs that have been submerged in water for a period of time and have lost the chalky surface have a good chance of successfully hatching if they were not chilled or soaked for too long. A fertile egg must be returned to a nest for parent rearing no later than the entry of the chick's bill into the air cell.

INITIAL CARE AND STABILIZATION

Chicks being hatched in the incubator/hatcher should be allowed to dry and fluff before being moved to the brooder. The dense down of the newly hatched chick provides excellent insulation, but even so, the newly hatched chick may easily chill. A brooder temp of 85–90°F (29.4–32.2°C) is a starting point. The chick will indicate its comfort level by open-mouth breathing if too hot or shivering if too cold. A feather duster as brood surrogate provides a place for the chick to feel secure.

At hatching, the chick's legs will be pink and puffy. This edema will reduce over the first few days, and the skin on the legs will gradually change to black over the first 2 weeks. Initially, the chick will not be able to stand, but within a day will be able to push itself around. By day 3, the chick will be able to stand for short periods, and by 5 days of age it should be able to walk clumsily.

Hydration is critical for both newly hatched chicks and those pulled from the parents. Initial feedings of water or very dilute formula should begin within 12 hours of hatch or immediately for chicks pulled from the parents. Newly hatched chicks quickly respond to liquid dripped onto the tip of their bills from a syringe. Chicks that have been with their parents will take more time to adjust to feeding from a syringe. As a chick ages, tube feeding with a stainless steel ball-tipped feeding needle (ACES) becomes much more efficient both in terms of time commitment and the ability to regulate and document food intake.

Feces of newly hatched chicks will be liquid and bright orange. Within a few days, the fecal matter will change to dark green/black as yolk reserves are used up and digestion has begun. If fecal output becomes less frequent and/or the texture is drier, the chick will need a more liquid formula or subcutaneous fluids to improve hydration.

Hand-reared and parent-reared chicks follow the same developmental time lines, although parent-reared chicks generally have a faster growth rate.

COMMON MEDICAL PROBLEMS AND SOLUTIONS

The greatest concern with chicks is maintaining hydration. Weight gain for hand-reared chicks is usually slower than for parent-reared but is generally not a concern. Hand-reared chicks will ultimately catch up to parent-reared counterparts. Occasionally, a chick will be stunted and will develop more slowly than other chicks. Sometimes these chicks will have short, occasionally bowed legs. The etiology of this is unclear and there does not seem to be any way to correct the problem when it occurs.

Flamingos are susceptible to common mosquito-borne diseases such as avian malaria, avian pox, or West Nile Virus. Malaria does not seem to have deleterious effects. Pox may be significant in chicks if it affects their ability to walk or see. Some institutions vaccinate their flocks against West Nile virus, but the vaccine's effectiveness is unclear. It is unknown what effect avian influenza will have on captive flamingos. Hand-reared chicks are likely to be protected from mosquitoes during the rearing process if they are maintained indoors or behind screened enclosures.

HAND-FEEDING RECIPES

Hand-rearing diets for flamingos vary widely between institutions. Some institutions have complicated mixes that change over time as the chick grows. Others are quite simple, with the most significant change over time being formula consistency and volume. Most diets contain a fish-based ingredient (fish, krill, shrimp) along with a protein source (low-protein primate biscuits [Mazuri], chicken crumbles, hard-boiled egg). In all cases, the first feedings of chicks are typically lactated Ringer's Solution, followed by very dilute formula until the feeding response is established and both chick and handler have mastered the feeding technique. Two typical formulas are listed below. For young chicks, small amounts of formula may be mixed and frozen in ice cube trays for use as needed. More or less water can be added, depending on the chick's acceptance and digestion of the formula.

Formulas

Audubon Park Zoo in New Orleans (personal communication):

- 12 parts water
- 4 parts low-protein primate chow biscuits
- 4 parts Layena (Purina) mash
- 4 hard-boiled egg yolks
- 5 eviscerated smelt (no fins or heads)

Perry and Atkins, 1997:

- 75 g krill
- 75 g capelin (heads, tails, fins removed)
- 75 g hard-boiled egg yolk
- 2 C dry Gerber Oatmeal baby cereal
- 1/2-tsp (approximately 900 mg) calcium carbonate
- 1200 cc water

Kunneman and Perry, 1992:

For the first 30 days, use the Perry and Atkins diet with the addition of 1 C soaked Mazuri Flamingo Complete maintenance pellets (Mazuri).

Bronx Formula 2003 (Ellen Dierenfeld and Christine Sheppard):

- Whole hard-boiled egg (1–2 whole eggs), 50 g
- Hard-boiled egg yolk (4–7 yolks), 100 g
- Water, 150 ml
- Calcium Carbonate (high purity), 2 g
- Corn oil, 6 g
- Vitamin E supplement, 20–25 IU

Riverbanks Zoo Formula (based on Bronx Formula):

- 50 g Whole Egg Powder (Honeyville) mixed with 150 g warm tap water
- 174 g Egg Yolk Powder (Honeyville) mixed with 226.4 g warm tap water

Add water, and then powder and mix together in blender. Then add the following:

- 600 ml water
- 8 g calcium
- 100 IU vitamin E
- 24 cc corn oil

Mix thoroughly.

FEEDING PROCEDURES

Newly hatched chicks require a very liquid diet. Initially, the chick's head needs to be supported and guided to the syringe. Within a few days, the chick will be able to hold its head steady and the only support needed will be a hand around the body to keep it from moving. At this point, changing to tube feeding makes the feeding process cleaner, faster, and more easily documented. Chicks pulled from the parents will be more difficult to teach to feed from a syringe. Tube-feeding is the preferred method for older chicks, and they will quickly learn to accept the tube. However, chicks may be fed directly with a syringe, but this method generally is more time-consuming and messier (see Figure 8.2). Chicks may be fed by hand for as long as necessary to maintain a positive weight gain.

From hatching, chicks are capable of picking up items in the environment and swallowing them. Once chicks are walking, well after about a week of age, self-feeding may be encouraged by providing a

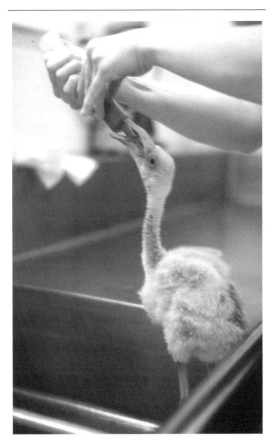

Figure 8.2. Feeding a 36-day-old flamingo chick with a catheter-tip syringe.

water dish for chicks to wade in along with a second pan filled with soft food items for the chick to pick at.

As chicks get older, they should be increasingly self-feeding and the hand-feedings may become less frequent. Some chicks may be completely self-feeding at 6 weeks of age. Others will remain dependent much longer. Housing multiple chicks together helps accelerate the development of feeding behaviors.

EXPECTED WEIGHT GAIN

The feeding regimen varies dramatically between institutions. Depending on the needs of an individual chick, feedings typically occur during daylight hours and once in the evening. A chick's weight is expected to drop for the first few days. Weight loss should level off by day 4. A 6-day-old chick should be back to its hatch weight and on an upward gain curve. From this point, a chick's weight should double every 10 days until about day 80 when it reaches a plateau. Some weight gains will continue after this age, but very slowly. As long as the chick continues to gain weight, the number of feedings may be reduced as the volume of formula increases and as the chick becomes self-feeding.

HOUSING

Housing should be in a small warm space with a feather duster or other comfort item next to the chick initially until the chick becomes mobile. Once the chick is mobile by the end of the first week, exercise will be increasingly important and the space available needs to expand accordingly. Extremes of temperature should be avoided until the chick is well-feathered.

Chicks are able to float and swim by the time they would normally be leaving the nest, at a week of age. Facilities should be available to provide swimming opportunities as early as possible to promote exercise and appropriate weight gain. Housing several chicks of similar age together helps promote activity, but care must be taken to ensure a larger chick does not unduly bully a smaller chick.

By 1 month of age, chicks should not require any supplemental heat as long as their enclosure maintains a comfortable, moderate temperature. Until the chicks have developed contour feathers, they should not be left overnight with access to deep water.

Flooring should be nonabrasive but provide secure footing. Outdoor exercise areas with grass provide good footing and the encourage self-foraging.

WEANING

Flamingo chicks will begin ingesting items on the nest before they can stand. At hatching, they have a predisposition to feed themselves. Typically, the items ingested will be eggshell pieces or bits of debris pulled onto the nest structure by the adults. Once they leave the nest, the chicks will continue to pick up items. Some adults will substantially wean their chicks (or perhaps more accurately, abandon their chicks) within 4–6 weeks of hatching. This may be a period of concern and should be monitored. If this occurs, the other parent will usually take on the full responsibility of rearing the chick. If this does not occur, intervention may be necessary, either to pull the chick for hand-rearing or to provide supplemental feeding to the chick if it remains with the flock. Chicks at this age are more difficult to feed, but usually quickly learn to accept insertion of the feeding tube. The bill structure for filter feeding is not developed at this stage, so all self-feeding is done by picking up food items.

Some adults will continue feeding their current chick into the following breeding season. Weaning appears to be performed by the adults, not the chicks. Once the adult stops responding to the insistent begging of the chick, the chick eventually gives up and is forced to forage for itself.

Food should be available to hand-reared chicks at all times between feedings to encourage self-forage. As soon as a chick shows a predilection to pick up food on its own, this behavior should be encouraged by reducing the daily hand-feeding. Daily weights should be the guideline for reducing hand-feeding. As the feedings are reduced, as long as the weight gain continues weaning may occur quickly.

Imprinting does not appear to be a serious concern in flamingos. However, efforts should be made to wean the young off hand-feeding as quickly as possible to reduce a dependence on caregivers. Raising several chicks together helps reduce this dependence.

PREPARATION FOR INTRODUCTION TO CAPTIVE FLOCK

During the hand-rearing process, exposure to adults during exercise periods may be beneficial but is not required. If the chicks are not raised near adults, it is ideal to construct a pen adjacent to, or within, the adult enclosure where the young birds can see and hear the flock. Once the birds are completely weaned, they should be fed using the same pans as are in the adult enclosure because they will need to be able to recognize the food pans that will be used to feed the flock.

When introduced to the adult enclosure, the chicks will be at the bottom of the pecking order initially, but flamingos are prone to bickering and the chicks should soon learn how to escape attacks from the adults. Although they will stand apart from the adults, chicks will eventually integrate themselves into the social order of the flock.

ACKNOWLEDGMENTS

Thanks to the many zoo colleagues who have collaborated over the years in an effort to improve our collective management of flamingos around the world.

SOURCES FOR PRODUCTS MENTIONED

ACES Animal Care Equipment and Services, Inc., 4920-F Fox St, Denver, CO 80216, (303) 29-287 (worldwide), (800) 338-ACES (North America), (303) 298-8894 (Fax), www.animal-care.com.

Gerber Products Co. Fremont, MI 49413, www.gerber.com.

Honeyville Grain Inc. 11600 Dayton Drive, Rancho Cucamonga, CA 91730, (888) 810-3212, ext. 107, www.honeyvillegrain.com.

Layena, Purina Mills, 555 Maryville University Drive, St. Louis, MO 63141, (800) 227-8941, www.purinamills.com.

Mazuri Flamingo Complete and Mazuri Maintenance Primate Biscuit (low protein), Mazuri, P.O. Box 66812, St. Louis, MO 63166, www.mazuri.com.

REFERENCES

Flamingo Husbandry Guidelines. A joint effort of the American Zoo Association and European Association of Zoos and Aquariums in cooperation with the Wildfowl and Wetlands Trust. Currently available only to AZA members.

Kunneman, F. and Perry, J. 1992. Hand-rearing the Caribbean flamingo *Phoenicopterus r. ruber* at the San Antonio Zoo. Proceedings of the 1990 Flamingo Workshop, AAZPA Western Regional Conference, Sacramento, CA, pp. 30–40.

Ogilvie, M.A. 1972. Large numbered leg bands for individual identification of swans. Journal of Wildlife Management 36: 261–1265.

Perry, J. and Atkins, V. 1997. The weaning, socialization, and breeding history of hand-reared Caribbean flamingos at the San Antonio Zoo. Proceedings of the 24th National Conference of the American Association of Zoo Keepers, pp. 15–23.

Shannon, P.W. 2000. Social and reproductive relationships of captive Caribbean flamingos. Waterbirds Vol 23 (Special Publication 1): 173–178.

9
Shorebirds

Libby Osnes-Erie

NATURAL HISTORY

Shorebirds are found on every continent except Antarctica. Numbering 214 species worldwide, about a third of these species touch down in North America on their intercontinental travels, and of these, 49 species breed here regularly. Five major shorebird families found in North America include Scolopacidae (sandpipers), Charadriidae (plovers), Haematopodidae (oystercatchers), Recurvirostridae (American Avocet and Black-necked Stilt) and Jacanidae (Northern Jacana). Shorebird migrations are among the most spectacular animal movements in the Western Hemisphere, spanning up to 15,000 miles (25,000 km), much of it over inhospitable oceans (Thurston 1996). Not all shorebirds are long-distance migrants. Many species winter in coastal and interior areas of the United States and Mexico. The majority, however, reach the Neotropics, in Central and South America.

Shorebirds usually occur near water but can be found in a wide variety of habitats, from tundra to grasslands to forests to open oceans. They spend two-thirds to three-quarters of their year on migration routes and wintering grounds, largely in tidal environments where they feed on marine invertebrates. The far-flung network of coastal and interior wetlands, rich in invertebrates, is critical to their ability to complete their annual cycle (Thurston 1996).

The variability in bill morphology of shorebirds results in a wide variety of feeding niches. Where a shorebird species is likely to be found feeding, in relation to the tide line and other birds, is determined by the length of its bill and, to a degree, the length of its legs (Thurston 1996). They generally feed by picking, probing, or scything.

Shorebirds are gregarious. On their migratory stopover sites and wintering grounds, they congregate in flocks varying in size from a few individuals to hundreds of thousands. During the breeding season, however, they disperse. These species display a great diversity of mating systems that seems to relate to the best use of available resources, including monogamy, polygyny, polyandry, and sequential polyandry (Thurston 1996).

The incubation period for most shorebirds is relatively brief (17 to 39 days, depending on the species). Shorebird chicks are extremely precocial that is, they are capable of moving around on their own very soon after hatching. As soon as they dry, they stumble from the nest and begin pecking for insects. On day 1, the chicks preen, exercise their wings, and crouch when warned by parents. With the exception of oystercatchers, shorebird parents do not feed their young but rather lead them to foraging areas. Oystercatcher young are fed by their parents for up to 1 month or more and may stay with adults for up to 6 months before becoming fully independent (Petersen 2001a).

Brooding is especially important during the first 2 weeks of life when the young cannot maintain a proper body temperature on their own (Petersen 2001b). In North American species, fledging can occur anywhere from 14 to 63 days after hatching and in some cases, the young may remain with their parents for even longer.

CRITERIA FOR INTERVENTION

Human disturbance of nesting sites and severe weather conditions are the most common reasons for shorebird eggs and chicks being brought into captivity. Shorebird parents may abandon their nests if humans or their pets remain in close proximity for an extended period of time. Nesting site conditions may change due to weather, with nests being temporarily flooded by extremely high tides or heavy rain or covered by sand, dirt, or debris in strong winds. Abandoned eggs may survive to hatching, even those moved by high tides, if found in time and incubated properly.

Shorebird chicks that become temporarily separated from their parents may be captured by well-meaning rescuers. If the chick is brought immediately to a wildlife rehabilitator and is in good condition, it may be possible to reunite it with the parents if the location where it was found is known. However, chicks are often kept by the rescuer for a day or more before being brought to a rehabilitator, in which case the bird will need immediate attention.

Orphans also may be the product of asynchronous hatching if the last chick or egg is left behind by the parents. Predation or injury of parents may also create orphans.

RECORD KEEPING

Detailed information on the location where the bird was found should be recorded. This will serve as a guide for suitable habitat for release.

Wildlife regulatory agencies have minimum standards for record keeping that require tracking of individual animals undergoing rehabilitation. Check with your regulating agencies for further information. See Appendix 1 for a list of North American resources for locating licensed wildlife rehabilitators or regulatory agencies. As a minimum, the following information should be kept: species, age, location found, reason brought into captivity, medical problems, final disposition, and release location.

A detailed medical record should be kept on each animal, with results of the initial examination recorded and any updated information added as it happens. This should include daily body weights, progress of treatments, and pertinent notes on behavior. Temporary plastic leg bands may be used to identify individual chicks (National Band and Tag Company). Leg bands used for identification should be regularly checked for correct fit, because many shorebirds have a substantial increase in leg size between hatching and fledging.

INCUBATION OF EGGS

Proper incubation temperature is critical for ensuring the maximum hatchability of the eggs as well as the best physical condition of the chicks that hatch. For more detailed information on incubation of eggs, see Chapter 3.

The Brinsea Octagon 20 Digital incubator is very user-friendly and reliable. The Octagon 20 Wet Bulb Thermometer (sold separately) is important for monitoring incubator humidity. For shorebirds, use the setting that is recommended for quail, which is 99.6–100°F (37.6–37.8°C). Moisture normally should be about 40–55% relative humidity, with an increase to 65% or more the final 3 days of incubation. Incubation time is species-dependent.

Fine cracks appear at the large end of the egg up to 4 days before hatching (these cracks are difficult to see without magnification). Regular tapping can be heard 2 days before hatching and regular peeping can be heard 1–1.5 days before hatching. Encourage the chicks by peeping back to them during this time. Eggs can hatch at any time of the day or night. A distinct hole is usually not present more than 4 hours before chick emergence. The time from a very distinct hole to emergence is approximately 20–30 minutes.

Once the chick has made the initial obvious hole and it is showing evidence of hatching difficulty (no progress after an hour, little movement from the chick, difficult respirations, etc.) it is safe to help the chick out of the egg. Carefully remove small pieces of the shell above the air cell with a blunt forceps to help free the chick. Lightly moisten the membrane if needed. A distressed chick may give up and could die before getting out of the egg on its own. Chicks that have a difficult hatch are often exhausted and may need extra time in the incubator.

Partially unretracted yolk sacs at the umbilicus usually resolve within hours on their own without assistance and are fully absorbed within a few hours of hatching.

Allow the chick to dry completely, fluff up, and gain strength inside the egg incubator. The yolk sac provides nourishment for the transition period from the time the bird hatches until it becomes active enough to seek food. This may take 6–24 hours. At this point, the chick may be moved to a brooder.

INITIAL CARE AND STABILIZATION

New patients should be allowed to rest for 15–20 minutes in a warm, dark, quiet container before examination. If the bird is not able to stand, it should be placed in a soft support structure. Do not allow the chick to lie on its side or other abnormal positions.

Baby birds should be placed in a climate-controlled intensive care unit or brooder if available.

Once the bird is warm, if it is active, offer live food items in shallow dishes. The best first live prey to offer are tubifex worms (in water) and small fly larvae (*Musca domestica*). These food items are active and the movement attracts the chicks. Chicks should begin pecking at the food almost immediately.

If the chick will not eat on its own after being warmed to normal body temperature, is not freshly hatched, and appears too weak to eat on its own, it should be rehydrated orally. Place a drop of unflavored electrolyte solution (such as Pedialyte) or lactated Ringer's solution (LRS) very carefully on the tip of the bill and allow it to roll down the bill for the chick to swallow. If needed, gently open the mouth slightly and insert a drop in the side of the bill. Be careful so that the chick does not aspirate. Repeat this a few times. Follow the drops of electrolyte solution with drops of 50% dextrose or Ensure (Abbott)—something to raise its blood glucose level.

Repetition of the fluids and dextrose or Ensure drops every 15–30 minutes may be needed until the chick becomes active enough and has the energy to start eating on its own. See the essay "Hatchling Killdeer Intensive Care" for tips and tricks to get hatchlings to start eating.

Hatchling Killdeer Intensive Care

Kappy Sprenger

WARMTH

Almost all killdeer chicks (*Charadrius vociferous*) are less than 5 days old when presented for care. Weighing around 10 g at hatch, these chicks are usually seen 1 to 3 days later at weights of 7–9 g. Many have become chilled. When cold, a precocial chick becomes inactive and lies down. Some killdeer also lie down when frightened. However, within 15–20 minutes in a quiet, warmed place these birds should be up and running around. Chilled young take considerably longer to become active.

Immediately upon admittance, killdeer chicks should be placed in a heated container or incubator and allowed to rest and get warm. If the chick is lying down or appears weak, the best temperature is 92–95°F (33.3–35°C). After warming, the chick can be weighed. Those that are weak or were chilled should remain at that temperature. Strong young up to 12 g can safely be kept at 90–92°F (32.2–33.3°C); those above 12 g, at 90°F (32.2°C). Until they are self-feeding, these temperatures should be maintained.

HYDRATION AND LIQUID NUTRITION

Until a chick has become warm and is strengthening, it should not be hydrated. The author generally uses lactated Ringer's solution or Pedialyte (Abbott), but any good hydrating solution will work. The warm fluid is offered from a 0.5 or 1.0 ml syringe, eyedropper, or a saturated cotton swab. This is much safer than attempting to gavage. One drop of fluid is drawn along the edges of the bill and repeated until drinking occurs. As it swallows, the bird's throat will move and the drop of liquid will disappear; however, the mouth will not appear to open. Each chick may be offered as much as it will drink, one drop at a time. Repeat every 30 minutes until definite strengthening is seen, and then hourly until the chick defecates. Defecations are quickly noticed if a white paper towel is used as a smooth-cover bedding. Next, warm liquid nutrition may be started using the same method. Vital High Nitrogen (Abbott) or Formula V Enteral Care (High Protein) (PetAg) are suggested. Initially, alternate diluted liquid nutrition with hydrating solution every 1–1.5 hours. Do not mix hydrating solution with liquid nutrition. As the chick continues to strengthen, this routine should be maintained, with the liquid nutrition at full strength until the chick is reliably self-feeding.

MONITORING

Be sure each chick's bottom is clean at all times. Until it is self-feeding and especially on a younger chick that has been chilled, a small bit of dark fecal matter may be noticed stuck to the white down just outside the vent. Remove this gently using a cotton swab dipped in warm water, carefully rolling the swab away from the vent area until it is clean, but not saturating the down. If the fecal matter appears again, clean it off. Left untended, this could build up and clog the vent, causing an obstruction and death.

GETTING THEM TO START EATING

When a chick is steady on its feet and running around, a very shallow dish or lid with water may be provided. This should be less than 3 in (1.2 cm) across, no more than 0.5 in (1 cm) deep, and easily stepped into and out of without tripping. Sometimes a chick will drink from this dish, but it shouldn't be depended upon for hydration. Once warm and hydrated, killdeer quickly learn to feed themselves if they are offered live foods of appropriate sizes. As a chick wades and stands in the little water dish with live creatures wiggling around its toes, it can hardly resist eating them and will learn to feed itself much faster than if food is given separately. Tubifex worms are the right size, naturally live in water, and are very wiggly. Available in some aquarium shops, they are also nutritious and easily cared for until being fed. Tiny white mealworms (just having shed) are a good initial food as well. Although these may not live very long, if the water is just barely covering the bottom of the dish they might remain active long enough to catch the chick's attention. They may also be placed in a small container immediately beside the shallow water dish. Do not risk using mealworms with hard, light brown skins. The skins are difficult to digest and can cause obstruction in debilitated, dehydrated, or very young birds. Live adult brine shrimp may be taken, as may very small earthworms. The diameter of any one item of food should not exceed the diameter of the bird's lower mandible. Once a plover chick starts feeding itself, it will quickly learn to eat nonliving foods as well.

Chicks seem to learn faster if small amounts of food are provided rather than large "clumps" where individual "bites" are not so readily noticed. Live guppies might be offered. Because the dish is shallow and temperatures high, the water will evaporate in just a couple hours. These shallow water feeding dishes will need to be replenished several times a day. Calcium carbonate powder should be lightly sprinkled on a chick's food at least once a day.

Live food is not always available. Frozen or freeze-dried products available in aquarium shops or tropical fish departments of large pet shores may be used. Before feeding, frozen foods should be defrosted and freeze-dried products soaked a few minutes until saturated with water. Put a small amount of food in the shallow water dish. If the water is stirred gently for a moment causing the food bits to slowly swirl around, the chick's interest may be aroused. When it sees the movement of the bits of food it usually will pick at them and quickly learn to eat. A slow drip of water into the water dish from above also creates movement to catch attention. If neither of these tricks work, try gently opening the chick's mouth after it has been given liquid nutrition or hydrating solution, and put in one small piece of food. This step may be repeated a couple times at each feeding until the chick gets the idea. Once plover chicks have started eating, they are quite willing to take a variety of foods, and have surprisingly large appetites. Among the frozen foods, "bloodworms" (sometimes called "red mosquito larvae") are a favorite and nutritious starter food, as are adult brine shrimp. Of the freeze-dried products, tiny krill or ocean plankton, tubifex, and tiny shrimp may be taken. Soon, processed foods may be added to the diet. Cichlid minipellets are small enough for very young killdeer, beginning with just a few placed in the shallow water dish, and later offered dry. It is usually only a day or two until the chicks that will recover are on their feet and running around, hungry and ready to grow.

After hatching, briefly examine the chick once it is dry to make sure the yolk sac is retracted and there are no obvious deformities. Make sure new arrivals are warm and well hydrated before proceeding with a thorough physical exam. During their time in captivity, birds should be briefly examined each time they are weighed for feather condition, vent cleanliness, foot condition, injuries, or signs of illness.

Always hold a bird by reaching around from the back. Birds must expand their chests to breathe and if they are held from the front you may restrict their breathing. Chicks are very fragile so be gentle, taking care that a chick does not suddenly jump out of your hand and fall to the floor. Because shorebird chicks must be able to run shortly after hatching, their legs are well developed from the start.

It is important to limit human contact so that birds do not become imprinted or habituated to humans. Whenever possible, raise chicks with conspecifics of similar size or use surrogate parent birds. This may mean sending the chick to, or getting a chick from, another rehabilitator. It may be difficult to raise a single chick from hatching for successful release. It may become imprinted or habituated to humans if it does not have the opportunity to interact with other shorebirds. If you are unable to match a chick with a conspecific, try putting it with other shorebirds of similar size so that it at least has another chick for companionship. Although aggression does not seem to be a problem between shorebird chicks, when putting different chick species together it is important to be wary of larger chicks accidentally stepping on smaller chicks. It is not recommended to raise shorebird chicks with other precocial chicks, such as quail, because disease transmission, such as avian pox, may occur.

COMMON MEDICAL PROBLEMS AND SOLUTIONS

Stilts and avocets seem to be particularly susceptible to foot problems, such as drying, cracking, and pressure sores. Keeping the substrate clean and soft and offering clean wading dishes and pools are important factors in preventing foot problems.

Wing abnormalities in the carpometacarpal area commonly called *slipped wing* or *angel wing* may occur for several reasons: deficiencies in one of several nutrients, such as vitamin E, vitamin D3, or manganese; excessive dietary protein; or overfeeding (Flinchum 2006). If this occurs, the chick should be moved into a larger enclosure to increase its activity level. Adjusting the diet so that a greater percentage is chitinous food, such as crickets and mealworms (waxworms and fly larvae are higher in fat), also may help. Food should be supplemented with powdered calcium carbonate and avian vitamins (Nekton-S). The wing should be wrapped into normal position and checked daily for improvement in its alignment. If attempts to correct this problem are made promptly, correction may occur within 3–5 days.

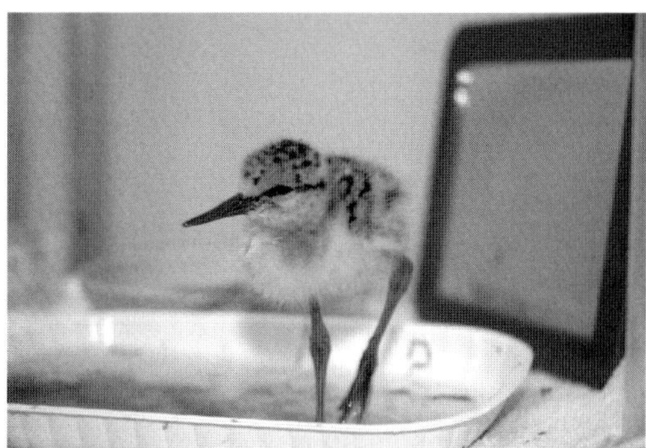

Figure 9.1. American avocet chick. Note shallow food dishes and mirror (photo courtesy of Marie Travers IBRRC).

DIET

Hatchlings

Chicks will instinctively be interested in objects of possible experimentation. Once newly hatched chicks are dry and walking around they will begin to peck at things.

Tubifex worms and small fly larvae (*Musca domestica*) play a critical role in getting chicks to begin eating. Different suppliers may ship different size larvae; the author uses "Tiny Wigglers" from Arbico. When placed in front of them, these two prey items seem to attract the chicks' attention and they begin feeding almost immediately. Their first attempts at feeding are awkward, but they quickly get the hang of it.

Use small jar lids or small shallow dishes for food and water so that chicks can easily walk in and out of them and if chicks fall, they can easily get out of the dish (see Figures 9.1, 9.2).

While chicks are in brooders it is best to feed small amounts of food frequently (at least four times a day) because food will die from the heat after a few hours and shallow water will evaporate. Adding ice chips to the wet food (tubifex worms) may help it stay alive longer. Open-top containers, such as aquariums or terrariums with a heat bulb, can be partially covered to create a shaded area where temperatures are somewhat cooler and the food stays alive longer.

Older Chicks

Consider the age and size of chicks when choosing food, water, and bathing/wading dishes. Chicks

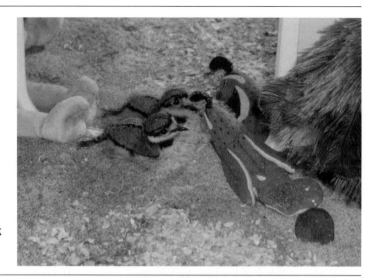

Figure 9.2. Puppets and stuffed animals may provide needed comfort to solitary chicks. Shown is a killdeer chick with a quail puppet in front of a mirror.

always should be easily able to get in and out of dishes. Flat or shallow dishes, such as planter bases, work well.

Food items should also be chosen based on the size of the chicks. Prey items will be eaten whole, so they must fit in the mouth of the chick. Shorebirds can be offered tubifex worms, fly larvae, mini-to-medium mealworms, small crickets, waxworms, and small or chopped krill. Food should be replenished two to three times per day.

Once chicks are in outdoor enclosures, feed some "dry" food (fly larvae, mealworms, and waxworms) in dishes and also begin to sprinkle some dry food onto the sand to encourage more normal foraging behavior. "Wet" food (tubifex and krill) is always put in dishes. Toss crickets onto the sand. Within a few days if chicks are easily finding food on the sand, sprinkle all of the dry food on the sand in several locations.

FEEDING PROCEDURES

Have food and water containers in more than one area so all chicks have access and get enough to eat. If you need to put chicks of different sizes in the same enclosure, make sure the smaller chicks are able to stay out of the way of the larger chicks so they don't get stepped on or outcompeted for food.

It is important to lightly sprinkle food with powdered calcium carbonate and avian vitamins (Nekton-S) throughout the rehabilitation process to help prevent nutritional deficiencies. Avoid using Nekton on tubifex worms as they seem to have an adverse reaction to it and crawl out of the dish.

EXPECTED WEIGHT GAIN

Chicks should steadily gain weight from hatching to fledging. If a chick is losing weight or not growing as rapidly as its cagemates, this may indicate a health problem or that the bird is not getting enough food or its access to food is being limited by larger birds. Weigh each chick every day until it has been outside for a few days, and then twice a week or every 4 days after that, and again on release day (see Figure 9.3).

HOUSING

There are many factors to consider that may influence how shorebirds are housed, such as the local ambient temperature, financial resources, and supplies and equipment available. At each step along the way, attention needs to be paid to each individual bird and how it is progressing in its development to determine when it is ready for the next step. If a chick seems overwhelmed, i.e., hiding/sitting in one spot for hours, not eating, or demonstrating other changes in its normal behavior when placed in a larger enclosure, it is advisable to reduce the enclosure size until the chick seems comfortable with its surroundings.

Shorebird parents brood their chicks for warmth at night and when not foraging during the day for at

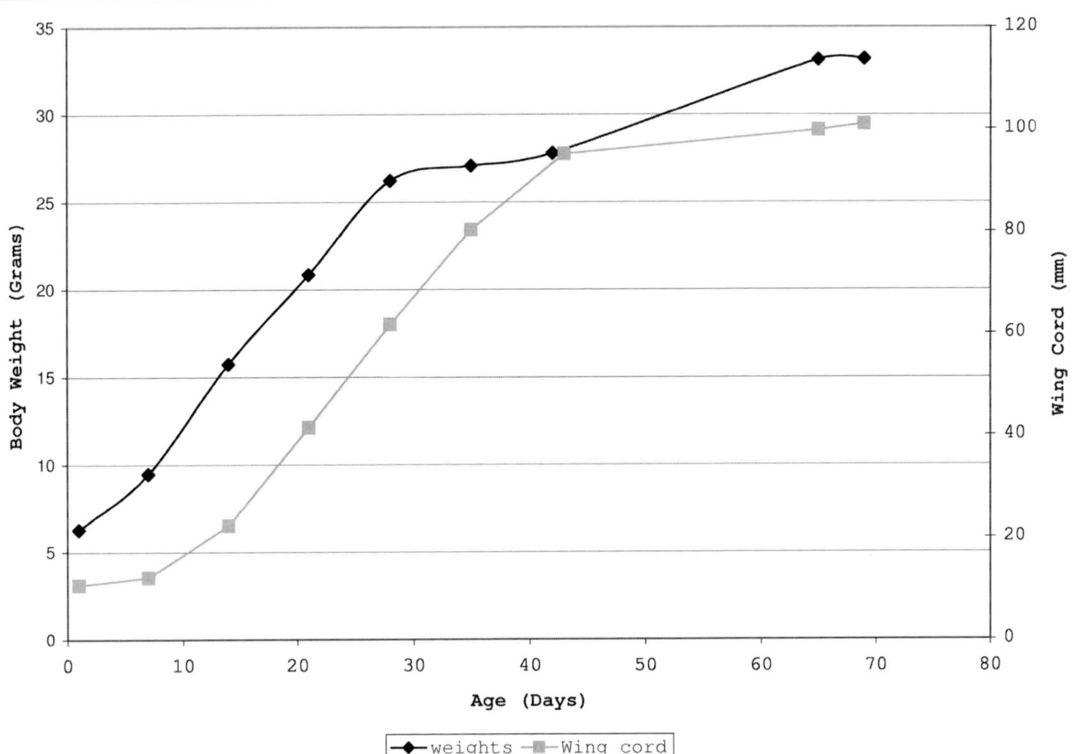

Figure 9.3. Weight gain and wing cord growth in snowy plover chicks (n = 12) (data courtesy of Meryl Faulkner).

least the first 1–2 weeks of life. Throughout the hatch to prefledge interval, a heat source will be needed to mimic what the chicks would have with a parent in the wild.

Hatchlings

Hatchlings and chicks less than a week old may be kept in an Intensive Care Unit (ICU, such as Lyon AICU Electronic Large Digital Intensive Care Unit), incubator, brooder, aquabrooder (see Figures 10.2 and 10.3), or aquarium/terrarium. The initial temperature of ICUs and incubators should be 99–100°F (31.6–32.0°C) and the temperature reduced by 1–2°F (0.5–1.0°C) each day, depending on the needs of the chick. Containers that are not fully enclosed should contain a heated section (warmed by a heat lamp) that is around 98–99°F (31.1–31.6°C) and an unheated section in case the chick gets too warm. Food dishes can be put at the cooler end. Use a dry air thermometer placed at the level of the chicks to determine correct temperature. A variety of spot heat bulbs may be used to create a warm area, such as a 100–150 watt spot incandescent nocturnal black heat lamp (such as ESU Reptile NightLight Spot, available at pet stores). The distance the heat lamp is above the brooder will need to be determined by the individual setup. Watch for signs of hypothermia (shivering, fluffed feathers) and hyperthermia (lethargy, open-mouth breathing) in chicks and adjust the temperature accordingly.

If the top of the brooder needs to be open to accommodate a heat bulb, cover as much of the top with a towel or solid cover as possible to help contain humidity. A partial cover will also create a shaded area under which food dishes can be placed.

Try to keep humidity at 40–55% for of the first few days, although ambient humidity may be adequate if different than this. Use a small container with a wet cloth or sponge inside to hold water. Make sure chicks cannot get into the container and

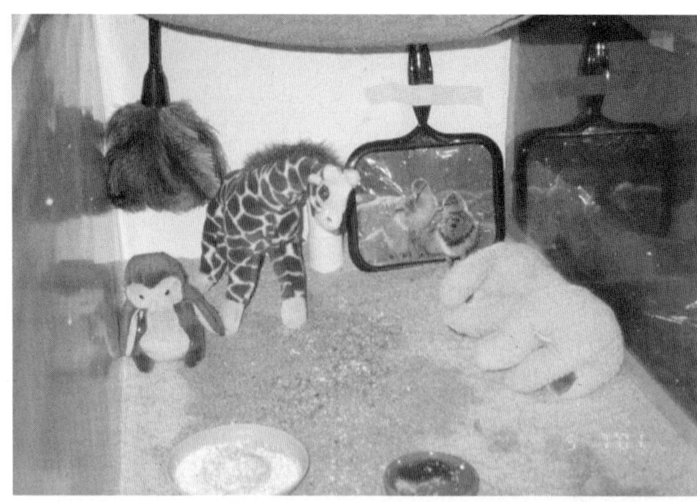

Figure 9.4. Avocet chick with mirror, stuffed animals, and shallow food dishes. Note sand scattered in the brooder.

drown. It can be difficult to control humidity if the top of the brooder is uncovered to accommodate a heat lamp. Change any wet material frequently to prevent mold growth in the brooder.

Flannel pillowcases work very nicely for the top layer of cage substrate; they have some traction but are smooth so toenails do not catch. Use a thin towel, pillowcase, or something that provides some padding (1–2 in [2.5–5 cm] thick) underneath the top layer. Change the pillowcase daily and coordinate with weighing to keep handling at a minimum and chicks contained during cleaning.

Hang a feather duster (preferably made with ostrich or natural feathers) in the corner of the container so that the chick(s) can hide underneath it. Place small stuffed animals, driftwood, and real and artificial plant material in the container that chicks can sit next to, climb on, or hide under (see Figure 9.4).

For single chicks, it is important to put a mirror against a wall so that the chick sees its reflection and thinks it has a buddy. Some chicks will exhibit pacing behavior in front of the mirror, in which case the mirror should be removed for a day or longer, if needed so the chick does not needlessly expend energy it should be investing in foraging activities.

Nestlings and Fledglings

Chicks more than a few days old may be kept in a large aquarium/terrarium, long container, or human infant playpen, depending on size and activity level of the chicks (see Figure 9.5). Similar-sized shorebird species may be housed together. Containers may range in size from 34–64 in (86–162 cm) long × 14–22 in (36–56 cm) wide × 14–20 in (36–51 cm) high.

Another caging option would be to make an enclosure up on legs off the floor with plywood walls, mesh flooring, and light fabric sheeting covering the top. The mesh bottom allows feces and urates to pass through, but mesh must be small enough to not risk entanglement of toes or feet.

Place a heat lamp as previously described over one portion of the enclosure to create an area that is approximately 95°F (29.7°C) while the rest of the enclosure is at indoor ambient temperature. Again, use a dry air thermometer at the level of the chicks to determine correct temperature. To provide artificial sunlight for chicks indoors, place one or two full-spectrum light bulbs, such as Reptisun 5.0 UVB (available at pet stores), across the top of the enclosure. See the manufacturer's specifications regarding the proper distance for placement of bulbs above the chicks.

Sand substrate is recommended. Use clean, kiln-dried, mesh #30 sand, at least 1 in (2.5 cm) thick. Monitor the temperature of the sand below the heat bulb to ensure that it does not become too hot. If sand is unavailable, use flannel sheets or smooth fabric with padding underneath, such as towels or more sheets. Obviously, for mesh-bottom cages the mesh forms the substrate. It is important to keep the substrate clean. Use a small hand broom and dustpan to sweep the debris off the sand and into a bucket. Sweep the sand once or twice a day depending on how many chicks are in the cage. Clean the water/wading dishes two or three times daily.

Comfort objects and cage furnishings are as for hatchlings but may be more naturalistic to reflect the ability of these somewhat older chicks to cope with a more complicated environment.

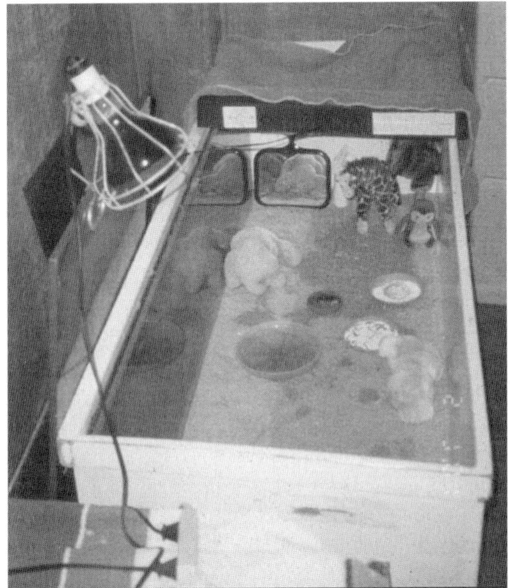

Figure 9.5. Large indoor tank set up for young chicks.

It is important to offer wading and bathing dishes of appropriate depth. Wading dishes should be deep enough to cover the birds' feet, and bathing dishes should allow birds to get in the water and splash water on themselves. Planter bases and cat litter pans work very well for many species. Surround dishes with sand or create sand ramps so that birds can easily get into dishes. It is advisable to create a ramp or step, such as a stone, smooth rock, or driftwood, inside the dish for birds to climb out on if needed.

Chicks more than 1–2 weeks old may be kept in an outdoor aviary, depending on ambient temperature and the size and activity level of the chicks (see Figure 9.6). Aviaries range in size from 8–25 ft (2.4–7.6 m) long × 5.5–24 ft (1.7–7.3 m) wide × 6–16 ft (1.8–4.9 m) high, depending on the size of the species. For minimum recommended sizes for waterbirds, see Miller (2000). Aviaries should be designed as naturalistic enclosures, offering ample opportunity for birds to explore and forage.

Sand substrate outdoors also should be clean, kiln-dried, mesh #30 but must be at least 2 in (5 cm) thick. The larger the shorebird species the thicker the sand should be. Additional substrate can include small smooth stones, mud, grasses, and a shallow sloped bottom pool covering a portion of the floor.

Clean the water and wading dishes once or twice daily and continue to sweep up soiled sand as needed. Pools should be drained and refilled as

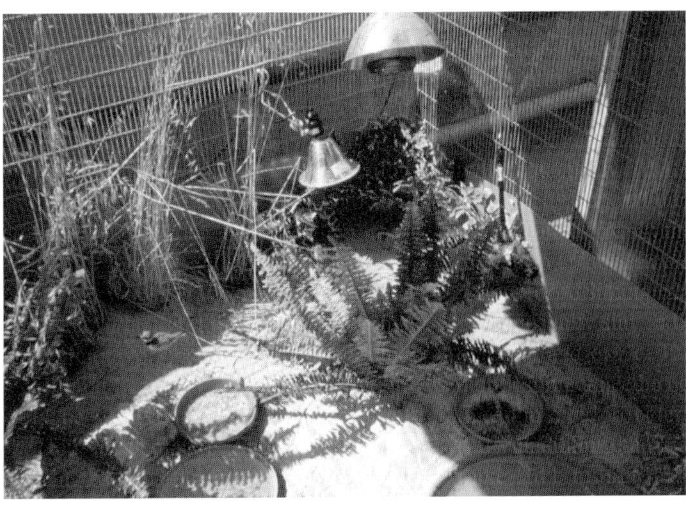

Figure 9.6. Killdeer in outdoor aviary with ample vegetation, heat lamps, sand substrate, wide flat food dishes, and large flat water pan for bathing. Note visual barrier at bottom of narrowly spaced cage wire walls.

needed to maintain high water quality if filtration is not available. Scrub driftwood with a brush and water once a day or every other day as needed to remove droppings.

Feather dusters, mirrors, and stuffed animals can be used as with younger birds until the birds cease using them. For single chicks, leave the mirror in the aviary until release. Continue to offer, as needed, a heat lamp in one portion of the enclosure to create a protected area that is about 95°F (29.7°C) while the rest of the enclosure is at ambient temperature. Remove the heat source just prior to when the birds begin to fly.

Use a disinfectant footbath and rinse before entering and after exiting outdoor aviaries to decrease the chance of tracking contaminants from shoes into and out of aviaries. Clean and disinfect aviaries thoroughly after birds have been released before refilling with new birds.

PREPARATION FOR WILD RELEASE

Find out the local wild fledging age to get an approximate time frame for release. Release birds a week or so after the normal fledging age, when they are flying well. Each bird should be in excellent health, waterproof, and an excellent flyer. Make sure the bird is well muscled and can fly well enough to avoid predators and travel with conspecifics. Wing chord length also can help determine approximate release date by comparing to a normal adult's wing chord length. This information may be available from field research studies from local biologists or government reports. Fledglings may not weigh as much as an adult, so find out what is normal for that species.

Birds should exhibit appropriate foraging behaviors and wariness of humans. Release birds in areas where there are conspecifics. They will do better if they can join a flock or groups of other fledglings.

Apply a federal leg band, if possible, prior to release. It is beneficial to work with researchers that may be studying shorebird species in the wild to gather postrelease data.

Captive placement of nonreleasable shorebirds in zoos and aquariums is possible. Make sure the facility (and captivity) is appropriate for the animal before placing it there. Nonreleasable shorebirds may be considered for use as surrogate parents if they can be maintained in an appropriate enclosure that allows proper foot health and general well-being. Either sex can be considered as a surrogate; however, if one sex is the primary caregiver in the wild, that sex may make a better surrogate.

ACKNOWLEDGMENTS

I would like to thank the many participants in the Snowy Plover Conservation Project, headed by Point Reyes Bird Observatory (PRBO) Conservation Science, for their tireless efforts to monitor, protect, rescue, raise, and rehabilitate snowy plovers along the California Coast. PRBO researchers also banded and monitored released chicks, which provided valuable postrelease information. I also would like to thank the remarkable shorebird eggs and chicks that were instrumental in the development of the rehabilitation methods described in this chapter. A special thank you to "Snowy" (a.k.a. The Little General), my favorite snowy plover who was an ambassador for his species and a great dad to orphaned chicks.

SOURCES FOR PRODUCTS MENTIONED

Leg bands: National Band and Tag Company, 721 York St, Newport, KY 41072-0430, (800) 261-TAGS (8247).

Incubators and ICUs: Double-R Discount Supply, 4000 Dow Road, Suite 8, Melbourne, FL 32934, (321) 259-9465, Fax (321) 259-2500.

Crickets: Bassetts Cricket Ranch, Inc., 365 S. Mariposa, Visalia, CA 93292-9242, (800) 634-2445 or (559) 747-2728, Fax 559-747-3619, www.bcrcricket.com.

Mealworms: Rainbow Mealworms, Inc., P.O. Box 4907, 126 East Spruce Street, Compton, CA 90220, (310) 635-1494.

Fly larvae: Arbico Environmental (tiny wigglers), P.O. Box 8910, Tucson, AZ 85738-0910, (800) 827-2847, Fax (520) 825-9785.

Waxworms: Grubco, Box 15001, Hamilton, OH 45015, (800) 222-3563.

Tubifex worms: Pan Ocean, 23384 Foley Street, Hayward, CA 94545, (510) 782-8936.

Krill: MST Enterprises (Superba, Pacifica), Nova Scotia, Canada.

Nekton-S: Guenter Enderle Enterprises, 27 West Tarpon Avenue, Tarpon Springs, FL 34689, (727) 938-1544.

REFERENCES

Flinchum, G.B. 2006. Management of waterfowl. In Clinical Avian Medicine. Harrison G.J. and Lightfoot, T.L., eds. Spix Publishing, Palm Beach, FL, p. 846.

Miller, E.A., ed. 2000. Minimum Standards for Wildlife Rehabilitation, 3rd Edition. National Wildlife Rehabilitation Association, St. Cloud, Minnesota, 77 pp.

Petersen, W.R. 2001a. Plovers and lapwings. In Elphick, C., Dunning, Jr., J.B., and Sibley, D.A., eds. The Sibley Guide to Bird Life and Behavior. Alfred A. Knopf, New York, pp. 257–264.

———. 2001b. Oystercatchers. In Elphick, C., Dunning, Jr., J.B., and Sibley, D.A., eds. The Sibley Guide to Bird Life and Behavior. Alfred A. Knopf, New York, pp. 265–267.

Thurston, H. 1996. The World of the Shorebirds. Sierra Club Books, San Francisco. 117 pp.

10
Gulls and Terns

Meryl Faulkner

NATURAL HISTORY

Laridae (gulls and terns) are represented in North America by 25 species of gulls, including two called kittiwakes, and eighteen species of terns, including two called Noddies. Gulls and terns are closely related to skuas, jaegers, and skimmers, and are grouped in the order Charadriiformes. Gulls and terns are colonial breeders nesting on the ground, on and around beaches, marshland, and abandoned salt works. Some gull species nest on rocky cliffs, but Western Gulls also may nest on man-made structures such as hotel, apartment, and office building roofs in many coastal cities. Nests may be a shallow scrape or structure lined with grass, twigs, pebbles and debris. Incubation typically lasts 21–27 days, depending on species.

Gull and tern chicks are semiprecocial. They hatch with their eyes open, covered with down, and able to walk, but remain at or near the nest for the first 2 or 3 weeks. Depending on the species, chicks fledge at 21 days (Least Tern) to 42 days (Western Gull), but are fed by parents for additional time. In the case of Western Gulls, this may last for 11 to 12 weeks posthatch.

Although both gulls and terns have webbed feet and have waterproof plumage, only gulls swim and float on the water for extended periods of time. Terns have shorter legs and smaller feet and do not spend any extended time paddling.

Adult gulls and terns eat fish; however, gulls are more likely to take invertebrates and human refuse, particularly if not feeding young or if environmental conditions change and fish are scarce.

Gulls and terns range in weight from the 40 g Least Tern to the 1000 g Western Gull. Young terns and gulls are fed primarily fish of the appropriate size on the day of hatching by the parent. Least Terns feed their chicks fish 28 cm and larger approximately twice an hour. Western Gull males feed chicks every 2–3 hours, with females feeding every 3–4 hours by the fledging period. Fish is offered whole by terns, but gulls regurgitate a bolus of food such as small fish or shrimp into young chicks' mouths or drop larger fish onto the ground for chicks older than 10 days to pick up.

CRITERIA FOR INTERVENTION

Terns and gulls may be brought to rehabilitators by state or federal agencies in cases where endangered or threatened species have been disturbed at nesting sites and the young abandoned. In addition, in some areas gulls may nest inappropriately on the roofs of commercial or residential buildings and because of aggressive behavior, the USFWS or state agencies may give permission for removal of the chicks.

Fledglings may be presented when predators have attacked nest sites, or fledglings have fallen from nest sites on roofs. Least Terns nest on rooftops in Florida and have been successfully replaced with parents. Replacement may be attempted if access to the correct nest site on the rooftop is possible. Chicks should be checked for injuries before this is attempted, and parental care should be observed after return to the nest site before the chick is left there.

RECORD KEEPING

State agencies require record keeping, which may vary from state to state. Minimum requirements are species, age class, location found, name and address of finder, reason for removal from nest site, medical problem, final disposition, and release location.

Endangered or threatened species may require additional detailed record keeping, which usually is mandated by the biologists managing the species' recovery.

INITIAL CARE AND STABILIZATION

As with other avian species, young gulls and terns should be warmed, hydrated, and then fed. Fluids can be given orally (by gavage) or subcutaneously at 5% of body weight if the bird is thin, underweight, or injured. Small species such as the endangered California Least Tern have fragile skin and often struggle when the subcutaneous route is attempted. The author prefers giving small terns appropriate amounts of lactated Ringer's solution or Pedialyte orally for the first feeding, and then both large and small species can be given Multimilk (PetAg) diluted 1 part powder to 2 parts water, or, alternatively, Isocal (Mead Johnson) or Ensure (Abbott), for another two feedings if the birds are thin or unsteady. Multimilk contains milk proteins; however, Multimilk is low in carbohydrates (which are not normally ingested by seabirds), is available in powdered form, and is tolerated well by sea and shore birds. Warming the fluids helps raise the core body temperature in hypothermic chicks and adult birds.

Young gulls and terns should be placed in a warm container and kept in a quiet area. Hatchlings (downy young chicks that would still be brooded) should be kept in a climate controlled incubator and be given fur, fabric, or some other "tented" product to hide under as a surrogate parent.

If the chick is orphaned but healthy, one feeding of fluids can be followed by solid food. Fish should be offered to terns, and shrimp, cat food, or chopped fish to gulls. Gulls and terns can be fed on demand every 90 minutes to 3 hours depending on age and size.

Hatchlings and young chicks may be kept in homemade aquabrooders or commercial incubators on paper or cloth towels (see Figures 10.1–10.3). Older chicks of larger species may be kept in cardboard or plastic pet carriers placed on heating pads on "low" setting to keep the interior warm.

COMMON MEDICAL PROBLEMS AND SOLUTIONS

Hatchlings collected by biologists from breeding sites may be abandoned chicks suffering from malnutrition or injury from predator attacks. In older fledglings, lacerations and fractures of wing and leg can be caused by fishhooks and fishing line.

Occasionally, adults feed chicks a bait fish with a hook attached. These juveniles present with a small length of line hanging from the bill. Usually because

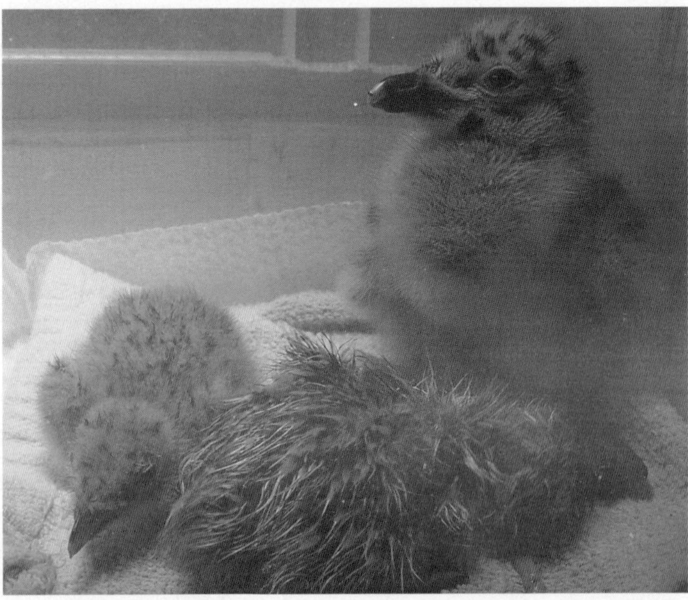

Figure 10.1. One Forster's Tern and two Western Gull hatchlings in aquabrooder.

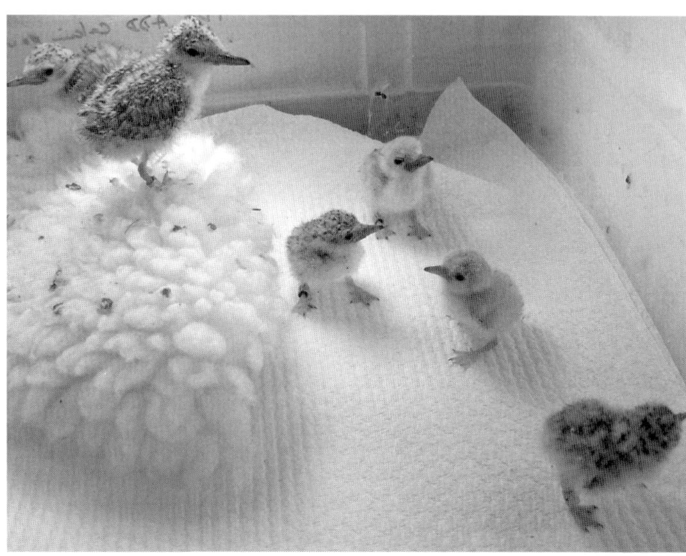

Figure 10.2. Least Tern chicks in aquabrooder.

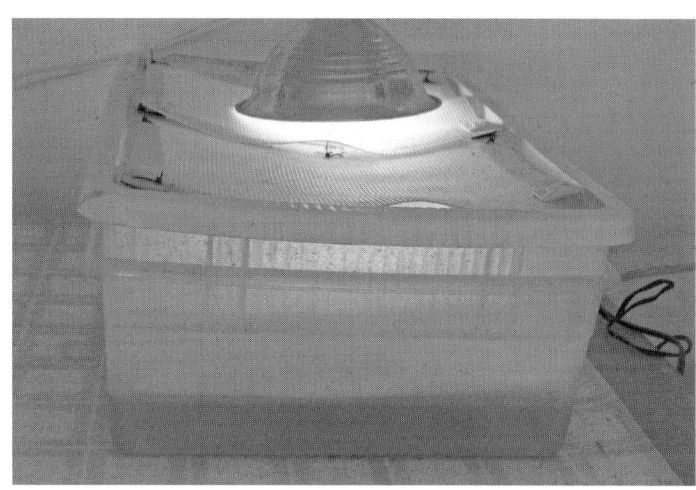

Figure 10.3. Outside view of aquabrooder. Note heat lamp placement. Water inside outer container is heated with an aquarium heating element. Top is fiberglass screening.

of emaciation of the chick and possible peritonitis, these birds may die before any treatment or surgery can be attempted.

Head injuries are infrequently seen in juvenile gulls and seem associated with sibling or adult attacks in crowded nesting conditions. Falls from rooftops may result in injured legs and wings. Tern species in San Diego (Least, Forster's, Elegant, Royal and Caspian) nest and roost on beaches. Injuries are often caused by predators such as raptors, but coyotes and raccoons often invade beach and lagoon nesting sites and cause adults to trample and injure young in their haste to escape.

Superficial wounds are treated by cleaning, disinfection, and the application of silver sulfadiazine cream. Oil-based ointments are not recommended because they contaminate feathers and allow water to penetrate the feathers.

Wing and leg fractures may be lightly splinted with appropriate material and Micropore paper tape (3M) or a light stretch fabric wrap. Unlike in adult gulls with closed fractures of the humerus, downy Western Gull chicks with closed near-midshaft fractures heal well when the wing is splinted and wrapped, and they have a good prognosis for being able to fly postrecovery.

Tern species with wing fractures should be assessed on the basis of postrelease flying ability because perfect flight is necessary for foraging.

Because plumage has to be intact prior to release for waterproofing purposes, veterinarians should be apprised that sticky or adhesive wraps directly on feathers are contraindicated in these species. The author prefers using nonadhesive materials such as Vetrap or Coban (3M) in a "figure of 8" format to wrap wings of larger species of terns and gulls. Small tern species' wings can be wrapped with light Micropore paper tape (3M), or narrow strips of non-adhesive materials.

Both juvenile gulls and terns with unilateral foot trauma (over half the foot missing) or an injured hock, knee, or hip joint have a poor prognosis. As the chicks or fledglings grow, the increasing weight is borne on the uninjured leg or foot, and the healthy limb becomes unable to bear weight either from pododermatitis or joint deformity.

Young gulls and terns treated with antibiotics should also be medicated with an appropriate anti-fungal medication, such as Itraconazole (Janssen) at 15 mg/kg orally once daily to prevent opportunistic fungal infections. As with most seabirds, these species are vulnerable to Aspergillosis.

Small tern species are particularly prone to pododermatitis, which presents as reddening and swelling on the underside of the foot webbing. This may occur when underweight or injured fledglings have to be maintained indoors on fabric or paper toweling. Foot lesions are difficult to treat and often result in systemic infections and death. Damp and wet conditions with debris (feces or dirt or gravel) on flooring increase the chances of damage to delicate foot webbing (see the section "Housing," later in this chapter, for suggested substrates).

In captivity, beak damage may occur in older juvenile gulls when housed temporarily in kennels because they may abrade their beaks on the metal door. The lesions heal once the bird is placed in an aviary setting. Gulls may also damage their feathers when placed in wire cages for even short periods of time.

DIET

Small tern chicks (Least, Common, or Forster's) can be fed silversides (Menidia) or lance fish (Ammodytes spp.). Many retail and online pet food suppliers carry these items frozen. Larger terns and Western Gull chicks can be fed small whitebait, lake smelt, or other whole fish. Gull chicks less than a week old can also be fed shrimp. Whole food items are better than chopped fish, because fish oils may sometimes remain on the beak, causing contamination of body plumage and the vent area when birds preen. Fish or shrimp or other food items should be offered fresh at each feeding. Older gulls can be offered dry cat food, cooked eggs, and bread as an introduction to the later miscellaneous diet that many gulls subsist on from humans. Least Terns and other small tern species will also eat large or giant mealworms when they are old enough for outdoor housing. For larger terns and gulls, whole lake smelt or night smelt (Canadian origin) are often available at local Asian markets fresh or frozen.

FEEDING PROCEDURES

Gull and tern chicks can be fed within a few hours of hatching. Parent birds of these species feed chicks on the day of hatch, although the yolk sac can nourish the bird for the first 48 hours if necessary. Chicks sit quietly until they become hungry and then begin soliciting for food by vocalizing. Food items can be given to the bird using a pair of forceps or by hand. Juvenile gulls and terns advance toward the handler and grasp offered fish after calling and gaping. Do not allow beaks to become sticky or dirty with food. Clean the beak and nares if this should become necessary. Food should be freshly thawed the day of feeding and kept refrigerated until an hour or two before feeding.

Hatchlings

Feeding frequency of hatchlings will depend on the species and size of the hatched chick. Hatchling gulls and terns eat readily, but less frequently on the day of hatch (see Figure 10.4). By the second day, chicks should eat approximately every 60–90 minutes. Feed every 90 minutes (9–10 times daily) until the chick is satiated, for 12 to 14 hours a day. If a chick seems reluctant to eat, it may be gently force-fed a moistened fish.

If the chick refuses to gape or beg for food, give fluids, skip the next feeding, and check that stool color and consistency are normal for the species and diet. Fish diets usually result in dark grey fecal material in a splash of white urates. Gray granular stools may indicate illness or dehydration. Birds that do not defecate regularly after every one or two feedings should be checked for cloacal impactions by

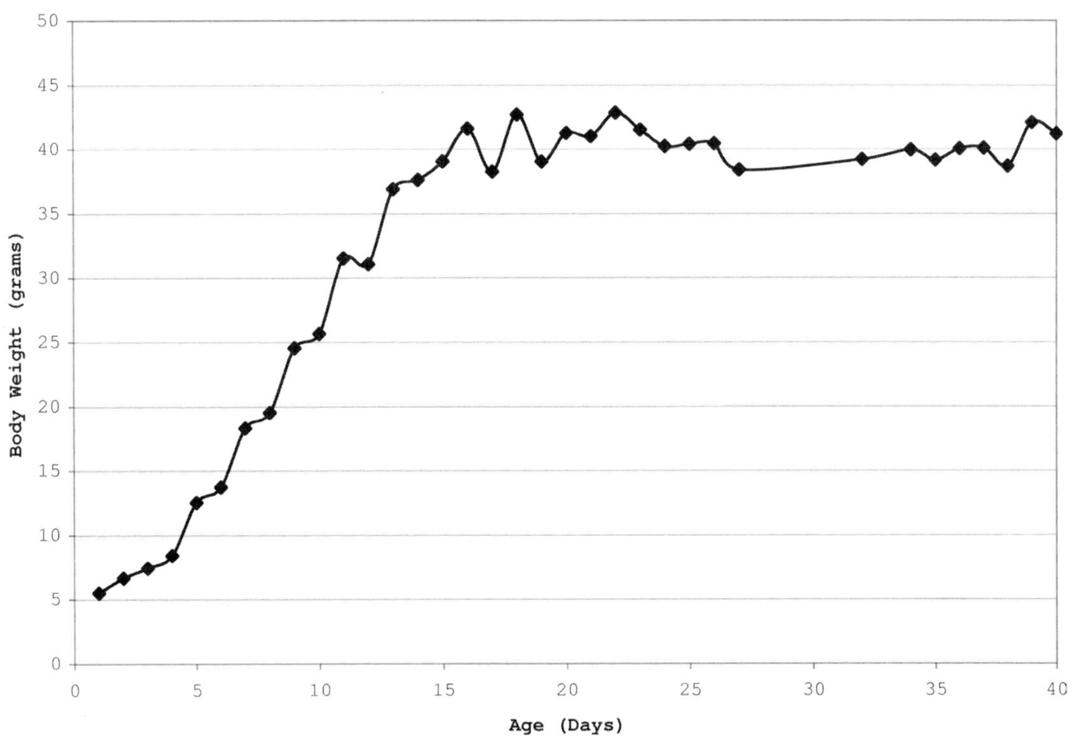

Figure 10.4. Weight gains of Least Tern chicks (n = 17).

inspecting the vent area for chalky or granular concretions. A gentle stream of warm water on the cloacal area may stimulate the bird to defecate. The bird should then have additional fluids added to its diet by tube-feeding fluids between solid feeding.

Nestlings and Fledglings

Nestlings and fledglings can be fed about every 90 minutes for 12 to 14 hours a day. After the first week, time intervals can be lengthened to every 3–4 hours for gull species, and every 90 minutes to 2 hours for terns. Small terns may need feeding every 2 hours until they are picking up food items from a dish. Larger tern and gull species will start picking up food from a dish after about 1–2 weeks, and at that stage food dishes should be refilled with fresh food at least four times daily.

EXPECTED WEIGHT GAIN

After hatching, gull and tern chicks may remain at the same weight for the first 48 hours. After this time, period weight gain should be steady and fairly linear (see Figures 10.4, 10.5) until about 3 weeks of age, at which point weight gain will slow, while feather growth continues. Individual variation is normal, but weights vary if taken fasted or nonfasted. Weigh birds at the same time each day because these species can hold a significant amount of their body weight in food within their digestive tract.

HOUSING

Hatchlings should be kept between 90–100°F (32–38°C) on hatch. Incubator floor temperature should be approximately 93°F (34°C), with a 40 watt light over one end of the incubator. A 4 in (10 cm) square piece of synthetic fur fabric is placed at the lighted end in one corner for small tern chicks to huddle under or sit on. The author uses an incubator (aquabrooder) for smaller terns and gull chicks less than 5 days old, which allows the chick to choose from a temperature gradient in the brooder (see Figures 10.1–10.3). As the birds start to grow in size,

1200
1000
800
600
400
200
0

Body Weight (grams)

6/23/06 6/30/06 7/7/06 7/14/06 7/21/06

Date

Gull 81 Gull 82 Gull 83 Gull SC

Figure 10.5. Weight gains of four Western Gull chicks.

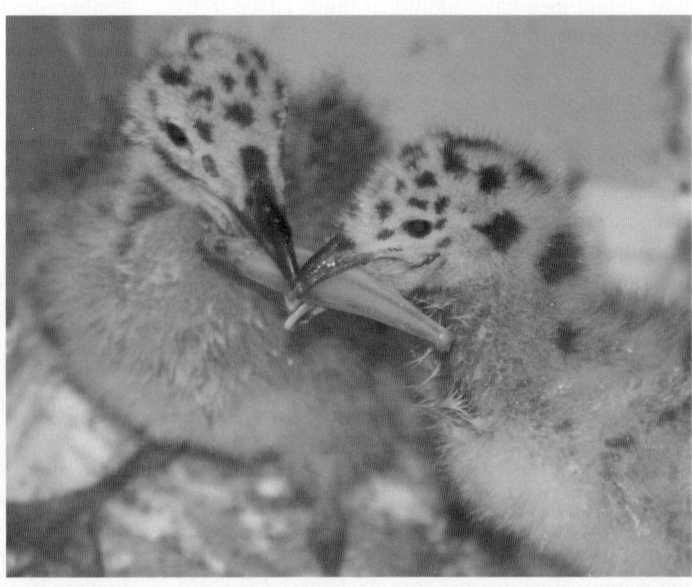

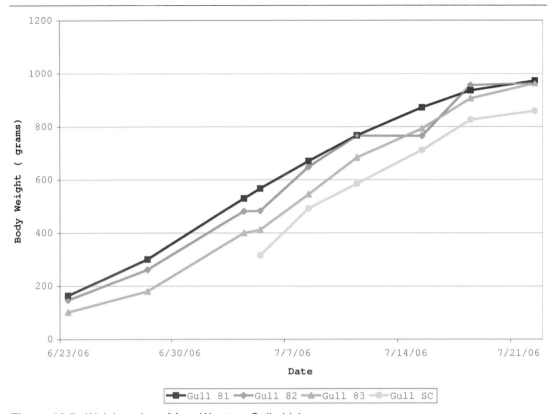

Figure 10.6. Two Western Gull chicks competing for lunch (photo courtesy of Mary F. Platter Rieger).

smaller species can be kept in an incubator; larger species can be housed in a kennel with a heating pad under one end to maintain a temperature between 85–95°F (29–35°C).

Hatchlings of California Least Terns and Forster's Terns can be housed on several layers of paper towels or cotton velour towels, changing the towel or paper when soiled. Another option is to use sterilized play sand 0.25 in (0.5 cm) deep, removing debris from the surface daily and changing the sand as needed.

After the chicks are able to thermoregulate at about 1 week of age for gulls, or 2 weeks for smaller tern species, the overhead tungsten light can be replaced with a full spectrum light. In tern and gull species metabolic bone disease is rare, but since the birds are reared indoors, full spectrum lights over the incubator (or though the door of the kennels) are prudent to provide chicks with adequate vitamin D production.

Once chicks are able to thermoregulate, the ambient temperature in their enclosure can be decreased gradually, and they can be moved to a larger enclosure.

At about 3 weeks of age for terns, or 4 weeks for gulls, the chicks should be near 80% of normal adult weight and have primary feathers at least half grown. Small terns will have lost most or all of the downy tufts on the head and back, larger gull species may still have some down. Gulls and terns at this stage of development are completely self-feeding, and can be transferred either to a small 6 × 8 ft (1.8 × 2.4 m) enclosure with a sand floor and small pool or directly into the final flight aviary.

When first placed outdoors, birds should be monitored to check that they do not get wet or become hypothermic. Monitoring is especially important if the weather is cool or if any birds are not completely waterproof. Heat should be provided in a protected corner of the aviary until it's certain that all birds are doing well at ambient outdoor temperatures.

Flight cages should have sand floors that are swept of surface debris several times a week. Fresh sand should be added when necessary. Pools (either concrete or with PVC liners) within the aviary should have a gradual slope, and they should be drained daily and filled with fresh water or allowed to overflow to constantly remove any floating potential plumage contaminants. Pools should be of a size and slope that allows birds to walk in and out to bathe. The minimum access to water recommended for these species is one 45 in diameter, 10–12 in deep pool for every 4–6 birds (Miller 2000).

WEANING

Most terns will start picking up food within 2 weeks of hatch. Some species (Western Gulls) will pick up dropped food at 3 days of age; some may take a little longer. Individuals may be slower to self-feed; several chicks grouped together will self-feed more rapidly and are less likely to become habituated to a human caregiver (see Figure 10.7, 10.8). The caregiver should feed smaller, weaker individuals if

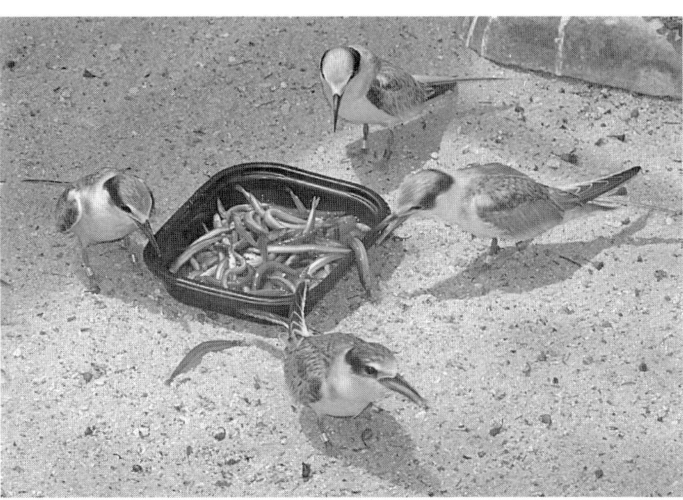

Figure 10.7. Four Least Tern fledglings in outdoor caging with dish of fish (photo courtesy of Mary F. Platter Rieger).

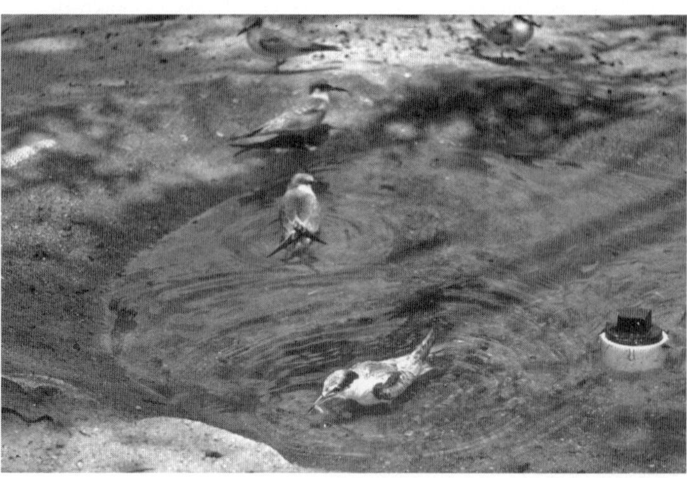

Figure 10.8. Least Terns in outdoor aviary with pool.

older birds in the group are more aggressive. Older juvenile terns are less likely to attack younger birds housed with them than are gulls. Overcrowding (or simply aggressive personalities) can cause Western Gull chicks to peck at the heads of younger birds and cause feather loss and sometimes lacerations.

Encouraging Foraging Skills

Western Gulls feed on land and water, but do not usually dive for food. These birds require no particular training to pick up food.

For terns, first place the usual food dishes (see Figure 10.7) in the aviary near the pool. After a few days, place the fish at the edge of the sloping pool. The pool should be about 4 ft (1.2 m) in diameter and 1 ft (30 cm) deep in the center so that the birds are used to picking up fish in the shallow area. Then toss the fish in a little deeper, and encourage the birds to wade into the water. Terns will not jump into deep water, so the slope needs to be gradual. If birds are reluctant, feed at 8 a.m., and then withhold food until 3–4 p.m. After several more days the fish can be placed somewhat deeper, and the birds should wade and then fly in and pick them up. Finally, feeder (live) goldfish should be placed in the food dishes for a day or two so the birds are accustomed to catch the feeders, and then the live feeders placed in the pool itself. Sometimes the birds have to be left with the feeder fish all day before they will forage, but hunger will usually prove adequate to overcome the reluctance to enter the water (see Figure 10.8).

PREPARATION FOR WILD RELEASE

Prerelease conditioning aviaries for small terns should minimally be 10 × 12 × 8 ft high (3 × 3.6 × 2.4 m high) with predator proof plastic mesh netting (0.25 in/0.5 cm mesh) to prevent feather damage. Larger terns should be housed in an enclosure at least 10 × 16 × 8 ft high (3 × 4.9 × 2.4 m high), but this is not really tall enough to provide practice plunging. Aviary size for large terns such as Caspian Terns should be at least 8 ft (2.4 m) wide, 32–50 ft (9.6–15 m) long and 12–25 ft (3.6–7.5 m) high. Large gulls can be safely housed in 0.5 in (1.25 cm) wire mesh "hardware cloth" enclosures. Flooring should be sterilized play sand to a depth of 1 in (2.5 cm) and the surface brushed once weekly to remove debris. Wire mesh under the cage may be necessary to prevent burrowing predator attack.

Birds should be held until they are able to make sustained flights, and in the case of gulls fly up to a perch 6 ft (1.8 m) above the ground. Terns and gulls should be capable of sustained flight without panting for several circuits of the flight cage and land with wings folded.

Terns should walk or plunge into water to capture and swallow live feeder fish of appropriate size. Gulls should readily eat a variety of foods, including fish, bread, cat or dog food (dry or soaked), and human "refuse" (fast food leftovers).

Gulls and terns reared in groups rarely become imprinted on humans; however, gulls reared with close human contact may never develop an appropriate fear of humans and may become a nuisance or a danger to the public.

In the case of Western Gulls and California Least Terns, it is the author's experience that fledglings of these two species can be safely housed with an adult conspecific in an aviary during the breeding season. Least Terns tolerate Least Tern chicks in a recovery cage or aviary; Western Gull adults have sometimes regurgitated food for Western Gull chicks when housed in an aviary. A recovered adult then can be released with a group of chicks.

California Least and Forster's Terns raised from hatch or brought in for rehabilitation beg for food from the caregiver and may appear tame. However, once in the fledgling stage when food is no longer offered by hand, these birds lose their "tameness" and quickly become apprehensive of human contact if weighed and measured once or twice prior to release.

Chicks of varying ages can be housed together, but older gull chicks may show aggression to younger smaller birds. This is manifested in aviaries by the appearance of reddened areas and missing feathers at the back of the head where they have been pecked. The younger bird should be separated into a younger group, or the aggressive bird detected and separated from the group. Adult terns of various species do not seem to attack juvenile conspecifics or other tern species but do vocalize during competition for food and give warning calls.

Chicks of most tern species remain with the parent and have been observed receiving supplemental food for extended periods of time. Little is known about the survival of hand-reared birds. However, Western Gull chicks released at 12 weeks of age have been observed surviving successfully 1 year postrelease in San Diego.

Criteria for Release

Birds should be wary of humans, able to sustain flight without panting, bank and turn circles in an aviary, and land smoothly. The birds' primary, contour, and tail feathers should be full length, and the birds should be able to bathe and emerge from the water looking dry (i.e., waterproof). Fledglings should achieve the minimum weight for their species, and have no foot or beak abnormalities. Birds should readily enter the water to bathe and pick up food.

Release Sites

Terns and gulls reared in captivity should be released in an appropriate habitat where there are others of the same species. Because some tern and gull species migrate, if birds are reared or rehabilitated late in the season and the others of that species have already migrated, they may need to be overwintered in suitable rehabilitation facilities.

ACKNOWLEDGMENTS

Thanks to Mary F. Platter Rieger for her enthusiasm, interest and support, and the generous use of her photographs. Thanks also to the many endangered species monitors working at California Least Tern breeding sites, in particular Elizabeth Copper, Brian Foster, Robert Patton and Shauna Wolf. Many thanks to Project Wildlife in San Diego, its wonderful volunteers, and to my late husband Dr. John Faulkner, who always encouraged me to pass on my knowledge through publication.

SOURCES FOR PRODUCTS MENTIONED

Vetrap, Coban, and Micropore paper tape: 3M Corporate Headquarters, 3M Center, St. Paul, MN 55144-1000, (888) 364-3577.

Ensure: Abbott Laboratories, Abbott Park, IL.

Multimilk PetAg 255 Keyes Avenue, Hampshire, IL 60140, (800) 323-6878.

Itraconazole: Janssen Pharmaceutica Inc. P.O. Box 200, Titusville, NJ 08560-0200, (609) 730-2000.

REFERENCES

Grabboski, R. 1995. Simple Things That Make a Difference: Making Water-Based Incubators. Journal of Wildlife Rehabilitation 18(2): 16–17.

Miller, E.A., ed. 2000. Minimum Standards for Wildlife Rehabilitation, 3rd Edition. National Wildlife Rehabilitation Association, St. Cloud, Minnesota, 77 pp.

Pierotti, R.J. and Annett, C.A. 1995. Western Gull (*Larus occidentalis*). In Birds of North America,

No 174, Poole, A., and Gill, F., eds. The Academy of Natural Sciences, Philadelphia, PA, and the American Ornithologists' Union, Washington, D.C.

Terres, J.K. 1980. The Audubon Encyclopedia of North American Birds by John K Terres. Alfred A. Knopf, Inc., New York.

Thompson, B.C., Jackson, J.A., Burger, J., Hill, L.A., Kirsch, E.M., and Atwood, J.L. 1997. Least Tern (*Sterna Antillarum*). In Birds of North America, No 290. Poole, A. and Gill, F, eds. The Academy of Natural Sciences, Philadelphia, PA, and the American Ornithologists' Union, Washington, D.C.

11
Alcids

David A. Oehler

NATURAL HISTORY

The family Alcidae, or auk, is a group of marine, neritic, and pelagic birds with a circumpolar range, found exclusively in the Northern Hemisphere. The name *auk* was derived from the Norse word *ālka,* given to describe the calls of these seabirds. Alcids have been divided into 11genera represented by 22 species. All members of this group are highly specialized, wing-propelled, diving birds with thickset, torpedo-shaped bodies and short wings and tails. Typical morphology consists of plumage that is mainly black or gray above and white below. This plumage is dramatically altered during the winter months, with certain species obtaining gray-and-white plumage. The specific diving abilities of particular species, coupled with variations in prey items from zooplankton to fish, alleviate competition among species. Diet is closely correlated to body mass and bill type (Strauch 1985, del Hoyo et al. 1996).

Due to their prey selection, alcids are normally found in the waters of the continental shelf located in low and Arctic waters, with only members of the genus Synthliboramphus located in subtropical waters. Foraging entails remaining on the water for a majority of the year and coming to land only to nest and propagate. Alcids normally use islands and sea cliffs to establish breeding colonies of up to more than one million birds in size. Nests within these colonies usually are found within rocky substrates, earthen burrows, or inaccessible cavities, with only one species utilizing an arboreal platform nest.

CRITERIA FOR INTERVENTION

Very few alcid chicks are encountered by rehabilitation facilities, which may be due to the inaccessibility of most breeding colonies and nest sites. Logging activities have resulted in a small number of Marbled Murrelets, *Brachyramphus marmoratus*, requiring intervention, since this species nests on the branches of old-growth conifers (Hamer & Nelson 1995). Murres and Razorbills have an intermediate developmental strategy, allowing the chicks to depart the colony at 2 to 3 weeks of age. These chicks then remain with the adults at sea for up to 8 weeks, being fed by a parent. Synthliboramphus chicks depart the nest with the parents shortly after hatching. These strategies likely reduce the energetic costs of chick rearing (Sealy 1973, Varoujean et al. 1977). The majority of alcids that need assistance are fledglings of the larger species and are found along the coastline. These puffin, murres, or guillemots are usually underweight and often have compromised plumage.

RECORD KEEPING

The importance of maintaining detailed records for each bird cannot be emphasized enough. For reporting requirements, general background information will be needed, such as species, age, locale of rescue, reason brought into captivity, medical information, final disposition, and/or release location. Monitoring each individual bird requires a systematic and consistent means of evaluation to ensure its health, and to provide data for future use. Recording environmental conditions, exposure to infectious agents or toxins, diet, feed intake, physical condition, and body mass are essential in the care of alcids in a captive situation.

INITIAL CARE AND STABILIZATION

Every attempt should be made to obtain a complete history of a bird upon arrival. This will assist in the evaluation of the bird and provide information designating proper release sites. Observe the bird and record the attitude, respiration, and plumage condition. A physical examination is required to ascertain body weight, general condition, and possible trauma. The examination and suitable medical treatment should be conducted as quickly as possible to reduce the stress to the bird.

Usually, alcids arrive as fledglings and are dehydrated and undernourished. Supportive care should be provided as part of a standard protocol for incoming birds. Begin rehydration of the bird by administering oral or subcutaneous fluids: 40–50 ml/kg of lactated Ringer's solution (LRS) or a similar balanced isotonic solution. A broad-spectrum antibiotic may be administered if indicated after an initial examination or preliminary diagnostic testing. This therapy should be prescribed by a veterinarian and may be altered, based on clinical signs, diagnostic tests, and culture and sensitivity results. Prophylactic antifungal therapies are often recommended for captive alcids because secondary fungal infections are common in seabirds. The initiation of itraconazole therapy is recommended within 48 hours of arrival, although only after the bird has been rehydrated to minimize the risk of potential toxic effects on the kidneys. Vitamin B complex, A, D3, and E supplementation should also be provided (ASLC 2006b, Huckabee personal communication).

Blood collection and analysis may be utilized to assist in the diagnosis of medical problems. If the fledgling is strong enough, a sufficient volume of blood can be collected for a packed cell volume (PCV), total protein, white blood cell count, and biochemistries.

Evaluate the plumage of each specimen to determine the level of waterproofing. Birds with good plumage, which properly sheds water, may be placed directly into an enclosure with pool facilities. Plumage that is excessively worn, oiled, and/or absorbs water precludes the introduction of the bird to open water. These birds with compromised feathers must be transferred to suitable holding areas, where supplemental heat can be provided. Poor plumage may indicate underlying and/or long-term health problems that may be investigated further. Screen each bird for ectoparasites, which are common in larger alcids.

A direct fecal analysis should be performed to evaluate for endoparasites.

COMMON MEDICAL PROBLEMS

Ectoparasites, such as lice and ticks adversely affect alcids, reducing growth rates and the condition of the plumage (Muzaffar & Jones 2004). A water-based pyrethrin spray can be used to eliminate these infestations. Any spray or other substance used on the feathers must not damage or leave a residue on the plumage that will interfere with the waterproofing capabilities. Oil- or petroleum-based products must be avoided.

Alcids, along with other seabirds, are susceptible to a fungal infection, aspergillosis, particularly when held indoors. Loss of body mass, without the presence of inappetence, may be one of the first clinical signs that this condition exists. Itraconazole therapy, maintaining a clean environment, fresh air, and proper ventilation (10–12 air exchanges per hour) are the best preventative measures that may be enacted.

Vitamin deficiencies occur regularly in piscivorous birds, due to the loss vitamins in the freezing and thawing process in the fish that are fed to these birds in a captive situation. Vitamin supplementation, mixing vitamin powder on smaller feed items or placing tablets in feed fish prevents these deficiencies (Mejeur et al. 1988).

Pododermatitis or *bumblefoot* is an inflammatory or degenerative condition, common in the feet of seabirds that are forced to stand on hard, smooth cement surfaces for extended periods of time. Preventative measures (see the section "Housing," later in this chapter) should be incorporated into any holding enclosure provided to alcids. Resolution of bumblefoot is slow and may require intense management. While on land, murres stand on tarsi or lower legs rather than on their feet. The ankle joint should be monitored frequently for swelling or heat, and birds demonstrating these clinical signs should be placed into water for as long as possible. It is far better to prevent the development of foot lesions than to attempt treatment after they have progressed to the point of bumblefoot.

DIET RECIPES

Small Alcids

The base auklet formula consists of 85 g Cyclop-eeze® (decapod microscopic crustaceans), 85 g superba krill, 30 g mealworms, and 60 cc Pedialyte (Abbott), with 5 g of Mazuri Alcid vitamin supplement added (Mazuri Company; see the section "Sources for Products Mentioned" at the end of this chapter). On short notice, substitute mysis shrimp from your local freshwater and marine pet store for Cyclop-eeze®. Additional Pedialyte (total of 100 cc) is utilized for chicks less than 3 days of age. All ingredients are processed in a blender until smooth, with caution not to blend long enough to heat the mixture. Upon completion, refrigerate the formula and make a fresh supply daily. The formula must be able to pass easily through a modified syringe and 14 French catheter tube (Oehler et al. 2003).

Feeding tubes may easily be produced using a 50–60 ml catheter tip syringe. A 14 French feeding tube or urethral catheter tube is attached. The tube is cut to a length of approximately 4 in (10 cm) at a 45° angle. The cut is heated with an open flame to remove any sharp edges. Similar pet-quality feeding syringes and tubes can be found at most larger pet stores. It is important to make sure that the tube is secured properly onto the syringe. Over the years, we have used this type of feeding tube in thousands of feedings, and once in a while the tube will become separated from the syringe and is swallowed by the chick. With patience and some manipulation, the tube can be removed, but this adds unnecessary stress to the bird and to the person attempting the removal.

Larger Alcids

Upon hatching, larger alcids, such as the guillemots, puffin, and murres are hand-fed sand lances, silversides, herring, smelt, or capelin, whole or sliced fish, up to five times per day. Murrelets, which normally prey upon smaller fish and fish larvae require small sand lances or thinly sliced fillets of larger fish. Soak fish in Pedialyte prior to each feeding.

ARTIFICIAL INCUBATION

Artificial incubation of eggs is not required on a routine basis. Late-term incubation parameters indicate that a dry-bulb temperature of 99.5°F (37.5°C) with a relative humidity of 60% is sufficient to accomplish a successful hatch (see Chapter 3).

Hatchlings

Although the dietary requirements for hatchlings vary between species, the brooder requirements may be interchanged. Chicks should be weighed each morning and volumes of feed should be recorded, along with brooder temperature, attitude of chick, and medical notations.

ThermoCare Inc. Portable ICS Units and/or Dean's Model II Brooders have been used as brooders for chicks under 3 days of age. A thermoregulating pad, set at 98.0°F (36.7°C) is rolled into a cylinder and placed at one side of the brooder. A feather duster is suspended from the ceiling of the brooder, providing the chicks with an insulated, dark, and secure area next to the heat source. Each brooder is covered with a towel to keep the interior darkened further. Although these high-tech brooders work well, we have been forced to improvise during excursions in the field. A shoebox, lined with lichens and moss with heat supplied by refilling a water bottle with warm water has been used successfully to rear day-old auklet and puffin chicks. Chicks greater than 3 days of age are moved to a cool room with an ambient temperature of 50°F (10.0°C). Although in the wild chicks may be brooded initially by the adults, after hatching we maintain a heat source for up to 2 weeks. A hot water heat source remains with the chicks and they are allowed access to the warmth and will self-regulate. At 21 days of age chicks are removed to an air-conditioned holding room with an ambient temperature of 55.0–60.0°F (12.8–15.6°C). Individuals remain separated from each other, using solid wall dividers between brooder sections to prevent aggression and to allow for monitoring of food intake (see Figure 11.1). The wire- or net-bottomed brooders are furnished with a 1 × 1 × 1 ft (30 cm × 30 cm × 30 cm) cardboard box, waxed on the outside, with a small opening approximately 4 × 5 in (10 × 12 cm) cut in the front of the box.

Paper towels line the bottom of the boxes and are cleaned at each feeding. Monitor chicks for dehydration and overheating throughout the day. Dry eyes and pinched skin that remains tented are signs of dehydration, and increased fluids in the formula may be required. Labored respiration, inappetence, or feet that radiate excess heat are clinical signs of heat distress and require a reduction in brooder or room temperature.

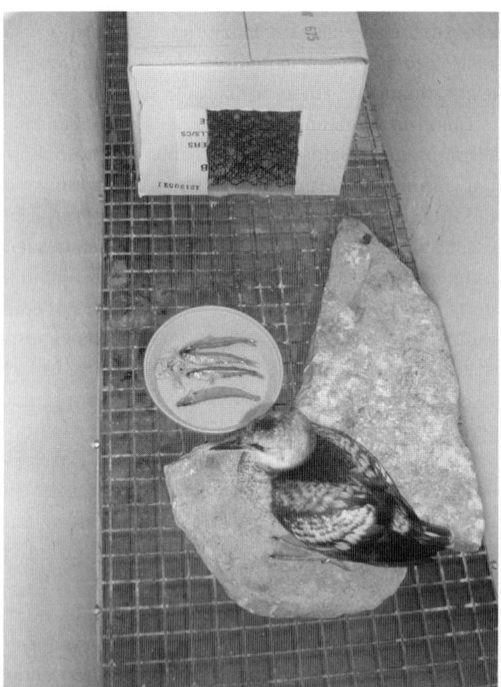

Figure 11.1. A 5-week-old Pigeon Guillemot fledgling is readied for transfer to open water. Note the use of a typical alcid brooder with solid wall dividers, cardboard box retreat area, and wire mesh substrate (photo by David Oehler).

HAND-REARING DIETS AND FEEDING RECOMMENDATIONS

Providing the proper nutrition to captive avifauna, even for commonly held taxa, is challenging. Improperly provided diets may lead to vitamin deficiency, fragile plumage, low bone density and many other life-threatening problems. Commercially formulated diets are not available for alcids in general, and the difficulty of duplicating the diet of the various auklets compounds the challenges we face.

Current recommendations for alcid diets parallel the diet of their wild counterparts as closely as possible. Small alcids, such as Whiskered and Least Auklets are exclusively planktivorous; Dovekies, the remaining auklets, and murrelets consume zooplankton and fish. Large alcids, the puffins, murres, and guillemots are mainly piscivorous, with nearly 95% of their diets consisting of fish, the remainder of invertebrates (Ewins 1993, Hatch and Sanger 1992, Hunt et al. 1993). The main difference between the diets of larger and small alcids is that the smaller birds feed on meals rich in wax esters (more than 60% of their total energy intake). This selection in prey items means that wax esters (long-chain fatty alcohols esterified to long-chain fatty acids) are the dominant dietary neutral lipid (Roby 1991, Roby et al. 1986). Many birds, especially seabirds, have a unique capacity for assimilating wax esters with higher efficiencies (greater than 90%) than that attainable by mammals (less than 50%) (Place 1992). Piscivorous species, the large alcids, rely on lipid-rich prey items, such as sand lances, Atlantic cod, Artic cod, and Pollock, to maintain their dietary requirements and in chick rearing (Ainley et al. 2002, Gaston and Hipfner 2002, Litzow et al. 2002, Piatt and Kitaysky 2002).

Small Alcids

Alcid chicks demonstrate a rapid growth rate, given the short Arctic summer. As a result, these chicks need to take in a higher percentage of calories than most neonatal birds. Crop content of auklets in Alaska indicates that they forage for krill, small medusa, fish, and copepods, although this varies greatly for each species (Day and Byrd 1989, Harrison 1990). The more diminutive auklets rely more heavily on smaller zooplankton and do not take fish. Copepods appear to be a major component of auklets in the wild, but availability of copepods as feed for captive specimens is limited. Frozen cultured copepods have been successfully incorporated into the hand-rearing formula to increase the calorie content per volume fed.

Using a warm-water bath, heat an appropriate amount of the small alcid formula required for one feeding and discard any unused portions. Chicks are fed approximately 10% of their initial morning body weight for each feeding. Placing the tube to the side of the bill and extruding a small amount of formula onto the bill may elicit a feeding response. As the chick tastes the formula, place the tube into the chick's mouth and allow the chick to swallow the tube on its own. Depress the plunger of the syringe with a slow and constant pressure, ensuring the chick continues to swallow (see Figure 11.2). If the chick stops swallowing or pulls away from the tube, discontinue the feeding. If the chick refuses to give a feeding response, do not force-feed, place the chick back in the brooder and try again in 1 hour. It cannot be stressed enough to allow the chick to

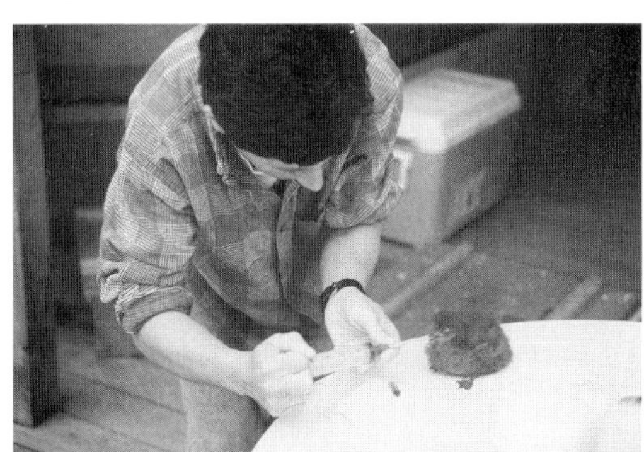

Figure 11.2. Aviculturist Sue Schmid, of the Cincinnati Zoo & Botanical Garden, hand-feeds a 25-day-old Whiskered Auklet (photo by Mark Alexander).

dictate how much food it will take at each feeding (Oehler et al. 1995, 2001) (see Table 11.1).

Large Alcids

Larger alcid hatchlings, such as the guillemots, puffins, and murres, are hand-fed sand lances, silversides, herring, smelt, or capelin, whole or sliced fish, up to five times per day. Murrelets, which normally prey upon smaller fish and fish larvae, require small sand lances or thinly sliced fillets of larger fish. Soak each fish in Pedialyte prior to each feeding. Chicks less than 5 days of age are fed approximately 40% of their initial morning body weight divided into five feedings over a 12-hour span. A feeding response may be elicited by placing the fish to the side of the bill, although these birds quickly recognize feed and will move toward the fish when the brooder is opened. At 5 days of age, begin to offer whole fish on a plate instead of hand feeding. Ensure that this feed is removed if not taken within the first 20–30 minutes. When chicks begin to consistently feed from the plates, larger amounts of fish may be placed upon the plates on beds of ice and left in the brooder. Feeding schedules will fluctuate between species, but as a general rule the number of feedings may be reduced to three when chicks are 21 days of age (ASLC 2006a, Thompson 1996) (see Table 11.1).

Fledglings

Feed is provided twice daily to better mimic their natural foraging habits in the wild and to ensure that the feed items are fresh. To maintain a safe supply of feed, these items may be placed in the water or on plates, with ice. Do not allow feed to remain in the enclosure for extended periods. Because a majority of the feed items are stored frozen, vitamin supplementation is required. These food items should be provided in clean, nontoxic, shallow bowls or plates. Water is provided only through the pool, and standing containers of water should never be offered to any of the alcids.

Due to commercial availability, or unavailability, and given the specific requirements of each taxon, careful examination must be given as to the choice of food items. Many of the alcids' food items are not commercially available, so choice in prey items is severely limited. Boiled superba krill has been proven to maintain auklets in captivity and makes up the bulk of their diet. This diet is deficient in extra long-chain fatty acids, a major component of their natural diet. Supplementation with live aquatic and nonaquatic invertebrates, along with cultured copepods has been attempted to offset this deficiency with success. The addition of live mealworms and Cyclop-eeze® has been effective in supplying the specimens with an abundance of medium to extra-long chain fatty acids and caloric intake. Superba krill is shipped both in boiled and raw forms; but the raw krill, being high in water content, spoils faster and tends to soil plumage. Because of its larger size, superba krill must be cut down for smaller auklet species, such as the Least and Whiskered Auklets. Sand lances should never be provided to these auklets, because the high protein content and the high-energy requirements associated with the assimilation of these proteins places the individuals in a negative calorie situation. Boiled krill may be thawed overnight and stored in a refrigerator for 3 to 4 days. Never feed krill that has turned brown or that smells rancid, and remove food from the enclosure within 15 hours, or less if housed in an environment that is conducive to accelerating the decomposing processes. Sand lances are the preferred food item of puffins, murres, and guillemots, forming the bulk of the diet for these larger alcids, and they can be diced for the smaller taxa.

During the freezing and thawing process, vitamins and nutrients naturally denature; therefore, vitamin supplements must be added daily. A multivitamin mix is essential to replace missing elements in the diet due to both the limited types of food that can be offered and the freezing and thawing process. Mazuri Auklet Blend (Mazuri) is a supplement

Table 11.1. Outline of the development of alcids in the wild and hand-rearing in captivity with suggested feeding schedules.

	Common Murre[1]		Thick-billed Murre[2]		Pigeon Guillemot[3]		Marbled Murrelet[4,5]		Parakeet Auklet[6,7]	
	In situ	Ex situ	In situ	Ex situ	In situ	Ex situ	In situ	Ex situ	In situ	Ex situ
Hatch wt (g)	55–95		65–70		34–43		33		27–32	
Feeding schedule: days 1–7	4–5/day over 15 hours		2–6/day over 15 hours			5/day over 12 hours		5/day over 12 hours		12/day over 22 hours
Growth rate: days 1–7			5–10 g/d		8–15 g/day	15%/day				25%/day
Feeding schedule: days 8–14	4–5/day over 15 hours		10–15/day over 15 hours			4/day over 12 hours		4/day over 12 hours		8/day over 20 hours
Growth rate: days 8–14			5–10 g/d		10–20 g/day	10%/day			9 g/day	15%/day
Feeding schedule: days 15–21		3/day over 15 hours		3/d over 15 hours		4/day over 12 hours	6/day over 12 hours	4/day over 12 hours		6/day over 12 hours
Growth rate: days 15–21	15 g/day					8%/day				8%/day
Fledge age (days)	14–21		18		35–42		27–40		33–36	
Fledge wt (g)	200		200–250		400–500				208–237	
Release wt (g)		> 700				> 400				> 200
Adult wt (g)	945–1044				450–550		220		238–247	

Hatch wt (g)	25		12–14		12		48		64	
Feeding schedule: days 1–7	1–4/day over 15 hours	12/day over 22 hours	hours	12/day over 22 hours	3/day over 15 hours	12/day over 22 hours	3/day over 15 hours	5/day over 12 hours	2–4/day over 15 hours	5/d over 12
Growth rate: days 1–7		25%/day	4–5 g/day	25%/day	5–6 g/day	25%/day	11 g/day	15%/day	16 g/day	15%/d
Feeding schedule: days 8–14	1–4/day over 15 hours	8/day over 20 hours		8/day over 20 hours	3/day over 15 hours	8/day over 20 hours	3/day over 15 hours	4/day over 12 hours	2–4/day over 15 hours	4//d over 12 hours
Growth rate: days 8–14		15%/day	4–5 g/day	15%/day		15%/day	11 g/day	10%/day	16 g/day	10%/d
Feeding schedule: days 15–21		6/day over 12 hours		6/day over 12 hours		6/day over 12 hours	6/day over 15 hours	4/day over 12 hours	2–4/day over 15 hours	4/d over 12 hours
Growth rate: days 15–21	11–13 g/day	8%/day		8%/day		8%/day		8%/day		8%/d
Fledge age (days)	27–36		39–42		29		37–46		49	
Fledge wt (g)	260		106		82		408		496	
Release wt (g)		> 230		> 100		> 80		> 375		> 450
Adult wt (g)	260		120		85		612		773	

[1] Ainley et al. (2002).
[2] Gaston and Hipfner (2000).
[3] Ewins (1993).
[4] del Hoyo et al. (1996).
[5] Kappy Sprenger, personal communication.
[6] Jones et al. (2001).
[7] Oehler et al. (1995).
[8] Jones (1993a).
[9] Byrd and Williams (1993).
[10] Jones (1993b).
[11] Oehler et al. (2001).
[12] Piatt and Kitaysky (2002).
[13] Wehle (1983).

containing essential vitamins and minerals, developed specifically for alcids at the Cincinnati Zoo & Botanical Garden. It is not always possible to have this type of vitamin mix available. A good quality multivitamin for birds, such as Quickon's Multivitamin or an equivalent will supplement the birds' nutritional requirements while the birds are being held. These mixes are placed on the food daily, in prescribed amounts.

Vitamin supplementation for the smaller alcids can be challenging, due to the minute size of the items provided. To overcome this obstacle, supplements are produced or ordered in a powdered form. Feed items are placed in a clean feed bucket, in a predetermined quantity, and a set amount of vitamin powder is added to the total supply of feed. The prescribed ratio of Mazuri Auklet Vitamin mix to feed has been determined to be 1.6g of vitamin powder to 1.0kg of feed. The vitamins are mixed into the provisions to ensure a homogenous blend prior to placement in feed dishes.

Birds that have compromised plumage, such as oiled feathers, or do not have access to a pool, should be offered feed plates placed on ice. If a pool is provided, fish and krill may be tossed into the water to promote diving behavior. Discontinue feeding into the pools when the bird(s) show no further interest in feeding (IBRRC 2006).

In emergencies, frozen shrimp and live baitfish may be substituted as feed items for these alcids. The shrimp must be diced into small pieces for the small alcids because they cannot break larger feed items apart. Live baitfish, placed in a small plastic pool, will provide larger alcids with food until alternative arrangements can be provided. Supply the pool with a source of fresh water that will create an overflow. This will remove any oils from the surface and maintain the condition of the birds' plumage.

EXPECTED WEIGHT GAIN

Small alcids should gain approximately 25% of their body mass each day during the first week after they hatch (see Table 11.1). Daily growth rates slow to 15% at 7–14 days of age, 8% at 15–21, and 5% at 22–34. For example, a Least Auklet with a weight of 12.0g at day 1 should gain approximately 3.1g on day 2, 3.8g on day 3, 4.7g on day 4, and so forth, slowing to 15% of their daily body mass gain by about 7 days of age.

Large alcids vary, although approximate growth rates for the first week should be around 15%, slowing to 10% at 7–14 days of age, 8% at 15–21, and 2% as they reach 34 days of age (see Table 11.1). Weight losses after fledging are not uncommon.

HOUSING

As with other pelagic avifauna, alcids in a captive situation are colonial in nature and share the intricate behaviors of their wild counterparts. An assemblage of alcids must not only address their requirements for congregation, but also must respect their needs for spatial segregation.

Exacting environmental conditions are the first requirements in maintaining any alcid. Vigilant monitoring of environmental conditions eliminates possible pathogens, environmental stresses, and physical sources of trauma that would endanger the health of the specimens held in any facility.

Facilities created for the housing of alcids indoors must condition the air to reduce the threat of overheating. Temperatures no greater than 40.0–50.0°F (4.4–10.0°C) are recommended for most alcids, although they are capable of withstanding temperatures well below these points. Air should be prefiltered to remove all particles greater than three microns in diameter.

Pool areas should provide chilled water, a surface skimmer (either physical overflow or protein skimmer), multifaceted filtration system, and an easy haul-out area. Maximum water temperatures of 40.0–50.0°F (4.4–10.0°C) provide a suitable aquatic environment. Due to the delicate nature of the alcids' plumage and the diminutive body mass of specific taxa, it is imperative for these birds to be able to bathe and maintain perfect plumage to ensure thermoregulation. All oils ascending to the surface of the water must be removed quickly to prevent these contaminants from building up on the outer contour feathers. If oils cannot be properly removed, low-lipid fish must be provided to prevent loss of waterproofing. Water filtration may be achieved through various filtration methods, including sand and gravel filters, bag filters, UV filtration, and ozone filtration. Chlorination should be avoided to prohibit degradation of the feathers that are in contact with the water.

Use of fiberglass, urethane, rock, and gravel substrates affords the birds with a solid surface that allows proper maintenance of plumage and prevents foot lesions. All deck areas should be well-drained in a manner to prevent contamination of pool and feeding areas. The abrasive alkaline nature of a cement deck is possibly the most detrimental surface that can be provided for alcids and seabirds in general.

Pelagic avifauna, due to their access to an abundance of UV light in their natural environment, requires greater amounts of supplemental lighting in a captive situation. Hypovitaminosis of vitamin D3 may occur in birds reared in indoor or shady enclosures, resulting in rickets. Augmentation of UV lighting, via an adequate lighting scheme, must be provided for any colony or individual alcid housed in an artificial environment.

WEANING

Small alcids are more difficult to acclimate to feeding on their own than the larger alcids. Initial steps should be made to encourage these birds to feed from plates. Most of the smaller alcids will not begin to feed on their own until after fledging; larger alcids do so prior to fledging. Once they begin to feed off of plates, the same techniques may be employed to condition all alcids to forage in the water.

Appropriate feed items may be tossed in front of the birds and into the pool throughout the day. Measures should be taken to prevent the birds from seeing the person providing the feed so that released birds do not associate people with food. Once the feed has been placed in the water, continue tossing small amounts of feed in front of the bird. If the bird ignores the feed, discontinue this activity for an hour. When the bird begins to dive and eat the feed provided, continue feeding until the bird has had its fill. If possible, maintain like species of alcids together when conditioning them to forage and feed on their own. Once one bird becomes proficient in feeding, others follow quickly.

Problem birds may be fed with hanging or floating feed plates. Live feed may also be used to stimulate foraging behavior. Feed, such as brine shrimp and baitfish can be easily obtained and will attract the attention of the bird.

PREPARATION FOR WILD RELEASE

Fully waterproof plumage is critical for alcid survival in the wild. Birds that have obtained proper plumage to survive in open water, are near adult weight, and are in good health, based on physical condition and blood parameters, are good candidates for release. Loss of body mass or inappetence at this stage along with a sudden aversion toward their caregiver, are indications that the fledgling is ready for release. At this time, any remaining down may be preened off overnight. Release sites should be determined by revisiting the original location of the rescue or known locations of like species in the area.

RELEASE

Once a release site has been chosen, make sure the weather conditions and the area are conducive for a successful release. The weather forecast should be for stable, clear weather for a 24-hour period. Alcids have difficulty becoming airborne and require long running starts to take flight. Make sure that the release site is open and free of immediate obstacles that the birds may collide with and that there are no gulls or other predators in the vicinity. A boat may be used to transport the released bird further from shore. Sun-filled skies along open shorelines will give each bird ample opportunity to go out to sea, maintain good plumage, and with luck find birds of their own kind.

ACKNOWLEDGMENTS

Thanks to Tasha DiMarzio/Alaska Sea Life Center; Karen McElmurry/Center for Wildlife, Maine; Cindy Palmatier/Bird Treatment & Learning Center, Alabama; and Mark Russell/IBRRC, California for providing valuable insight into the rehabilitation aspects of alcids. In particular, I am grateful to Dr. John Huckabee, DVM/PAWS Wildlife Department, Washington, Kappy Sprenger, and Fritz Haas/ Cincinnati Zoo, who critically read all or parts of the manuscript, providing information and improvements through their reviews.

SOURCES FOR PRODUCTS MENTIONED

Cyclop-eeze®, Argent Chemical Laboratory, 8702 152nd Ave, N.E., Redmond, WA 98052, (800) 426-6258, www.argent-labs.com.

Mazuri Auklet Vitamin Mix (5M25-3M), Mazuri, 1050 Progress Dr, Richmond, IN 47374, (800) 227-8941, www.mazuri.com, Product information at http://www.mazuri.com/PDF/52M5.pdf.

Quikon Multivitamin, Orchid Tree Exotics, 2388 County Road EF, Swanton, OH 43558, (866) 412-5275, www.sunseed.com.

ThermoCare Portable ICS Units ThermoCare Inc., PO Box 6069,

Incline Village, NV 89450, (800) 262-4020, www.thermocare.com.

Pedialyte Abbott Laboratories, Columbus, OH 43215, www.abbott.com.

Portable Brooder, Dean's Animal Supply. PO Box 701172, St. Cloud, FL 34770, (407) 891-8030 www.thebrooder.com.

REFERENCES

Ainley, G.G., Nettleship, D.N., Carter, H.R., and Storey, A.E. 2002. Common Murre (Uria aalge). In The Birds of North America, No. 666. Poole, A. and Gill, F., eds. The Birds of North America, Inc., Philadelphia.

ASLC. 2006a. Alaska Sea Life Center, Seward, Alaska, ASLC Alcid Rearing Protocol (in house publication).

———. Alaska Sea Life Center, Seward, Alaska, ASLC Marine Bird/Mammal Rehabilitation SOP-AVIAN (in house publication).

Byrd, G.V. and Williams, J.C. 1993. Whiskered Auklet (Aethia pygmaea). In The Birds of North America, No. 76. Poole, A. and Gill, F., eds. Philadelphia: The Academy of Natural Sciences; Washington, D.C.: The American Ornithologists' Union.

Day, R.H. and Byrd, G.V. 1989. Food habits of the whiskered auklet at Buldir Island, Alaska. The Condor 91: 65–72.

del Hoyo, J., Elliott, A., and Sargatal, J., eds. 1996. Handbook of the Birds of the World. Vol. 3. Hoatzin to Auks. Lynx Edicions, Barcelona.

Ewins, P.J. 1993. Pigeon Guillemot (Cepphus Columba). In The Birds of North America, No 49. Poole, A. and Gill, F., eds. Philadelphia: The Academy of Natural Sciences; Washington D.C.: The American Ornithologists' Union.

Gaston, A.J. and Hipfner, J.M. 2000. Growth of nestling Thick-billed Murres (Uria lomvia) in relation to parental experience and hatching date. The Auk 119(3): 827–832.

———. 2002. Thick-billed Murre (Uria lomvia). In The Birds of North America, No. 497. Poole, A. and Gill, F., eds. The Birds of North America, Inc., Philadelphia.

Hamer, T.E. and Nelson, S.K. 1995. Characteristics of Marbled Murrelet nest trees and nesting stands. Pages 69–82, In Ecology and Conservation of Marbled Murrelet. Raphael, C.J. and Piatt, J.F. eds. U.S. Department of Agriculture, Forest Service General Technical Report PSW-GTR-152.

Harrison, N.M. 1990. Gelatinous zooplankton in the diet of the parakeet auklet: Comparisons with other auklets. Studies in Avian Biology 14: 114–124.

Hatch, S.A. and Sanger, G.A. 1992. Puffins as samplers of juvenile Pollock and other forage fish in the Gulf of Alaska, Marine Ecology Progress Series, Vol. 80: 1–14.

Huckabee, J.R., DVM. 2006. The Progressive Animal Welfare Society (PAWS), PO Box 1037, Lynnwood, Washington, Personal Communications.

Hunt, G.L., Jr., Harrison, N.M., and Piatt, J.F. 1993. Foraging ecology as related to the distribution of planktivorous auklets in the Bering Sea. Pages 18–26, In Vermeer, K., Briggs, K.T., Morgan, K.H., and Siegel-Causey, D., eds. The Status, Ecology and Conservation of Marine Birds of the North Pacific. Can Wildl Serv Spec Publ, Ottawa.

IBRRC. 2006. International Bird Rescue Research Center; Common Murre, Enclosure and Feeding (in house publication).

Jones, I.L. 1993a. Crested Auklet (Aethia cristatella). In The Birds of North America, No. 70, Poole, A. and Gill, F., eds. Philadelphia: The Academy of Natural Sciences; Washington, D.C.: The American Ornithologists' Union.

———. 1993b. Least Auklet (Aethia pusilla). In The Birds of North America, No. 69, Poole, A. and Gill, F., eds. Philadelphia: The Academy of Natural Sciences; Washington, D.C.: The American Ornithologists' Union.

Jones, I.L., Konyukhov, N.B., Williams, J.C., and Byrd, G.V. 2001. Parakeet Auklet (Aethia psittacula). In The Birds of North America, No. 594, Poole, A. and Gill, F., eds. The Birds of North America, Philadelphia.

Konyukhov, N.B., Zubakin, V.A., Williams, J., and Fischer, J. 2000. Breeding Biology of the Whiskered Auklet (Aethia pygmaea): Incubation, Chick Growth, and Feather Development, Biology Bulletin, Vol 27, No. 2, pp. 164–170.

Litzow, M.A., Piatt, J.F., Prichard, A.K., and Roby, D.D. 2002. Response of pigeon guillemots to variable abundance of high-lipid and low-lipid prey. Oecologia 132: 286–295.

Manuwal, D.A. and Thoresen, A.C. 1993. Cassin's Auklet (Ptychoramphus aleuticus). In The Birds of North America, No. 50, The Birds of North America, Inc., Philadelphia.

Mejeur, J.H., Dierenfeld, E.S., and Murtaugh, J.A. 1988. Development of a Vitamin Supplement for Puffins and Other Alcids, AAZPA 1988 Regional Proceedings, pp. 696–700.

Muzaffar, S.B. and Jones, I.L. 2004. Parasites and diseases of the auks (Alcidae) of the world and their ecology—A review. Marine Ornithology 32: 121–146.

Oehler, D.A., Schmid, S.C., and Miller, M.P. 1995. Maintaining parakeet auklets at the Cincinnati Zoo & Botanical Garden: Handrearing protocol with development and behavioral observations, Vol: 101, No. 1, pp. 3–12.

———. 2001. Maintaining Least Auklet, Aethia pusilla, at the Cincinnati Zoo & Botanical Garden: Hand-rearing protocol with field, development and behavioral observations. Zool Garten N.F. 71: 316–334.

Oehler, D.A., Campbell, C., Edelen, C., Haas, F., Huffman, B., Kinley, R., Lewis, C., Malowski, S., and Schmid, S. 2003. Auklet Husbandry Manual (in house publication; The Cincinnati Zoo and Botanical Garden).

Piatt, J.F. and Kitaysky, A.S. 2002. Horned Puffin (Fratercula corniculata). In The Birds of North America, No. 603, The Birds of North America, Inc., Philadelphia.

Place, A.R. 1992. Comparative aspects of lipid digestion and absorption physiological correlates of wax ester digestion. American Physiological Society 1990 Proceedings, pp. 464–471.

Roby, D.D. 1991. Diet and postnatal energetics in convergent taxa of plankton-feeding seabirds. The Auk 108: 131–146.

Roby, D.D., Place, A.R., and Ricklefs, R.E. 1986. Assimilation and deposition of wax esters in planktivorous seabirds. The Journal of Experimental Zoology 238: 29–41.

Sealy, S.G. 1973. The adaptive significance of post-hatching developmental patterns and growth rates in the Alcidae. Ornis Scand 4: 113–121.

Sprenger, K. 2006. Personal Communications.

Strauch, J.G. 1985. The phylogeny of the Alcidae. The Auk 102: 520–539.

Thomson, T. 1996. Hand Rearing a Tufted Puffin Chick, Animal Keeper's Forum, Vol: 23.

Varoujean, D.H., Sanders, S.D., Graybill, M.R., and Spear, M.R. 1977. Aspects of Common Murre breeding biology. Pacific Seabird Group Bulletin 6: 28.

Wehle, D.H.S. 1983. The food, feeding and development of young tufted and horned puffins in Alaska. Condor 85: 427–442.

12
Ducks, Geese, and Swans

Marjorie Gibson

NATURAL HISTORY

Ducks, geese, and swans are well known in every part of the world, and have a long history of association with humans. They often are the subject of literature, music, and art of all forms, and are an intimate part of human culture (Stromberg 1986). From ancient writings to Shakespeare's sonnets to children's literature, references to these magnificent birds that both fly and swim hold a unique place in our lives (Price 1994). Several species of geese and ducks have been domesticated and bred as farm flocks. Some are legally hunted during certain seasons.

Order Anseriformes, family Anatidae, includes 154 species of swans, geese, true ducks, and whistling ducks. The group is commonly referred to in North America as "waterfowl" and "wildfowl" in Britain (Weller 2001). Species vary dramatically in size, posture, plumage, diet, and breeding habits. Adult body weights range from 230 g to over 13 kg.

Members of the Order Anseriformes are easily recognized as waterfowl even when newly hatched. Young are down-covered and leave the nest immediately or within a few days of hatching (see Figure 12.1). Many species share similarities of structure and form, including large heads, horizontally flattened blunt beaks, long necks, heavy bodies, and webbed feet (Altman 1997; Weller 2001). Smaller species fledge in 6 weeks; the larger ones do not fledge for 10–12 weeks. There is great diversity in natural history and diet, and therefore substantial variation of the manner in which these species are cared for as patients in a captive state.

Waterfowl live in aquatic habitats that include lakes, streams, rivers, oceans, and estuaries. In recent years, several species have shown great adaptability of nesting habitat, expanding their territories into highly urban areas. This adaptability comes with mixed success. A generation ago, urban nesting ducks and geese were rare and generally regarded with fond curiosity. As urban nesting increased, public opinion gradually reflected less fondness, and more concern for sanitation and inconvenience (Erickson 2006). Accommodating territorial adults near a nest site becomes annoying and downright risky. Many species of waterfowl, including swans, have become comfortable with the manicured landscaping of corporate campuses or other urban sites. This is particularly so when landscaping includes a lake or other water elements designed to replicate nature. Rehabilitators become involved when nesting sites are placed too near humans, an adult becomes territorial, or when young have hatched within enclosed courtyards or similar areas that have no foot access to natural habitat.

These species have strong wings, necessary to carry their heavy bodies into flight. The wings are also used effectively for defense. Swans and geese are well known for aggressive defense of their territories and protection of young. Aggression also occurs outside of breeding season in birds that are imprinted to humans. Swans, the largest of the anseriformes, can be dangerous and have been known to break ribs and arms, cause concussions, and even render human captors unconscious with brutal wing beating. They should not be underestimated in terms of strength and tenacity. Do not attempt to rescue an adult or nearly grown swan that is still swimming, because they have the advantage in the water. It is a good idea to work as a team when rescuing any large waterfowl.

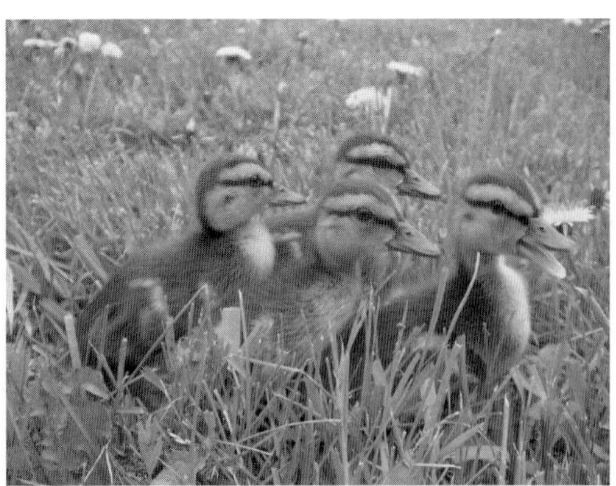

Figure 12.1. Anseriformes such as these mallard ducklings are easily recognized as waterfowl at hatch. Large heads, flattened beaks, and webbed feet are structures common to all species.

Several species have declined significantly in population in recent years; others have responded to conservation habitat restoration and nestbox development efforts (Erickson 2006). With endangered species, captive breeding and reintroduction continue to be utilized. The rehabilitator must be able to recognize species within the region that are of threatened or endangered status, in case one is admitted for care. Special permits are often required by state or provincial government to work with threatened and endangered species.

Waterfowl of various species have been kept and captive bred by aviculturists for many generations throughout the world (Tarsnane 1996). Because of this, a wealth of information on captive care is available online through waterfowl breeders associations, including housing and veterinary care for common species (Wobeser 1981). Excellent age- and species-specific commercial diets can be obtained through

American Coots: Diet and Housing Considerations

Marie Travers

NATURAL HISTORY

Coots and rails belong to order Gruiformes along with cranes, but they are included here with waterfowl due to lifestyle similarities. These are shy wetland species that build floating nests, with chicks precocial at hatching. American Coot hatchlings are quite distinctive in appearance, with blackish down on the back and wings but a bright reddish-orange crown. Feet are large with semilobate toes, as shown in Figure 12a.1. (compare to lobate grebe foot in Figure 7.1).

DIET

Coots and rails are omnivorous and may be offered a wide variety of food items. Very young birds may be more inclined to eat live food, because they are attracted to the movement. Live food items include mealworms, tubifex worms, and minnows. Nonlive food items that can be offered are seed, brine shrimp, krill, duckweed or other greens, small slices of fish, and a small amount of soaked waterfowl starter (or other kibble) mixed with other food items. All of their food should be sprinkled with vitamin B1 and calcium powder.

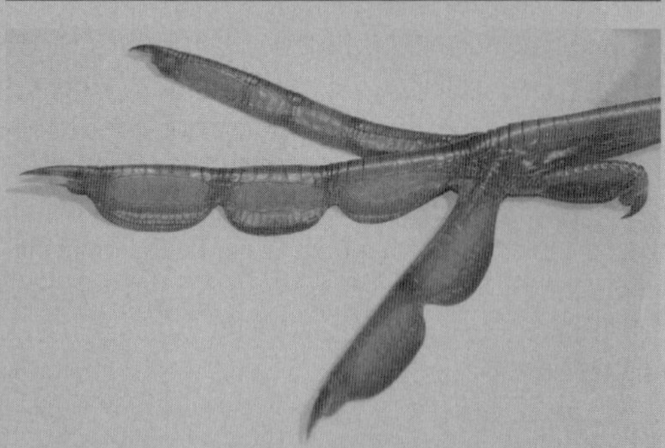

Figure 12a.1. A close look at a coot foot. (Photo Courtesy of David Bozsik)

FOOD PRESENTATION

Food should be offered in shallow dishes such as jar lids, ashtrays, or shallow pans and made to look as natural as possible. Food items that will not contaminate feathers (such as greens) can be offered in a pool.

HOUSING

As somewhat secretive birds, young American Coots can be given plants and/or feather dusters to hide behind. Very young coots should be kept in a 100°F (37.8°C) incubator, and once they are thermoregulating, can be moved to an environment that is half water and half land. Chicks should be monitored closely when introduced to water to make sure they do not get hypothermic. A heat lamp over the land area of their enclosure will help with thermoregulation and with drying after swimming. A shallow pan (less than 1–2 in (2.5–5 cm) deep) can be used in place of a pool so that the birds have an opportunity to swim and become waterproof. Duckweed can be added to the pool so they can eat in the water. Care should be taken to provide an environment where coots do not catch their long toenails. Use of towels can be dangerous because of this, so pillowcases or a nonfabric substrate will help minimize the risk of their nails being caught.

OTHER CONSIDERATIONS

Coots and rails are secretive and high strung, so contact with humans should be kept to a minimum. They are also incredibly fast, so care should be taken when handling them. Once flighted, they are exceptional escape artists.

most farm feed stores. Mazuri brand makes several commonly used products. Due to the wide variation in species requirements, it is important to have good references in one's library to anticipate specific habitat, behavior, or diet questions. Protein, mineral, and fiber requirements vary by species.

It is imperative to stay current on emerging wildlife diseases and local or regional pockets of disease or infection. State or provincial wildlife health agencies have resources that are usually easily accessible.

Waterfowl rely on clean water to maintain health. Most spend their lifetime in or near water. If their habitat is polluted with toxins, bacteria, algae overgrowth, or an oil spill, the birds that utilize the contaminated water will become sick and die. In short, the birds reflect the condition of their habitat.

This chapter focuses on the rehabilitation of wild anseriformes, with emphasis on releasing the birds rather than giving lifelong captive care. Challenges exist for sensitive species that do not thrive well. Much of the literature deals with domesticated rather than wild waterfowl, so allowances have to be made. Chicks, both domestic and wild, do best with the companionship of others of their species. Networking with other wildlife rehabilitators that care for waterfowl is a good idea for the best survival and success.

By Any Other Name

Ducks, geese, and swans are commonly known by the following terms for gender and age:

- *Ducks:* The female is a hen, the male is a drake, and young are ducklings.
- *Geese:* The female is a goose, the male is a gander, and young are goslings.
- *Swans:* The female is a swan, the male is a cob, young are cygnets.

CRITERIA FOR INTERVENTION

Reasons for young waterfowl to be admitted to rehabilitation include "kidnapping" by people, separation from parent shortly after hatch, cat or dog bite, or hypothermia with cold weather hatch. Baby waterfowl attract people. The small size and soft downy appearance of a hatchling contributes to many wild young being taken from nature into human homes. Most of these will be stressed, hypothermic, and starving when admitted to rehabilitation.

Calls from the Public

If a caller is seeking advice about youngsters that are still in the wild, it is important to tell them to give the adult space and privacy in order to come back to a site if they have been startled and scattered due to disturbance. Suggest that the caller observe from a safe distance for at least an hour, unless the youngster is in immediate danger. Offering natural history information about the species will be helpful in determining whether the chick is actually an orphan. If the youngster is already captive but still at the capture site, urge the finder to locate the family with the purpose of reuniting if possible. If the finder and the youngster are away from the capture site, stress that the youngster must remain warm and dry. People are often not aware of the need for supplemental heat, particularly with precocial young that are downy, mobile, and appear self-sufficient. Reinforce that the young are brooded by the adults in nature and are not able to maintain body heat on their own for several weeks after hatch or until contour feathers grow in.

A complete history is important. Ask specific questions such as where was the chick found? What type of habitat? This will give information for species identification. Were adults in the area? The chick may be a species that can be reunited with the adults. What were the circumstances of the finding? There may be injury or other young at the site. How long has it been in captivity? The time away from adults will indicate the degree of starvation or hypothermia. Who has handled the chick? If children are involved there may be unintentional internal injuries to the patient. What is the behavior at the present time? Is it peeping loudly, lying still, or gasping? Has it been in contact with domestic fowl during captivity? If so, isolation may be necessary.

Reunion with Parents

Reuniting families can be successful, but must be done with care and follow-up observation. Some species are agreeable to reuniting and even adopting foster chicks; others will reject chicks and even kill them, usually by drowning. The general rule is if the family or area from which a youngster was taken is known, reunion can be attempted within the day. Some rehabilitators have had success with species such as the Canada Goose accepting foster chicks if the adult has goslings of the same age, but other rehabilitators report unhappy experiences with the same. The same variation is shown with swans. Wild counterparts often reject human-imprinted waterfowl.

Transportation to Wildlife Facility

The chick should be transported as soon as possible. A transport box no more than twice the size of the bird will lower stress and keep the youngster secure. A cardboard box with air holes works well. A towel or dry grass on the bottom of the box will prevent chicks from sliding and possible leg splaying from poor traction. Do not transport with a water bowl. Spilled water will wet the chick and cause hypothermia. Provide supplemental heat during transport, such as from warmed rice bags, hot water bottles or the equivalent. Pad with towels so the chick is not directly in contact with the heat source. A stuffed animal, feather duster, or calm and gentle holding may comfort the youngster during transport.

INITIAL CARE AND STABILIZATION

Newly hatched waterfowl, regardless of the species, have the following common needs: heat, water, and nutrition, given in that order. A young waterfowl patient that is hypothermic is always critical and must be tended to immediately. It is important to bring the temperature up quickly or death will result. Before a physical exam can be done, the bird must have a normal core body temperature. Hypothermic chicks should not be given oral food or water. The digestive system does not function until the core body temperature is restored. Massage the patient with a warmed towel to stimulate response and increase circulation. To warm a chilled bird, a heating pad set on low setting can be used. Nonresponsive patients should never be left on heat without constant monitoring. Heating pads and lamps can overheat debilitated patients unable to move from the heat. Death may result.

Once the chick is stabilized, offer warmed electrolyte fluid such as human infant rehydration solutions to the tip of the beak. In small species, this can be from the tip of a finger. A spoon or syringe will work with larger birds. The action of swallowing when accompanied by fluid will stimulate intestine function. Once hydration is complete, tube-feed with a weak mixture of baby cereal and water. Use small amounts at first until the chick defecates. Long red rubber catheters make excellent feeding tubes, with an appropriate diameter used based on body size of the chick. The tube-feeding amount should be as small as 0.1 ml for the smallest ducklings to 2 ml for a cygnet. Initial tube-feedings are meant to further stimulate peristalsis rather than filling the crop, because once these species are stable they should eat and drink on their own. When the birds are stable and mobile, they can be put into a brooder set up as described below.

Be sure the birds are eating. Do not assume the youngsters are eating and drinking unless directly observed swallowing water and with food disappearing down their beak. Young birds often nibble at food and move it around, giving the appearance of eating, but they are not ingesting enough or any at all. Weighing chicks and documenting weight gain is important during the first 2 weeks of life. Stimulation that mirrors circumstances that occur in the wild may be needed for sensitive species in order to get them eating and drinking. Mallard ducklings are low-stress birds, eat eagerly unless injured, and can be used as models to encourage more sensitive species to eat. Young Canada geese can provide the same service for larger waterfowl.

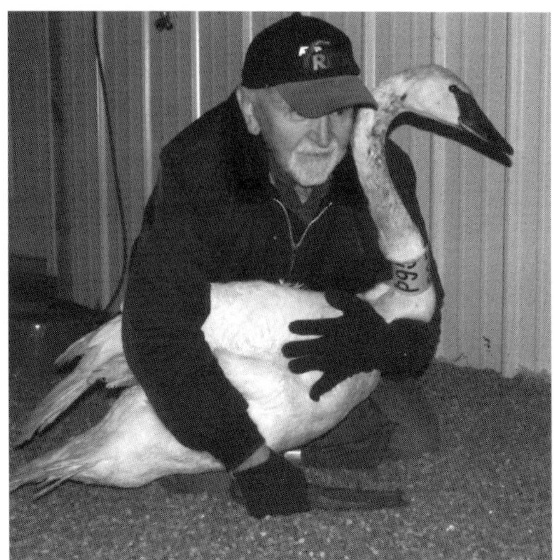

Figure 12.2. A trumpeter swan being restrained by Don Gibson. It is very important to restrain the wings and provide support to the feet when picking up a swan. These birds may be fractious.

Tips on Teaching to Drink and Eat

Ducklings and other newly hatched waterfowl do not drink or eat easily on their own once separated from their parents. Observe the young bird. If it does not drink on its own take it in hand and gently tip its beak into the water dish. After a few efforts the chick should began to drink on its own. If it does not, repeat the process until it drinks on its own. Offering electrolyte solution alternately with water is a good practice for the first week of life.

Cavity-nesting ducks have natural techniques to stimulate eating. By their natural history it is known that within the first day, these ducklings take their first step out of the nesting cavity and tumble to the ground. This tumble is sometimes from impressive heights, without apparent injury. Their first meal follows this event. The most common cavity-nesting ducks in North America are Wood Ducks, Mergansers, Buffleheads, and Common Goldeneyes. All are considered high-stress and difficult to raise in captivity. When orphaned, these nervous species go into stress overload. To help them over the trauma we can simulate a new start in life. Taking a hint from their natural history, the best thing to do with a newly hatched cavity-nesting species is to literally "drop" it from several feet into the brooder. When the chick lands, life begins anew. Use freshwater as opposed to saltwater—even if the bird is an ocean or marine species such as the King Eider. The salt gland, which enables marine birds to excrete excess salt, is poorly developed in ducklings (Weller 2001). Saltwater will be fatal until chicks are nearly feathered. This may seem like a crazy method, but it works for most youngsters. Be certain of the species before attempting this method of stimulation. Ground-nesting species are not made for "taking the plunge" into life.

Restraint

Young waterfowl are often very active and can escape even a firm grasp. A towel dropped over the top of the back of a patient and wrapped under the legs is helpful in securing the bird and preventing damage to the legs and developing wings.

Adult birds can be restrained in the same manner as chicks. Adult waterfowl use their wings as a method of defense. It is important to maintain control of the wings, keeping them firmly against the restrainer's body as well as the legs to prevent injury to the bird and the rehabilitator (see Figure 12.2).

COMMON MEDICAL PROBLEMS AND SOLUTIONS

Infectious Diseases

Waterfowl carry many types of parasites, not all of which are dangerous to them, as well as viruses, bacteria, and other disease-causing agents (Altman et al. 1997; Ritchie 1995; Wobeser 1981). Wild birds should be prevented from contact with domestic birds. Disease transference can occur and spread during migration (Ritchie 1995). See Chapter 17, "Domestic Poultry," for more in-depth information on common diseases and parasite problems in domestic anseriformes. Many treatments are good for one species and harmful to another. It is therefore important to consult an avian veterinarian with waterfowl experience. Some states have required testing for diseases such as Newcastle's, duck plague, avian influenza, and others. Check governmental requirements before networking with rehabilitators out of state or transferring birds to out-of-state migratory areas for release.

Bumblefoot

Foot problems are common with wildfowl that are raised or kept in captivity. In natural habitats, waterfowl live and rear young around lakes, wetlands, and ocean estuaries. Water, muddy, or bog areas effectively massage the foot constantly as the bird walks or swims. Hard or harsh substrates are unnatural to the footpad and contribute to callusing and bumblefoot (pododermatitis), particularly in heavy-bodied waterfowl. Bumblefoot is a serious disease in large waterfowl and is fatal in many cases. For this reason, birds should not be kept on cement floors without padding. Substrates used in housing waterfowl should allow the foot to sink into the substrate with each step (Ritchie et al. 1994). Appropriate substrate includes carpet (when housed indoors), artificial turf, pea gravel, sand, and natural soil.

Waterfowl in captivity should be examined monthly for signs of footpad calluses or lesions. As a preventive measure in addition to appropriate substrate, massage of the foot with lanolin cream (udder balm) is suggested once per month or whenever the bird is handled. Soaking the foot in canola oil may also be beneficial. If calluses are visible, warm-water pulse massage and foot massage treatments with lanolin cream should be done twice per week to prevent bumblefoot from developing. Prevent feathers from contacting oil or udder balm.

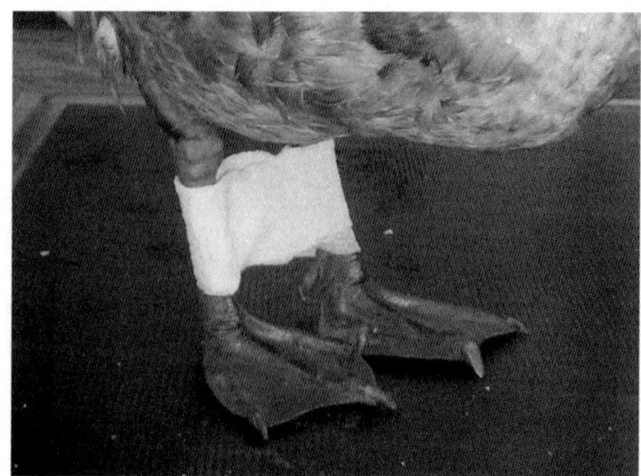

Figure 12.3. This juvenile Canada Goose suffered splayed legs from impact injury to the back. Note the soft splint that holds his legs in a normal position while allowing him to function while healing.

Splayed Legs

Leg splaying can result when a young bird slips on unstable substrate, stretching ligaments beyond normal range. If caught early, it can be corrected by using Vetrap (3M) or similar material to "soft-splint" legs in a natural position (this is also sometimes called "hobbling"). The feet should be separated by normal standing/walking distance. The bird should be able to walk and maintain normal behavior with the splint on its legs. Standing and walking while splinted is important to maintain muscle tone and development (see Figure 12.3). Depending on the severity of the problem, the legs should remain splinted for a few days to a week. Adjust the splint daily in a newly hatched bird to accommodate the rapid growth (Altman et al. 1997).

Mud-balling

Mud-balling occurs when material, such as mud or feces, adhere and form a ball around the foot of a young bird. If the problem becomes severe the bird may be unable to walk or move naturally. Mud-balling sometimes occurs in nature in habitats with clay soil and in brooders during captive rearing. Most cases that develop in brooders are due to wet feces sticking to the feet and combining with wood shavings or other substrates. Early intervention is important to prevent foot or leg deformity or death from exhaustion. See Chapter 18, "Wild Turkeys,

Quail, Grouse, and Pheasants," for photographs and more information on mud-balling (Welty and Baptista 1988).

Trauma

Damage to the wings, face, and beak may occur when a bird comes into contact with wire fencing or occasionally in a territorial dispute with another bird. Injuries can be very severe, causing blindness and even death of a patient. If a bird is observed pacing a fenced area in escape attempts or coming into physical contact with it, remove the bird from the pen immediately until privacy screening or solid barrier on the perimeter fence can be installed. If bleeding or injury is evident, stop bleeding with pressure, wash the area, and apply topical water-soluble antibiotic cream to prevent secondary infection.

Angel Wing

Geese and swans in particular should be watched carefully for development of *angel wing,* a condition thought to be nutritionally based. In this condition, the flight feathers at the wingtip flip up and out, giving the appearance that suggests its name. It is also referred to as *airplane, reversed, slipped, or sword wing*. There are several dietary factors that may contribute to the malady. Diets high in sulfur-producing amino acids, deficiency of vitamin E and manganese, plus high protein for some species, have been cited as factors (Ritchie et al. 1994). The physical problem begins when the weight of the flight feathers and gravity pulls the carpal joint down and out. Angel wing can be corrected if intercepted early. Wrapping the wing to itself in a natural position for a few days should correct the problem. Untreated, the wing will be permanently deformed.

Lead Poisoning

Lead poisoning is a serious but unfortunately common problem in waterfowl coming into rehabilitation. In the United States alone it is estimated 2.4 million waterfowl die yearly from lead poisoning (Ritchie et al. 1994). Birds come into contact with lead in the wild in various ways, including swallowing lead sinkers commonly used for fishing, lead shot from bullets, or ingestion of mine wastes. The possibility of lead poisoning should be considered with all swans and, to a lesser degree, geese.

Birds admitted with lead poisoning may have a variety of symptoms that include low weight, weakness, inability to walk or use legs well, wing droop, and the signature grass-green feces. Often feathers on the chest and crop area may be soiled due to vomiting. Patients with lead poisoning also will be generally lethargic, anemic, and dehydrated. Not all symptoms need to be present and will vary with patient, species, amount of toxicity, and source of lead. Many will be unable to digest food. Vomiting is common. In these cases, fluids should be given subcutaneously. Oral tube-feeding in small amounts can be attempted, keeping in mind that aspiration may result if the bird regurgitates the oral diet. If the crop empties and the bird is defecating, more liquid diet can be fed (see the section "Emaciation Diet for Debilitated Waterfowl," later in this chapter). Offer the bird water, but do not allow it to eat grain or solid food until the digestive system is functioning normally.

Blood testing and diagnostic imaging play an important role in diagnosis of lead poisoning, and early diagnosis and treatment is imperative. If metallic densities are observed on x-ray, gastric lavage or endoscopic removal of metal pieces (Ritchie et al. 1994) may be required. Consult an avian veterinarian in lead poisoning cases. Calcium sodium versenate or dimercaptosuccinic acid (DMSA) are often used to chelate lead from the blood stream.

Many states have banned the use of lead for waterfowl hunting, but lead shot is often used in small and large game hunting as well as fishing. Lead does not degrade in the environment. Swans in particular encounter lead pellets when water levels are low and they eat material from the bottom of lakes or streams. Conservation groups often have material available on nontoxic alternatives to lead sinkers and lead shot that may be helpful to create an awareness of the problem.

Botulism

Young waterfowl may present with botulism. *Clostridium botulinum* grows in anaerobic conditions, when bodies of water become warm and have poor flow. This bacteria produces a toxin that paralyzes the neuromuscular junctions of affected animals. Birds are exposed when they eat invertebrates in the water that have the toxin in their tissues. Affected birds display varying degrees of paralysis of the neck, legs, and wings, and often have odorous diarrhea. Severe cases may have difficulty breathing.

Mild to moderately affected birds have an excellent prognosis. Unlike lead poisoning, this disease may result in dozens or even hundreds of birds of mixed species presenting at once, often from a particular water source.

Because this disease is an intoxication rather than an infection, antibiotics are of no use. Provide birds with supportive care, including frequent tube-feedings of small amounts of oral fluids to flush any remaining invertebrates from the intestines. After 24 hours of frequent tube-feedings, switch to a more nutritious tube-feeding formula, such as the emaciation diet given in this chapter. Keep birds clean and comfortable, with heads elevated above the body to reduce regurgitation and ease respiration. A laundry basket with a towel over thick bedding of shredded paper makes appropriate temporary housing for affected birds to prevent problems with pressure sores on legs. Apply eye ointment several times daily because some birds may be unable to blink. Unlike mammals, birds recover from botulism very quickly, often within 1–2 weeks. Many birds will regain the ability to hold their heads up within 2–4 days and will be able to stand and eat within a week.

DIETS

Diet variation is a huge issue when rearing waterfowl. One species may do very well on commercial duckling starter; the next species may need live food to survive. It cannot be stressed enough that birds coming into care at a rehabilitation facility must be correctly identified in order to care for them successfully (Baicich and Harrison 2005). There are a few "first" foods that waterfowl young respond to universally. These "first" foods are not meant to be the only food offered. The health of young waterfowl requires a varied diet (see Figure 12.4).

First Foods

After stabilization feedings, introduce wild growing duckweed or watercress. It is one of the best first foods for young waterfowl. Duckweed contains tiny invertebrates important for rapid growth. Wild ducklings, goslings, and cygnets readily eat natural greens (Stromberg 1986). Duckweed can be legally collected from lakes or streams and maintained under refrigeration for a week or more. With fresh water, gently rinse as much as needed for a day's feeding until water runs clear but most natural material remains. Natural greens have organisms that occur naturally in the wild. In the past, some sources have expressed concern about introducing potentially pathogenic organisms to young waterfowl. That concern may be valid for those birds that are domestic or remain captive; however, this author suggests rehabilitated birds will experience these upon release and it is better to do that with a natural immunity developed from hatch.

Float the greens in a shallow pan of water and place it in the brooder box. Water dishes should have a ramp to facilitate access into and out of the pan for

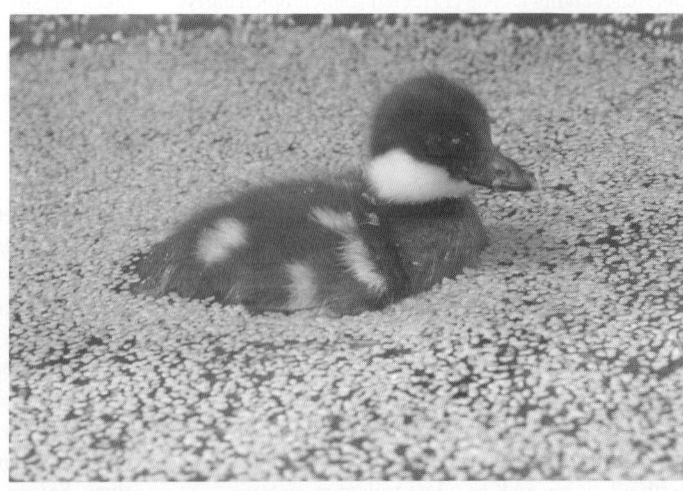

Figure 12.4. This young Common Goldeneye is enjoying fresh duckweed and working on waterproofing plumage at the same time.

small species. Change water and rinse greens frequently, or when soiled with feces. If there is no access to natural duckweed, finely chopped romaine lettuce can be used. Small amounts of dried bloodworms available in pet store tropical fish departments, human baby cereal available in grocery stores, or Waterfowl Starter (Mazuri) crushed into a powder can be added to the duckweed water to increase protein and food taste experience. More advanced chicks will appreciate the addition of small minnows and insects to the duckweed water.

Many young birds refuse to eat dry food. Wetting food may increase success. However, wet mash sours easily and should be changed at least twice per day. Commercial starter pellets come in a variety of sizes. They can be crushed into a powder for very young waterfowl. For reluctant eaters, the powdered starter can be sprinkled over the youngsters' backs. While preening, the chick will naturally get some of the powder into its mouth and may begin the eating process. Soaked feline and canine growth pellets such as Science Diet (Hills), and crushed hard-boiled egg can be used as part of a successful starter diet for young waterfowl.

"Shoveling" best describes the method of eating for anseriformes. The beak works as a strainer to take in tiny invertebrates and grasses. Dry mash can be a hazard to swallow when it forms a paste with the bird's natural saliva. Water must be in close proximity to the food to allow normal food intake. Pellets are preferred to mash in most species, because it is easier to eat.

Listing foods for all anseriformes is a nearly impossible task due to the great variety in diet. The best information available for species not addressed in this chapter is a field guide that includes diet information (Elphick et al. 2001). As a general rule, youngsters eat mostly insects or invertebrate protein their first few weeks or month of life and graduate to the wide variety of foods references list for adults as they develop to maturity. Local natural areas will be the guide as to what insects, invertebrates, or other listed diet items are available during nesting season and therefore used as food for waterfowl. General foods are minnows, crayfish, insects including grasshoppers, crickets, and mealworms, as well as a variety of grains and grasses.

Shallow dishes or saucers make appropriate dishes for ducklings. Cake-pan size and depth dishes are needed for goslings and cygnets. Water founts, available in most farm equipment supply stores for domestic fowl, may be used. Whenever using smooth dishes the birds may enter or smoothly surfaced floors, be sure to cover the bottom with sand or pea gravel to assure stable footing. This will prevent the legs from slipping and splaying out (see the discussion on splayed legs in the "Medical Problems and Solutions" section earlier in this chapter). Include marbles or gravel in the bottom of water founts to prevent the youngsters from entering the water and possibly drowning. As odd as it sounds, waterfowl young do drown in shallow water. Water must be changed often and dishes disinfected to prevent bacterial growth and subsequent illness.

Aggressive behavior at the food dish suggests that more food or a different variety of food is needed. Increased urgency in "peeping" occurs when chicks are hungry or lonely. If the feces are normal consistency and the chick is eating, it may not be eating adequately. It may be advisable to supplement tube-feedings a few times to see whether the vocalizations calm, and offer new food variety such a small minnows or active insects. Examine the vent if chicks appear fluffed and tired or are avoiding other chicks. Soft feces can dry and build up on down near the vent and not allow the chick to defecate. In this case, wash the area with warm water until the material is removed.

Emaciation Diet for Debilitated Waterfowl

The following is a recommended diet for emaciated waterfowl:

- 2 oz (56 g) human baby mixed grain cereal, such as Gerber's brand
- One 2.5 oz (71 g) jar of Gerber's baby meat food (beef, chicken, turkey or veal)
- One 2.5 oz (71 g) jar water
- One 2.5 oz (71 g) jar human infant electrolyte replacer such as Pedialyte

Whip ingredients together, adding more water if needed, until the diet will pass through an appropriately sized French red rubber feeding tube (catheter tube). Make the diet thinner for very weak patients.

Diet should be prepared fresh each feeding in the amount needed. Feed the amount that fills the crop and is able to be moved out of the crop in an hour. If the chick regurgitates or fluid comes up, cut back the quantity given. Continue tube-feedings until the chick is eating on its own. Offer food items when the chick is able to stand. The diet must be warmed to 90°F (32°C) when administered, but it should not be hot or crop burns will result. Microwave heating is not recommended due to uneven heating of the food particles. Feeding cold diet may well put a fragile patient into shock and result in death.

HOUSING

Waterfowl vary greatly in size. As another general rule, chicks of the same size and age can be put together even with species variation. Mixed housing has advantages and disadvantages that must be weighed. A singleton of any species will likely not survive. If it does, the chick may imprint on the caregiver and not be releasable to the wild. Older chicks may suffocate, injure, or not allow newly hatched young to feed. Use care if this is the only option for housing. Older chicks that have begun to eat on their own may encourage and teach younger ones how to eat and drink. Observe the birds carefully for any aggression and separate immediately if it occurs, especially if mixing age groups. Networking with other waterfowl rehabilitators is suggested and very helpful with housing multiple species or varied ages.

Brooders

Brooder boxes can be made from a variety of materials. Dry brooders have no option for swimming; wet brooders do. Each has benefits and drawbacks. Experience, including what species is most common in the region and numbers of patients expected, will be the best method of selecting which box and brooder type will work for a particular facility (see Figure 12.5). Many breeders use a "walk-in" wooden box about 6 ft (1.8 m) high to accommodate highly active cavity-nesting duck species as well as geese and swans. Other breeders find that a rectangle-shaped plastic storage container makes a very good brooder for most young waterfowl. A large cardboard box works well as a dry brooder. The size of the container will vary according to species and numbers of chicks.

A box 42 × 24 × 36 in (1 × 0.6 × 0.9 m) will accommodate up to eight newly hatched ducklings. Some species of ducklings, "jumpers," or larger waterfowl require taller containers. Cardboard can be used to increase the height of the brooder box. Do not use wire, because some species of cavity-nesting ducks hatch with toenails and will use the wire as a "stairway" to escape. Larger waterfowl may injure their beaks on wire. Pea gravel, course sand, or carpet sample pieces all make good substrate for the bottom of the brooder. Wood shavings, straw, and newspaper may be ingested by chicks and should not be used as substrate. Wet carpet and towels can harbor fungus and must be replaced when they are wet or soiled. Fine sand many irritate the eyes of hatchlings. Hard substrate such as cement will cause foot problems and should not be used. For

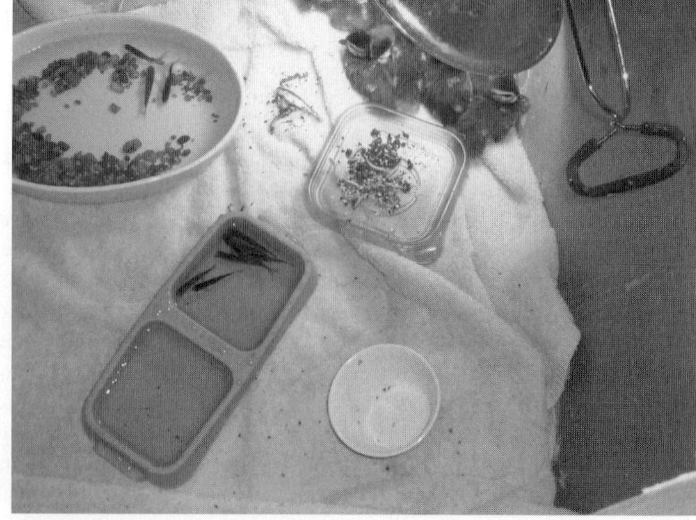

Figure 12.5. A brooder can be a simple box, with nonslip substrate and a clip-on reflector lamp secured in one corner. Temperature under the lamp should be 95—99°F (34.7—37.4°C).

the first few days of rehabilitation, place a white muslin cloth or towel on top of the substrate. A white background will allow the rehabilitator to assess the dropping of the young birds, both for color and consistency, indicating problems from not eating or digestion issues (Rupley 1997).

A heat lamp firmly fixed to one corner of the brooder box should keep the temperature under the lamp between 95—99°F (35.0—37.2°C). In the case of rearing only a few chicks, the lamp can be as simple as a reflector-style clip-on lamp with a 40—60 watt bulb. Raising or lowering the lamp can easily adjust the heat. Commercial brooders and heat lamps are available at farm supply stores if caring for larger numbers of hatchlings.

Observation of behavior will be the best guide to several factors including whether heat lamp is adequate, too cold, or too warm; whether brooder box space is adequate or a larger area is needed; and whether enough food is available. Chicks that huddle under the heat lamp are cold and need increased heat. Chicks that stand away from the heat lamp or have their wings hanging are overheated. Chicks should have ample room to walk and exercise without being crowded (Tarsnane 1996; Ritchie et al. 1994; Altman et al. 1997).

If caring for a single youngster, a clean cotton mop head (Ritchie et al. 1994) or feather duster and a mirror in combination with a windup alarm clock that ticks may offer the chick security. If using a feather duster, check for preservatives on the feathers that may give off toxic fumes when wet.

Access to Swimming

Anseriforme young are nidifugous (i.e., leave the nest shortly after hatching), and when with their parents can eat, swim, and dive soon after hatch (Ritchie et al. 1994). Having said that, chicks are not waterproof when hatched and depend on their parents or parent to waterproof them, preening on oil from the adult oil gland. Putting young chicks that have not had parental assistance in waterproofing into the water will be fatal, due to hypothermia or drowning. Once the chicks are stable and eating, usually several days after admission, begin to expose young birds to brief warm-water swims for a minute or two, and then put them back into the dry brooder under heat. If the chicks begin to shiver in the water, take them out immediately and put them under the brooder at 95—99°F (35.2—37.2°C). Short periods of swimming will encourage preening, which is necessary to repel water from the chicks. Dry brooders should be used for 10—14 days, or until the young birds are eating well and comfortable with finding the heat lamp when chilled. Supplemental heat will be required for most waterfowl young until they are feathered. However, heat lamp temperatures can be gradually lowered to 75°F (24°C) by age 3 weeks and maintained at that temperature, allowing the young to choose heat if they desire.

Feather development varies by species and even between broods. Young waterfowl that have undergone physiological stress from starvation, injury, or even captivity itself in very sensitive species, may have delayed development and need more time in a dry brooder. As a general rule, young waterfowl should be maintained in a confined area with the option of a heat lamp until fully feathered. Due to the wide range of problems that may affect development with birds in rehabilitation, the rehabilitator will be the best judge of when it is safe to move young from an indoor brooder to an outdoor pen. Weather including rain or other inclement conditions will be a factor.

Outside Pens

Intermediate pens housing juvenile birds should have both indoor and outdoor access. The inside area should be protected from the elements and have a heat lamp, food, and water available. The size of these areas depends on how many young are in care. An outdoor grassy area 20 × 20 × 6 feet (6 × 6 × 1.8 m) will accommodate eight juvenile ducks. Overcrowding waterfowl can cause stress and disease. Pens made to raptor specifications work well because the young have access to natural sun and rain and protection from predators (Gibson 1996). A solid visual barrier 2—5 ft high from the ground, depending on species, lowers stress and injury due to contact with fencing.

Water is a common requirement for waterfowl (see Figure 12.6). All need access to some form of pond or swimming pool prior to release to the wild. Swimming will assure that feathers are waterproofed as well as provide needed exercise and experience. A children's swimming pool works well for a small number of birds. Use a ramp to assist chicks in and out of the water. Larger ponds should be used for larger species or large numbers of ducklings. Waterfowl are messy eaters and defecate frequently. Food and feces often end up in ponds. Water must be kept clean, with pools being drained and water changed

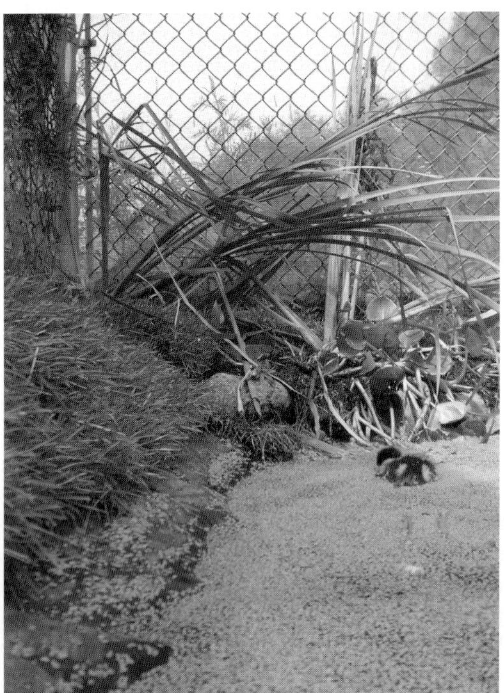

Figure 12.6. A young merganser in an outdoor aviary pond, with ample vegetation and duckweed over the water surface.

often. A good filtration system should be installed in larger ponds.

Keeping Predators Out

Predator guards must be in place on all outdoor pens. There are several methods to prevent predators from accessing patients. Multiple methods, including buried fencing, electric fencing, humane trapping of persistent predators, or other techniques may be required on a single enclosure in order to adequately protect wild patients. It will be necessary to customize the protection of enclosures to the predators and type of soil native to the region. This information will be best obtained from wildlife agencies within each region.

The best approach to protecting patients from predation is to take steps not to attract predators to the pens. This will involve not leaving excess food lying about and cleaning up spillage of grain outside the pen should it occur. Solid barrier fences will block visual attraction. Trees near or bordering enclosures may allow avian predators to perch or climbing predators to use as a launching platform to access the enclosure; these should be eliminated. Digging animals such as skunks can be discouraged with buried 1 × .5 in (2.5 × 1.3 cm) galvanized wire. The wire should be buried 2 ft (0.7 m) straight into the ground and angled outward from the pen another 2 ft (0.7 m). The use of galvanized moderate- to heavy-gauge wire is wise because less substantial wire will deteriorate in the ground and require costly maintenance or replacement every few years. Some rehabilitators have success using multiple strands of electric fencing on the outside of the perimeter fencing. This technique will discourage climbing predators such as raccoons, mink, and fishers. Several strands of electrical fencing starting inches from the ground and going to approximately 5 feet (1.5 m) from the ground are generally adequate to discourage most predators. Check with local wildlife officials for a list of predators that frequent the area and for regulations for legal means to control them. Humane trapping using live traps or other methods may be needed for persistent predators. Local regulations affect the translocation of live-trapped predators. Under no circumstances should poison be used to control predators. The chance of poisoning non-target species is great, including the patients being protected. For the most complete protection, the enclosure should be covered or enclosed to prevent avian predation, wild visitors that may bring parasites or other problems to pens, and premature release.

HUMAN IMPRINTING

Waterfowl, particularly geese and swans, imprint easily on humans. Raising a single bird of these species without a foster parent, adult model, or conspecifics almost assures the bird will be imprinted. Large-bodied imprinted waterfowl can be dangerous to humans and should be kept with care and never be allowed to range freely.

RELEASE

Youngsters remain with the adult until fully feathered and, in some cases, through the first winter. Fully feathered juvenile ducks, familiar with natural food, can be released into a natural habitat, preferably with wild birds of the same species. Waterfowl releases ideally are done away from human activity. Release should be done in the morning to allow young birds time to adapt, integrate with the wild population, and find cover for the night.

Larger species may stay in family groups through the first winter. If migratory flocks can be located, most species of geese can be successfully released into the flock. If larger numbers of geese of the same species are reared together at a rehabilitation center, they form a "family group" and do well released together. Rehabilitated adults can be integrated with juvenile birds and released with the young birds.

Swans can be aggressive with cygnets not their own. A close working relationship with state and federal wildlife agencies is important to develop a release plan for larger species that may require overwintering and a spring release for better success.

EXOTIC SPECIES

Aviculturists, game farms, and zoos care for and breed a vast array of waterfowl species, not all of which are native to a region or even a given continent. Because many of these birds can fly, escape is always possible and does occur. Some species may adapt well and thrive while others die from starvation or exposure in an environment to which they are not suited. Exotic species compete and often conflict with native species. If a facility admits a patient that is not native to the area, do not release it even if it was found in the wild. Finding captive placement for the bird with a zoo or game farm is the best solution for the individual bird and for the future of native wildlife.

ACKNOWLEDGMENTS

In honor of E95, a Trumpeter Swan, an early member of the State of Wisconsin Trumpeter Swan reintroduction program and frequent Raptor Education Group patient. He changed our world and will always have a place in our hearts. Many thanks to the men and women of our state and federal wildlife agencies, particularly Pat Manthey and Sumner Matteson of State of Wisconsin BER. Thanks to aviculturists and conservation groups that continue to contribute to habitat and species preservation, assuring a place for our magnificent waterfowl.

SOURCES FOR PRODUCTS MENTIONED

Mazuri Waterfowl Starter: Mazuri, P.O. Box 66812, St. Louis, MO 63166, (800) 227-8941, www.mazuri.com.

Science Diet: Hill's Pet Nutrition, Inc., Consumer Affairs, P.O. Box 148, Topeka, KS 66601-0148, (800) 445-5777, www.hillspet.com.

REFERENCES

Altman, R.B., Clubb, S.L., Dorrestein, G.M., and Quesenberry, K. 1997. Avian Medicine and Surgery. W.B. Saunders Co., Philadelphia, pp. 944–959.

Anderson Brown, A.F. and Robins, G.E.S. 2002. The New Incubation Book. Hancock House Publishing Ltd., Blaine, Washington, pp. 206–213.

Baicich, P.J. and Harrison, C.J.O. 2005. Nest, Eggs, and Nestlings of North American Birds, Second Edition. Princeton University Press, Princeton, New Jersey, 347 pp.

Elphick, C., Dunning, J.B., Jr., and Sibley, D.A. 2001. The Sibley Guide to Bird Life and Behavior. Alfred A. Knopf, Inc., New York, pp. 73–77, 190–211.

Erickson, L. 2006. 101 Ways to Help Birds. Stackpole Books, Mechanicsburg, Pennsylvania, pp. 43, 166, 217.

Gibson, M. 1996. The ABC's of housing raptors. Journal of Wildlife Rehabilitation 19(3): 23–31.

———. 1997. Natural history: Square one for wildlife rehabilitation. Journal of Wildlife Rehabilitation 17(1): 3–6, 16.

Price, A.L. 1994. Swans of the World in History, Myth and Art. Council Oak Books, Tulsa, Oklahoma, pp. 14, 131–153.

Ritchie, B.W. 1995. Avian Viruses: Function and Control. Wingers Publishing, Inc., Lake Worth, Florida, pp. 50–73, 329.

Ritchie, B.W., Harrison, G.J., and Harrison, L.R. 1994. Avian Medicine: Principles and Application. Wingers Publishing Inc., Lake Worth, Florida, 1384 pp.

Rogers, L.J. and Kaplan, G. 2000. Songs, Roars and Rituals, Communications in Birds, Mammals, and Other Animals. Harvard University Press, Cambridge, Massachusetts, pp. 20, 83, 90.

Rupley, A. 1997. Manual of Avian Practice. W.B. Saunders, Philadelphia, pp. 265–291.

Sibley, D.A. 2000. The Sibley Guide to Birds. Alfred A. Knopf, Inc., New York, pp. 70–103.

Stromberg, L. 1986. Swan Breeding and Management. Stromberg Publishing Company, Pine River, Minnesota, 95 pp.

Tarsnane, S. 1996. Waterfowl Care, Breeding and Conservation. Hancock House Publishing Ltd., Blaine, Washington, 288 pp.

Weller, M.L. 2001. Ducks, Geese, and Swans. In The Sibley Guide to Bird Life and Behavior, Elphick, C., Dunning, J.B., and Sibley, D.A., eds. Alfred A. Knopf, Inc., New York, 588 pp.

Welty, J.C. and Baptista, L. 1988. The Life of Birds, Fourth Edition. HBJ College Publishing, pp. 95, 103, 393, 379.

Wobeser, G.A. 1981. Diseases of Wild Waterfowl, Second Edition. Plenum Press, New York, pp. 153–157, 165–187, 223.

HELPFUL WEBSITES

http://www.npwrc.usgs.gov/resource/1999/woodduck/wdnbox.htm.

http://www.nwwildfowl.com/Veterinary-care.htm.

Loon Watch: http://www.northland.edu/loonwatch.

Raptor Education Group, Inc., http://www.raptoreducationgroup.org.

State of Minnesota Pollution Control Agency, http://www.cleancarcampaign.org/GettingLeadOUT.pdf.

13
Eagles

Nancy A. Lang

NATURAL HISTORY

There are 68 species of true eagles found in the order Accipitriformes and family Accipitridae. They include the following numbers of species: 10 fish and fishing-eagles, 22 snake and serpent-eagles, 4 harpy eagles, 1 Indian black eagle (*Ictinaetus malayensis*), 9 Aquila eagles, and 22 hawk eagles (Ferguson-Lees and Christie 2001). The majority of species build stick nests, but nest types vary even within a species and may include cliff or ground nests. Incubation length increases with egg size. Smaller eagles produce smaller eggs. The larger eggs take longer for embryonic development. Two species of eagles breed regularly in North America, the bald eagle (*Haliaeetus leucocephalus*) and the golden eagle (*Aquila chrysaetos*). Their incubation periods are 35 days for the bald eagle and 41 to 45 days for the golden eagle. Both species fledge from the nest in approximately 11 weeks.

Eagles generally have strong beaks and feet. The shape of the bill is similar to that of the talons, and both are adapted for foraging. The feet, which have four toes and talons, are powerful and allow eagles to efficiently catch and carry prey. Foot strength varies according to dietary adaptations (Ferguson-Lees and Christie 2001).

Adult diets consist of everything from nest contents of other species, including eggs, taken by the Indian black eagle, to primates taken by the Philippine eagle *Pithecophaga jefferyi* (Ferguson-Lees and Christie 2001).

Because there are numerous species of eagles and because there are many differences in natural history, it is critically important to understand the dietary, social, and behavioral needs of the birds that come into your care. Ferguson-Lees and Christie (2001), provide a concise, up-to-date, accurate accounting of all 68 species. They also provide an extensive bibliography that will allow animal managers find more in-depth information about the eagles they rear.

CRITERIA FOR INTERVENTION

Eagles are hand-reared for a variety of reasons. They are brought into captivity when nests are abandoned or one or both parents die. Eagle chicks that jump or fall from nests prior to fledging may be placed back in nests if they are healthy and not injured. If they leave the nest on a subsequent occasion or if they sustain injury as a result of the jump or fall or are found to be ill, they will require hand-rearing. Abandoned eggs may be incubated, and the subsequent hatchlings are then hand-reared. Some eagle chicks are hand-reared after being illegally removed from nests by members of the public, who realize the difficulties of caring for eagle chicks and will bring them into rehabilitation centers or zoos for rearing. Finally, eggs or eaglets are removed from nests for hand-rearing for propagation or education programs.

RECORD KEEPING

Detailed records are imperative for hand-rearing programs. They aid the animal management team in assessing the progress of individuals. Over time, records are vital for improving rearing techniques for each species encountered.

It is important, whenever possible, to gather information on the exact location from which the chick was taken. The name, address, phone number, and email address of the person that found or took the bird should be entered in the chick's permanent record. If the person providing you with the eaglet is not the same as the person that found or took the bird, every effort should be made to obtain the above information on the individual who first acquired the bird. As questions arise about the eagle's health or future disposition, information obtained by the person who first acquired the bird may be helpful. Upon admission, a complete medical examination should take place. An admission form is useful for gathering information on chicks that need to be hand-reared.

Once the eaglet is received, whether it is acquired or it hatches at your facility, a detailed daily record must be kept. The records become a vital part of the daily and weekly communication system between staff members, and more importantly they become a part of a critical data base for improving each species' hand-rearing program as more individuals are raised over time.

Each day, and with each observation or interaction with the chick, written records should be kept. Weigh the chick each morning prior to the first feeding and record the weight. To properly monitor the chick's development, record the following information: medical problems and treatments; behavioral and unusual postural changes, including attitude toward food; dietary consumption; and unusual feces. If possible on a weekly basis, measure growth parameters that include wing and tail length, bill width and depth, tarsus length, and foot length. The growth measurements are helpful for a number of reasons. If the diet is altered, it is possible to analyze how diet affects growth rate. The growth rate of males versus females (including weight) is different and should be documented so the disparity between the sexes may be ascertained.

There are programs available that allow the information described above to be entered into a data base. The author utilizes the International Species Inventory System (ISIS). It is a database used by zoos and other facilities where large numbers of eagles are raised. The program allows member facilities to share information that is beneficial to all. The ISIS database is expensive, and alternative resources are available. Recording systems using Excel and statistical data bases including Minitab (Minitab Inc.) may be used. It may be necessary to find an information technology (IT) expert to help set up a simple system to enter your information. The data gleaned over time will be well worth the initial investment.

INITIAL CARE AND STABILIZATION

A quiet place should be prepared for eagle chicks. They need to be kept calm and usually need to be warmed and hydrated. Eagles are visually oriented. Visual stimuli may cause stress. When examining the chick, covering the eyes with a cloth or a falconry hood should calm it. Before covering the eyes, a protective ophthalmic ointment may be applied. Initial care and stabilization often requires treating for hypothermia, especially in young eaglets that are unable to thermoregulate. If the chick is damp, it may be towel-dried. If it is wet, a blow drier set on low is effective in drying the feathers. The bird should then be exposed to a heat source. In cases of extreme temperature loss, the bird should slowly be warmed. This may be facilitated in a number of ways. For slight temperature loss, the chick may be placed in a brooder, isolette, or on a heating or K-Pad (Thermocare). If a heating pad is used, it should be on the low or medium setting with a blanket or towel between the eaglet and the heat source. Infrared heat lamps and light bulbs are often used, but they are a source of fire if they come loose. They should be designed such that the bird cannot come in contact with them. In all cases, the eaglet should have the ability to move away from the heat source to a cooler environment.

Chicks that have gone into shock require fluid therapy. Many other eaglets will arrive dehydrated and in need of fluid therapy. Two types of fluid therapy are utilized: oral and subcutaneous. For oral therapy, use Pedialyte (Abbott) or a similar oral electrolyte solution. A French catheter (Tyco) attached to a luer-tipped syringe facilitates administration of the warm fluids. To avoid aspiration, administer fluids when the crop is empty or only minimally full. Initially, administer an amount that fills the crop to approximately one-quarter of its capacity. As the eagle begins to defecate and the crop empties completely, fluids may then be administered in a manner that fills the crop to half its size. Severely dehydrated and depressed birds may receive up to 10% of their body weight in oral fluids over a 24-hour period. In this case, the birds will not be given food until they are stable. For subcutaneous therapy, your veterinarian will prescribe warmed fluids such as lactated Ringer's or a solution of sodium chloride. Eagles may receive up to 10% of their body weight in injected fluids over a 24-hour period. The site of injection should be changed each time fluids are administered. Once the bird is quiet, warm, and hydrated, food may be offered.

If limbs are broken, they may need to be splinted until they are tended to by qualified veterinary staff.

COMMON MEDICAL PROBLEMS

Mites and lice are controlled with an injection of ivermectin at the appropriate dosage.

Toes that curl should be splinted and taped. Carefully place the toes in the normal position on the splint and then secure with tape. Splinting supplies vary depending upon the age of the bird and the materials available. Effective splints may be made from everyday objects, such as coffee stirrers (plastic and wooden), tongue depressors, or several layers of plastic cable ties, taped together. Ensure the splint does not have sharp edges that might cut the bird's toes. Tape may consist of a conforming bandage (Vetrap, 3-M) further anchored by surgical tape, or the splint may be secured with gauze and fastened with surgical tape. Cardboard shoes may be cut to the size of the bird's foot. The foot is placed on the "shoe" and fastened with surgical tape. Ensure that the tape is bound to the toes or foot in such a way that it holds the toes solidly in place but does not cut into the foot or toes or stop circulation. All splints and tape should be checked every few hours and changed at least every 24 hours. After the curl has been corrected, it may require an additional 24 to 48 hours to ensure that the problem does not recur.

Legs that bow and wings that curl may be corrected using techniques that are somewhat similar. Legs are placed in a normal position and one leg is wrapped with a strip of conforming wrap material. (Vetrap, 3-M). One to two wraps should suffice. A small piece of tape should be used to secure the first wrap. Without cutting the Vetrap, continue to the second leg, ensuring that the distance between the legs is normal. Wrap that leg in the same manner and secure with tape. The bird's legs should return to normal position within a few days.

Wings that droop or curl should also be placed in the natural position with Vetrap and secured as described above. Wraps should be removed daily to check for progress and ensure that circulation is not compromised. Again, after the desired correction is attained, it may require an additional 24 to 48 hours or rewrapping to ensure that the problem is not repeated.

DIET RECIPES

Eagles of all ages may be fed diets that simulate their natural diets. Food items may consist of rabbits, rodents, chicks, and quail. Because of potential thiamine problems associated with fish, do not feed fish until after the eagles fledge.

FEEDING PROCEDURES

During the hand-rearing phase, if the birds are being reared for release or propagation, it is critical to avoid human imprinting. This can be facilitated by feeding all nestlings with a puppet (Horwich 1989; Wallace 1994). Latex puppets may be easily sanitized. The latex puppet should have a head that is the same size, shape, and color as an adult, allowing for proper socialization (Wallace 1991) (see Figure 13.1). The arm of the human puppeteer

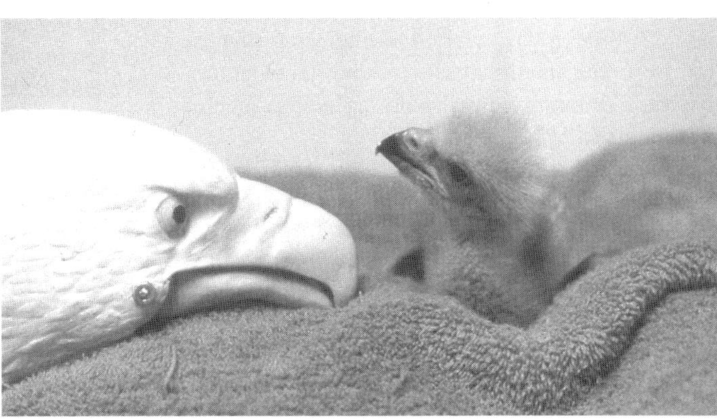

Figure 13.1. Bald eagle chick with puppet head.

should be covered with material such as a black felt sock. Forceps that fit through the bill facilitates passing bits of meat from the puppet to the chick. The forceps may touch the beak of the bird to elicit a feeding response. As the chick begins to self-feed, the puppet should be present for imprinting purposes. Following each feeding the forceps and the puppet must be sanitized. This may be done by scrubbing them with a 1:30 dilution of chlorine bleach:water. Following the scrubbing, soak them in the same dilution for 15 minutes or more before thoroughly rinsing and finally drying the puppet.

The chicks should be fed bits of muscle meat using the puppet until the crop is approximately three-quarters distended. Each chick must be examined prior to feeding, and food should be offered only to chicks that have a completely empty crop. Feeding birds that have food in the crop may cause sour crop, resulting in a chick that becomes ill and vomits.

Hatchlings

New hatchlings are not fed for the first 12 to 24 hours. After that time, they are offered tiny bits of muscle meat that have been dipped in an electrolyte solution such as Pedialyte (Abbott). At the first feeding of each day, the Pedialyte-moistened food may be dusted with a vitamin mixture that consists of Superpreen brand avian vitamin-mineral mix and dicalcium phosphate. The first few feedings should be small. The crop should barely expand. The young eagles from hatching to 5 or 7 days may be fed every 3 to 5 hours, but only after the crop has completely emptied.

Nestlings

Once the chicks begin to grow feathers they may be fed three times a day, every 4 to 5 hours during the day. Depending on the species, as they get older they may be fed during normal working hours, such as 0800 hours to 1700 hours.

The eaglets may be fed using a protocol adapted from that used by the Peregrine Fund for raising young raptors (Heck and Konkel 1991). At this age, diets consisting of quail and rodent may be fed either fresh or previously frozen and thawed to just below room temperature. To reduce the risk of bacterial infection, fresh food should be fed immediately, and thawed food should never sit out after thawing without refrigeration. The food animals may be prepared by gutting and removing appendages. In the case of quail, three-quarters of the feathers should be plucked when feeding young chicks. As the chick develops, the amount of feathers left on the quail may gradually increase. When the eaglets are about halfway through development, quail with about one-quarter of the feathers removed may be fed. All feathers may be consumed shortly thereafter. In all cases, the food animals should be pounded to rupture bones and then cut into bite-sized chunks. Super Preen brand avian vitamin-mineral mix (Arcata) and dicalcium phosphate should be added once daily to the diet, according to the veterinarian's prescription.

As the chicks reach the self-feeding stage, they may be offered the diet described below that is used for fledglings. The puppet should still be used whenever food is placed in the nest.

Fledglings

A balanced diet was provided for the birds by maintaining the following feeding schedule:

Sunday	Chicks or rodents
Monday	Fish
Tuesday	Chicks or rodents
Wednesday	Chicks or rodents
Thursday	Rodents
Friday	Rodents/Rabbit
Saturday	Rodents

Food animals may be acquired commercially or from laboratories. Commercially purchased food will probably be primarily fish and it should be suitable for human consumption. The fish (which may be fed once the birds reach fledgling stage) should be flash-frozen when caught and purchased as close to the catch date as possible. Fish should be used within 6 months of catch date.

Eagles that are being prepared for release should be allowed to capture live prey. Prey items, if domestic, should be as closely related as possible to what the bird would encounter in the wild.

WEIGHING CHICKS

Chicks from 2 weeks to 1 month of age may be weighed daily to analyze the effectiveness of the diet and ascertain the health and development of the chick. Weighing should take place just prior to the first feeding of the morning.

HOUSING

Specialized housing is required for eagles. Chicks are normally housed in self-contained brooders or in units with heating devices, such as K-Pads (Thermocare), until they are able to thermoregulate. As they feather out and develop the ability to thermoregulate, they may be placed in man-made nests in a chamber or solid enclosure. If the time of release is after fledging, the juveniles can fledge into these chambers.

CHICK HOUSING

Young birds of prey are unable to thermoregulate at hatch. Thermoregulation starts as a result of weight gain, the development of fat deposits, and the initiation of feather growth (Gill 1995). Very young birds (from hatch day to 2 or 3 weeks, depending upon health and behavior) may be successfully raised in one of two types of brooders. One is a standard hospital isolette used for premature human infants. Hospitals will often donate used isolettes to wildlife facilities. The other is a standard-sized, plastic restaurant bus tub fitted with a K-Pad brand heating pad (Thermocare). A custom-made plexiglass brooder with a heating pad may also be used (see Figure 13.2). The heating pad, developed for use in human medicine, is made of a soft, malleable rubber and there is warm water circulating within the pad. Rolled towels or jars may be laid along the center of the tub and the K-Pad may be draped over this ridge to provide a warm side and increase heat within the unit. This also allows for rearing two chicks in one unit. Young eaglets must have a physical barrier when being hand-reared because fratricide may be problematic among captive-reared raptors. The bottom of the rearing tub may be filled with corncob litter to a depth of 2 to 3 in (5 to 7.5 cm).

For young chicks, the brooder should provide warmth. The behavior of the individual bird dictates the exact temperature in the brooder. If the bird shivers, the temperature should be raised until it is comfortable. If the chick sprawls out or is panting, it indicates that the unit is too warm and the temperature should be lowered. At the proper temperature, chicks should sleep quietly in a sternally recumbent position with the legs tucked under the body and the wings held loosely against the chest cavity. As birds age, the temperature is gradually decreased until the chick is comfortable in an ambient temperature room. Halfway from hatch to fledge, they should be able to withstand the outdoor temperature full time without artificial heat.

The following alternative method allows eagle chicks to be placed outdoors at a younger age. In moderate climates, birds as young as 2 weeks old may be placed outdoors in man-made nests. The nests may be placed in the chambers that the eagles will eventually use for fledging. They birds can be warmed with the K-Pad heating pads and overhead heat units. The nest may be lined with pine needles and branches or other appropriate vegetation that allows the birds to complete grabbing exercises like those observed in wild eaglets.

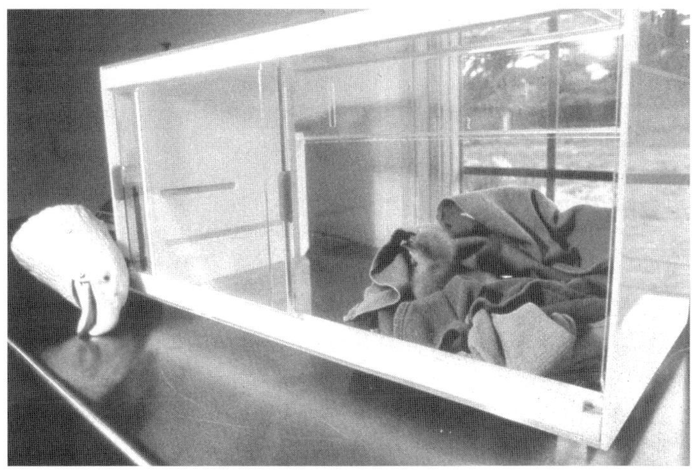

Figure 13.2. Bald eagle chick in a custom brooder with a puppet head at the far end.

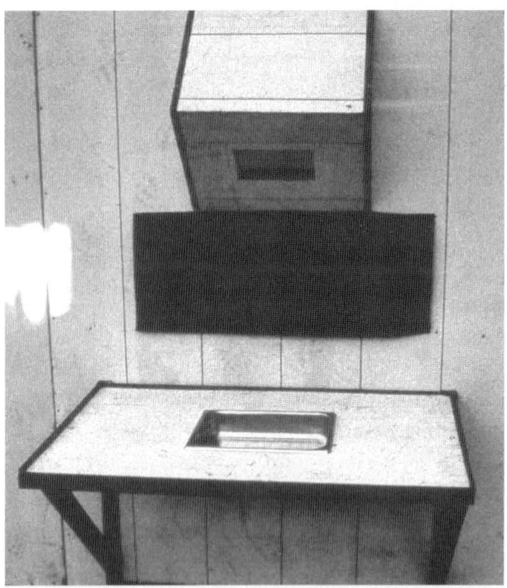

Figure 13.3. The feeding port is covered with a soft artificial turf (Astroturf) panel to provide the nestlings a visual screen from the feeder.

WEANING

In preparation for fledging, young eagles that are halfway developed should be moved outdoors and put in chambers. An appropriate size for bald or golden eagles has proven to be 11.6 × 4.9 × 3.0 m (38.05 ft × 16.07 ft × 9.84 ft). The chambers should be outfitted with nests and multiple branches so that once the birds fledge they can get an adequate amount of exercise. The size of the sticks may vary, but the length and diameter should be species-appropriate. The sticks are important in that they allow the birds to grab and grasp, thereby strengthening their feet in preparation for hunting. For birds being prepared for release, it is convenient to have a method of feeding and observing them without having them see you. The feeding port seen in Figure 13.3 is covered with a soft artificial turf (Astroturf) panel to provide the nestlings a visual screen from the feeder.

PREPARATION FOR WILD RELEASE

If possible, the timing of release of eagles should coincide with the time they are about to fledge. At that time, the eagle should be banded, and if possible, fitted with a radio telemetry device such as a tail-mounted transmitter or a back pack. Banding of eagles is often (especially in the United States) permitted only with a special license through the federal government. Patagial markers may be used with eagles to aid in ease of identification after release.

When eagles are ready to propagate, they tend to return to their natal area or the area where they were released. If possible, release the eagle where it was originally found. The locale of the release of hand-reared eagles should be carefully researched. There must be enough appropriate breeding habitat including nest trees or cliffs, and night roosts. There must also be enough prey to sustain the eagle at the time of release and when it returns years later to nest and rear young. Some states and federal agencies such as the United States Department of Fish and Wildlife, the Bureau of Land Management, and the United States Forest Service, may have a jurisdiction over when and where eagles are released. Release on private land does not generally have these restrictions, but chances are that birds released on federal lands will have a better chance of using the same location for breeding for generations to come.

Birds reared in captivity, or those that are products of rehabilitation programs, must be behaviorally fit for life in the wild. They must be able to recognize and catch appropriate prey. Birds that are not behaviorally suited for a release program will likewise be unsuitable for release to the wild.

RELEASE

Common methods of releasing eagles include hacking and fostering. The process of hacking was developed by falconers. Hacking became an important conservation tool for bald eagles and other raptors in the 1970s and 1980s. Birds of prey released from hack sites tended to return to the areas from which they were released. Bald eagles were therefore hacked from areas that managers wanted to repopulate with breeding bald eagles. Hacking involves the traditional falconry method of hacking birds into the wild. Young eagles can be placed in an artificial nest from which they will fledge. The nest is in a hack box and the birds are placed in the nest at the fledging stage. They are fed in the nest from which they can see their surrounding environment. When they are ready to fledge the box is opened. The birds are continually fed after fledging. The feeding process is continued until the birds are self-sufficient and independent of the nest.

Hacking raptors is helpful in habituating released birds to a natal area that it is hoped will become their future breeding grounds, but though the human hack site attendants provide the birds with food, they cannot teach them to hunt. As a result, mortality rates are higher for hacked birds than for those that fledge out of nests.

If at all possible, foster chicks in nests where birds are of the same age. Birds can be aged in the field. As described by Carpenter (1990), in his 1987 draft of *An Illustrated Guide for Identifying Developmental Stages of Nestling Bald Eagles in the Field,* and by Bortolotti (1984), bald eagle chicks can be aged by plumage. Age determinations can be made in the field without disturbing the chicks. By using a spotting scope, age can be readily determined by an observer at 10 ft (3 m) from a nest. Birds that fledge out of foster nests become imprinted on the area from which they fledge and their surrogate parents teach them to hunt. Birds that are fostered also have the best chances of developing behaviorally in a manner that will ensure that they become future breeders.

ACKNOWLEDGMENTS

Special thanks to Betty Nudelman, Jennifer Sheehan, and Kimberly Robertson for their assistance and support.

SOURCES FOR PRODUCTS MENTIONED

Astroturf, Solutia Inc., PO Box 66760, St. Louis, MO 63166-6760, (800) 723-8873, www.astroturfmats.com.

Feeding Tube and Urethral Catheter available from Tyco Healthcare/Kendall, (800) 962–9888, www.kendallhq.com. Sizes 8 through 18 French.

Heating pads available from Gaymar Industries, Inc., (716) 662-2551; International (716) 662-8636, www.gaymar.com.

K-Pad (Distributor Thermocare), (800) 262-4020, www.thermocare.com.

Minitab Inc., Quality Plaza, 1829 Pine Hall Road, State College, PA 16801–3008, (814) 238-3280, www.minitab.com.

Pedialyte, Abbott Laboratories, 100 Abbott Park Road, Abbott Park, IL 60064-3500, (847) 937-6100, www.abbott.com.

Syringes with catheter tip available from Tyco Healthcare/Kendall, (800) 962-9888, www.kendallhq.com. Monoject, 60 ml.

Vetrap (3-M) available from Jeffers, (800) 533-3377, www.jefferspet.com. Sizes: 2 in wide × 5 yd and 4 in wide × 5 yd.

Super Preen, Aracata Pet Supplies, (800) 822-9085, www.arcatapet.com.

REFERENCES

Bortolotti, G.R. 1984. Criteria for determining age and sex of nestling bald eagles. Journal of Field Ornithology 55(4): 467–481.

Carpenter, G. 1990. An Illustrated Guide for Identifying Developmental Stages of Nestling Bald Eagles in the Field. San Francisco Zoological Society, San Francisco.

Ferguson-Lees, J. and Christie, D.A. 2001. Raptors of the World. Houghton Mifflin Company, New York, 992 pp.

Gill, F.B. 1995. Ornithology, Second Edition. W.H. Freeman and Company, New York, 766 pp.

Hartt, E.W., Harvey, N.C., Leete, A.J., and Preston, K. 1994. Effects of age at pairing on reproduction in captive California condors *Gymnogyps californianus*. Zoo Biology 13: 3–11.

Heck, W.R. and Konkel, D. 1991. Incubation and rearing. In Weaver, J.D. and Cade, T.J., eds., Falcon Propagation. The Peregrine Fund, Boise, Idaho, pp. 34–76.

Horwich, R.H. 1989. Use of surrogate parental models and age periods in a successful release of hand-reared sandhill cranes. Zoo Biology 8: 379–390.

Wallace, M.P. 1991. Methods and strategies for the release of California condors to the wild. Proceedings American Aquarium and Zoological Park Association, San Diego, California, pp. 121–128.

———. 1994. Control of behavioral development in the context of reintroduction programs for birds. Zoo Biology 13: 491–499.

14
Hawks, Falcons, Kites, Osprey, and New World Vultures

Louise Shimmel

NATURAL HISTORY

There are several types of birds that make up the very large diurnal (daytime-active) raptor group: 313 species worldwide of hawks, harriers, eagles, falcons, kites, osprey, and vultures. Although this classification changes from time to time, especially with DNA analysis rather than morphological attributes, generally accepted categories are as follows: the order Accipitriformes includes osprey (1 species in its own family), kites (23 species), Old World vultures (15 species), harriers (15 species), hawks (120 species), and eagles (68 species covered in a separate chapter).

The order Falconiformes includes the falcons (54 species), Caracara (9 species), and Secretary Bird (1 species). The seven species of New World vultures, technically now classified in the order Ciconiiformes (with storks), are typically included in listings of raptors and are so treated in this chapter.

Raptors are obligate or absolute carnivores that (except for the scavengers) typically catch their food with their well-adapted feet, which have long, sharp, curved talons and strong toes. Their hooked beak is designed for ripping and tearing flesh, whether it's a small animal they have caught alive or a carcass into which they are tearing as scavengers. The vultures and many of the buteonine hawks and eagles scavenge already dead animals as at least part of what they eat. All or part of the diet of any one species may be insects, reptiles, amphibians, fish, birds, small rodents and other mammals, or carrion of any animal.

However, there are lots of other avian species not considered raptors that are obligate carnivores and eat the same type of prey items as do the raptors. Thus, it is actually anatomy rather than diet that determines which species are considered raptors or birds of prey. Like any rule, there are often exceptions, and although vulture feet do not carry the same equipment as a typical raptor, their powerful hooked beak and diet do match those aspects of the raptor profile.

Hawks

Among the hawks, there are two general, distinctively different types. The "true" hawks or *accipiters* tend to be long-legged, long-toed, long-tailed, short-winged birds whose sprintlike speed and maneuverability in a typically wooded habitat allows them to make birds a high percentage of their diet. The soaring hawks or *buteos* (typically called "buzzards" outside the Americas) are birds whose long, broad wings allow them to be relatively hefty, in a bird sense, because they are built for gliding and soaring, but otherwise tend to be perch-and-pounce predators.

In North America north of Mexico, the hawks routinely found include three species of accipiters: Sharp-shinned Hawk, Cooper's Hawk, and Northern Goshawk. There are also 11 species of buteos: Red-tailed Hawk (having the largest range), Rough-legged Hawk, Red-shouldered Hawk, Broad-winged Hawk, Ferruginous Hawk, Swainson's Hawk (the next most widespread, at least during certain times of the year), plus Short-tailed Hawk, Zone-tailed Hawk, White-tailed Hawk, Black Hawk, and Roadside Hawk, all of which have ranges that barely extend into the southern United States. Harris' Hawks are a *parabuteo* hawk found in the Southwestern U.S. and down into Central and South America.

Hawks are typically tree-nesting birds that build nests of sticks. However, Harris' Hawks are fascinating communal raptors that nest on cactus. Where hawks reuse nests in subsequent seasons, the nests are typically well-constructed and are refurbished as needed. Orphaned hatchlings or nestlings come in most often because of windstorms blowing whole nests down or breaking branches, or from logging or landscaping that take out trees.

Harriers

Harriers are long-winged, slender birds that typically course back and forth over fields searching for food using their owl-like facial disks, it is thought, to help locate their prey by sound. The one representative of this group of birds in North America is the Northern Harrier. This bird nests on the ground, making a rough nest of trampled grass and some sticks, in tall grass or under a small shrub. Most eggs, hatchlings, or nestlings come in from accidents with mowers, as the field is hayed or mown by someone not knowing that this secretive bird has a nest there. Even food exchanges, where the male is bringing food to his mate and offspring, take place away from the hidden nest.

Osprey

Osprey are found worldwide, always near water, and their diets are almost exclusively fish. Though remains of a wide range of other prey items have been found in nests, such nonfish prey typically represent a very small percentage of their diet. Osprey nests can be very bulky affairs, placed on the very top of dead trees, power poles, or platforms introduced specifically for their nesting. Awkward birds, except in the air, they seem to require clear access to their nests, rather than hiding them down in the branches, as most other raptors make some effort to do. Hatchlings or young nestlings are sometimes blown down with a nest, and returning them can sometimes be difficult when the nest is at the very top of a snag whose overall condition may make it dangerous to climb. If it does not overburden a nest or place a nestling with much younger or much older adoptive siblings, fostering into nests of a different pair placed on lower, often man-made platforms is a viable alternative to returning them to their own nest. In captivity, this species is particularly difficult to condition for release, so maximal efforts should be made to reunite uninjured fallen chicks with their parents.

Kites

Kites are most typically found in the southern states in the U.S., although the White-tailed Kite has recently expanded its range north into Oregon from California. In North America north of Mexico are Mississippi Kites, Swallow-tailed Kites, the White-tailed Kite (with the widest distribution), and the Snail Kite and Hook-billed Kite whose ranges barely touch Florida and the southernmost tip of Texas, respectively. As tree or woody vegetation nesters, young kites are most likely to be presented for care due to windstorms, landscaping, or other nest disruption.

Falcons

Falcons found in North America north of Mexico consist of the Gyrfalcon, Peregrine Falcon, Prairie Falcon, Merlin, and American Kestrel primarily, with the Aplomado Falcon the subject of reintroduction efforts in south Texas. Falcons are typically open-country or edge habitat birds that do not make a nest; they are either cliff- or cavity-nesters, or will take over an old corvid nest (Merlins). Kestrels and Peregrines have adapted to human habitats, with Peregrines found in many cities nesting on tall buildings, industrial towers, or bridges where suitable platforms can be found or are placed. Kestrels opportunistically use any cavity of a suitable size, and very young birds present typically from human disruption of a nest site or because of a fall from a poorly chosen nest site.

New World Vultures

New World Vultures found in North America north of Mexico are the Black Vulture, Turkey Vulture, and California Condor. California Condors are covered in Chapter 15, "Condors," but are realistically unlikely to be presented for hand-rearing outside a small number of specialized institutions. However, if the population continues to grow in the wild, it may eventually become possible that a juvenile condor would be presented for temporary care, such as if an injured fledgling was found by a member of the public.

Turkey and Black Vultures often nest on the ground, under windfalls or in caves, and occasionally in broken top snags or hollow stumps. Eggs or young birds may be brought into care due to logging or development, or other type of nest disturbance.

It is strongly encouraged that Turkey Vultures, of all birds, be reunited with parents or placed in wild foster nests, if at all possible, because they are extremely difficult to raise in captivity without excessive socialization to people. Given their highly developed sense of smell, it is very difficult to avoid having them associate humans with food.

CRITERIA FOR INTERVENTION

As with many other species of wild birds, both parents are actively involved in rearing young. The loss of one parent may or may not be cause for intervention. The death of a brooding female could lead to the death of youngsters, because most males will not brood. In cold weather the death of a male while the female is incubating or brooding may lead to the death of the young, because the female could certainly provide food for the young but not also keep them warm.

Young found on the ground that are cold, injured, dehydrated, caught by a cat or dog, or emaciated should be presented for captive care. If the condition can be corrected quickly (e.g., cold or dehydrated), the nest location is known and reachable, and the parents are obviously still present, the young can often be replaced in the nest within a day or two. If other young are known to be in the nest and the chick can be replaced in the nest at fledging age, a delayed reunion with the natural parents remains a possibility even after treatment for a more severe condition such as a broken bone or wound.

Long-term captive care due to the loss of the whole nest or even the nest tree may at times be avoided by placing the nestlings in a replacement nest such as a basket or an open-topped wooden box with drainage holes. The young need to be old enough to thermoregulate and vocalize and thus be found by the parents. Nestboxes for kestrels can also be put up. Kestrels are the most likely to require intervention due to inappropriate nesting sites, such as in an old barn about to be torn down. If, however, the nest or nest tree is lost due to larger scale destruction at a logging site or new development or mowed field, intervention may be necessary. Even though both parents are still present, continuous disturbance or lack of a nearby tree or other appropriate nest site may preclude the return of the nestlings.

Healthy fledglings of any species found on the ground should be left alone or perhaps put nearby, somewhere safe from domestic predators. Though essentially full grown, they cannot yet fly. Their parents will continue to feed them wherever they are.

RECORD KEEPING

Detailed information on the location where the bird was found should be recorded. This will serve as a guide for suitable habitat for release and also will place the bird back with its relatives, which may still recognize the young bird.

Wildlife regulatory agencies have minimum standards for record keeping that require tracking of individual animals undergoing rehabilitation. Check with your regulating agencies for further information. See Appendix 1 for a list of North American resources for locating licensed wildlife rehabilitators or regulatory agencies. As a minimum, the following information should be kept: species, age, location found, reason brought into captivity, medical problems, final disposition, and release location. Each nestling in care can be given a unique log number and its leg banded with temporary materials in order to track its growth. To avoid placing sticky tape directly on the bird's leg, the lower tarsus can be wrapped first with a layer of nonsticky elastic bandaging material, and then with a white cloth tape on which the log number can be written. There are also plastic poultry bands available in different colors or with distinct numbers or blanks on which numbers can be written. Care should be taken, however, that hard edges of such bands will not cut into the bird's skin when the nestling is back on its hocks or will not trap inquisitive beaks while preening. All bands, cloth or otherwise, need to be checked daily as the bird is growing and must be removed before release.

A detailed medical record should be kept on each animal, with results of the initial examination recorded and any updated information added as it happens. This should include daily body weights taken at the same time each day, whether the bird has cast (regurgitated a pellet of indigestible materials such as hair and bones), any unusual droppings, whether the crop is emptying, what has been fed at what times and how much was eaten and any medications given, as well as progress of treatments and pertinent notes on behavior.

INITIAL CARE AND STABILIZATION

The main rule of initial baby bird care for any species is warmth, rehydration, and feeding, in that order. Warm chicks before giving fluids, and then hydrate them until they start passing droppings. Only then is it safe to commence feedings. Feeding a cold or dehydrated baby bird before it is warm and hydrated will probably kill it.

New patients should be allowed to rest for 15–20 minutes in a warm, dark, quiet container before examination. If the bird is not able to stand, it should be placed in a soft support structure such as a rolled cloth "donut" or paper nest not much larger than the bird's body. For larger species, an upside-down cloth toilet seat cover with a towel rolled and placed under the elastic edges makes a good substitute nest. The whole thing can be covered with another towel to minimize how many towels need to be changed at each feeding. This provides the legs with needed support to avoid splaying.

Do not allow the bird to lie on its side or other abnormal positions. Hatchlings and nestlings should be placed in a climate-controlled incubator if available. When the animal is warm and calm, it may be hydrated orally and/or subcutaneously (SQ). If there is any sign of blood in the mouth or droppings, or extensive bruising of the abdomen, any of which might signal injuries from the fall from the nest, SQ administration of fluids is advised. A gentle palpation of the abdomen will indicate whether there is food or casting material in the ventriculus.

Warm sterile fluids such as 2.5% dextrose in 0.45% sodium chloride or lactated Ringer's solution may be administered SQ at 5% of body weight once, although repeated administrations every 2 or 3 hours may be needed for extremely dehydrated birds.

Because raptors do not gape, active hatchlings or nestlings should be orally hydrated via gavage until they produce droppings. Human infant electrolyte fluids (unflavored) are excellent for oral rehydration of baby birds. Again, ensure that the bird is warm before administering fluids, and that the bird is both warm and well-hydrated before receiving food. Start the bird on a small piece of clean meat dipped in warm water after it begins passing droppings.

If the bird is depressed or not swallowing well, oral rehydration must be done—very carefully, because there is a greater risk of aspiration of fluids into the respiratory system. It may be better in this circumstance to use SQ fluids, rather than to give oral fluids. If SQ fluids are not an option, give tiny amounts of oral fluids deep into the mouth by tube (into the crop if possible) and ensure that the bird swallows everything before giving more.

If a young bird does not begin passing droppings within 3 hours of giving the fluids, begin feeding the appropriate diet. However, keep the diet very moist and the meal size small until droppings are seen.

COMMON MEDICAL PROBLEMS

Steroids or nonsteroidal anti-inflammatory drugs (NSAIDs) may be of use in treating head injuries, although steroid use is controversial. Many wildlife veterinarians prefer the newer NSAIDs such as meloxicam (Metacam, Boeringer-Ingleheim) at 0.1–0.2 mg/kg orally once or twice daily or Celecoxib (Celebrex, Pfizer) at 10 mg/kg orally once daily (Carpenter 2005) to using dexamethasone for head injuries due to concerns of the steroids causing a depression of immune system function. Do not overheat a bird with head injury, because this may aggravate brain swelling.

Metabolic bone disease is seen unfortunately often in young birds that have been in the hands of the public for even a few days on an inadequate diet. Though recognizing a young raptor as a meat-eater, people fail to understand that a diet of hamburger, organ meat, or muscle meat creates a severe imbalance of calcium and phosphorus, at a very vulnerable time when young birds are growing at an astronomical rate. The severely unbalanced calcium-to-phosphorus (Ca : P) ratio in such meats causes stripping of available calcium from the bones, leading to deformities such as bowing of the long bones or outright fractures. When these birds come into care, often because the finders finally realize that something is wrong, this situation can only sometimes be corrected. Providing a diet with the correct Ca : P ratio of 2 : 1 plus oral calcium supplementation for as long as the inadequate diet was fed can sometimes overcome the problem if the birds do not yet have any fractures or major deformities. A veterinarian should be consulted for help in such cases. Once fractures have occurred, little can be done because the cortices of the bones are usually so thin that they will break somewhere else if an attempt is made to immobilize or pin the fracture site. Feather development will usually be severely compromised in these cases as well.

Young birds without wing feathers to slow their fall can be badly bruised in a drop from a high nest. If very young, their abdomen tends to be the center of gravity, and bruising there can lead to impactions of pellet material. Fecal matter in droppings may look like a string of small beads rather than a typical fried egg appearance. Appetite may be low and a hard mass may be palpated between the legs in the abdomen. Fluids and a small amount of Metamucil can help correct this over time. Clean meat supplemented to correct the Ca : P ratio can also be dipped in Metamucil and then fed. This will provide nutrition without adding to the casting burden. This condition sometimes takes up to 3 days to resolve.

Wounds can be treated as in adult birds but if antibiotics are deemed necessary for, say, a cat bite, check with an avian veterinarian. Broad-spectrum antibiotics frequently used in injured raptors include cephalosporins such as Cephalexin at 40–100 mg/kg orally (PO) or intramuscularly (IM) three to four times daily, or Cefazolin at 50–100 mg/kg PO or IM twice daily, or penicillins such as Ampicillin at 15 mg/kg IM twice daily or Amoxicillin/clavulanic acid at 125 mg/kg PO twice daily (Carpenter 2005).

Severe infestations of external or internal parasites are sometimes found in young raptors. Pale mucus membranes or emaciation should lead to further diagnostics such as a blood smear or fecal analysis, if not done routinely. Coccidia infections may be severe enough to cause anemia and a failure to thrive, as can leukocytozoonosis, especially in older postfledging birds. Coccidiosis is best treated with Toltrazuril (Baycox, Bayer) at 10 mg/kg once daily for 3 days (Carpenter 2005). Leucocytozoon infection is treated with both Primaquine given once PO at 0.75–1.0 mg/kg and Chloroquine at 25 mg/kg at 0 hour, and then 15 mg/kg at hours 12, 24 and 48 (Carpenter 2005). Ectoparasites, which may also lead to severe anemia or feather damage if not controlled, can be treated with a pyrethrin-based powder. Treating all birds for external parasites upon admission is a good practice to help limit disease and blood parasite transmission between birds.

Additionally, young birds in the hands of the public are frequently malimprinted on humans, which, though not a medical problem, nevertheless leads to a nonreleasable bird. This may become a lethal problem if placement in permanent care is not available. Euthanasia may be the only option in such cases, because these birds cannot be released.

RE-NESTING

Usually, the best choice for an uninjured, displaced wild raptor is returning it to its nest. Local tree services, arborists, utilities, and state or federal forest service offices may have tree climbers willing to assist in returning youngsters to nests. Occasionally, due to extremely aggressive parents nesting close to human activity, governmental authorities authorize taking eggs or young from the nest, sometimes even killing the parents. This should obviously be an absolute last resort.

FOSTERING

Placing uninjured, displaced hatchling or nestling raptors in a foster nest is also an option preferable to raising them in captivity. Care should be taken in regard to the following: that the orphan and his surrogate nestmates are old enough to thermoregulate in case the brooding adult female is flushed from the nest for a prolonged period of time by the activity of adding a new youngster; that a nest is not overloaded, jeopardizing the ability of the parents to care for the expanded number of young; that nestmates are neither so much older nor so much younger than the introduced youngster that it would either outcompete the natural young or be outcompeted. Maximum number per nest is dependent on the normal number of young for each species: A kestrel nest might do well with 4–5 chicks, whereas 2–3 would be maximum for an osprey nest. Prey availability in each given season should be taken into account as well. If local raptors are having a tough year, fewer young per nest is warranted. Consult local natural history sources to find out the normal clutch size of each species.

CAPTIVE FOSTERING

Using captive, nonreleasable adults as foster parents is also an option to be considered before hand-rearing. Some adults, either male or female, will foster any young of their species that makes an appropriate sound; the only way to find out whether an adult will foster is to test it. To keep the young safe during the initial introduction, it is recommended that they be in sight of the adult but protected. For example, the nestling can be placed inside the captive adult's mew in a box or airline kennel with wire front, so that the adult can see the young and vice versa. Ideally, the box could have a rear door through which the human caretakers can feed the young without entering the enclosure. If the adult starts sitting near the nestlings, or tries to shove food through the wire in response to the begging calls, access can be provided (see Figure 14.1).

If the adult takes no interest in the young, it can

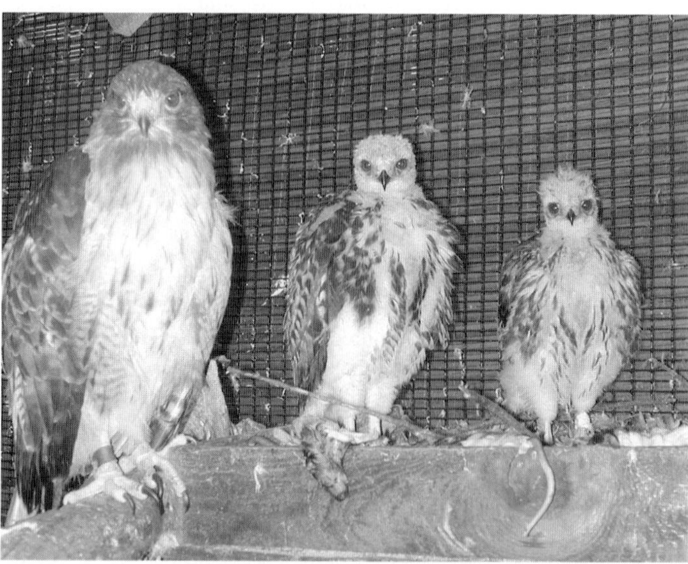

Figure 14.1. Education Red-tailed Hawk acting as a foster parent for two orphans.

still fulfill the important role of a visual model. Once the youngsters are eating cut-up food off a plate, food can be placed in the box or kennel through a slot, while the young has 24-hour visual contact with the adult. Once at branching or fledging age, the two can be put together. If introducing them in the adult's territory gives rise to aggression, consider moving them both to neutral territory while taking the young through live prey training.

Renesting and Fostering Caveat

When renesting or fostering, the introduction of the young to the adults should be done as soon as possible, and all precautions to avoid imprinting on humans (e.g., feeding puppets, ghost costumes, feeding through a chute or slot) should be taken in the meantime. If the young bird reacts inappropriately to the adult by showing fear or aggression, it may be killed. If the youngster has been presented for care and it is not known how long the finder has had the bird, safely testing the youngster with a captive adult or conspecifics could be critical.

HACKING

Hacking is an appropriate technique, especially for a lone chick (that is most at risk of malimprinting) and for the bird-catching falcons and accipiters for which it is really impossible to provide adequate live prey training in a cage. A hackbox is a wooden box, the size of which varies depending on the type of bird for which it is designed (see Figure 14.2). The front of the box is a door that is opened when the bird is old enough to begin exploring its environment. The primary considerations are (1) that the box be mounted such that the bird has a wide view of its surroundings (which should be habitat appropriate for the species, obviously, because the bird will be released there), (2) that the bird be protected from the elements and predators, and (3) that the back of the box must be solid except for a feeding slot so that the bird does not associate humans with food. For example, to meet the first criterion, the front and half the roof and sides can be slatted. For the second, the remaining part of the roof and sides would be made of solid wood for shade and protection from rain, and consideration should be given depending on the location of the box, to add predator barriers such as wire on the outside of the slats or flashing around the base of the tree to prevent climbing. For the third, human access to the hackbox and the entire approach to the box should be from the back or blind side to avoid even a conditioned response that the approach of a human means food.

The young bird must be placed in the hackbox at nestling age, as soon as it is thermoregulating and eating cut up food from a plate. The hackbox is its nest, and it must have the opportunity to branch and fledge from there. It is of little use to place an older brancher or fledgling in a hackbox. There is typically

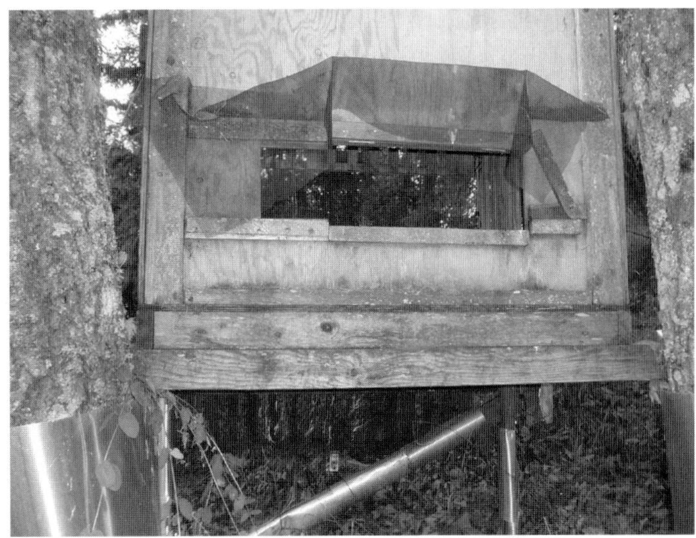

Figure 14.2. Back of hackbox, showing sliding door for food, flap door for water, and screening for mosquitoes and yellow jackets.

not enough room to give it the exercise needed for flight and as soon as the door is opened, the bird may just disappear as there has been insufficient developmental time for it to imprint on the hackbox as its nest. A bird that is imprinted on the box as its home nest will continue to return for food while exploring the area and attempting to hunt on its own. To this end, a *hack board* or consistent feeding tray is used. Whether it is white or black or a plastic plate or board, it is important that it be something consistent and recognizable that the young bird will associate with food. The bird will come back less and less as it becomes competent at hunting.

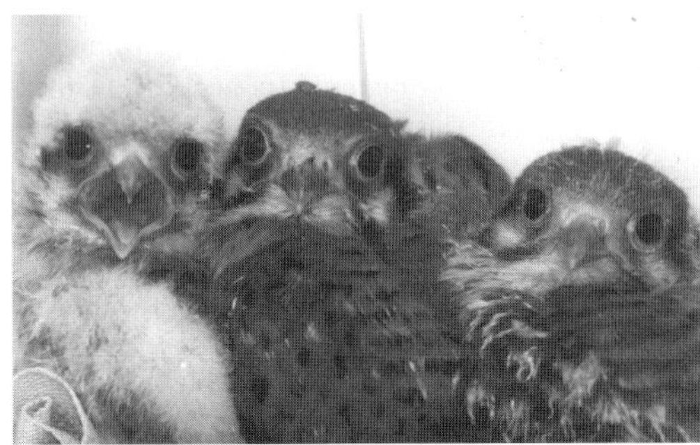

Figure 14.3. Young kestrels, and other orphans, benefit from being with conspecifics, despite an age difference.

CONSPECIFICS AND FEEDING PUPPETS

In the unfortunate event that none of the above is possible (for example, the nestling is injured and needs daily medication or bandage changes, there is no way to return the bird to its own or another nest, or no hackbox is available) hand-rearing will be necessary. Wherever possible through networking with others in the area, babies should be placed with conspecifics, because it will help limit the risk of human imprinting to be with other young of their own kind (see Figure 14.3). These conspecifics can be older, if the single youngster can at least have visual contact with them, even when actually placing them together would put the nestling at risk.

If feeding puppets are available, their use can make a huge difference when used as the youngsters' eyes are opening and beginning to focus (see Figure 14.4). Providing 24-hour visual access to the puppet or to a study skin placed over a bottle of water, or taxidermy mount of an adult, can also be an important aid in appropriate imprinting. Human voices should be kept to a minimum, especially at feeding time.

Even without puppets, "ghost" costumes (shapeless white or camouflage coverings to hide the human face and form) should be worn for feeding, as well as carefully facing the very young birds away from the person feeding.

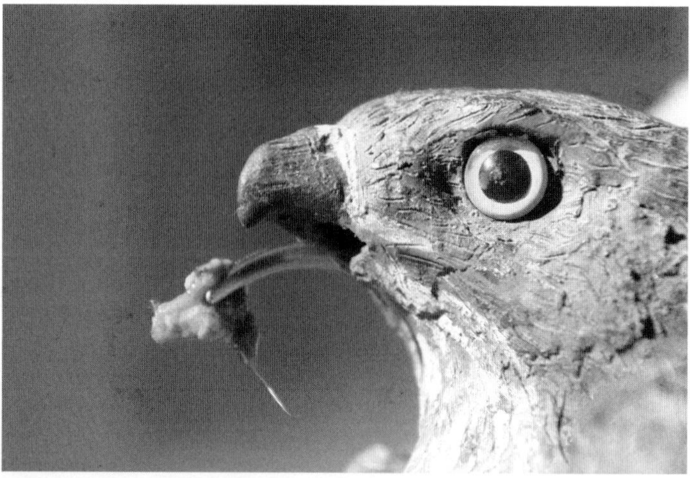

Figure 14.4. Hawk puppet with hemostat holding food.

DIET RECIPES

With raptors, there is no substitute for a whole small animal diet. The age of the bird will determine how much, if any, casting material (bones, fur, feathers) should be given. The species of bird and its natural diet can help determine a substitute food while in care, but typically quail or mice are a good place to start with very young birds that do not yet have or need a search image of what appropriate food for their species looks like. Day-old chickens can be fed to young raptors if the Ca:P ratio of the chicks is augmented. It is generally felt that the undeveloped bones of such young chickens are not sufficiently mineralized to provide enough calcium or phosphorus, even if what is there is in a low but balanced ratio (Ca:P of 1:1 is the typical ratio of a day-old chick). Although bone meal is not often recommended as a calcium supplement for birds, this supplement may be combined 1:1 by weight with calcium carbonate powder to form a powder with a C:P of 4.5:1. This powder may then be used to sprinkle on all calcium-deficient foods.

If large numbers of young birds need to be fed, quail can be plucked; head, feet, wings and lower intestine removed; and the remains then placed through a meat grinder. The resulting paste can be made into patties and frozen in a thin layer between sheets of waxed paper for later thawing as needed. Mice, too, can be easily skinned and ground. Remove heads prior to grinding. Leave the tails because they form an excellent source of calcium and, indeed, may be one the first casting materials fed to chicks, because they are not as sharp as other bones. Using whole adult animals as food allows the nestling raptors to get the minerals from the bones they would otherwise be too young to handle whole.

FEEDING PROCEDURES

Hatchlings

Blunt forceps or hemostats can be used to pick up very small pieces of warm, clean meat (e.g., quail breast meat) dipped in warm water. The hemostat should touch the beak to elicit a feeding response: the hatchling will grab the food from the instrument as it would from the tip of its mother's beak. It will be quickly obvious if a piece is too large or an awkward shape. Four or five very small pieces are probably all a hatchling can handle at a feeding before it falls back asleep. It is easy to see the food in the crop and easy to see or palpate when the crop is empty. Hatchlings should be fed every 2 hours or so during daylight hours, if the crop has emptied, the bird is hungry, and droppings have been passed. Very small bits of bone, carefully broken or ground can be included by 3 days of age, casting material by day 5. The food should be warmed to approximately body temperature by placing it in a container that is then placed in or above hot water (to avoid bacterial growth, do not soak the food in the hot water while thawing). Dipping the individual pieces of food in the warm water as they are fed provides the extra moisture needed by hatchlings.

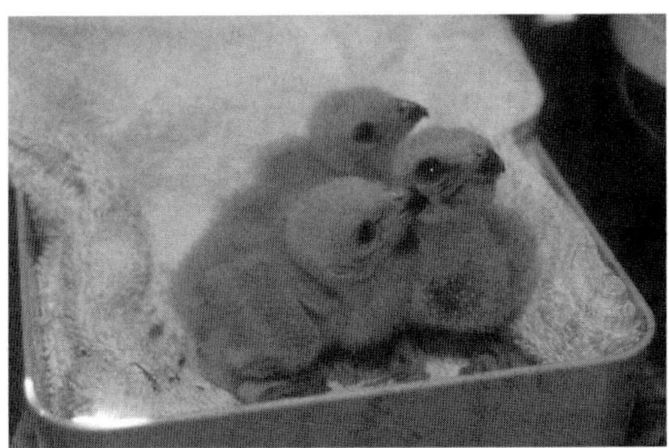

Figure 14.5. Nestling harriers.

Nestlings and Fledglings

Blunt forceps or hemostats may continue to be used to feed, until the nestling recognizes cut-up food on a small plate or lid and starts to pick it up on its own. This can be encouraged by placing the lid or small plate of food directly in front of the nestlings and picking the food up from the lid while they watch. Typically, younger nestlings dropping food seem to think it has simply disappeared; once they start to discover the food that has fallen to their feet, they are often ready to start picking it up themselves from a plate. The sooner they eat on their own, the less the risk of socialization to humans. Picking up small pieces of food from a plate should be expected by at least 2 weeks of age, usually before they can stand, though holding food down with their feet and ripping it up takes quite a bit longer, of course.

Once the birds' eyes are open and focusing, a puppet should be used for feeding, "ghost" costumes to disguise human caregivers should be worn, and the babies carefully faced away from the human feeder during meals. If at all possible, do not house a baby alone. Place it with or in sight of conspecifics or in sight of adult surrogates, if an actual foster parent is not available (see Figure 14.5).

EXPECTED WEIGHT GAIN

Weight gain in the first few days after hatching can be expected to be slow but should be steady. Hatch weight should double within 5 to 7 days, and will rise very rapidly after those first few days. With the smaller species like the kestrel, approximate adult weight can be reached before they are even off their hocks and have much of their feather tips out of the sheath, at around 2 weeks of age. With the larger species, like the Red-tailed Hawk or Turkey Vulture, it may take 5 to 7 weeks to reach adult weight. Again, each species varies, but they should be able to pick up cut-up food from a plate or lid on their own within 10–14 days and should be placed in a hackbox at that point, if that is the method of choice.

It is important to chart weights daily, weighing them at the same time each day, preferably before their first meal.

HOUSING

Hatchlings should be kept at 85–90°F (29–32°C) and around 40% humidity; however, more important than an absolute temperature and humidity level is watching the comfort of the birds. A cold baby will be reluctant to eat; a hot one may pant or be splayed out in the nest. These birds all have some natal down but cannot usually maintain their own body temperature until the secondary down comes in. This secondary down is very wooly in texture and provides excellent insulation.

For young chicks, towels (without holes or stringy edges) provide the best substrate. The towels should be arranged to surround them, as in a nest, giving them something to grip with their feet and to support them in an upright position with their legs tucked under them (see Figure 14.6). The hawks, osprey, harriers, and young kestrels *slice* their droppings: that is, shoot them either out or up or both. This creates an obvious challenge to keep their enclosure clean! Caging should be cleaned thoroughly at least once a day, wiped down with a disinfectant such as dilute chlorhexidine, towels or papers changed, or the chicks moved to new housing as necessary to maintain a hygienic environment. It is critical that the young growing feathers be kept clean, including those around the mouth, which can be soiled during feeding. Whereas adult birds that slice are usually given a tail sheath while in hospital cages, this is not possible when the feathers are growing in, because the birds need to be able to preen the feather sheaths off.

As the birds come off their hocks and start to flap their wings in practice flight, they should be allowed to *branch,* i.e., leave the nest and move around a safe environment. If thermoregulating and eating on their own, being outside with access to ambient temperatures and correct photoperiods, as well as sunlight, is important.

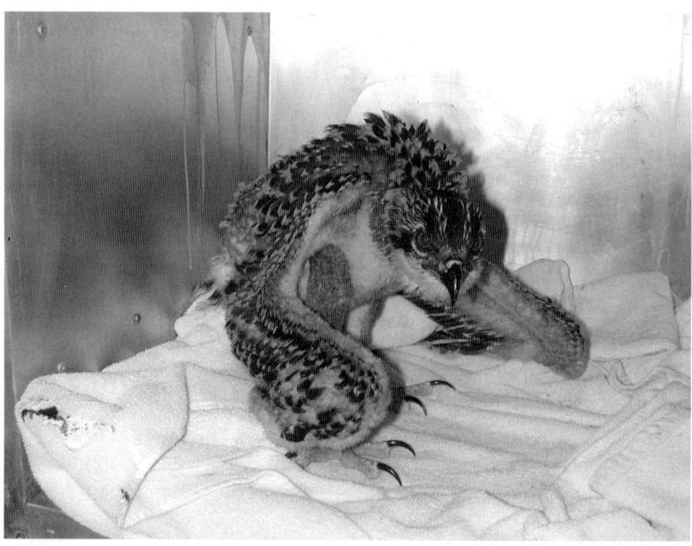

Figure 14.6. The gawky age: a nestling osprey in an incubator.

Minimum required cage sizes for prerelease conditioning can be found in Miller (2000). Recommendations vary widely in relation to the size and needs of the species, from 8 × 16 × 8 ft high (2.4 × 4.9 × 2.4 m high) for kestrels, small kites and merlins, to 20 × 100 × 16 ft high (6.1 × 30.5 × 4.9 m high) for Turkey and Black Vultures, Ferruginous Hawks, osprey, and Peregrine and Prairie Falcons. Walls should be constructed of wood or narrowly spaced wood slats, with no chain link or wire used anywhere the birds have access for clinging or climbing. Ample clean drinking and bathing water must be available at all times. Plastic artificial turf or indoor-outdoor carpeting must be used to pad round dowel or plastic pipe perches to help prevent pododermatitis (bumblefoot). Natural branches with bark make excellent perches. Provide at least two perches of varying height and angles. Many rehabilitation centers suspend perches from pulleys such that when raised they form a "swing," which provides excellent exercise and practice landing on moving objects, and when lowered they allow easier cleaning or capturing of birds.

WEANING

For raptors, catching live prey is obviously a critical skill. Presentation of whole food items should begin as soon as the birds learn to hold food down and tear it up. Darkly colored mice make an excellent starting point for most species. With kestrels and the insectivorous kites, mealworms make a good starting food because their movement attracts the birds' attention. Adding live crickets is often the second step, then young mice, then older mice, and then providing the mice with hiding places. There is no way to really provide sufficient experience in captivity to prepare them for the real-world difficulties of wild prey, so releasing them at a time when, and in a place where, naive young prey are available is important.

PREPARATION FOR WILD RELEASE

A kestrel or harrier, possibly a merlin, and most of the buteos can probably receive adequate tuition in a large flight cage with a live prey arena. Live prey arenas are typically large, secure, open-topped containers placed within the aviary, where live prey is presented to the birds for hunting practice. These can be set into the ground or placed on the surface. These can be constructed of plywood with a secure bottom that cannot be dug through, or be a large premade container such as horse trough. Important aspects are that they must be rodent escape-proof and must be large enough for the birds to maneuver to capture their dinner.

For several species, however, live prey arenas are not sufficient. Assuming renesting or wild fostering was not an option, hacking is the method of choice for accipiters, large falcons, and osprey. The latter should also be released in an area with other osprey, so as to provide models for fishing. The larger falcons and accipiters are best transferred to licensed falconers, if they cannot be hacked. The amount of practice, experience, and skill needed to catch birds on the wing needs to be learned with a backup system in place that can really be provided only by one of these two systems.

RELEASE

Besides flight conditioning and live prey training, finding an appropriate release site is critical. A cavity nester like a kestrel is best released into a nestbox rather than simply allowed to fly off. Being hidden in a box adds a level of security and provides extra time for birds to recover from the stress of transport and handling. They can then look out of the box and get used to their surroundings rather than simply taking off for the horizon.

The timing of release is also critical. Ideally, release would coincide with the independence of wild young in the area, because that is designed to be optimal. If a migratory species, release must precede the earliest migration dates by at least 2 or 3 weeks for the bird to orient itself and practice hunting in a familiar place, before linking up with others of its species.

ACKNOWLEDGMENTS

Thanks to Carol Lee, South Plains Wildlife Rehabilitation Center, Lubbock Texas, for information on kites; to members of RaptorCare for generously sharing information, trials, and tribulations over the last 7 years; and to the great team of volunteers and staff at Cascades Raptor Center for tolerating me in all my moods.

REFERENCES

Brown, L. and Amadon, D. 1968. Eagles, Hawks and Falcons of the World. McGraw-Hill, Inc., New York, 945 pp.

Carpenter, J.W., ed. 2005. Exotic Animal Formulary. Third Edition. Elsevier Saunders, St Louis, pp. 135–344.

Ehrlich, P.R., Dobkin, D.S., and Wheye, D. 1988. The Birder's Handbook: A Field Guide to the Natural History of North American Birds. Simon and Schuster, Inc., New York, 785 pp.

Ferguson-Lees, J. and Christie, D.A. 2001. Raptors of the World. Houghton Mifflin, New York, 992 pp.

Fox, N. 2000. Nutrition, The Bird of Prey Management Series. Faraway Films Productions.

International Wildlife Rehabilitation Council. 2000. Basic Wildlife Rehabilitation 1A/B, An Interpretation of Existing Biological and Veterinary Literature for the Wildlife Rehabilitator. International Wildlife Rehabilitation Council, San Jose, California.

Johnsgard, P.A. 1990. Hawks, Eagles & Falcons of North America. Smithsonian Press, 403 pp.

Miller, E.A., ed. 2000. Minimum Standards for Wildlife Rehabilitation, 3rd Edition. National Wildlife Rehabilitation Association, St. Cloud, Minnesota. 77 pp.

Palmer, R.S., ed. 1988. Handbook of North American Birds, volumes 4 & 5: Diurnal Raptors. Yale University Press, New Haven, Connecticut. 898 pp.

Poole, A. and Gill, F., eds. 1992–2004. The Birds of North America. Philadelphia: The Academy of Natural Sciences; Washington, D.C.: The American Ornithologists' Union.

Weidensaul, S. 1996. Raptors: The Birds of Prey. Lyons & Burford, New York, 382 pp.

15
Condors

Susie Kasielke

NATURAL HISTORY

The New World vultures, including the California Condor (*Gymnogyps californianus*), Andean Condor (*Vultur gryphus*), King Vulture (*Sarcorhamphus papa*), Turkey Vulture (*Cathartes aura*), Black Vulture (*Coragyps atratus*), Greater Yellow-headed Vulture (*Cathartes melambrotus*) and Lesser Yellow-headed Vulture (*Cathartes burrovianus*), are classified in the family Cathartidae, under the order Falconiformes. Although there is significant evidence to indicate that Cathartid vultures are more closely related to storks, in the order Ciconiiformes, they have not yet been reclassified as such.

As with their Old World counterparts, Cathartid vultures are obligate scavengers, spending much of their time soaring at high elevations to watch for activity on the ground that might indicate a feeding opportunity. They often feed together in large numbers in a guild of avian scavengers that may include other Cathartids, golden eagles, and ravens. They also compete with mammalian scavengers such as coyote, fox, and bear. Condors and King Vultures are the largest and typically the dominant birds at feeding sites, and often the only ones with bills powerful enough to open bigger carcasses, allowing all to feed. Their foraging strategy relies on a high degree of learned behavior, with young birds remaining with their parents for a year or more as they absorb the foraging traditions of the population. These large vultures are long-lived, with both species of condor as well as the King Vulture often living more than 40 years in captivity. The California Condor is the largest flying bird in North America with a wingspan of up to 2.7 m (9 ft). Sexes are indistinguishable, although males are typically heavier, weighing 9–11 kg (20–24 lb); females weigh 8–10 kg (18–22 lb). Juveniles have brownish-black plumage, which is lighter under the wings, dark skin on the bare head and neck, and tan colored irises.

California Condors nest in caves and potholes in steep mountain cliff faces. Only one egg is laid. Both parents share incubation duties for the 57 days (±1 day) of incubation. Once the chick has hatched, the parents take turns brooding and feeding the chick continuously for the first 3 weeks and then only at night for an additional 3 weeks. After 6 weeks, neither parent may be in attendance in the nest, although one is usually nearby for the remainder of the 5.5–6 month nestling period. Once the chick has fledged, it will continue to follow and be fed by its parents for months until it is able to feed successfully alongside adult birds. Because the entire nesting and rearing process usually takes more than a year, wild condors usually nest only every other year at most and less often when resources are scarce. California Condors reach sexual maturity at 5–6 years. The species is critically endangered, having reached an all-time low of 22 birds in 1982, but due to intensive management efforts there are now over 300 birds, nearly half of which have been released to the wild.

With a wingspan of up to 3 m (10 ft), the Andean Condor is the largest flying bird in the Americas. Juvenile plumage is an overall dark brownish grey color until the young birds reach sexual maturity at 6–7 years of age. The sexes are dimorphic from hatch because males have a fleshy caruncle along the top of the bill, which is lacking in females. This caruncle increases in size as the bird ages, as do the folds of skin around the face and neck, allowing some inference of age from a bird's appearance. Adult males weigh 11–15 kg (24–33 lb) and adult females weigh 8–11 kg (18–24 lb).

The nesting strategy of the Andean Condor is similar to that of its northern counterpart but with an incubation term of 60 days (±2 days) and a nestling period of 6.5–7 months. The species is also considered endangered, but numbers are believed to be in the thousands. Over 60 Andean Condors that were captive-bred and reared in U.S. zoos have been released to the wild in Colombia and Venezuela.

King Vultures are the most colorful of all vultures. Young chicks have dark heads and white down, and juvenile plumage and skin are overall dark gray. They are essentially monomorphic, although males tend to develop a larger caruncle and typically outweigh females. Adults weigh 3.00–3.75 kg (6.6–8.25 lb) and have a wingspan of 1.8–2.0 m (5.9–6.6 ft). Their nesting habits in the wild are virtually unknown, with nests thought to be in tree stumps or on the ground, without added nest material. They produce a single-egg clutch, with the parents taking turns incubating the egg and caring for the chick. The incubation term for King Vulture eggs in captivity is typically 55 days (±1 day). King Vultures are not considered endangered or threatened with extinction at this time.

Vultures of the genus *Gyps* are classified in the family Accipitridae, along with the other Old World vultures, hawks, and eagles, with whom they share more characteristics than do the Cathartid vultures. All are highly gregarious when feeding and roosting, and often nest colonially. They are found in a variety of open habitats including woodlands, savannahs, and steppes. Like their New World counterparts, they are monomorphic, nest in pairs, remain with the same mates indefinitely, rear one chick per nesting effort, and are long-lived. In contrast to the Cathartid vultures, females are larger than males in all Accipitrid vultures.

In recent years, populations of the three Asian species (Indian White-backed Vulture, *Gyps bengalensis*, Long-billed Vulture, *Gyps indicus*, and Himalayan Griffon Vulture, *Gyps himalayensis*) have been reduced almost to extinction. Captive breeding facilities are being developed to aid with the recovery of these ecologically and culturally important species.

All seven species in this genus have been kept in captivity, with the three African species, the African White-backed Vulture (*Gyps africanus*), Ruppell's Griffon Vulture (*Gyps rueppellii*) and Cape Griffon Vulture (*Gyps coprotheres*), being the most common in the United States.

The African White-backed Vulture is the smallest of these three at 4.2–7.2 kg (9.2–15.9 lb). The pair builds a stick nest in the crown of a tree, either separately or in small, loose colonies of up to 13 pairs. The single egg is incubated for 56 days (±1 day), and chicks fledge at 4 months.

Adult Ruppell's Griffon Vultures weigh 6.8–9.0 kg (15.0–19.8 lb). The pair builds a stick nest on a cliff ledge in the midst of a large colony consisting of 10 to 1,000 pairs. The single egg is incubated for 55 days (±1 day), and chicks fledge at about 5 months.

Cape Griffon Vultures are the largest of the *Gyps* species, weighing 7.1–10.9 kg (15.6–24.0 lb) as adults. The pair builds a stick nest on a cliff ledge in the midst of a large colony. The single egg is incubated for 55 days (±1 day), and chicks fledge at about 4.5 months.

Although this chapter addresses California and Andean Condors, King Vultures, and *Gyps* vultures specifically, the methods described should work equally well with other vulture species, with adjustments for incubation and rearing periods and proportionate feeding and weight gain amounts.

CRITERIA FOR INTERVENTION

Eggs or chicks that are neglected or compromised and cannot be returned to the parents, whether due to poor parenting, interference by enclosure mates, accident, or weather extremes, are candidates for hand-rearing. It is generally not advisable to hand-rear vultures to produce handleable animals for educational programs as these birds invariably become quite aggressive when they reach sexual maturity, greatly limiting their usefulness and diminishing their breeding potential. Whether the choice to hand-rear is intentional or as a rescue, use of the isolation-rearing methods described below will prevent malimprintation on humans and produce behaviorally healthy adults.

Determining that an egg or chick requires intervention is usually straightforward, but the need for this can often be avoided through good husbandry and subtle management techniques.

If given an appropriate, private nesting area, most vultures will prove to be excellent parents. Even so, it may be desirable to artificially hatch and rear chicks, allowing multiple clutching to increase production, as in the case of endangered species being reared for release to the wild. Occasionally, parent birds are not able to care for the egg or chick. This is more often the case with inexperienced, young parent birds and those that were hand-reared without adequate socialization with conspecifics. Individual birds, usually males, may be overly aggressive with their mates despite proper rearing and experience. In any of these situations, birds may fail to incubate consistently or brood and feed chicks adequately. They may also fight over these duties, risking egg breakage or cannibalization of the chick. Tensions are highest and the risk of injury is greatest around the times of egg laying and chick hatching. Parent birds that feel they must defend their nest site will be more aggressive with each other in general and are more likely to break eggs or injure chicks.

A good nestbox (or platform in the case of some Old World species) design will allow close monitoring of eggs and chicks through one-way glass or closed circuit video, while ensuring a sense of privacy and security for the parents. Adults can be accustomed to feeding in a specific area at a specific time, ideally one in which they can be secured and that is out of view of the nest area, thereby allowing eggs and chicks to be checked directly without the parents' awareness of this activity. This may facilitate removing eggs and replacement with dummy eggs, fostering eggs or chicks to more reliable parents, monitoring eggs and chicks, and providing supportive care to chicks until parents can fully care for them. For example, these techniques allowed a male-male pair of Cape Griffon vultures that had built and defended a nest to foster-hatch and rear a chick. The chick was given supplemental feedings for 3 weeks before morning and evening weights demonstrated that the parents were feeding it adequately. After that, no further intervention was needed.

RECORD KEEPING

Detailed records are essential to ongoing improvement of rearing methods and future successes. Careful recording of quantitative data, although it may seem tedious at the time, will facilitate later analysis. Even in facilities where large numbers of chicks are reared with limited staff, key data may be captured easily with an efficient record-keeping system. Active records should be kept in the rearing area so that information is captured while it is fresh in one's mind.

Chicks are considered to be 0 days old on the day of hatch. Daily weights, diet and amounts consumed, feeding frequency, type of enclosure, enclosure mates (if any), and brooder temperature and humidity are the most essential data to record. Weights should be taken each morning before the first morning feeding. It is useful to record the percent gained each day and/or to track weights graphically. Diet ingredients, including supplements and size of pieces offered, should be noted and the actual amount consumed recorded. This may be complicated by the fact that water or other fluids are usually offered, but solids and liquids offered should be weighed separately, both to guide others in the future and to allow nutritional analysis. After each feeding, the weight of any remaining food is subtracted from the total offered, giving the amount consumed. An alternative way to determine the amount consumed is to weigh the chick before and after each feeding. This second method is less easily done when isolation rearing methods are being used. The brooder temperature and humidity, or those of the room or chamber once the chick is no longer brooded, should be recorded at each feeding and when the chick is handled for other reasons, such as a veterinary check.

Other quantitative information recorded at each feeding includes an estimate of crop fullness (0–100%) before and after feeding, duration of feeding/puppeting session, and feeding response. A scale of 0–4 is used for the feeding response, with 0 defined as no feeding response and 4 as lunging eagerly and eating very quickly. Basic information about examination, treatment, and/or medication (including method of administration and acceptance) should be recorded, even if separate medical records exist. This ensures that the chick-rearing record provides a complete picture.

In addition, narrative comments, especially detailed descriptions of behavior and developmental stages, as well as both successful and unsuccessful feeding and handling techniques, are particularly useful for future chick-rearing and for training new staff. Comments such as "ate well" and "looks good" may be helpful to the person on the next shift, but do not provide useful information for the future. Photographic documentation of California Condor chicks at all stages of development is proving especially valuable for determining whether chicks being reared by condors in the wild are developing normally.

INCUBATION OF EGGS

California Condor eggs are incubated at 98.0°F (36.7°C). Humidity is set at 50–60% relative humidity (RH) to start. As with all artificially incubated eggs, eggs should be weighed on a regular schedule to monitor egg weight loss, adjusting incubator humidity to increase or decrease weight loss. (See Chapter 3, "Incubation.") Eggs from this species, particularly from older females, may have difficulty losing sufficient weight even in a dry incubator running at 40% RH or less. If left under the incubating parent for 7–14 days before being removed for artificial incubation, such eggs usually establish an appropriate weight loss trend that can be maintained in the incubator with sufficient care. Rarely, eggs that have not received parental incubation or otherwise do not lose sufficient weight and may require drastic measures, such as sanding the shell. (See Chapter 3.) In addition to machine-turning every 2 hours, eggs are hand-turned through ~180° twice daily in opposite directions.

Signs that the hatching process has begun may be observed as early as day 49 but more typically on day 50–51 with the air cell beginning to draw down. Between this stage and the internal pip, the egg is transferred to a separate hatcher set at 97.5°F (36.4°C) and 50% RH and is no longer turned. Internal pip usually occurs on day 53 and external pip on day 54. Once the egg is externally pipped, humidity is increased to 80% RH or more to prevent the shell membranes and extraembryonic membranes from drying out during the protracted hatching process. Hatching usually occurs on day 57. Healthy self-hatches have occurred in as little as 45 hours or as long as 96 hours after external pip. Condor eggs are easily candled, which facilitates frequent monitoring during the entire hatching process at intervals of 2–6 hours depending on the stage and progress of the egg. Chorioallantoic vessels may be seen gradually receding and yellowing. Unlike most bird species, California Condor embryos typically defecate in the shell shortly before hatching. This may also be visible on candling, and along with absence of active vessels, is a good indicator that hatching should be imminent. The embryo will respond to tapping and vocalization as it would to the parent during this stage. This can encourage the embryo to make progress toward hatching. Embryos that do not make sufficient progress at this stage may require assistance.

Andean Condor eggs are also incubated at 98.0°F (36.7°C) and started at 50–60% RH, and hatched at 97.5°F (36.4°C) and ≥70% RH. Because this species has been reared at many different facilities, incubation temperatures of 97.5–99.5°F (36.4–37.5°C) have been used with success, but incubating at 98.0°F (36.7°C) gives the most consistently healthy hatches. Their incubation term is 60 days ±2 days, with a similar pattern of internal pip 4 days prior to hatching and external pip 3 days prior. The incubation term for eggs from specific females is usually consistent from egg to egg. In other words, a female whose egg hatches at 59 days of incubation will likely have future eggs that hatch on day 59.

Both King Vulture eggs and *Gyps* vulture eggs are incubated at 98.5°F (36.9°C) and started at 50–60% RH and hatched at 98.0°F (36.7°C) and ≥70% RH. Their incubation term is 55 days and 55–56 days ±1 day, respectively, with a similar pattern of internal pip 4 days prior to hatching and external pip 3 days prior. Both Andean Condor and King Vulture eggs are also easily candled; Accipitrid vulture eggs, like all eggs from this family are difficult to candle. *Gyps* vulture eggs are white and unmarked, so early embryonic development may be readily observed, although this will appear less distinct than in Cathartid eggs. By one-quarter to one-third of the incubation period, the progression of the chorioallantoic membrane lining the inside of the shell will make the egg virtually opaque below the air cell. It is difficult to assess viability after this. One method, for eggs past midincubation, is to place the egg on a hard, flat surface, guarding it carefully to prevent rolling, and watching for movement. This may take up to 2 minutes. Another option is the use of a heartbeat detector made for eggs, such as the Egg Buddy (Avian Biotech). A negative result from either of these tests cannot confirm mortality, so eggs should be left in the incubator at least to full term unless obvious signs of death are present. Lastly, eggs of any species may be radiographed to confirm a full-term embryo and determine whether it is in the correct hatching position.

Andean Condor and *Gyps* vulture eggs, like those of California Condors, may have difficulty losing sufficient weight and should be treated similarly. King Vulture eggs, however, rarely present this challenge, perhaps because they come from a climate with much higher humidity.

Once the chick has hatched, any pieces of membrane adhering to the chick, as well as feces or urates, should be gently removed with a moistened cotton swab or gauze sponge while the chick is still wet. This material is nearly impossible to remove when it dries without damaging the chick's down or skin. Residual umbilical vessels, if present, may be cut to a length of 1 cm. The umbilical seal should be swabbed with a povidone iodine solution, such as

Betadine Solution (Purdue). This is repeated about every 6 hours for the first 72 hours. Betadine ointment, which is water-based, may be used instead of solution after the first swabbing because it stays longer without keeping the area too moist as would a petroleum-based ointment.

The newly hatched chick is allowed to rest and dry off on a fresh sterile towel in the hatcher. Once it is able to maintain sternal posture, will give a feeding response, and has defecated, it will be moved to the brooder.

INITIAL CARE AND STABILIZATION

Artificially hatched chicks that have met the above criteria for moving to the brooder may be fed 6–12 hours after hatching. Feeding may be delayed longer for chicks that have a particularly large yolk reserve. Meals are initially kept small, dilute, and frequent to allow the digestive tract to adapt gradually to processing food.

Chicks pulled due to parental neglect, illness, or injury may be chilled and/or dehydrated. Most chicks may be warmed in a preheated brooder set at 96.0–97.0°F (35.5–36.1°C), but severely hypothermic chicks may benefit from additional contact heat from a hot water bottle or similar mild heat source. As with any hypothermic animal, care must be taken to warm it gradually to ensure that the core temperature rises along with that of the extremities. Dehydrated chicks should be given fluids subcutaneously, usually in the inguinal web. Injectable antibiotics may be given to treat or prevent infection in wounds or systemically. Rocephin (Roche) has been preferred for use with chicks in recent years, particularly since it is less likely than some other products to damage immature kidneys.

Compromised chicks may have difficulty feeding and may suffer from GI stasis. Small, dilute meals given more frequently are safest in this situation. Mouse pinks (newborn mouse pups) may be minced finely enough and mixed with distilled water to pass through a standard syringe if necessary. Oral feeding is preferred whenever possible, but gavage feeding is also an option. For dehydrated chicks, an electrolyte solution such as unflavored Pedialyte (Ross) or lactated Ringer's solution, may be used instead of distilled water to moisten and dilute the diet. Great care must be taken to ensure that the chick is swallowing well when fed a liquid diet or supplemental fluids so that the chick does not aspirate these into its lungs. This is especially true of weak chicks. If the chick does not swallow readily, it is better to continue injectable fluids and/or gavage feeding until it can safely be fed by mouth.

COMMON MEDICAL PROBLEMS AND SOLUTIONS

Condors and other large vultures are exceptionally hardy and resilient birds, and their chicks are no exception. Given appropriate rearing conditions and diet, illness is rare. Of 40 California Condor chicks artificially hatched and hand-reared over the most recent 10-year period, during the first 30 days after hatch, morbidity was 10% and mortality was 5%. A chick whose unretracted yolk sac was amputated at hatch was given extensive supportive care and successfully treated for opisthotonis (or *stargazing*). Another chick developed sour crop and was also successfully treated. Six chicks that required hatching assistance were treated prophylactically with antibiotics but were never clinically ill. One chick was euthanized due to congenital deformities and neurological problems and another due to a severely infected yolk sac.

Chicks that required hatching assistance are at higher risk of infection. They may have been unable to self-hatch due to preexisting infection, edema, or dehydration. Eggs of these large vulture species that are assisted to hatch may have been opened to the air 3 or more days before hatching, with the exposed extraembryonic membranes and open umbilical seal being ideal substrates for opportunistic microbial growth. It may be useful to treat such eggs prophylactically with antibiotics. Rocephin (Roche) has been given to the embryo in ovo if an injection site is accessible or, if not, dripped onto the inner surface of the chorioallantoic membrane. The dosage for a California Condor embryo, which will weigh on average 183 g (6.5 oz) at hatch, is 12.5 mg twice daily. If the chick is normal and vigorous, with a good umbilical seal at hatching, antibiotics are discontinued. If, however, the chick has an open seal, exposed yolk sac, or is otherwise compromised, the antibiotics are continued until the condition resolves.

Although it is unusual in these large vultures, the most common illness and potential cause of death in any chick is umbilical and/or yolk sac infection. Symptoms may include diarrhea, GI stasis, redness/inflammation around the seal, discoloration of the yolk sac visible through the skin, lethargy, and/or swelling of the limb joints. When some or all of these symptoms are present, the prognosis is likely to be poor, but some chicks may recover with antibiotic therapy and supportive care.

One chick whose yolk sac was completely unretracted and partially necrotic at hatch required complete removal of the yolk sac as part of the assisted hatching procedure. Immediately following the procedure, the chick weighed 99 g (3.5 oz), 84 g (3.0 oz) lighter than the average hatch weight of 183 g (6.5 oz) of a healthy California Condor chick. This chick was given frequent fluid meals as described above and treated with antibiotics. Within 8 days it was indistinguishable from other chicks of the same age and was eventually released to the wild.

Edema due to insufficient egg weight loss may severely compromise the chick's mobility initially, particularly when the head is very edematous and difficult for the chick to lift. Although this usually dissipates through pulmonary respiration within 24–48 hours, special care and feeding assistance will likely be required during this period. Administration of a diuretic, such as furosemide, (Lasix, Aventis) may be necessary if the edema is severe. The chick may need to have its head slightly elevated and supported to ensure normal respiration while at rest and during feeding. If the edema in the head is such that creases are formed on the neck, frequent, gentle massage of these folds seems to help reduce the swelling more rapidly.

From 1991 through 1993, three unrelated California Condor chicks presented with opisthotonis immediately following hatching. Their heads were pulling sharply backward at rest and occasionally chicks would flip over onto their backs. Most of the time, chicks could bring their heads into a normal posture for a few seconds to a minute, such as for feeding, but would immediately revert to the head-back position when the effort ended. This condition may be caused by thiamine deficiency in the egg. Each of these chicks was treated with both injectable and oral thiamine in varying doses within the first 24 hours and all made a full recovery, one within 15 hours and the other two within a few days. They were able to feed relatively normally during treatment, with some steadying of their heads. Although the cause of the thiamine deficiency that resulted in the dams producing thiamine-deficient eggs could not be pinpointed with certainty, a simple diet change seems to have eliminated the problem. Prior to producing these affected chicks, adult birds were fed previously frozen, thawed trout once every 2 weeks. Because condors tear up their food rather than swallowing it whole as entirely piscivorous birds do, the fish could not be adequately supplemented to compensate for the deficiency of vitamin E and thiamine, and the presence of thiaminase that is well documented in frozen, thawed fish (Barnard and Allen 1997). The small proportion of fish in the overall diet was not expected to be harmful to the adults, and indeed it was not, but the effect on egg formation was not anticipated. Since the fish was removed from the diet of breeding birds, no further incidences of stargazing in chicks have occurred.

Sour crop is more common in true raptors, but has occurred in large vulture chicks. It may be evident immediately by a strong, sour odor coming from the chick, or the chick may regurgitate its malodorous crop contents. The feces are also likely to be strong-smelling. The smell of sour crop is much stronger than that of normal castings or other regurgitant and is almost unmistakable. It may be a side effect of systemic infection in which the digestion is otherwise slowed, or it may result from overfeeding or feeding of spoiled food. Left untreated, crop and gut stasis may follow. Treatment may be as simple as emptying the crop contents and flushing it with normal saline solution (Heidenreich 1997). Great care must be taken with these procedures to prevent aspiration of fluid into the lungs. Additional treatment for systemic infection may also be indicated.

Splayed legs may be caused by the chick slipping on a substrate that does not provide enough traction, such as toweling that is laid flat and smooth. In a normally developing chick, the knee joints should be vertically aligned with the hock joints and the feet hip-width apart. Failure to promptly correct splaying will result in permanently deviated legs. An early, mild tendency to splay may be corrected by keeping the chick tucked into snug folds of the toweling or in a towel-lined, straight-sided nest bowl for a few days. More severe cases require hobbling the legs in the normal posture. The hobbles can be made with a nonflexible bandaging tape that is doubled over to prevent sticking to the chick's skin at any point. Hobbles are placed just below the hocks, around the tarsometatarsi, and should be loose enough that circulation is not compromised, but not so loose as to allow the hobbles to slip over the hock or foot or allow toes to get caught. They must be changed daily or every other day as the chick grows.

King Vulture chicks may develop constriction bands around the toes. This syndrome is also seen in parrot chicks but has not been documented in condors or Accipitrid vultures. The cause remains unclear, but the constriction may be so severe as to restrict blood flow and cause necrosis of the distal part of the affected toe(s). Ensuring that the humidity in the brooder remains high (≥50–60% RH) will usually prevent this condition. If it does occur and is detected early, immediately increasing the humidity, maintaining a very light coating of an oil-based lubricant such as triple antibiotic ointment, and frequent massage of the toes can prevent permanent damage. If the condition is advanced, surgical intervention may be indicated (Romagnano 2003).

Condor and King Vulture chicks usually develop flaky skin on the head at some point during the brooder stage. This appears to be a normal process and not a result of low humidity or nutritional deficiency. It resolves without intervention. Condors have an extensive system of air sacs that extend under the skin of the neck and head, allowing inflation for dramatic effect. A few California Condor chicks have developed a large, persistent air "bubble" along one side of the head, which is not considered problematic and disappears by 6–8 weeks of age.

Since the arrival of West Nile Virus (WNV) in North America, large numbers of birds have become infected and died. Although Cathartid vultures fortunately have not been proven to be one of the more susceptible groups, a few California Condors, both adults and chicks, have died from the disease. In addition, two adult Andean Condors became severely ill but recovered from WNV infection, and some California Condors are showing titers far too high to have been vaccine-induced. As might be expected with an Old World species, there have been no reports of WNV morbidity or mortality in *Gyps* vultures in the U.S., but the majority of them, along with most birds in zoological collections, have been vaccinated with the equine vaccine (Fort Dodge). California Condors have been included in the DNA vaccine testing program conducted by the Centers for Disease Control. The product has not been made available commercially at this writing. Regardless of species, chicks are vaccinated beginning as early as 30 days and definitely before being placed in outdoor environments. Parent-reared birds are vaccinated at 30 days.

DIET AND WEANING

For the first 72 hours, chicks are fed mouse pinks, well minced and moistened with distilled water. Typical amounts and feeding frequencies for California Condors are shown in Table 15.1. Over the next 72 hours, the diet is converted from pinks to fuzzies (partly furred mouse pups) and then from fuzzies to adult mice (skinned, with heads, tails, and feet removed), so that by day 9, chicks are receiving 100% skinned mouse torsos (SMTs), chopped more coarsely. The ratio of solids to liquids is 2 : 1, and the mixture is warmed to body temperature before feeding. This initial diet, without supplementation of calcium or vitamin D, works well for these slow-growing vultures, but might result in metabolic bone disease if used for true raptors and other fast-growing species.

By day 12, some fur is left on the mice, which will help chicks to cast properly. Chicks will not cast every day, especially early on, and there is considerable variability in frequency, quantity, and consistency. Casts will not be pelleted as with raptors, but should be moist and semiformed. Some will produce small balls of material the size of BBs or may pass indigestible material in the feces. Wet, pasty castings and those with a sour odor indicate that chicks are not receiving sufficient casting material to cast as often as they should. At 2 weeks, chicks are often able to consume 100% furred mice, chopped but including some of the heads, tails, and feet. By 4 weeks, chicks can usually consume mice cut in quarters or halves, and by 6 weeks may easily swallow whole mice. Although parent-reared chicks would have little or no exposure to whole carcasses until fledging, hand-reared chicks at this age will also begin to eat from rat carcasses that have been cut open for them and presented when other food is not available. Encouraging this ability to self-feed makes food preparation more efficient and less costly for the remainder of the rearing period, and it helps the chick master feeding skills at an early age.

By 12 weeks, if chicks are feeding well on rats, leaving little but the skins and heads, mice may be gradually eliminated from the diet and other adult items gradually introduced. During the nestling period, this includes adult rabbits once per week and horsemeat (or beef), cut in strips and supplemented with calcium carbonate ($CaCO_3$) at 6 g $CaCO_3$ per 1 kg of meat, also once per week. The latter would be a poor diet alone, but in combination with whole prey items, it is another small economy and ensures that birds will eat this readily available product in case of interruption in the supply of rats or rabbits.

By fledging, nestlings should be established on the adult diet. The diet for one California Condor would include 1 rabbit 1 day per week, 600 g (1.25 lb) chunk horsemeat (unsupplemented) 1 day per week

Table 15.1. Los Angeles Zoo—California Condor chick rearing guide.

Age, days	Diet	Supplements	Solids, amount per feeding, gm (average)	Liquids, amount per feeding, gm (average)	Number of feedings per day and interval	Brooder temperature	Other
0	Pinks (finely minced)	—	4	2	7–2$\frac{1}{2}$ h	95°F	Distilled water in diet, sterile towel substrate, Betadine ointment to seal q 6 h × 72 h
1	Pinks (finely minced)	—	4	2	7–2$\frac{1}{2}$ h	94°F	Introduce puppet
2	Pinks (finely minced)	—	6	3	7–2$\frac{1}{2}$ h	93°F	Full isolation
3	Pinks 2:1 fuzzies (minced)	—	7	3	6–3 h	92°F	
4	Pinks 1:2 fuzzies (1/4″ pieces)	—	8	4	6–3 h	91°F	
5	Fuzzies (1/4″ pieces)	—	9	4	6–3 h	90°F	
6	Fuzzies 2:1 SMT (1/4–1/2″)	—	10	5	5–3$\frac{1}{2}$ h	89°F	
7	Fuzzies 1:2 SMT (1/4–1/2″)	—	11	5	5–3$\frac{1}{2}$ h	88°F	
8	SMT (1/2″ pieces)	—	13–14	6	4–4 h	87°F	
9	SMT (1/2″ pieces)	—	15–16	6	4–4 h	86°F	
10	SMT 1:1 mice (furred, 1/4 s)	—	29–30	12	3–5 h	85°F	
11	SMT 1:1 mice (furred, 1/4 s)	—	30–38	12	3–5 h	84°F	
12	Mice (1/4 s)	—	33–45	12–13	3–5 h	83°F	
13	Mice (1/4 s & 1/2 s)	—	37–52	12–13	3–5 h	82°F	
14	Mice (1/4 s & 1/2 s)	—	43–62	13–17	3–5 h	81°F	

15	Mice (1/4 s & 1/2 s)	—	58–90	13–17	2–10 h	82°F	
16	Mice (1/2 s)	—	66–106	18–24	2–10 h	80°F	
17	Mice (1/2 s)	—	72–102	18–24	2–10 h	79°F	
18	Mice (1/2 s)	—	80–124	20–26	2–10 h	78°F	Tap water in diet
19	Mice (1/2 s)	—	88–130	20–30	2–10 h	77°F	
20	Mice (1/2 s)	—	98–138	22–30	2–10 h	76°F	
21	Mice (1/2 s)	—	110–160	26–30	2–10 h	75°F	Move to tub (18–21 days)
35	Rat (slit open)—am mice (1/2 s)—pm	—	1 @ 265 g	— 30–38	2–10 h	75°F (room)	
42	Rat (slit open)—am mice (whole)—pm	—	1 @ 265 g	— 30–38	2–10 h	Outdoor w/heat lamp	Move to outdoor rearing chamber
60	Rats (whole)	—	4–5 @ 125 g	—	1	Outdoor w/heat lamp	
75–80	Rats Su·M·Tu·Th·F·Sa horsemeat (cut in strips) W	0.60 gm $CaCO_3$/ 100 gm meat	4–5 @ 125 g	—	1	Outdoor	
150–180	Feline diet M rabbit Tu horsemeat (chunk) W rats Su·Th·F·Sa	—	500 g 1 @ 570 g 4–5 @	—	1		

and 4–5 rats daily for 3–5 days per week. Adults feeding chicks and recently fledged, hand-reared juveniles are fed daily until the youngest bird is 9–10 months old, when 1–2 fast days per week are implemented.

FEEDING PROCEDURES

To elicit feeding by the parent, the chick will reach upward toward the parent's beak, wing-begging by pumping its wings rapidly up and down. The parent then regurgitates partially digested food, which is very liquid for a new chick but more solid later on, and the chick may reach part way into the parent's mouth to feed. For hand-reared chicks, this feeding response can be elicited in the chick by placing the thumb and forefinger alongside the beak. Initial feedings are best delivered using a small plastic spoon to slowly slide the diet into the chick's mouth. It is important to get all the fluid into the chick to ensure good hydration. Most new chicks will stop feeding and turn away if they bite down on anything hard, such as the spoon or a bone fragment, so care should be taken to avoid this. Some feeders prefer using their fingers to using a spoon, but it is difficult to get all the liquid into the chick by this method. In either case, coordination of this process with an eager but uncoordinated chick takes practice. Chicks may eat so fast that they expel fluid from their nares, which should be promptly blotted away. As long as the chick is feeding voluntarily, aspiration of fluids into the lungs is rare, but the chick should be monitored for a few minutes to ensure that this has not occurred.

Chicks can learn to self-feed from a small cup as early as the first day, but most will take 2–3 days to master this. It is essential that chicks be able to do this by about 72 hours of age in order to implement an effective isolation-rearing protocol at this stage (see Figure 15.1). A shallow, light-colored, plastic measuring cup of 50–75 ml (.25–.33 C) capacity works well. Chicks are naturally attracted to the red color of the food and will quickly reach for it when the cup is held at just the right angle. This takes practice for both chick and feeder. Again, care should be taken to ensure that the fluids are consumed, using the spoon at the end of the feeding if necessary.

Amounts fed are not limited to a prescribed amount or percentage of body weight because excessive weight gain has not been a problem with these species. Records from healthy chicks provide a guide for expected intake. The chick's crop should empty to no more than 5–10% fullness between feedings and should empty completely overnight. If this does not occur, the scheduled feeding should be delayed or skipped until the crop clears. Chicks that are overfed or are slow to process may develop sour crop and subsequent crop stasis, requiring intervention.

Once chicks are out of the brooder and housed in a tub, food is presented in a small, shallow ceramic crock. Plastic crocks have also been used but are more lightweight and easily spilled by the chick.

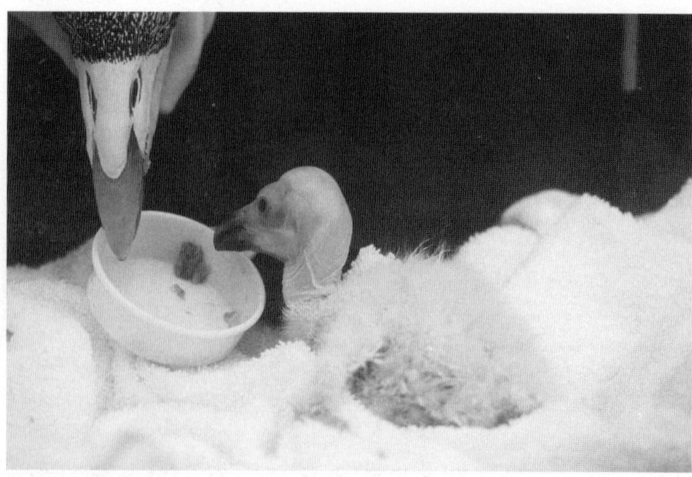

Figure 15.1. Feeding a 36-hour-old California Condor chick with a puppet (photo by Mike Wallace, courtesy of the Los Angeles Zoo).

When chicks have moved and adjusted to an outdoor nestbox chamber, food and water are delivered in larger crocks placed in a shallow tray, such as a small cat litter box. This tray slides into a custom-made fixed plywood box with a sliding lid, allowing food and water to be changed from outside the enclosure. This system also minimizes the chicks' ability to remove the crocks to out-of-reach areas of the chamber.

After fledging, juveniles and adults are usually fed only in the holding enclosure, which is about 2 × 4 × 2.5 m (6 × 12 × 8 ft) high and attached to the main flight enclosure. This conditions birds to routinely enter this enclosure, the door of which may be closed from the outside, allowing staff to capture birds easily for physical exams and moves. Food is delivered by way of a chute, made from a section of 20 cm (8 in) diameter PVC pipe, painted black and mounted through the fence on a downward angle at a height of 2 m (6 ft). The tube is covered with a PVC cap when not in use. The holding area and adjacent enclosure walls are covered with solid material, such as corrugated metal sheets, to provide a sight barrier. This virtually eliminates the birds' associating humans with food, as long as staff members are especially quiet and stay out of view when feeding.

EXPECTED WEIGHT GAIN

Chicks should be weighed daily before the first morning feeding to provide the most consistent basis for comparison. This is easily done while chicks are still housed in brooders or in open tubs indoors. Chicks usually do not gain weight the first day and in fact lose 1% of their hatch weight on average. Initial weight gain is slow, from 3–5% daily for days 2 through 5, but jumps dramatically to an average of 12% ± 5% for days 6 through 18 (see Figure 15.2). From day 19 through 35, weight gain averages 7% daily but varies from 2–16% each day.

Once they have been moved to outdoor rearing chambers or nestboxes, weighing is more difficult because chicks are no longer handled directly on a daily basis. Weights may be taken opportunistically during this period, such as when chicks are

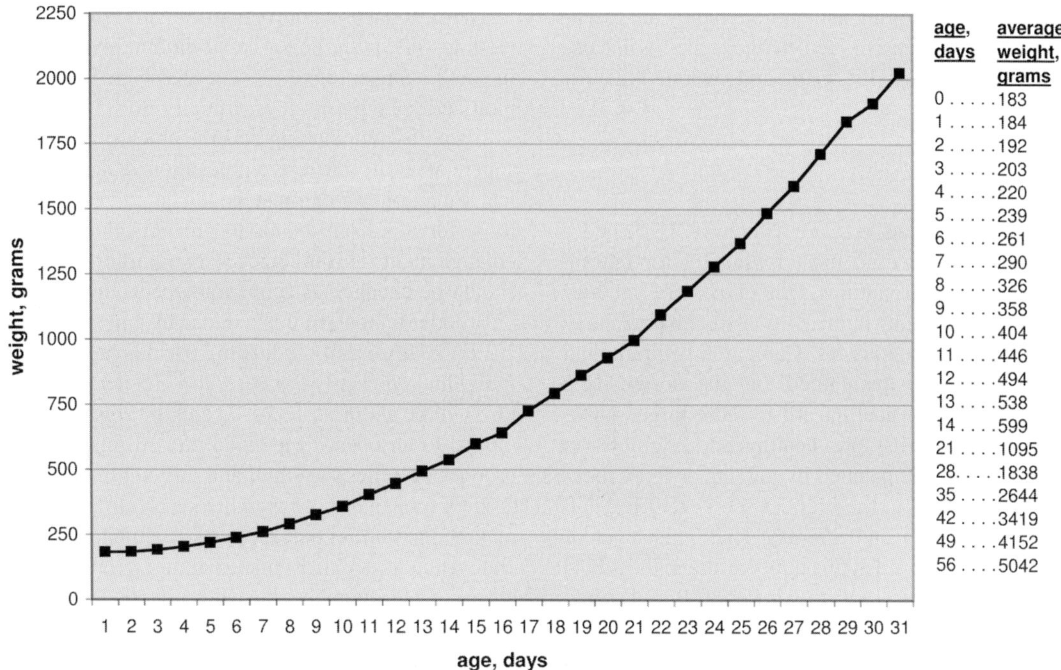

Figure 15.2. California Condor chick growth graph (courtesy of the Los Angeles Zoo).

vaccinated. Once they are old enough to jump up on a low perch, 30–40 cm (12–15 in) high, a sturdy spring scale (Pelouze model 10B60 heavy duty receiving scale, 27 kg/60 lb capacity), on which a protective plywood box housing is attached to replace the weighing platform, may be mounted inside the rearing chamber. Placed where it is likely to be a favored perch, this scale may provide weights on a fairly consistent basis without the need to handle the chick. Scales may also be placed in outdoor flight enclosures, mounted high on a sturdy post to serve as a preferred perch, to provide weight information on fledged juveniles and adults. Because the birds tend to bounce heavily on the scale, the plywood box housing should be mounted to the scale platform brackets using nuts and bolts designed for aircraft. These may take a bit of effort to find, but hang-gliding shops and light aircraft mechanics are good places to start. Similarly, the lightweight metal ferrule that secures the clear cover over the face of the scale must be secured with screws to prevent the birds from systematically tearing it off and destroying the face of the scale. Electronic scales have been tried with condors on a limited basis but have not proven to be practical because both the birds and the environment are too hard on the scales.

Unlike many smaller bird species, Cathartid and *Gyps* vulture chicks may not achieve or exceed adult weight before fledging and, although they are essentially at adult stature when fledged, they will continue to increase bone mass and overall bulk for more than a year.

HOUSING

The Animal Intensive Care Unit (AICU) brooder (Lyon) has been used most frequently for rearing condors and other vultures. Other types of forced-air brooders, including human infant incubators, may also be used as long as stable temperature and humidity can be maintained and the design does not present a physical hazard to these large, active chicks. Chicks that are healthy and vigorous at hatching, whether hatched by parents or in an incubator, are placed in the brooder set at 95.0°F ± 1°F (35.0°C ± 0.5°C) and 35–40% RH. This level of humidity is achieved at this temperature in the AICU when the water reservoir tray is kept full of distilled water. Although low, it has proven appropriate for both species of condor and *Gyps* vultures. King Vultures will require higher humidity, at least 50% RH. Until the temperature begins to approach room temperature when ambient humidity will be adequate, using a second reservoir inside the brooding chamber helps increase humidity. A straight-sided, plastic food container, about 6–8 in (15–20 cm) square, partly filled with distilled water and paper or cloth towels (bunched up to increase the evaporative surface area), and securely covered with wire or plastic mesh, works well. Towels should be changed daily to limit microbial growth.

As with egg incubators, prior to placing a chick in a brooder, it is wise to do some temperature mapping by taking temperature readings in all parts of the chamber to ensure that there are no hot or cool areas, and if there are to compensate for them. AICU brooders run at temperatures over 86°F (30°C) will maintain more consistent and stable temperatures if a folded bath towel is placed on top for insulation and multiple layers of towel substrate are used under the chick.

Larger, more vigorous chicks may require slightly lower initial temperatures; small or compromised chicks tend to need a higher temperature. Chicks that are too hot will be sprawled or listless, may develop white salt accumulation around their nares, and may become dehydrated. Cold chicks will huddle tightly and may even shiver or feel cool to the touch. Their digestion will slow, potentially resulting in crop stasis and/or sour crop.

The brooder is bedded thickly with white terry-cloth towels, with the top layer thoroughly rumpled in small, snug folds to prevent the chick from slipping and splaying its legs. Initially, towels may be sterilized by autoclaving and the chick placed on a square of sterile gauze as a precaution against umbilical infection. Care must be taken to remove all loose threads from towels to prevent injury due to entanglement of the chick's extremities. Towels should be changed as soon as they become soiled.

Brooder temperature is reduced by approximately 1.0°F (90.5°C) daily, adjusting as indicated by the individual chick. By 3 weeks, the brooder temperature will be about 75°F (24°C) and the chick may be moved to an open, deep-sided tub. At this age, the brooder becomes too small and difficult to clean for a chick that may now weigh 1 kg (2.2 lb). The tub may be the bottom half of a plastic animal shipping crate, such as a Vari Kennel (Petmate), modified by covering the door opening with plywood or mesh, or a deep, rubber feeding tub (Fortex). The tub may be lined only with towels, or may have a 3–4 in (8–10 cm) layer of substrate such as decomposed granite or sand lightly covered with towels. *Gyps* vultures are reared in stick nests in the wild, so a stable arrangement of sturdy sticks under older hand-reared chicks may help with foot development. If a substrate is used, it must be changed at least weekly to prevent the buildup of ammonia from urates. Chicks should be monitored to ensure that they do not drag food through the substrate and ingest it. Chicks from this stage onward spend a lot of time manipulating objects in their immediate environment. Clean, molted feathers from adult birds and rocks or sturdy sticks too big to swallow make good nest "toys."

It is also possible to house chicks in open tubs a few days earlier if a contact heat source is provided. Towels should be the only substrate for these younger chicks. A heating pad set under half of the tub allows chicks that are able to move around to self-regulate their need for warmth. Heating pads should never be used directly inside the chick's enclosure due to the risk of electrocution should the wiring become exposed by the chick or due to wear. Chicks under 2 weeks of age are not mobile enough to self-regulate their temperature needs and should be kept in a forced-air brooder.

At 6–8 weeks of age, chicks may be transferred to an outdoor rearing chamber that allows them to see and hear adult birds. This may be an enclosure designed especially for this purpose or an unused nestbox. Nestboxes are usually 2 × 2 × 2 m (6 × 6 × 6 ft) high; dedicated rearing chambers may be only 2/3 this width, or smaller for King Vultures. These are plywood on all sides with a sturdy wire mesh covered opening, 0.5–1 m (1.5–3 ft) square, on the side adjacent to the flight enclosure. The bottom of this opening is about 0.6 m (2 ft) above the floor with a sturdy shelf perch just underneath that allows the chick to directly view the adult enclosure at will when it is old enough to jump up on the shelf. As with nestboxes for condors and King Vultures, the nestbox floor should be covered with clean sand 10–15 cm (4–6 in) deep. When chicks are first transferred from the indoor tub to the outdoor rearing chamber, a few of the terrycloth towels are also placed in the chamber as familiar things that help ease the transition. These are eventually removed and not replaced. If temperatures will drop below 65°F (18°C), supplemental heat should be provided by a heat lamp or other radiant heat source placed over one section of the chamber and protected by a wire mesh cover to prevent older chicks from having direct contact with it. Ventilation should be provided by an exhaust fan and/or mesh-covered windows around the top of the chamber.

A dark blind, made of plywood or dark, opaque tarp over a PVC pipe frame, is attached to the outside of the rearing chamber and all chick care is provided through small doors accessed through this blind. A small window, 10 × 30 cm (4 × 12 in), covered with dark automotive window tinting film to create one-way glass and installed above the access door about 10 × 20 cm (4 × 8 in)), allows staff members to continue to use the puppet surrogate to interact with the chick. Initially, food and water crocks can be put in and removed through this port, but chicks will soon begin dragging crocks out of reach. When chicks have adjusted to their new enclosure and are large enough to reach, a feeding box (described in the section "Diet," earlier in this chapter) may be used.

Closed-circuit video cameras are used to monitor chicks remotely from hatching through fledging and beyond. This may be a sophisticated, commercial system or a simple, inexpensive security camera.

PREPARATION FOR WILD RELEASE

Vulture chicks that will be hand-reared and later released to the wild must be carefully managed in strict isolation from human contact and socialized with adult conspecifics in order to have the best chance of survival and long-term success in the wild. Unlike most raptors, such as hawks, eagles, and falcons, vultures do not have a discrete, hard-wired window of imprintation as young chicks in which they form their species identity. With the high capacity for learned behavior and innate inquisitiveness required of these scavenging species, vultures very readily malimprint on humans. This tendency persists well beyond a year of age and disappears entirely only by the age of sexual maturity.

Visual and auditory isolation from human contact is implemented with chicks no later than 72 hours after hatching. No talking or whispering of any kind is permitted near chicks or juvenile birds, and a recording of nature sounds is played continuously in the brooder room to mask the sounds of people working. All feeding and other care is provided with the caregiver in a dark blind and the chick, whether in a brooder or later in a tub, in a well-lighted area. The blind is constructed using dark, opaque fabric curtains with openings at arm height and a shaded viewing window. The fabric of the armholes is overlapped to prevent gaps. The window, about 20 × 30 cm (8 × 12 in), is made of two or more layers of window screen or shade cloth and is covered with a

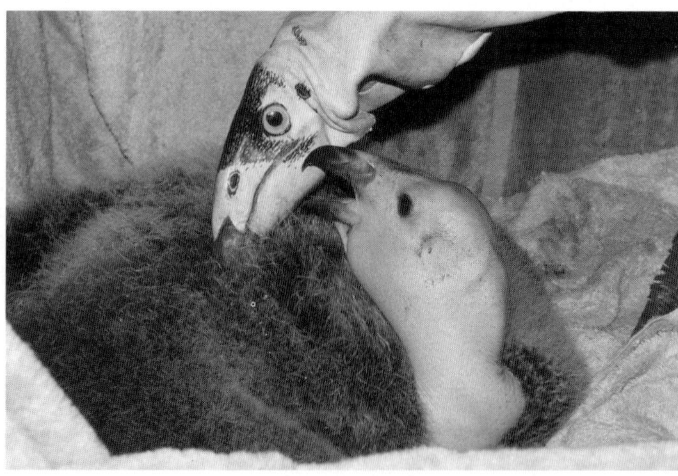

Figure 15.3. California Condor chick at 46 days of age interacting with a condor puppet (photo by Mike Wallace, courtesy of the Los Angeles Zoo).

dark fabric flap when not in use. The curtains are suspended from cables anchored to the walls or attached to PVC pipe frames. Dark fabric is also used for the ceiling of the blind.

A lifelike condor (or other vulture species) hand puppet is used to interact with the chick. The puppet is made with an acrylic molded skull, glass taxidermy eyes, and elkhide skin, attached to an artificial fur sleeve that reaches the caregiver's upper arm (see Figure 15.3). The puppet rarely offers food to the chick but rather functions in social interactions, behaving and responding as much like a parent condor as possible, including preening the chick, chastising it when it is too assertive and reacting to external noises. The caregiver's other arm is covered with a loose, closed-ended lightweight black fabric sleeve of equal length. This allows good dexterity for handling the chick and materials around it.

To remove the chick from the brooder for daily weighing and cleaning or for medical procedures, a dark drape is first loosely placed over the chick by the puppet and sleeve. The caregiver can then move the curtain aside and place the covered chick in a deep container for weighing. It is very important to ensure adequate ventilation for these young chicks, which have a naturally low carrying capacity for oxygen in the blood. Isolation can be maintained if the weighing container has numerous ventilation holes on one side and is always kept facing away from the caregiver, with the drape placed loosely over the top of the container.

A newer method of maintaining visual isolation during routine procedures is to use the loose sleeve as a hood. Chicks will naturally probe and push, so the caregiver uses the sleeved hand to gently cover the chick's head and then inverts the entire sleeve over the chick's neck. The open end is gathered with a soft elastic insert that helps secure it. As with a drape, the time a chick is hooded should be kept brief and adequate ventilation must be ensured. As long as the fabric is lightweight, the elastic end is slightly loose, and the chick is not agitated, ventilation should be adequate. Chicks that are draped or hooded behave much as they do when brooded or when it is dark, remaining very relaxed. They will, however, continue to probe and poke their heads out from under a drape or through a curtain if given the opportunity. This might seem like a minor problem, but chicks very rapidly become habituated with just this limited exposure to humans, so caregivers must be vigilant to prevent this.

Even with good isolation, chicks may become habituated to change of all sorts if they are handled too much or desensitized to many new experiences. Because of this, moves and other changes in the chick's environment, incidences of physical restraint, and exposure to other chicks are kept to an absolute minimum. For older chicks and juveniles, moves and exams are best done at night when the birds are less alert and there is no association with routine, daytime activities.

As chicks get older and are moved to outdoor chambers, the puppet is less and less suitable to fill the role of an adult condor, so use of the puppet is decreased over time. Chicks may become overly aggressive with this surrogate parent, which is not appropriate chick-to-adult behavior. At this stage, visual and auditory access to one or more adult condors provides more appropriate role modeling for the chick. For California Condors, a single adult male mentor is housed adjacent to the hand-reared chicks and they are later fledged, one at a time, into the enclosure with him. Males have proven more tolerant with chicks than females who are often far too aggressive with them, especially if there is an adult male nearby. Females have been good mentors for juveniles over 1 year of age. Mentors are chosen for their appropriate behavior in response to human activity, primarily avoidance or at least lack of interest. Birds that are inquisitive about human activity and novel events are not suitable mentors even if they have previously been in a flock situation or have been good parents. The goal is for young birds to be wary of new things and to develop the skills and confidence necessary for social interaction in a competitive, hierarchical population.

This rearing method, conscientiously carried out, produces chicks that are as wild as their wild-reared counterparts. Although this is a good thing that will serve them well once released, it requires careful management during the remainder of their time in captivity. A fledged juvenile that is suddenly frightened may fly into the enclosure mesh, attempting to climb it to gain height, but eventually putting so much pressure on its beak that the beak cracks or breaks, requiring major repair. In order to prevent this, the beak tips of chicks are blunted by filing with an emery board before fledging.

California Condor juveniles, whether hand-reared or parent-reared, remain with their initial adult mentor until they are about 14–18 months old. When it is determined that all juveniles in the cohort have developed appropriate confidence and social behavior, they are ready to be transferred to the prerelease enclosure in the field. This enclosure is similar to the captive breeding enclosures. The juvenile cohort stays in this facility with the adult mentor for several weeks to months, adjusting to the diet and environment they will find after release. Once released, biologists continue to place carcasses in or near the enclosure, ensuring that the birds find food while they are adapting to the wild and providing a ready means of recapture.

PREPARATION FOR INTRODUCTION TO CAPTIVE FLOCK

Birds that are hand-reared for captive breeding or display purposes should also be reared by the above methods, but they require less stringent precautions to avoid exposure to human activity after fledging. The primary consideration should be to avoid the chick's developing a strong association with humans as a food source because this will lead to aggression. It is not necessary to deliberately habituate juveniles to any particular aspect of captive life. If staff members conduct routine activities, such as cleaning and maintaining enclosures, without encouraging interaction with the birds and discouraging their approaches, juveniles will not feel rewarded by human attention and will naturally acclimate to the captive environment.

BEHAVIORAL TRAINING FOR EDUCATIONAL PROGRAMS

Birds intended to work in educational programs should be parent-reared or isolation-reared up to the age of fledging. Hand-reared birds with which no isolation precautions have been taken are very affectionate and relaxed with human caregivers well into their juvenile stage. As these birds approach sexual maturity, however, they will become increasingly aggressive, particularly with people other than those who reared them. Even parent- or isolation-reared birds, especially males, tend to become increasingly challenging to work with at this age. These large vultures are best prepared for educational programs by individuals with a strong animal-training background, ideally in both falconry methods and general operant conditioning with a variety of species. Vultures that have been used in educational programs may also become good breeding birds later if managed consistently well. Adult birds that were not handled properly when young may become unmanageable and dangerous, necessitating their removal from programs. They are likely to be poor display birds, lacking the social skills to integrate with other vultures, and will be unlikely to be good parents. Given the long life spans of all these species, careful and informed management from the beginning is essential.

ACKNOWLEDGMENTS

Thanks to the many people with the California Condor Recovery Program, as well as the staff at the Los Angeles Zoo. Their work with California Condors and all our other vultures is the foundation of this chapter. They include Animal Keepers Mike Clark, Chandra David, Debbie Sears, Dawn Swalberg, Marti Jenkins, Laurie Ahlander, and Nancy

Thomas, along with Veterinarians Dr. Cynthia Stringfield, Dr. Janna Wynne, Dr. Leah Greer, Dr. Russ Burns, Dr. P. K. Robbins, Dr. Michelle Miller, Dr. Scott Amsel, and Dr. Ben Gonzales, and Veterinary Technicians Jeanette Tonnies and Julie Sweet, just to name a few. Mike Wallace, Ph.D., California Condor Recovery Team Leader and former Curator of Birds at the Los Angeles Zoo, has been a primary driving force of the recovery program. Their abilities are amazing and their passion inspiring.

SOURCES FOR PRODUCTS MENTIONED

Aventis (Sanofi-Aventis), 300 Somerset Corporate Boulevard, Bridgewater, NJ 08807-2854, (800) 981-2491, (800) 207-8049, http://products.sanofi-aventis.us/lasix/lasix.html.

Avian Biotech International, 1336 Timberlane Road, Tallahassee, FL 32312-1766, (850) 386-1145, (800) 514-9672, http://www.avianbiotech.com/buddy.htm.

Purdue Pharma L.P., Stamford, CT, (800) 877-5666, (203) 588-8000, http://www.pharma.com.

Fort Dodge Animal Health, West Nile Vaccine Product Manager, P.O. Box 25945, Overland Park, KS 66225-5945, (800) 477-1365 (U.S.), (800) 267-1777 (Canada), http://www.equinewestnile.com/index.htm.

Fortex Fortiflex, (800) 468-4460, http://www.fortexfortiflex.com/rubberpans.html.

Lyon Technologies, Inc., 1690 Brandywine Avenue, Chula Vista, CA 91911, (888) 596-6872, http://www.lyonelectric.com.

Pelouze Scales, Rubbermaid Commercial Products, 3124 Valley Avenue, Winchester, VA 22601, (800) 950-9787, (888) 761-8574, http://www.pelouze.com.

Roche Pharmaceuticals, Hoffman-La Roche, Inc., 340 Kingsland Street, Nutley, NJ 07110, (973) 235-5000, http://www.rocheusa.com/products/rocephin/pi.pdf.

Ross Consumer Products Division, Abbott Laboratories, 625 Cleveland Avenue, Columbus, OH 43215, (800) 227-5767, http://www.pedialyte.com.

Petmate, P.O. Box 1246, Arlington, TX 76004-1246, (877) 738-6283, http://www.petmate.com/Catalog.plx.

REFERENCES

Bernard, Joni B. and Allen, Mary, E. 1997. Feeding captive piscivorous animals: Nutritional aspects of fish as food. In Nutrition Advisory Group Handbook. Association of Zoos and Aquariums, Silver Spring, Maryland.

Clark, Michael, Wallace, Michael, and David, Chandra. 2006. Rearing California Condors for Release Using a Modified Puppet-rearing Technique. In press.

del Hoyo, Josep, Elliott, Andrew, and Sargatal, Jordi, eds. 1994. Handbook of the Birds of the World. Volume 2. New World Vultures to Guineafowl. Lynx Editions. Barcelona.

Ferguson-Lees, James and Christie, David A. 2001. Raptors of the World. Houghton Mifflin Co., New York.

Heidenreich, Manfred. 1997. Birds of Prey: Medicine and Management. Blackwell Science, Oxford.

Koford, Carl B. 1953. The California Condor. Dover Publications, Inc., New York.

Kuehler, Cynthia M., Sterner, Donald J., Jones, Deborah S., Usnik, Rebecca L., and Kasielke, Susie. 1991. Report on the captive hatches of California Condors (*Gymnogyps californianus*): 1983–1990. Zoo Biology 10: 65–68.

Ritchie, Branson W., Harrison, Greg J., and Harrison, Linda R. 1994. Avian Medicine: Principles and Application. Wingers Publishing, Inc., Lake Worth, Florida.

Romagnano, April. 2003. Avian Pediatrics. Proceedings of the International Aviculturists Society.

Snyder, Noel F.R. and Snyder, Helen. 2000. The California Condor: A Saga of Natural History and Conservation. Academic Press, San Diego.

Wilbur, Sanford R. and Jackson, Jerome A., eds. 1983. Vulture Biology and Management. U.C. Press, Berkeley.

16
Herons and Egrets

Megan Shaw Prelinger

NATURAL HISTORY

There are 65 species of herons, egrets, and bitterns in the suborder Ardeidae in the order Ciconiiformes, and 10 species of herons and egrets are found in North America. All species of herons and egrets nest in trees, although some may occasionally nest on the ground in treeless areas. All species hatch altricial, downy young. Herons and egrets are colonial nesters and typically hatch groups of nestlings at the rate of two to four per nest. Incubation lasts 17–28 days, depending on the size of the species, and young fledge in 21–30 days (Dent 1963). Some species may continue to support fledglings for a short period after they have left the nest.

Herons and egrets have anisodactyl feet, with three long toes pointing forward and one pointing back. Each toe is furnished with a sharp and pointed claw. The remarkable length and hensile strength of their toes and the sharpness of their claws enable them to firmly grip tree branches of varying thicknesses.

Adult diets are adaptable to available food stocks. Small fish and aquatic invertebrates are preferred foods, although all herons and egrets rely additionally in varying measures on small rodents and insects. Young are fed a regurgitated diet for their first few days of life, but they readily learn to pick up foods left for them on the floors of their nests.

CRITERIA FOR INTERVENTION

Herons and egrets are gregarious colonial nesters that are less sensitive to human population density than some other families of birds. Many young fall from nests in their early days or weeks of life. Fallen young hatched in colonies that are situated in remote environments may be fed on the ground by their parents while they hide in surrounding grasses. Fallen young hatched in urban or suburban colonies, however, are extremely vulnerable to predators such as birds of prey, cars, cats, and dogs, because such colonies tend to be situated above cropped grass or pavement rather than above tall natural grasses. Fallen nestlings are thus left entirely exposed. They are also subject to being harassed or "rescued" by passing children or adults. Such interventions are likely to end a young bird's life unless a subsequent intervention is made by a rehabilitator.

Nestlings and fledglings that fall from high branches are prone to skeletal injuries and soft-tissue bruising. Most critically, they are subject to life-threatening hypothermia, even on warm days. Additionally, placing even healthy and alert individuals back in their nests is often impossible due to the heights at which tree-nesting colonies are located.

RECORD KEEPING

It is important to keep records on individual orphaned and injured herons and egrets, so that developmentally alike individuals can be housed and cared for together. It is also important to track and note the progress of injury recovery and the key developmental stages as birds progress from rescue to release. Rescue events tend to be clustered around specific locations and seasons, so rehabilitators are more often faced with hand-rearing groups of animals rather than individuals. It is important to keep detailed notes on the progress of feather coverage on young birds' bodies, because the process of feather growth determines birds' abilities to thermoregulate and to begin to learn to fly. Together, these are the most important criteria by which young birds are graduated from stage to stage within the orphan-rearing process.

Such careful tracking will also allow age-appropriate clustering of patients, which will facilitate peer group socialization and insulate individuals from peer-to-peer aggression that may occur when young at different developmental stages are housed together.

INITIAL CARE AND STABILIZATION

The importance of addressing hypothermia in young herons and egrets cannot be overstated. Herons and egrets for their first 2 to 3 weeks of life are unable to thermoregulate outside their nests, even on warm days. Rehabilitators who are expecting young herons and egrets should keep on hand a prewarmed incubator or cage with heat lamp, set to maintain an ambient temperature of 100°F (37.7°C) and 40–50% humidity. Young birds should be placed within such an environment immediately upon arrival, even if they are alert (see Figure 16.1). New patients should be allowed 30 to 60 minutes to rest and warm up prior to any examination. If birds are sleepy or unresponsive, supplemental hydration should be provided during the warm-up period, using prewarmed sterile fluids such as lactated Ringer's solution administered subcutaneously (SQ) at 5% of body weight (50 ml/kg), or electrolyte solution offered orally. Subsequent hydrations and all nutrition should be withheld until after a complete examination has been performed.

Alert young herons and egrets are poor candidates for oral hydration. The ability to expand the throat and mouth very wide is required for young to ingest the sometimes large fish, insects, and rodents that parents may deliver to the nest. However, the ability to gape wide enough to swallow a whole 15 g fish provides these birds with an easy mechanism for rejecting oral hydration: they simply open their throats in a gape following fluid administration and the fluids fall right out of their proventriculus onto the floor of the cage in front of them. This scenario creates unnecessary risks of aspiration and can be avoided by sticking to subcutaneous methods of supplemental hydration.

Extremely young hatchlings arriving with only downy feathers may be placed in a shallow dish lined with a washcloth to support their bodies in an upright position. Herons and egrets that are old enough to begin developing contour or flight feathers on their bodies are generally able to hold their bodies up independently and look around.

When warm and alert, new arrivals should be given a thorough intake examination, consisting of a cloacal temperature check and a beak-to-toe physical exam. Digital human oral thermometers are adequate for monitoring body temperature. Be careful to insert only the tip of the thermometer into the bird's cloaca, as trauma to delicate tissue is a risk.

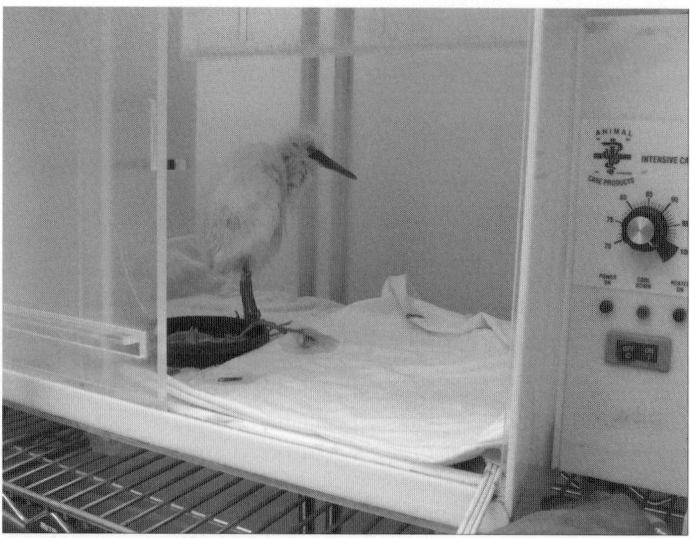

Figure 16.1. Snowy Egret fledgling warming up in an incubator with a supplemental heating pad.

Temperature checks of self-feeding animals should be made before food is offered: a hungry bird having feasted on a large meal of recently refrigerated fish will likely register a temporary drop in body temperature as its body warms up the meal it has just consumed, leading to inaccurate body temperature readings.

COMMON MEDICAL PROBLEMS AND SOLUTIONS

Young herons and egrets are vulnerable to bone injuries and malformations at all stages of rearing. Supplemental calcium is recommended in the form of crushed or powdered calcium carbonate sprinkled onto foods daily throughout care.

Throughout the orphan-rearing process young birds should be checked regularly for any signs of limping behavior or drooping wings that could indicate hairline fractures or bone softening. This is especially critical when oral supplementation of calcium is not available. Bone injuries are often subtle enough in their beginning stages that they may not be observable on a tabletop exam.

If a limp or a wing droop is detected on intake or at any time during the orphan-rearing process, the afflicted limb should be stabilized with a light supportive wrap, such as a figure-8 bandage made from Vetrap (3M) (for a wing) or a splint or light supportive wrap, using either SAM Splint (SAM Medical Products) or Vetrap, or both (if for a leg or toe). The affected animal should then be placed in a cage that restricts motion and inhibits exacerbation of the injury. For example, if a fledgling bird is found limping in either an indoor or outdoor flight aviary, the bird should be brought inside and placed in a cage that is tall enough to allow it to stand, but small enough to allow it to take no more than a few steps. If available, padding should be used on walls and floors to minimize the injury becoming aggravated by loss of balance. At the same time, the bird's calcium intake should be reassessed to assist the bone healing process. Vitamin D may also be given orally or intramuscularly to assist with uptake of the calcium supplementation. Consult your avian veterinarian for species-appropriate doses and combinations of supplements to assist bone development. Excessive vitamin D supplementation may result in mineralization of soft tissues.

Swollen joints can signal rickets, which is caused by insufficient calcium or vitamin D3, or inadequate dietary calcium-to-phosphorus ratio. For proper bone growth, the diet should contain twice as many milligrams calcium as phosphorus.

Many nestlings sustain bruising or lacerations during their falls from their nests. In some cases, these falls can result in organ damage or internal hemorrhage that is life-threatening. Bright light shown against the skin of the abdomen can reveal hemorrhage in the coelomic cavity. The severity of such damage is best revealed in a radiograph.

Superficial lacerations should be cleaned daily with a dilute solution of chlorhexidine or betadine. If lacerations are superficial, small, clean, and have already begun to heal through secondary intention, daily cleaning is generally adequate to result in quick resolution. Fresh lacerations, and larger or deeper lacerations, should be cleaned and then closed with a topical dressing such as Tegaderm (3M), Biodres (DVM Pharmaceuticals), or both in combination. Lacerations that involve exposed muscle, bone, or tendon, should be evaluated for surgical closure by a veterinarian. When evaluating lacerations on intake, special care should be taken to identify any puncture wounds that may be present, especially if there is suspicion of cat involvement in a bird's grounding. Patients with confirmed cat bites should be treated with an antibiotic such as Clavamox (amoxicillin with clavulanic acid) or Cephalexin that is effective on the virulent bacteria common to cats' mouths such as *Pasteurella multocida*.

Young birds that are rescued from rookeries situated near or over water are also susceptible to any of the injuries that generally befall waterbirds: fishhook and fishing line injuries, oiling, and boat collisions. Although these conditions are less likely to be seen in hatching-year birds than in adults of the same species, they should not be forgotten if a young bird has been rescued from an aquatic environment.

Herons and egrets are vulnerable to debilitation due to heavy parasite loads, and this may occasionally cause verminous peritonitis. Every intake exam of a young bird should include a gentle but thorough palpation of the abdomen to search for solid areas, and an oral examination to look for wormy patterns in the subcutaneous tissue proximal to the tongue. Peritonitis resulting from parasite overloads can often be identified by wormy ridges crisscrossing a firm, lumpy abdomen. Fecal flotation examination may confirm the species of endoparasite that is causing the infestation. This condition, once positively identified, needs to be treated aggressively with antihelminthic drugs, though any use of these medicines should be balanced against a consideration of the animal's overall metabolic strength. Some antihelminthics, such as praziquantel, can be fatal to nestlings and small fledglings. Additionally, fenbendazole may affect feather growth, and is contraindicated in hatching-year birds. Rehabilitators should consult an avian veterinarian for guidance when treating young or debilitated birds.

DIET RECIPES

Young herons and egrets in the wild eat a diverse diet that is based on fish but also includes small rodents and large insects. Great Blue Herons eat more small mammals than do smaller herons and egrets. Cattle Egrets are less oriented toward water than other egrets. Black-crowned Night Herons rely more exclusively on fish than other species. Within and across these generalities and specificities, a basic set of diet supplies can be stocked that will satisfy the nutritional needs of all herons and egrets. This basic set must include an adequate stock of frozen blocks of small fish (smelt or herring, in the 5–20 g size range), which comprise the basic captive diet, and stocks of frozen mice and live insects. Rehabilitators who grow mealworms (*Tenebrio molitor*) for other species can separate a group of mealworms into a separate container and allow them to mature into beetles. These bugs make excellent live forage practice for birds in prerelease flight aviaries. Because young herons and egrets can eat half their body weight per day, however, it is impractical to rely on live food for the bulk of their diet. At all stages of orphan rearing, food should be sprinkled with crushed calcium tablets.

Thawed, quartered mice should be introduced into the diets of all herons and egrets as a complement to the basic diet of fish: one mouse per bird per day will give the birds a chance to sample these nonfish foodstuffs. Rehabilitators can assess additional quantities based on species preferences.

FEEDING PROCEDURES

Hatchlings

Hatchling birds should be offered small pieces of fish that have been soaking in water or electrolyte solution and sprinkled with powdered calcium. It is very important for the fish to be sliced diagonally, so that each sliver has two pointed ends. Young birds learn to navigate food in their mouths by instinctively finding "head" and "tail" ends of food items, and only diagonally sliced fish slivers can substitute effectively for whole small fish. Hands should be disguised in a sock or puppet of appropriate appearance to discourage habituation to humans. Herons and egrets are less vulnerable to imprinting than many other species of birds, but it is always best to err on the side of caution. Birds should be offered food hourly throughout the day until they begin self-feeding.

The size of the fish pieces offered should correspond to the size of the hatchling. Hatchling Green Herons can be as small as 100 g, and should be offered small slivers, about the size of a 10 g smelt sliced into four pieces. At the other end of the size spectrum, Great Blue Heron and Great Egret chicks can eat whole 10 g fish even at the hatchling stage. Snowy Egrets and the Black-crowned Night Herons may be fed 5 g fish halves at the hatchling stage, and as nestlings will progress quickly to whole fish.

Hatchling herons and egrets do not gape, and must have their mouths opened in order to be fed. Often their mouths can be opened by the suggestive tap of a fish on the side of the beak. Weaker, less precocial individuals may need to be force-fed at first until they learn to respond to the sight of fish.

As they become aware of their surroundings, nestlings will look to the cage floor for food left for them by their parents. A food dish should therefore be left in the cage with young birds, to familiarize them with the appearance of the food presentation. At feeding time, every effort should be made to entice young birds to notice the fish dish that is in front of them and encourage them to self-feed. Fish slivers left in cages for free feeding should be presented in dishes 0.5 in (1 cm) deep, submerged in fresh water and covered with a light "snowfall" of calcium powder. Self-feeding birds can absorb adequate hydration through picking up a mouthful of water with each fish that they eat from the dish. Young herons and egrets may begin self-feeding at a remarkably early age, before their bodies are covered with down. Do not underestimate the amounts they can eat! Black-crowned Night Herons in particular are voracious eaters that can eat half their body weight per day in fish, distributed across several feedings. Herons and egrets will not necessarily produce a volume of droppings commensurate with the amount they are eating.

Table 16.1. Weights at admission, housing transitions, and at release.

Weight	Species		
	Green Herons	Snowy Egrets	Black-crowned Night Herons
Average arrival weight	156 g	252 g	477 g
Average weight on move to 75°F caging	198 g	316 g	584 g
Average days since arrival	3	5	3
Average weight on move to prerelease aviary	205 g	364 g	708 g
Average days since arrival	8.5	9	10
Average weight at release	233 g	380 g	755 g
Average total days in care	14	18	22

Nestlings and Fledglings

Partially and fully feathered herons and egrets should be able to self-feed. As soon as young birds are strong enough to stand up, they will begin looking at the cage floor for food, and there should be easily found fish dishes in the center of the cage floor in front of them. Nestlings can be introduced to self-feeding by having fish splashed in the dish in front of them (using a hemostat), and by having fish tapped on the side of their beak and then splash-dropped into the dish when they open their mouths for it. Fish dishes should be checked frequently and refilled when empty. There is no need to hesitate to graduate newly self-feeding birds to whole fish as soon as they will accept them.

EXPECTED WEIGHT GAIN

Birds should be weighed daily. Weight gains and losses within 10% of a bird's weight are normal on a daily basis, but any series of weight measures that shows a failure to increase, or a trend toward decrease over 3 or 4 days, should be addressed directly. Weights should be measured first thing in the morning to reduce variation due to ingested food, because young herons and egrets may eat as much as 20% of their body weight in a single meal. Additionally, individuals at the same development stage, as measured by feather growth, may vary considerably in size.

See Table 16.1 for average weights of some common species on intake and at three transition stages during the orphan-rearing process.

EXPECTED THERMOREGULATION PROGRESS

The development of thermoregulatory ability is the central benchmark in the hand-rearing of orphaned herons and egrets. They are extremely vulnerable to hypothermia throughout their first 8 to 12 days of life. Their normal body temperature ranges between 103–106°F (39.5–41.1°C). It is not unusual for newly arrived hatchlings and fledglings to register significantly lower body temperatures prior to stabilization. For this reason, prewarmed stabilization environments should be kept standing ready throughout the season.

Rehabilitators planning to rear orphaned herons and egrets should develop housing plans to allow for four main stages of thermoregulatory support:

- *Stage One:* 100°F (37.7°C) with 40–50% humidity environment for initial stabilization of hypothermic birds of all ages, and housing for hatchlings and nestlings (see Figures 16.1).
- *Stage Two:* 85°F (30°C) environment for fledglings in early stages of feather growth (see Figure 16.2).
- *Stage Three:* 70–75°F (21–24°C) environment (ambient indoor temperature) for fledglings that are developing feather growth throughout their backs, axillary regions, sides, hocks, and chests (see Figures 16.3, 16.5).
- *Stage Four:* Variable outdoor ambient environment for fledglings that have contour feathers covering their backs, axillary regions, sides, hocks, and chests (see Figures 16.4, 16.6, 16.7).

Caging at the first three stages should have heating pads and heat lamps available as accessories that can be added and removed as needed to create transitional stages of thermal support within the basic stages. At every transition point, birds should be monitored closely to ensure that they are comfortable in their new heat environment. Cloacal temperatures should be taken daily while birds are housed in stage one and stage two environments. When moved to stage three, birds should be provided with a heating pad or heat lamp in one corner of the cage for the first day, and they should have their temperatures checked daily for the first 2 days in the new environment, or every day until stable. Additionally, temperatures should be checked at any time that young birds exhibit behavior changes when

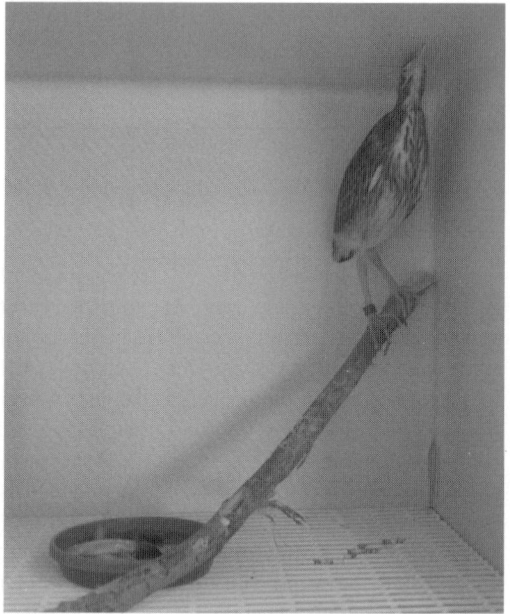

Figure 16.2. Green Heron chick in a standard veterinary animal cage.

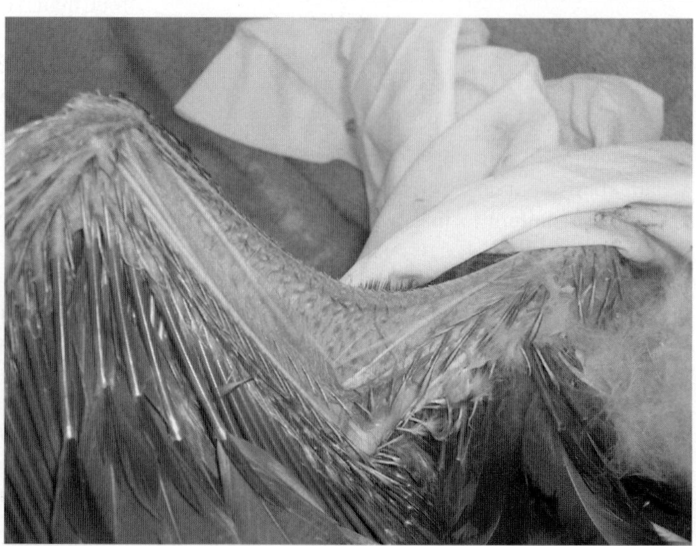

Figure 16.3. Ventral aspect of the right wing of a Black-crowned Night Heron chick. Note bald skin areas and that primary and secondary feathers are approximately half emerged from their shafts.

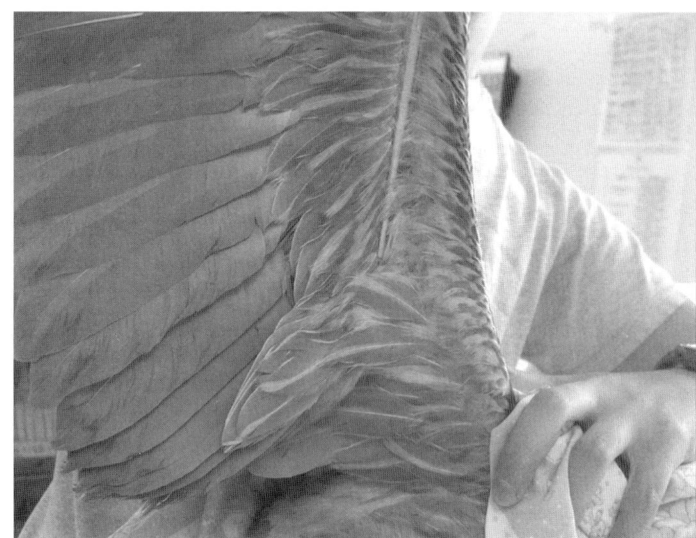

Figure 16.4. A release-ready Black-crowned Night Heron chick with axillary regions fully covered and flight feathers fully emerged.

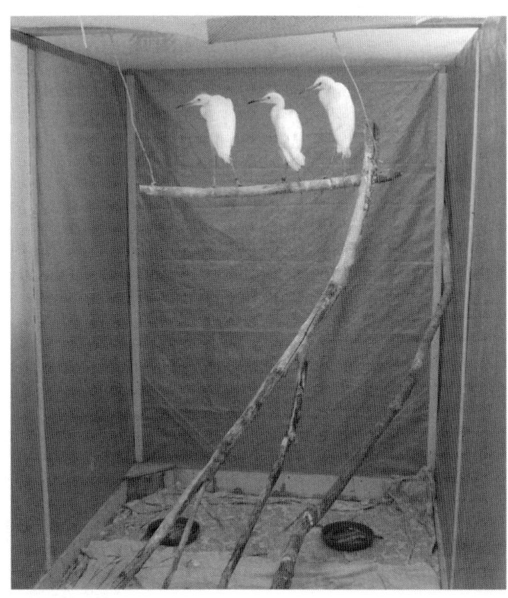

Figure 16.5. Indoor flight caging, interior view.

introduced to a new environment. Behavior changes such as anorexia, hunching, and sitting quietly are all indicators of possible thermoregulatory distress. Any bird that exhibits these signs or has a body temperature below 102°F (39°C) should be regressed one step and reevaluated for progress in 24–48 hours.

After birds have demonstrated consistent thermoregulatory ability over a period of 2 to 3 days at stage three, daily temperature checks can be discontinued, and thermoregulatory progress can be monitored visually on the basis of behavior changes. Warm birds will be alert, active, vocal, and self-feeding.

Before young birds are moved to variable outdoor ambient environments, they should have contour feather growth covering their axillary areas and backs. The axillae are the last part to become

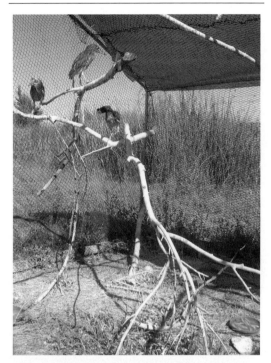

Figure 16.6. Black-crowned Night Herons in an aluminum frame flight aviary.

covered, and this is necessary to protect birds from ambient temperatures below 65°F (18.3°C).

At no point in time will young birds' abdomens become fully feathered. A fringe of powder down feathers will grow underneath coverts at the perimeters of the abdomen, but this area remains bare through adulthood.

HOUSING

Whenever possible, young herons and egrets should be housed together in groups matched by developmental age and species. They are gregarious in hatchling and nestling stages, and will be especially well supported to develop self-feeding habits if housed in a casually competitive caging environment. Cages should be monitored for aggressive competition, and aggressive individuals should be moved in with birds of like demeanor.

For birds at the first stage of thermoregulatory support, appropriate housing may consist of a neonatal incubator (Lyon Technologies, Inc.). This is a clear acrylic box with sliding front door and hinged roof (see Figure 16.1). Its side-mounted electric-powered heat unit is controlled by an exterior LED display and touch-panel. It also has a removable water trough that keeps the environment hydrated and an automatic alarm that sounds if the tempera-

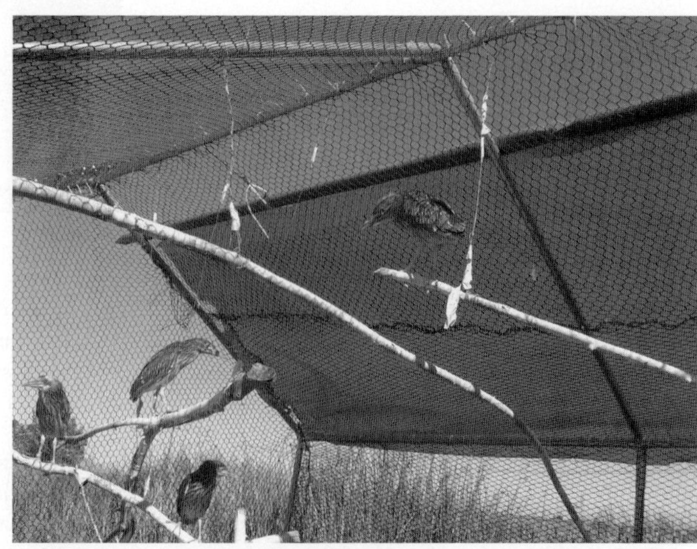

Figure 16.7. Detail of suspended perches in outdoor flight aviary. Note that the ends of the suspension wires are wrapped in tape to prevent injury to birds.

ture diverges from the level that has been set. Such incubators can be set to 100°F (37.7°C). Interior measurements of such units are typically 24 × 12 × 12 in (61 × 30 × 30 cm).

As mentioned earlier, at no point in time will young birds' abdomens become fully feathered. A fringe of powder down feathers will grow underneath coverts at the perimeters of the abdomen, but this area remains bare through adulthood.

Where such a premade device is not available, heat lamps and heating pads can be furnished in other forms of caging to create a 100°F (37.7°C) environment. In such cases, a thermometer should be placed inside the cage where it is easily visible from outside and monitored several times per day to check for temperature fluctuations.

Standard veterinary animal cages are well suited for housing fledgling herons and egrets at stage two (see Figure 16.2), and also at stage three when indoor flight caging is not available. Suggested cage sizes include interior measurements of 24 × 23 × 23 in (61 × 59 × 59 cm) for up to three individuals of smaller species, or 43 × 23 × 36 in (109 × 58 × 91 cm) for up to six individuals of smaller species. Cages should be furnished with branches to enable birds to practice grasping and balancing. Cage bottom inserts should be plastic-coated metal with no sharp edges, and should easily allow droppings to fall through to the cage bottom below. Cage bottoms should be lined with newspaper for easy cleaning. Cages should be cleaned daily and disinfected with an agent such as dilute bleach or chlorhexidine, and newspaper linings should be changed.

When possible, indoor flight housing should be provided to enable young birds to practice flying in advance of their thermoregulatory capacity allowing them to be moved outside. An example of indoor flight housing is a cage constructed of a wood plank frame with walls of canvas or tarpaulin, a fishing net ceiling that allows maximum light and air exchange, and a hinged door of canvas or tarpaulin that has a small window cut in it covered with fishing net to allow for visual checks of the animals. A good size for such a cage is 6 × 6.5 × 7.5 feet (1.5 × 2 × 2.25 m). Such flight housing should be furnished with swinging branches for young birds to practice balancing on unstable perches and navigating short distances between floors and perches. Such caging can be built on wheels with no flooring, to be rolled over whatever area of floor is convenient for its location. Flooring can then be covered with one or two layers of sheets or newspapers for easy cleaning. Ample perches should be provided to allow every individual housed to perch up off the floor. Up to 12 individuals can be housed in such a box, depending on species size.

Outdoor flight aviaries should be located in a shady area, and they should provide ample free-hanging branches or other swinging perches of varying thicknesses to allow young herons and egrets to practice perching, balancing, launching, and alighting from waving branches. One good size for an outdoor flight aviary for up to 20 birds, depending on species size, is 8 × 16 × 12 feet (2.5 × 5 × 3.5 m). Flooring may be of deep gravel or removable rubber padding. Aviaries can be constructed of wood or aluminum frame, with hardware cloth or nylon fishnet walls and ceiling, with shade cloth, plywood boarding, or other screen type surrounding the lower 5 feet (1.5 m) of wall area, to diminish animals' visual stress. Aviaries not situated in naturally shady locations should have shadecloth drapes over at least 50% of their ceiling area. It is essential that outdoor aviaries have hardware cloth flooring that is firmly attached to the walls at their bases. Otherwise, young birds may be exposed to tunneling predators.

In the prerelease aviary, young birds will be acclimating to outdoor ambient temperatures, developing their ability to balance on swaying branches, and learning to forage live food from the cage floor. The most economical live food is ambiently available invertebrates in the outdoor environment. These can be supplemented by mealworm beetles, and when available, live minnows or other feeder fish, pond bugs, and free-roaming mice.

Birds should be evaluated for release from the aviary on a regularly scheduled basis, usually every 2 or 3 days. During the evaluation, it will become apparent which birds are strong, competent flyers, skilled at balancing on swaying branches, and extremely alert and active. New arrivals will contrast with releasable birds by their relative clumsiness and uncertainty in the flight aviary environment. Release candidates should be organized in groups of three or more, due to these species' gregarious nature. When possible, young herons and egrets can be soft released into a semisupported environment where food is provided to them for a brief transitional period, usually 1 to 2 weeks. Young herons and egrets are less vulnerable to habituation than other species, and it is possible to soft-release them and provide them this transitional food support while they learn to self-feed, and have them still fly away and never return once they become fully confident self-feeders.

RELEASE

Most herons and egrets are not broadly migratory. Northern colonies may migrate south in the winter within North America; colonies in temperate regions may not migrate at all. Individuals do range over wide swaths of land and are not territorial. Great Blue Herons and Great Egrets are solitary as adults outside the breeding season, and young can be released singly. Smaller species are more gregarious and should be released in groups whenever possible. They can be released into any territory that is not already overcrowded with conspecifics, and where there is ample food available. The smaller the number of individuals to be released together on a given day, the more important it is to identify a release location where conspecifics are present to provide young birds with community upon release.

Releases of most species are best done in the morning, and during clear weather, to allow young birds maximum daylight hours and weather advantages to orient themselves to their new environment. Black-crowned Night Herons are nocturnal, and can adapt to either daytime or late-afternoon release times.

ACKNOWLEDGMENTS

Thanks to Jay Holcomb, Michelle Bellizzi, Marie Travers, Dr. Greg Massey, and Coleen Doucette for contributing to the knowledge base on which this chapter is founded, and to International Bird Rescue Research Center for its orphan-rearing program. Very special thanks to Katy Siquig and Ann Yasuda for research assistance.

SOURCES FOR PRODUCTS MENTIONED

Incubators: Lyon Technologies, Inc., 1690 Brandywine Avenue, Chula Vista, CA 91911, (888) 596-6872.

Vetrap and Tegaderm: 3M Corporate Headquarters, 3M Center, St. Paul, MN 55144-1000, (888) 364-3577.

SAM Splint: SAM Medical Products, 7100 SW Hampton St, Ste 217, Portland, OR 97223, (800) 818-4726.

BioDres: DVM Pharmaceuticals, Subsidiary of IVAX Corporation, 4400 Biscayne Blvd, Miami, FL 33137, (305) 575-6000.

REFERENCES

Davis, W.E., Jr. 2001. Herons, egrets, and bitterns. In The Sibley Guide to Bird Life and Behavior. Elphick, C., Dunning Jr., J.B., and Sibley, D.A., eds. ALfred A. Knopf, Inc., New York, pp. 170–176.

Dent, A.C. 1963. *Life Histories of North American Marsh Birds*. Dover Publications Inc., New York, pp. 101–218.

17
Domestic Poultry

Nora Pihkala and Patricia Wakenell

NATURAL HISTORY

Several species of birds in the orders Galliformes (chickens, turkeys, quail, pheasants, partridges) and Anseriformes (ducks, geese) have been domesticated for use as food, sources of feathers, or pets. All species covered in this chapter hatch precocial chicks that are fully covered with downy feathers and are able to run and eat on their own shortly after hatching. Although parents of these species do not regurgitate food for their young, they do show their chicks what to eat and provide warmth and protection from the environment and predators.

Duck and goose chicks have three toes facing forward that are fully webbed for swimming, with feet that are usually orange. The rear digit is reduced but present slightly above the plane of the foot. Galliform chicks have an anisodactyl toe arrangement with three toes facing forward and one back.

Because state and federal permits are required to be able to rehabilitate wild birds, it is critical to identify the species of the chick(s). Contacting your local wildlife rehabilitation center or avian veterinarian or even the Internet is a good option for positively identifying stray chicks. It often requires a professional eye to tell the difference between a domestic and a wild chick of similar species. As a general rule, chicks of most wild species have mottled or striped coloring, and are never bright yellow. Wild orphans are covered in Chapter 18, "Wild Turkeys, Quail, Grouse, and Pheasants," and Chapter 12, "Ducks, Geese, and Swans."

Domestication of Chickens

Chickens (*Gallus gallus domesticus*) belong to the order Galliformes, family Phasianidae, and were domesticated from the Red Jungle Fowl native to Asia. Chickens were originally domesticated for cockfighting, and it was for this purpose that chickens spread throughout the world (Smith 1976). At some point, chickens also became valued for their contributions to the table, namely in the form of eggs and meat.

Humans have bred chickens selectively for favorable traits, concentrating on livability and production, usually incorporating environmental considerations into breeding. This is apparent when studying the various classes of standardbred chickens, organized by world region by the American Poultry Association, an organization dedicated to advocating purebred poultry and their origins. The American class of chickens, for example, comprises 13 breeds of chickens, all of which characteristically have rounded bodies and thick, loose plumage to insulate against New England winters and provide a balance between egg production and meat quantity. These are currently classified as dual-purpose chickens. In contrast, the Mediterranean class of chickens encompasses 7 breeds of chickens characterized by a long, lean body shape and plumage held close to the body for hot summers, frequently dark plumage, high alertness to evade predators in year-round foliage, and keenness to forage widely while producing a high number of eggs. Most of these are categorized as laying-type chickens. Commercial broiler chickens are the best example of meat-type chickens, and their sole purpose is to produce meat. See American Poultry Association (2001) for further descriptions, illustrations, and breed histories of purebred domestic poultry.

It is not the intention of this chapter to address raising commercial meat and egg-producing chickens, because these birds and situations have specific management needs. An excellent reference for commercial poultry production is Bell and Weaver (2002).

Domestication of Other Galliformes

Because turkeys, pheasants, quail, and partridges were domesticated more recently than chickens, there are fewer domestic breeds of these game birds.

Turkeys are thought to have been domesticated from North and Central America's Wild Turkey (*Meleagris galapavo*) in Mexico by the Aztecs as meat birds. They were introduced into Europe in the mid 16th century (Richardson 1897). Varieties such as the Royal Palm and Narragansett were developed in Europe and North America and can still be found in hobbyists' yards and poultry shows. Today's modern meat turkeys are strains of the Broad Breasted White breed, developed for quick rate of growth and lack of visible feather tracts after processing. These birds are strikingly different from wild turkeys and exhibition turkeys. If left to grow to full size, strains of modern meat turkeys can weigh upwards of 50 lb (22 kg). Illustrations and descriptions of domesticated turkey breeds can be found in American Poultry Association (2001).

Pheasants were first domesticated in Asia Minor (Quarles 1916). Breeds include the Ringneck, Amherst, Reeves, Mongolian, Silver, and Golden. American breeders have crossbred pheasants to suit commercial purposes, but it is often difficult to distinguish pure breeds from cross breeds. Today they are popular birds raised for release at hunting clubs. Jumbo Ringnecks of 7 lb (3 kg) have been developed for the tables of many fine restaurants (Hayes 1995). In the early 20th century, Ringnecks were successfully introduced into many areas of the U.S., where wild populations continue to thrive or are replenished by regular releases.

The most commonly encountered domesticated quail breeds are Japanese and Bobwhite Quail. Japanese Quail (also known as Pharaoh Quail, *Coturnix japonica*) were domesticated in Japan in the 11th century, initially for their singing and as pets (Hayes 1995). These birds reach sexual maturity at 6 weeks of age, and are prolific producers of small eggs, for which they are currently raised. They have also been a popular bird for scientific research because of their quick growth, hardiness, and ease of rearing. Bobwhite Quail (*Colinus virginianus*) originated in North and Central America, and there are many subspecies found throughout the continent. It is not clear when they became domesticated, but they adapt easily to different environments. With many variations in color pattern, they are raised for hunting clubs just as pheasants are. A jumbo Bobwhite of 22 oz (620 g) has been developed for the table; wild and other non-jumbo breeds usually weigh 7 to 8 oz (225 g). Hayes (1995) is a good reference for more information on domesticated game bird rearing.

Domestication of Anseriformes

The wild Mallard (*Anas platyrhynchos*) is thought to be the first duck domesticated and is the progenitor of all domesticated ducks except the Muscovy (*Cairina moschata*). Evidence suggests that Mallards were domesticated around 500 BC in Southeast Asia or Italy. Muscovies are thought to have been domesticated in Colombia, likely over 1,000 years ago (Holderread 2001). Ducks spread throughout the world after their domestication because of their versatility in producing meat, eggs, and feathers. Common breeds of ducks include Pekins, Runners, Khaki Campbells, Rouens, and Swedish. Please see American Poultry Association (2001) and Holderread (2001) for descriptions and illustrations of domestic ducks breeds and their development. The latter also provides more detailed information about raising these birds.

Raising chickens, quail, and turkeys as a backyard hobby and for exhibition in poultry shows are popular pastimes. All manner of poultry are raised, from crossbreeds to purebred chickens, turkeys, ducks, geese, pheasants, and quail. Although many people choose to raise these birds in elaborate coops, poultry are hardy birds and do well under most circumstances provided that appropriate nutrition and environmental conditions are provided.

CRITERIA FOR INTERVENTION

Individual chicks are often brought to veterinary clinics or wildlife rehabilitation centers by good Samaritans or are found wandering neighborhoods or streets after becoming lost.

Chicks may be identified that do not eat or drink well, or that display other nonspecific symptoms of illness such as ruffled feathers, depressed posture and attitude, thinness, and pallor. Chicks suffering from gastrointestinal problems may present with diarrhea. Those with respiratory problems may present gasping for air, with open-mouthed breathing (be aware of concurrent causes of open-mouthed breathing, such as heat stress), and/or with *snicking* (quickly shaking head in one direction while making a sneezing or clicking sound). They may also cheep loudly if distressed; healthy chicks chirp in soft tones. More dramatic presentations include cannibalism, external parasitism, and traumatic injury.

INITIAL CARE AND STABILIZATION

Regardless of species or whether being cared for permanently or temporarily, the first thing a new chick requires is warmth. When examining chicks, use warm hands and avoid placing them on cold surfaces. Particularly cold chicks may shiver and may cheep loudly. In this case, chicks should be warmed under a heat lamp before further evaluation is attempted unless immediate action is required (such as significant bleeding). Because these species are precocial at hatching, they are able to thermoregulate within a wider temperature range than altricial species. However, chilling chicks stresses them, and they should be handled in a warm room.

When birds of apparently different species are presented, they should immediately be separated and raised apart from each other. Young game birds should not be raised with chickens, turkeys, ducks, or geese because they are very susceptible to diseases these other species may carry, and the larger birds may peck at the game birds, causing injury.

All young poultry need a source of heat until fully feathered. The least expensive option is to arrange a screen-covered heat lamp so that the distance from floor to lamp is 1.5–2.5 ft (0.5–0.75 m), depending on the lamp wattage. The bulb should be red rather than white to discourage cannibalism in older chicks. Floor temperature should be approximately 100°F (37.7°C) directly under the lamp. A round, 1–2 ft (0.3–0.6 meter) high brooder ring is placed under the lamp to act as a corral to keep chicks from straying too far from the heat source. It is unwise to use a square enclosure because some species will pile in corners and suffocate. This ring can be removed after the first week. The best rule of thumb for achieving the proper temperature is to observe the distribution of the chicks at rest under the lamp. Chicks should be in an even and fanned pattern outward from the lamp. If they are piled under the lamp, the temperature is too cold; if they are pressed against the brooder ring, the temperature is too hot or there may be a draft.

Solitary chicks may benefit from the addition of a feather duster or even a mirror in their enclosure, because many chicks of these species are stressed by being alone. Frequent handling of chicks destined to become pets will assist them in becoming socialized to humans, but chicks must be allowed ample time to eat and drink throughout the day. Children should be instructed about this because many children enjoy carrying chicks around, but may inadvertently prevent them from obtaining adequate nutrition.

Many chicks need some introduction to food and water. If the flock size is large, about 25% of the flock can have "formal instruction," and those can be counted on to "teach" the rest. Instruction consists of dipping the beak into the water and feed a few times. Waterers must have a small lip for the chicks to drink from; even smaller if the species has tiny chicks. Generally, waterers are a bell shape that allows water from the center holder to refill the lip as needed. Never use waterers that are big enough for the chicks to fall into. Newly hatched chicks are unstable on their feet and have trouble righting themselves if flipped over (see Figure 17.1). This can result in mass drowning if waterers consist of open dishes. If this is a concern, placing marbles or stones in the waterers reduces the depth of the water and the possibility of entrapment. Gradually, the waterers can be replaced with larger units to accommodate the growing birds (see Figure 17.2).

Healthy or mildly dehydrated chicks may begin drinking on their own or after a few turns of beak dipping. Weak chicks may attempt to swallow but may not be able to hold up their heads. In this situation, after dipping, tip the chick backward gently, using a thumb and index finger to gently support the beak; observe them swallowing. Once they have swallowed, dip their beaks into the water again. Repeat the dipping and tipping until they no longer drink.

The goal throughout initial treatment is to stabilize birds and reduce stress as much as possible. Stress causes depression of the immune system and otherwise weakens chicks' defense against disease (Saif 2003). Stressors include chilling, nutritional deficiency (including due to decreased appetite), dehydration, excessive handling (particularly of game birds), and overcrowding.

Physical Examination

General: Is the bird thin? Feel the bird's breast and note the keel bone; the more prominent, the more underweight the bird. Does the bird appear pale? Is

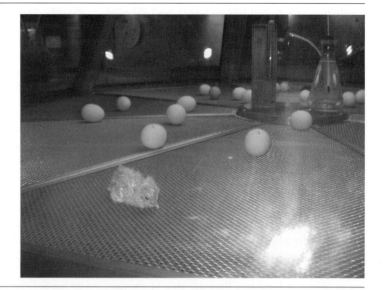

Figure 17.1. Domestic chicks are often hatched from an egg incubator, which automatically turns the eggs. Shown is a rotary model.

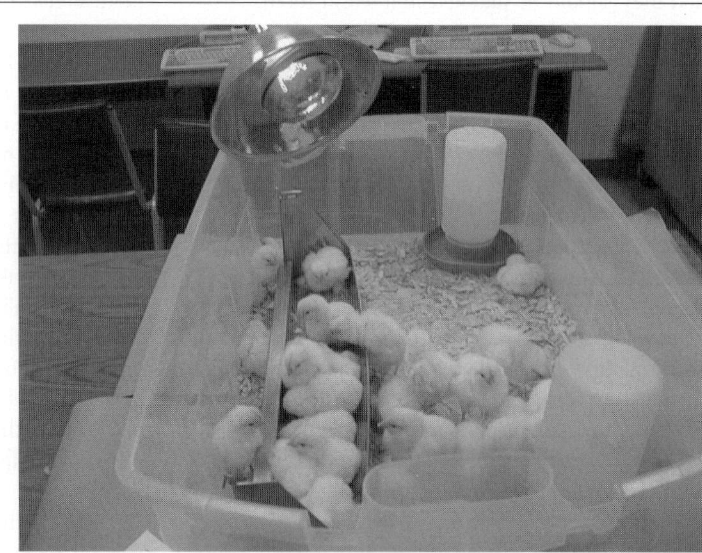

Figure 17.2. Simple brooder setup, with heat lamp at one end, ample feed for all chicks, and multiple shallow waterers. Some species of chicks can jump quite high, so ceilings on brooders should secure birds from escape (not shown).

the bird lethargic? Is the bird hunched over or showing an otherwise abnormal posture? Are there signs of trauma (puncture wounds, broken skin)?

Integumentary (skin and feathers): Is the skin dry and clean? Are there any cuts, scrapes, or abscesses on the body? Are there any bumps or nodules on the skin? Are feathers ruffled and held away from the body? Examine feet and legs. Do leg and foot scales lie flat and appear smooth, or are they raised and crusted? Are the pads of the feet clean and intact, or is there thickened skin or an apparent "scab"? Examine feathers and skin near the vent and tail base very closely for signs of external parasites. Use a magnifying glass to examine the base of the feathers and along the feather shafts and barbs. If legs and toes are feathered (a breed characteristic in some chickens), examine feathers there also. Examining feather plucks under a microscope can help identify the type of parasites. Lice and mites are the most common types of ectoparasites. Poultry have their own type of flea, the stick-tight flea, which is usually found on facial skin and on the comb. Poultry also have their own type of tick.

Eyes, ears, nose, throat: Hold the bird's mouth open and gently extend the head and neck so that the mouth and esophagus can be visualized. Note any lesions in the mouth, including in the choanal opening. Whitish masses may indicate a yeast or parasitic infection (possibly *Candida albicans* and *Trichomonas gallinae*, respectively). An avian veterinarian can differentiate these conditions. Shine a penlight or small flashlight down the trachea (or transilluminate across the trachea) and look carefully for tiny red worms known as gapeworms. Care must be taken during this procedure because gapeworms reduce breathing capacity, and added stress can asphyxiate the birds. Look carefully at the eyes and note whether the eyes appear clear or cloudy. Note whether the bird appears blind in one or both eyes. Is nasal discharge present, and if so, what does it look like (thick, frothy, bloody, watery, opaque)?

Cardiovascular: Heart rate is difficult to assess in chicks owing to birds' normally high heart rate. Examine mucous membranes of the mouth (or just inside the vent) and describe color. Pale pink color (in light pigmented birds) may indicate anemia, poor perfusion (blood reaching tissues), or blood loss. Birds with dark pigmented skin are difficult to assess.

Respiratory: Is the bird having difficulty breathing? Is it rasping, gasping, or coughing?

Gastrointestinal: Examine the vent area. Are there signs of diarrhea such as dried, crusted feces around the vent and adherent to surrounding feathers? Are there worms in any adherent feces?

Neurological: Is the bird able to walk? Does the bird exhibit gait abnormalities, incoordination, or leg weakness? When resting, does the bird have tremors (other than shivering)? Does the bird rest on its hocks? Is the bird *stargazing,* (turning its head so that it is looking toward the sky)?

When receiving many chicks, it may not be practical to perform physical exams on all birds. In this situation, observe all birds as a group before handling individual birds. Note their general appearance, behavior, and gait. Performing physical examinations on a few representative birds can provide a quick overview of what may be going on with other birds in the flock.

RECORD KEEPING

A detailed history should be obtained from the person presenting the chicks, if available. If the chicks were found, they should be asked where they found the chicks, how long they have had them, whether they attempted to feed or water them (and the results), and what environmental conditions they had been exposed to (such as cold nights). If an owner is presenting you with chicks that he or she is raising, finding out about the growing environment, feed, vaccination history, history of exposure to other birds, and history of avian disease on the premises can potentially yield helpful information about underlying causes of disease or injury. Specifically, ask about housing, feeding, and environmental conditions.

Housing: Are chicks raised in a brooder or loose with other birds? Of what material is the brooder made? If it is a nonporous material, do they clean and disinfect after each brood? With what disinfectants? If they use cardboard boxes to brood, do they reuse them for brooding? From what source do they get the cardboard boxes?

Feed: What are they feeding? Where do they purchase it? Does the feed ever have an "off" or musty smell? If so, do they feed it? How do they store the feed? Do they feed additional feed such as table scraps or scratch feed? What type of feeder is used? Does it appear that the chicks are having difficulty eating?

Environment: Are chicks brooded indoors or outdoors? If they are brooded outdoors, are they raised near or have access to other birds? If so, what species? Are chicks exposed to drafts? To direct sunlight? To rain? What type of litter is used? Is newspaper used during brooding? When is litter changed? Does litter ever get wet and caked? Is mold ever found when litter is changed?

COMMON MEDICAL PROBLEMS AND SOLUTIONS

Most pet poultry, unless used for show, rarely encounter the same intensity of disease exposure that commercial poultry do. Many "disease" conditions are actually the result of environmental or feed mismanagement or are unusual presentations of normal events (such as molt). Vaccinations, with a few exceptions, are unnecessary for backyard poultry and can be difficult to obtain in the proper dose size. Most vaccines are sold in bottles of 500–10,000 doses, and mixing errors can be devastating. In addition, medication is also frequently tailored for commercial flock sizes, and dilution errors for small flocks are common. Be sure to document all dilution calculations in case of possible overdosing. Due to space constraints, a thorough discussion of most infectious diseases will not be included here. Please see Charleton (2000) for an excellent and inexpensive resource for most avian diseases.

The following sections are not meant to be comprehensive, but include some of the more common conditions that are encountered in backyard poultry practice.

Cannibalism

Domestic galliformes are naturally cannibalistic; game birds especially should be observed for cannibalistic behavior. Cannibalism usually does not begin in earnest under 2–3 weeks of age. If observed in young chicks, it is generally the result of insufficient feed or diarrhea (soiled vents can be attractive pecking targets). In older birds, methods of controlling pecking include reducing lighting, reducing bird density, increasing the number of feeders, and trimming the beaks. Remove moderately to severely cannibalized birds and segregate them until their skin has healed completely. Avian skin regenerates quickly and with little to no scarring, particularly in younger birds. If an individual bird has been pecked severely but no isolation facilities are available, spraying the affected area with pruning tar (used for trees) is a good solution. The tar protects the skinless area from fluid loss, is nontoxic even when used on open wounds and has the advantage of identifying the perpetrators by staining their beaks black. If small numbers of birds are the aggressors, these birds can be given red spectacles that attach to their nares or be fitted with red contact lenses, which are available at most poultry supply stores.

Bumblefoot

Bumblefoot or pododermatitis occurs when the footpad is abraded or punctured, allowing *Staphylococcus* bacteria to infect the wound. Bumblefoot is readily identified on physical exam as a well-defined, thickened "callus" (granuloma) on the footpad. A granuloma is a collection of hardened inflammatory cells. Granulomas may be very large and when removed result in pain and expose underlying tissue to further infection. Consult an avian veterinarian, who will definitively diagnose the condition and may prescribe a course of antibiotics. Although more commonly encountered in older birds, bumblefoot can be seen in chicks. Keeping litter clean and dry, and not allowing it to get caked up, can reduce the incidence of this condition. Use soft yet supportive litter such as rice hulls or wood shavings. Avoiding exposure to sharp objects can reduce the chance of injury to footpads and prevent *Staphylococcus* infection.

Crop Impaction

Chicks are naturally curious and will peck at anything that interests them. When chicks ingest nonfood particles such as sand or sawdust, their crops may become filled with this nondigestible material. Birds may stop eating and the crop may appear pendulous and feel very full. In older birds, crop impaction may indicate Marek's disease, which can cause paralysis of the vagus nerve and loss of gut motility.

Infectious Diseases

When infectious diseases are suspected, an avian veterinarian should be consulted. He or she will observe the birds, perform diagnostic tests, and make specific treatment and prevention recommendations. If an avian veterinarian is not available, one or more birds may be submitted to the nearest veterinary diagnostic laboratory. Birds submitted will be humanely destroyed and undergo necropsy and pathology to determine cause of disease. This service, when provided at a university or state facility, is usually free or low cost to noncommercial individuals.

Ectoparasites

Two common mites of poultry are the Northern Fowl Mite and the Red Mite. The Northern Fowl Mite is most common around the vent, tail, and breast of the bird. They are easily observed and are a reddish-brown color. The Red Mite feeds only at night, making daytime diagnosis difficult. They can be found in cracks and seams near the bedding areas and appear as white fuzz balls or salt-and-pepper–like deposits. Red Mites will cause feather loss, irritation, and anemia. Insecticides are available for treatment of both mites. Effective insecticides, such as carbaryl powder (5% Sevin dust, GardenTech), may be used for treatment of both types of mite and are available at feed or home and garden stores. Apply the powder liberally, ensuring that it reaches the skin, paying special attention to the skin around the vent and base of the tail. Reapply in 4 weeks if needed. Keep in mind that the withdrawal period before slaughter is 7 days (Campbell 1914). Another insecticide is permethrin dust or spray; consult the label on specific products used for the withdrawal period. Other approved insecticides are listed in Beyer and Mock (1999).

There are several types of lice that live on poultry, and lice or nits can be observed at the base of the feathers. With severe infestations, growth and egg production can be affected. Again, carbaryl and permethrin are effective in treating lice.

Fowl ticks compromise a group of soft ticks, which parasitize many species of poultry and wild birds. Ticks are easily missed because they spend relatively little time on the bird. Heavy infestations can cause anemia or tick paralysis, and ticks can be vectors for *Borrelia anserina* (spirochetosis). Spraying of buildings with permethrin is the treatment of choice.

Endoparasites

Large roundworms and tapeworms are the most common poultry worms and are generally the result of soil contamination and poor management. Unless infestations are heavy, clinical disease is usually not evident. Piperazine can be used for roundworms (repeat in 10–14 days) and dibutyltin dilaurate for tapeworms. Do not use these compounds in laying hens. Proper litter management will reduce parasite loads and reinfection.

Control of coccidia is one of the more costly problems of commercial and backyard poultry raising. Coccidia are found primarily in the intestinal tract of most poultry, but occur in the kidney in geese. Coccidiosis is generally observed in young birds between the ages of 1 and 4 months. The disease causes diarrhea that is often bloody and frequently leads to death. Coccidia thrive in moist, heavily soiled litter, and disease is often a result of excessively high bird density. Prevention can be obtained by supplying coccidiostats in the feed. Outbreaks of disease can be treated, usually with sulfa drugs, but the outcome is frequently disappointing. Sulfa drugs should not be used in laying hens.

Viral Diseases

Marek's disease (MD) is a common viral disease of chickens. The primary lesions are tumors of the viscera, muscle, skin, and peripheral nerves. Nerve lesions can be an early indicator of the disease resulting in a condition termed "range paralysis." Birds with visceral tumors will often have only cachexia (wasting) as a clinical sign. Tumors of the muscles and skin are frequently palpable. Marek's disease cannot be treated but can be prevented by vaccination at hatch. When acquiring backyard poultry or hatching your own, every attempt should be made to vaccinate against MD. Vaccinations are not effective if applied to birds older than 1–2 weeks of age. Clinical MD generally affects birds between 4 and 14 weeks of age; however, it is not uncommon in older birds. If tumors are found in the viscera of deceased birds, carcasses should be submitted to a diagnostic laboratory for differential diagnosis between MD and another common lymphoid tumor disease, avian leukosis. Avian leukosis is found in birds older than 14 weeks and tumors are very similar to those found with MD. Avian leukosis has no treatment or vaccination.

Infectious bronchitis virus (IBV) causes a rapidly spreading respiratory disease in young chicks. Laying hens experience reduced production and eggshell abnormalities. Certain strains of IBV will also cause kidney disease. Chicks that are infected early in life may have permanent damage to the oviduct, which will prevent them from laying eggs. Although IBV is highly transmissible, most birds will recover with supportive treatment. Antibiotics can be applied to the water in order to prevent secondary infection. Vaccines are available; however, backyard chickens are usually not vaccinated unless they come in contact with other chickens (neighbors, shows).

Newcastle disease virus (ND) affects numerous species of birds and is the reason for establishment of quarantine regulations for birds entering the United States. Exotic ND is highly fatal and does not exist in the U.S. at this time, although outbreaks have occurred in the recent past resulting in the slaughter of thousands of birds. ND does exist in milder forms in the U.S., and is primarily characterized by respiratory disease and an egg production drop. Mortality is variable and depends upon the strain of the virus. As with IBV, vaccination is available, but is generally given only to pet poultry that are exposed to other birds.

Fowl pox virus causes nodular lesions primarily on the unfeathered portions of the bird's skin (dry form). Occasionally, pox virus can cause lesions in the mouth and trachea causing death due to suffocation (wet form). Once the bird recovers from the disease, immunity is generally lifelong. Not all pox outbreaks are caused by fowl pox virus but can be caused by related strains such as turkey pox, psittacine pox, quail pox, etc. Strains are usually species-specific but can occasionally affect other species. One strain may not cross-protect with another. Vaccination is available and should be applied to flocks on premises with a previous history of pox or with presence of pox in nearby birds. Poxvirus is transmitted through contact of infected lesions with open wounds and through insect bites (mosquitoes).

Avian Encephalomyelitis (AE) occurs in chickens, turkeys, pheasants, and quail and primarily affects young chicks 1–3 weeks old. Nearly all commercial flocks are infected but clinical disease is low due to maternal antibodies. AE can be transmitted vertically in eggs laid between 5 and 13 days postinfection, and it is an enteric infection under natural conditions. The spread is more rapid in floor-raised birds than in those cage-raised. There is no treatment, and vaccination of breeders (both chicken and turkey), so that maternal antibodies protect the young during early life, is critical to prevention. Because many specialty breeders, particularly those that sell stock to feed stores, do not vaccinate, AE is a fairly common viral disease in backyard birds. Vaccination should be given to hens after 8 weeks of age but by at least 4 weeks prior to onset of laying.

Bacterial Infections

There are many different species in the bacterial genus of Salmonella. Generally speaking, *S. pullorum* and *S. gallinarum* cause the greatest problem for poultry; *S. typhimurium* and *S. enteriditis* are important for the public health aspect. Pullorum (*S. pullorum*) is egg-transmitted and causes a diarrheal disease in young chicks and turkey poults resulting in high mortality. Adult birds are asymptomatic carriers. Diagnosis is based on disease history and isolation of the bacteria. Prevention is achieved by purchasing birds from disease-free flocks. Treatment is not recommended because it can cause birds to become carriers. Fowl typhoid (*S. gallinarum*) occurs in chickens, turkeys, and many other game and wild birds. Fowl typhoid is similar in disease presentation and diagnosis to pullorum, although mature birds can show clinical signs of fowl typhoid. Prevention is again achieved by obtaining disease-free stock. Clinical signs are infrequently observed in poultry infected with *S. enteriditis* and *S. typhimurium*. Flocks can be monitored by obtaining egg samples and environmental samples for culturing the organism.

Colibacillosis is caused by the organism *Escherichia coli* (*E. coli*) and is usually secondary to other infections such as IBV and Mycoplasmosis. A wide variety of clinical signs, both respiratory and enteric, can be observed, and the organism occurs in most species and age groups. Vigorous adherence to biosecurity and sanitation programs will effectively prevent the organism from causing disease. Many antibiotics can be used for treatment, and sensitivity to the antibiotic should be ascertained. Treatment is usually successful if the disease is in the early stages.

Chronic respiratory disease in poultry (primarily chickens and turkeys) is generally caused by *Mycoplasma gallisepticum* infection. Pathogenicity of the organism is enhanced by infection with other organisms. Clinical signs of respiratory disease develop slowly in a flock and feed consumption drops. Infection of the sinuses is common in turkeys. Serology and isolation and identification of the organism can be used for diagnosis. Prevention, as with the Salmonellas, rests with the establishment of a clean flock by eliminating the infected flock, complete sanitation, and obtaining clean stock. Vaccination is available on a state-by-state basis. Treatment is expensive, and the disease often recurs after cessation of treatment. Other important mycoplasmas in poultry include *M. synoviae* (infectious synovitis) and *M. meleagridis* (venereal infection and airsacculitis).

Fungal Diseases

Aspergillosis (brooder pneumonia) occurs in many poultry and nonpoultry species of birds. Birds under 3 weeks of age are most commonly affected, and infection is obtained from hatchers or brooders that are contaminated with fungal spores. Morbidity is variable and mortality can be high in clinically affected birds. Culturing the fungus or demonstration of typical fungal hyphae in fresh preparations from lesions are used for diagnosis. Prevention is obtained by thoroughly cleaning hatchers, incubators, waterers, feeders, and ventilation fans and by keeping litter clean and dry. Treatment is expensive and may not be effective. Ketoconazole and nystatin have been used.

When to Notify State Authorities

Reportable diseases are those diseases that cause severe morbidity and/or mortality, are economically harmful, or spread very rapidly. Veterinarians and rehabilitators are very important first lines of defense in identifying reportable avian diseases such as Exotic Newcastle Disease and Avian Influenza. It was a veterinarian in private practice who first discovered the presence of Exotic ND in California in 2002 and reported it to the state food and agriculture department.

The World Organization for Animal Health (OIE) is an international animal health group that has over 160 member countries. The OIE has several objectives, including collecting data on animal diseases. It has created a list of reportable avian diseases: IBV, avian infectious laryngotracheitis, avian tuberculosis, duck virus hepatitis, duck virus enteritis, fowl cholera, fowl pox, fowl typhoid, infectious bursal disease (Gumboro disease), MD, avian mycoplasmosis (*M. gallisepticum*), avian chlamydiosis, pullorum disease, highly pathogenic avian influenza, and ND (OIE 2006). Additionally, each state may have deemed additional diseases as reportable; contact the state Department of Agriculture for additional reportable diseases.

When suspecting that birds presented may have a reportable disease, immediately contact the state department of agriculture and instruct the owner to quarantine all their birds until authorities give more specific instructions. Time is an exceptionally important factor in controlling disease outbreaks, and state departments of agriculture urge anyone who suspects a reportable disease to contact them as soon as these diseases are suspected. Clinical signs of reportable (and nonreportable) diseases are often nonspecific and may include depression, lethargy, inappetance, decreased water intake, ruffled feathers, and decreased egg production. It is when a disease outbreak results in dramatic, acute morbidity and/or mortality, lasts for a prolonged period of time, and/or spreads rapidly within a flock that authorities should be notified.

DIET RECIPES AND FEEDING PROCEDURES

More is known about the nutritional needs of chickens than of any other animal, including humans. Specific dietary formulations are available for young, growing chicks; for young, growing turkeys, pheasants, and quail; and for ducks and geese. Feed may be purchased in 25–50 lb sacks at any feed store. In suburban areas, some hardware stores may sell feed in sacks as well as by the pound. Sacks of feed are very economical and practical when several chicks are being raised. However, when raising only one to two chicks, such large quantities of feed may grow stale before they can be consumed and are more likely to become moldy or parasitized. In this situation, purchasing 3–4 lb of feed at a time may be more expensive, but it will help ensure that feed is palatable and safe for consumption.

For very young chicks, a small handful of feed should be placed on a plastic or disposable tray with sides no higher than 0.5 in (1 cm). Disposable foam or cardboard trays are convenient and may be purchased inexpensively at craft and hobby stores. Foam trays that have been used to hold raw meat should not be used due to the risk of bacterial contamination. Egg carton tops may also be used if the sides have been cut short. Chicks are naturally curious and peck instinctively at objects around their toes. By placing chicks on top of the food they will become familiar with it. They also imitate one another; if one chick learns to eat the others will follow suit. If chicks do not seem interested in food, gently stir the feed with a finger as chicks observe. The movement will help stimulate them to eat. Observe that all chicks are eating and drinking before leaving them for any period of time. Usually by 1 week of age, chicks will be able to use a chick feeder. Introduce a chick feeder after the first few days. Chick feeders have the advantage of being covered to keep older chicks from scratching out feed and wasting it. As chicks grow they will learn to eat from the feeders, and the trays should be removed.

When feeding young chickens, a chick starter ration should be fed until 6 weeks of age, when they should be switched to a grower ration. Feed is available in dry mash, crumbles, and pellets. Pellets are often too large for chicks and should be avoided. Mash is very palatable but can be wasteful; chicks also tend to pick through the mash to ingest preferred grains (usually corn), potentially leading to nutritional deficiencies. Crumbles ensure nutritional adequacy and are usually small enough for even youngest chicks to easily ingest. If crumbles prove to be too large for chicks to eat easily, mash should be fed instead. If no mash is available, crumbles may be further pulverized by placing some crumbles into a resealable plastic freezer bag and grinding with a rolling pin. At 18–20 weeks of age, a laying ration should be fed to both male and female birds.

Young turkeys, pheasants, and quail have higher requirements for protein and calcium. These birds should be fed game bird starter feed until 6–8 weeks of age. Ideally, game bird conditioner or game bird developer ration should be fed thereafter until 16–20 weeks of age. Game bird layer ration may be fed thereafter. Although game bird diets are generally well-balanced nutritionally, individual species can have different nutritional needs. It is advisable to use a mineral mix in chicks' water until their species and breed can be established, and then feed accordingly. Use mineral mixes specifically formulated for birds; consult your feed store on their available products and follow instructions carefully.

An important exception to feeding game birds is the Japanese Quail. They reach sexual maturity rapidly and may begin laying eggs as soon as 6 weeks of age. They should be fed a game bird starter mash until 6 weeks of age. Game bird layer mash or crumbles should be fed thereafter.

Ducks and geese have their own feeds as well. Feed starter ration for the first 2 weeks, grower until 8 weeks of age, developer until 20 weeks of age, and a maintenance or laying ration thereafter. Waterfowl feeds are not as easily available as chicken and game bird feeds. Consult with knowledgeable feed store personnel or feed manufacturer representatives about which feeds are appropriate in the absence of waterfowl feed. A good description of feed substitutions and additions when waterfowl feed is not available can be found in Holderread (2001).

When raising young chickens with ducks, geese, and turkeys, an all-purpose grower feed such as Purina Mills® Flock Raiser® may be fed to all young birds after 8–10 weeks of age. However, it is vital that turkeys, pheasants, and quail be fed a game bird starter until 8–10 weeks of age. It is equally important that young chickens *not* be fed game bird starter, because this feed has excessive levels of calcium and protein, which may lead to problems with maturation of the long bones. Because there are dozens of feed millers in the U.S. and their formulations or feeding programs may vary, consult the feed dealer for recommendations on raising mixed flocks.

There are other considerations when selecting and feeding poultry diets. It is highly recommended to feed a diet containing a coccidiostat such as amprolium. Coccidiosis is a protozoal disease caused by species in the genus *Eimeria*, which inhabit the small intestine of most poultry. Coccidiosis is a leading cause of fatal diarrhea in young poultry. Coccidiostats prevent *Eimeria* from undergoing its normal life cycle in affected animals and are safe to use in even the youngest chicks. They should be used until 16 weeks of age (Smith 2007). Feeding diets containing premixed coccidiostats is the easiest and safest method to reduce or eliminate coccidiosis because only FDA-approved drugs are allowed in feeds. Follow the feed manufacturer's recommendations on drug withdrawal before consuming meat or eggs.

Antibiotics should not be used in chicks unless bacteria have been found to be the agent of disease. During the first few weeks of life, a chick's digestive tract is being colonized by many beneficial microflora. These microflora serve to aid digestion as well as to successfully compete with pathogenic bacteria such as *E. coli*. When antibiotics are given to young chicks without a specific therapeutic goal, beneficial microflora are destroyed, thus leaving the digestive tract open to colonization by pathogens.

When young chickens are eating well, dietary supplements should not be given because feeds are nutritionally complete. Feed stores may offer scratch feed, but this is more of a treat for adult birds. Scratch contains little nutritive value and may contribute to obesity if fed excessively. Feeding kitchen vegetable scraps is acceptable for adult birds but should not be fed to chicks because they may potentially cause diarrhea.

When chicks are ill they may refuse to eat dry food. In this case, they may prefer a wet mash. Wet mash (gruel) is highly palatable, contributes to hydration, and is simple to make. In a large saucepan or Dutch oven, place 3 parts water and 1 part mixed grains. Grains such as rolled oats, crushed wheat, milo, and wheat bran can be purchased in bulk at many grocery and natural food stores. Heat over medium-high heat, stirring occasionally. When it starts to boil, reduce heat to low and continue to stir occasionally until most liquid is absorbed, from 10–30 minutes depending on the amount made. Cool completely and add 1 teaspoon to 1 tablespoon of cod liver oil (depending on amount made), stirring thoroughly. If gruel is difficult to stir once cooled, add a little water until it is of a cooked oatmeal consistency. Because this gruel is not nutritionally balanced, it should be used only to nurse ill chicks to health until they can eat dry food on their own.

Poultry feed should be protected from the elements and from pests such as rodents and beetles. Depending on amount obtained, feed may be stored in sturdy containers ranging from plastic breakfast cereal storage canisters to plastic or metal trash cans. Lids should be tight fitting. In warm, humid climates, mold may be a problem, particularly when it cools at night and moisture condenses within the container. To prevent mold growth, feed should preferably be stored indoors or other areas in which there is not a wide variation in temperature. Moldy feed should *never* be fed to any animals because of its potential toxicity. Mold in feed may be identified by its appearance (green, black, or rusty-colored "fuzz") or by its musty odor.

Water is the most important nutrient. Ensure that fresh, clean water is available at all times and is changed daily or whenever it is soiled with feces, litter, or feed. When water is changed, the waterer should be scrubbed out using a sponge or brush, because algae and bacteria may accumulate quickly. Chicks will begin scratching behavior at 7–10 days of age. At this time, water availability should be verified several times per day because of chicks' propensity to kick feed and litter into their water.

A few types of waterers are available. Plastic founts are readily available at feed stores and are easy to use. They usually have an opaque white reservoir and red base (red attracts chicks' attention). They are easily disassembled for filling and cleaning, and the threaded screw-on type is most secure. For a small number of chicks, a quart fount waterer is preferable to a gallon size fount as the lip is shallower and narrower, discouraging drowning. To further discourage chicks from falling into water, clean aquarium gravel or marbles may be placed so that water depth is 1/8–1/4 in (3–6 mm).

EXPECTED WEIGHT GAIN

Because poultry come in many sizes, there is great variation in normal expected weight gain. A good indicator of appropriate growth and development for any poultry species is to simply feel the keel bone (sternum) and the musculature on either side. Ideally, the tip of the keel should be surrounded by full, round pectoralis muscles. A sharp keel with sunken pectoralis muscles indicates that a bird is very thin; nutritional and gastrointestinal parasitic causes should be investigated.

HOUSING

Preferably, brood chicks indoors until they are four to 5 weeks old or until the weather outside is relatively warm, at least 70°F (21°C). Brooding inside allows close observation and protection from predators and the elements should the heat lamp fail.

When brooding chicks, the most convenient housing is a sturdy cardboard box with high sides of at least 24 in (60 cm). For chickens, turkeys, ducks, and geese, this height should prevent chicks from jumping out. For game birds, placing a piece of cut wire mesh over the box should prevent chicks from jumping out (the wire can easily be cut to accommodate the heating lamp).

Space requirements vary depending on species and age of the chicks. These requirements are particularly important to consider when raising game birds, because they are easily stressed and are prone to cannibalism when too closely confined.

Appropriate litter material can include wood shavings or rice hulls. Avoid sand or sawdust because chicks may ingest these materials, causing crop impaction. Also, newspaper or other slick surfaces should never be used because young chicks' legs easily slide out underneath them. Because they are weak and their bones and joints are still very malleable, chicks may become permanently deformed if their legs are splayed out for extended periods of time. Deformed chicks may never walk or may walk abnormally, causing unnecessary joint problems throughout life.

A heat source may be set up as described above in the section "Initial Care and Stabilization." Caution must be used because there is a fire hazard with this setup due to the intense heat production from the 24-hour light. Make sure the lamp is sturdily affixed and that the lamp edges are at least 4 in away from any flammable materials. As mentioned previously, very young chicks should be observed for the behavior and comfort under heat lamps before leaving them unsupervised. Regardless of species, decreasing temperature by 5°F (2.8°C) each week results in comfortable chicks as the temperature drops to match the rate of feather growth.

BIOSECURITY

Losses from disease can be reduced substantially by adhering to biosecurity practices. The biggest single source of disease is other birds, both from the same species and from different species. No person or animal should be allowed to visit the flock unless they have not been around other birds. Frequent transgressors are domestic animals (dogs and cats) and rodents. These animals can mechanically transmit disease or be biological vectors. Attractants for animals need to be removed; feed must be kept in rodentproof containers and spilled feed rapidly cleaned up. Carcasses should be removed immediately and disposed of appropriately; observe local environmental regulations. If burial is chosen, carcasses can be covered with lime in order to reduce the likelihood of being dug up by animals. Good rodenticide and insecticide programs are essential. Waterers and feeders must be cleaned and disinfected at least every 2–3 days and houses cleaned when litter becomes moist. Store feed in containers that are not sun exposed, which can cause condensation when the containers cool at night and subsequent mold growth. Use feed rapidly and store no more than a 1-week supply. Foot pans filled with a dilute iodine solution can reduce the risk of carrying in organisms on boots; when the iodinated water becomes clear, it needs to be replaced. All equipment must be thoroughly cleaned and disinfected before use. Organic matter left on equipment can render even the best disinfectant useless. Again, species should not be mixed and in best conditions, ages should not be mixed as well.

All birds leaving the premises and encountering other birds (i.e., shows) should be quarantined for 6 weeks in a separate area. Be sure to not feed medicated feed during quarantine. Any equipment used at shows—such as cages, feeders, waterers, and egg flats—needs to be disinfected before storage or reuse. If housing birds being quarantined for any reason or that are ill, be sure to work with these birds last to avoid exposing healthy birds to potential disease organisms.

Additionally, in the U.S. many Cooperative Extension offices have pamphlets on specific poultry husbandry topics. These pamphlets are written by poultry scientists and veterinarians and are the most accurate and up-to-date sources of information, particularly regarding region-specific diseases and husbandry matters. Materials from Cooperative Extension are usually free.

BEHAVIORAL TRAINING FOR PET BIRDS

Many species of poultry make excellent, personable pets. Ducks and chickens in particular are often kept as beloved house pets. In order to raise a bird so that it is well socialized to humans, be sure to handle it frequently while it is growing up, as you would any pet. Young chicks that are exposed to close human contact and activity become very accustomed to people and often seek their company. Certain breeds lend themselves better to being pets; heavier breeds such as Plymouth Rocks and Cochins are generally calmer than high-strung Mediterranean breeds such as Leghorns. See American Poultry Association (2001) for more examples of "friendlier" breeds.

SOURCES FOR PRODUCTS MENTIONED

Purina Mills Poultry Diets: 2005, SunFresh Recipe Products Index Page, St. Louis, MO, http://www.rabbitnutrition.com/flock/index.html.

Sevin Dust: GardenTech, PO Box 24830, Lexington, KY 40524–4830, (800) 969–7200.

REFERENCES

American Poultry Association. 2001. The American Standard of Perfection. American Poultry Association, Inc., Mendon, Massachusetts, 372 pp.

Bell, D.D. and Weaver, Jr., W.D., eds. 2002. Commercial Chicken Meat and Egg Production, 5th ed. Kluwer Academic Publishers, Norwell, Massachusetts, 1365 pp.

Beyer, R.S. and D. Mock. 1999. Eliminating Mites in Poultry Flocks. Kansas State University Agricultural Experiment Station and Cooperative Extension Service publication MF-2387. Kansas State University, Kansas. http://www.oznet.ksu.edu/library/lvstk2/MF2387.PDF.

Campbell, J.B. 1914. Nebraska Management Guide for Control of Arthropod Pests of Poultry and Pets: Featuring: Poultry, Dogs, Cats, Rabbits, Birds, Guinea Pigs and Gerbils. Nebraska Cooperative Extension Circular EC89-1551. Nebraska Cooperative Extension, Nebraska. http://ianrpubs.unl.edu/insects/ec1551.htm.

Charleton, B.R., Bermudez, A.J., Boulianne, M., Halvorson, D.A., Jeffrey, J.S., Newman, L.J., Sander, J.E., and Wakenell, P.S., eds. 2000. Avian Disease Manual, 5th ed. American Association of Avian Pathologists, Kennett Square, Pennsylvania, 243 pp.

Hayes, L.B. 1995. Upland Game Birds: Their Breeding and Care. Valley Center, California, self-published, 350 pp.

Holderread, D. 2001. Storey's Guide to Raising Ducks. Storey Publishing, Pownal, Vermont, 288 pp.

Office International des Epizooties (OIE)/World Organization for Animal Health. 2006. Diseases Notifiable to the OIE. Paris, France. http://www.oie.int/eng/maladies/en_classification.htm.

Quarles, E.A. 1916. American Pheasant Breeding and Care. Hercules Powder Company, Wilmington, Delaware.

Richardson, E. 1897. The turkey: Its natural history and origin of name. In Myrick, H., ed. Turkeys and How to Grow Them. Orange Judd Company, New York, pp. 1–4.

Saif, Y.M., ed. 2003. Diseases of Poultry, 11th ed. Iowa State Press, Ames, Iowa, 1231 pp.

Smith, H.E. 1976. Modern Poultry Development: A History of Domestic Poultry Keeping. Spur Publications Company, Hampshire, England, 215 pp.

Smith, T.W. 1997. Feeding Game Birds. Mississippi State University, Mississippi State, Mississippi. http://www.msstate.edu/dept/poultry/bwqfeed.htm#nutr.

Smith, T.W. Accessed 2007. Feeding Chickens Properly. Mississippi State University Extension Information Sheet 1214. 2 pp. Available online at http://www.msstate.edu/dept/poultry/is1214.pdf.

18
Wild Turkeys, Quail, Grouse, and Pheasants

Marjorie Gibson

NATURAL HISTORY

Worldwide, there are 256 species and 7 families considered to be in the order Galliformes. In North America, there are only 4 families, but many species within those families. They include grouse, pheasants, turkeys, quail, and curassows.

These terrestrial birds have added much to human history and continue to play a huge role in life through art, literature, and, notably, economics. They are considered by many to be the single most important source of protein in the world today.

These species are terrestrial, meaning living and foraging on the ground, although they do roost in trees. Although equipped with strong wings, they are not known for their flight ability due to the round, short structure of the wing. Flight is in short, powerful bursts. These birds have chickenlike feet, which are feathered in some species and are equipped with hard nails for scratching the ground to expose food. They do not swim. The main method of escaping from predators is by running or taking evasive action. If forced to defend themselves, they use their strong legs, feet, nails, and occasionally spurs to thwart attackers. The wings can be used aggressively as clubs to beat enemies, or in some cases rehabilitators or rescuers (see Figure 18.1).

Most species have cryptic coloration, feathers that match their environment (see Figure 18.2). Some, like ptarmigans, molt and change color seasonally. This cryptic form of camouflage allows individuals to blend into the habitat, remaining inconspicuous to people and predators.

Wild galliformes most likely to be encountered in wildlife rehabilitation facilities include pheasants, quail, grouse, partridges, ptarmigans, prairie chickens, turkeys, peafowl, and jungle fowl. Due to widespread domestication and hybridization of several species, caregivers should make every effort to correctly identify the patient, as it may be a domestic fowl, an escaped exotic species, a native species, or even a threatened or endangered species. In some regions, populations of native species such as quail and Prairie Chickens have declined dramatically, causing the birds to be listed as threatened or endangered. Nonindigenous species have been introduced regionally in North American by sportsmen and organizations in attempts to establish new hunting opportunities. Some introduced species such as the Ring-necked Pheasant have become so common in regions of the U.S.A., that they are considered native by some. See Chapter 17, "Domestic Poultry," for information on hand-rearing chickens and other domestic galliformes.

Game birds hunted for sport and food are frequently raised commercially. Game birds are also known for their beauty, and are kept in zoos and private aviaries as ornamental birds. The most common species for commercial game farm production are pheasant and quail. These species adapt easily and do well with commercial game bird diet. Although many species are common and easy to raise, some in this order are among the most difficult birds to raise and maintain in captivity. Many are secretive in nature, fastidious, and difficult to study in the wild, so little is known about their life history and diet. Unfortunately, a native bird taken into wildlife rehabilitation is frequently one of the challenging species. Information on domestic fowl diseases and housing techniques may be helpful, but many aspects of rearing wild species differ, sometimes in dramatic ways.

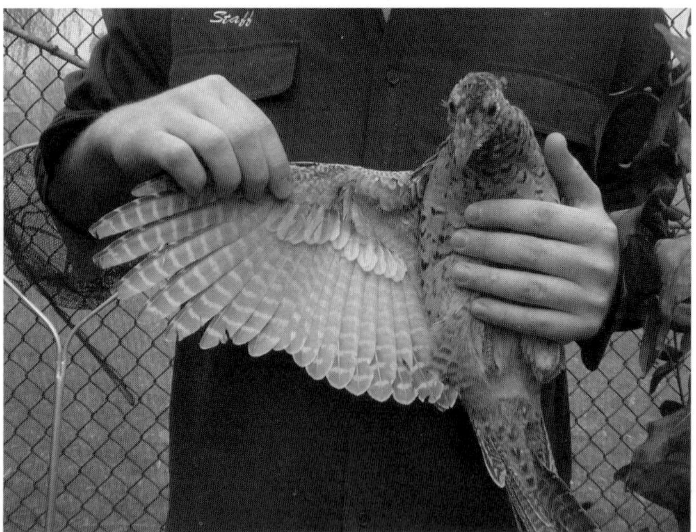

Figure 18.1. Galliformes have short broad wings, in relation to their body size, for short, strong flights rather than long distance movement.

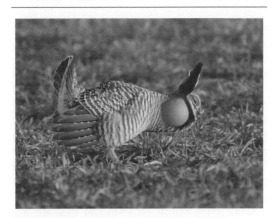

Figure 18.2. Adult male Greater Prairie Chicken displaying.

Identification Is a Must

Within the vast numbers of wild species within this order, many are specialists in terms of diet (Elphick et al. 2001) and disease sensitivity (Altman et al. 1997). Correct identification is therefore extremely important when a young galliform is admitted into care. Some field guides have descriptions of the young as well as habitat, range, nest, and eggs. One excellent resource is *A Guide to the Nests, Eggs and Nestlings of North American Birds* (Baicich and Harrison 2005).

Although obtaining a history is important to document with any patient, the specific habitat of grouse and other sensitive species makes the information of where the chick was found invaluable in identifying a wild patient, and may directly affect the successful rehabilitation of the individual bird.

It may be determined that a patient is an exotic species. It may have escaped from a local game farm or zoo. If that is the case, the bird can simply be returned to the owner. Or, the new patient may be a domestic chicken. Some breeds of chickens when hatched are striped and resemble wild grouse, pheasant, or quail. Because of the commercial nature of many galliformes, private ownership may be a factor. Depending on your city, state, or provincial laws, this may have legal ramifications, and attempts to find the owner should be made.

Many galliformes are legally hunted. It is beneficial to know hunting laws and have information available regarding legal hunting seasons. Some states or provinces may discourage rehabilitation of game birds. Be sure to check permits to clarify this status before a game bird is admitted as a patient.

Highly Precocial Chicks

Galliform chicks are highly precocial at hatch. Nests with rare exception are located on the ground, because these are terrestrial birds and the young leave the nest soon after hatching. At hatch, the primaries of many species are already formed (Sibley

2000; Ritchie et al. 1994). Chicks are downy, often striped or mottled in color and blend in with their surroundings. Although able to forage soon after hatch, chicks rely on adults to locate food (Williams 1991). Most chicks feed themselves; however, some species including turkeys, are known to place food directly into the mouth of their young (Skutch 1976). Chicks are sensitive to cold and require brooding by the adult until well feathered, and are capable of flight within 2–10 days. Many species have large families numbering up to 25 chicks per nest. The adult communicates with chicks before hatch and shortly after, cementing parental imprinting and voice recognition. Many species not only identify their mother's voice, but that of each sibling as an individual as well (Williams 1991; Skutch 1976; Gibson 1998). For this reason fostering can be difficult.

CRITERIA FOR INTERVENTION

Youngsters may be kidnapped by well-intentioned people or energetic children. Ground nests are sometimes located by buildings or agricultural projects. Often, eggs from these will be collected before the finder calls a wildlife center for advice. Wildlife personnel may be asked to come and remove eggs so a building project can advance on time. Nest disturbance is illegal for native species. It is important to be well versed in federal and state migratory bird laws before responding to such calls. Other reasons for admission include the death of a parent on the road or injuries from domestic dogs or cats. Chicks hatched in cold or inclement weather may be abandoned by parents due to low probability of survival.

The wildlife rehabilitator plays an important role keeping wild youngsters with their natural parents through dissemination of information to the public. Most galliformes hatch between 18–26 days. Once hatched, they are able to leave the nest area within hours, but need brooding from the adult to survive.

Offer natural history information to the caller. The fact that the eggs hatch within 3 weeks of being laid and the young leave the nest soon thereafter can be a comfort.

If a caller has questions about a hatchling that is not yet captive, urge the caller not to touch the chick unless it is in immediate danger. Reassure the caller that the adult is likely close by and will respond to the voice of her chick once human disturbance abates.

If the caller has the chick in captivity but is still in the area where it was found, urge the caller to release it and leave the immediate area, giving the adult bird an opportunity to reunite with the chick. Observation from a distance is suggested for a period of 1 hour.

If the chick is injured, or other reasons exist whereby reuniting with the adult is not an option, underscore the need to keep the chick warm and confined. Galliformes brood their chicks, keeping them close to their bodies. Situations that mimic brooding, such as wrapping a towel around the chick in a warmed environment, will lower stress and give the best chance for survival.

Adult birds of these wild species may appear "tame" and approach people. Grouse in particular occasionally show an odd behavior in which they appear very tame. They allow people to hand-feed them and even follow vehicles (Bump et al. 1947). These birds are not imprinted or raised in captivity, but exhibit a behavior that, although well documented, is poorly understood. If the bird is a native species and is not in immediate danger, the caller should be advised that it should be left in the wild. The behavior generally stops as quickly as it began. It has been reported, however, that individual birds have maintained "tame" behavior for up to 2 years. If the bird becomes territorial or aggressive, relocation should be considered.

Adult galliformes are most frequently injured when hit by cars, shot, or caught in a barbed-wire fence (Erickson 2006). Instruct the caller to gently remove the injured bird from the area, place it in a cardboard box with towel or leaf material on the bottom, and transport it as soon as possible to a wildlife rehabilitation facility.

Regulating agencies may have rules discouraging the rehabilitation of game birds or hatching eggs of disturbed nests. Check with officials in the area to clarify responses to the public.

Transportation to Wildlife Facility

The chick should be transported as soon as possible. A transport box no more than twice the size of the bird will lower stress and keep the youngster secure. A cardboard box with air holes works well. A towel or teeshirt on the bottom of the box will prevent chicks from sliding and possible leg splaying. Do not transport with a filled water bowl. Spilled water will wet the chick and cause hypothermia. Provide supplemental heat during transport. Heating pads, warmed rice bags, a hot water bottle, or the equivalent may be used when padded with towels so the chick is not in direct contact with the heat source. A stuffed animal or feather duster or being held may comfort the youngster during transport.

INITIAL CARE AND STABILIZATION

Chicks of these species are often tiny at hatch, sometimes weighing 1 g or less. They are very susceptible to stress and cold. The condition of a hypothermic patient is always critical. It is vital to bring the temperature up quickly or death will result. Before a physical can be done, the bird must have a normal core body temperature. Hypothermic birds should not be given food or water orally. The digestive system does not function until the core body temperature is restored. To warm a chilled bird, a heating pad set on low setting can be used or a heated box or incubator set at 97–99°F (36.1–37.2°C) (Anderson Brown and Robins 2002). Nonresponsive patients should never be left on heat without constant monitoring. Heating pads and lamps can overheat debilitated patients unable to move from the heat. Death can result. Massage the patient with a warmed towel to stimulate response and increase circulation.

Physical examination of chicks should be brief to avoid stress. Much of the exam can be done by observation in the brooder. Check for an egg tooth on the patient to determine whether the patient is a hatchling. The egg tooth assists hatching and remains visible only a few days. It is important to remember that many species hatch with primary feathers, and thus may be wrongly assumed to be older. Check the vent to make sure it is clean and not pasted. Soft feces can dry and build up on down near the vent and not allow the chick to defecate. If the vent is not clean, wash the area with warm water until all material is removed.

Offer a drop of warmed water or electrolyte fluid (Pedialyte, 0.9% sodium chloride, or lactated Ringer's solution) off the tip of a finger after the chick has opened its eyes and has a swallowing reflex. Allow the chick to drink in this manner. Once the chick is strong enough to stand, add a light mixture of protein to the fluid and continue to offer drops from a fingertip (see the recipe in Chapter 19, "Cranes," in the section titled "Emaciation Diet for Crane Colts"). Because many of these species are so tiny, syringe or pipette feeding can overwhelm their ability to swallow and they may drown. Continue feeding the light mixture until the chick defecates. Tube feeding should be initiated in small amounts (0.05 ml for quail). Initial tube feedings are meant to stimulate peristalsis rather than to fill the crop.

COMMON MEDICAL PROBLEMS AND SOLUTIONS

Wild galliform chicks, unlike their domestic counterparts, are very easily stressed birds. Those raised in captivity are more susceptible to disease and parasites. Stress of captivity likely plays a role. When raised with the parent in a natural habitat, they are more likely to die from predation than disease (Bump 1978; Woodward 1993). Although not clearly understood, wild-raised chicks and adults benefit from the large variety of natural insects and foliage available, perhaps by boosting their immune systems and providing natural remedies. Some naturally ingested plants have secondary compounds and chemicals that are toxic, and yet are easily digested and tolerated by species such as grouse (Elphick et al. 2001). For this reason, using litter from a forest floor or other habitat native to the patient may improve success rates. The treatment of parasites and disease in domestic Galliformes is covered in Chapter 17, "Domestic Poultry."

Preventing disease is much better than treating after it occurs. Due to their small size and the sensitivity to stress of galliform chicks, diagnosis through blood work is not practical, although older birds may have blood collected from the cutaneous ulnar vein when needed (see Figure 18.3). For the same reason, treatment is frequently not successful once the process has begun. The rehabilitator's focus should therefore be on prevention and early detection.

Bacterial diseases such as salmonellosis may develop through a contaminated water or food source. Water should be changed several times a day for young patients, and food should not be allowed to sour or become contaminated by feces. Observe the birds' droppings and respond to changes such as diarrhea quickly. Keep the vent clean and be alert for pasting that can occur with digestive problems. A bird with a pasted vent cannot defecate adequately and may die.

A single chick of any wild galliform species reared alone is unlikely to survive despite the best efforts of the rehabilitator. Reasons for this have been discussed earlier in this chapter. The chances of survival increase dramatically when another chick

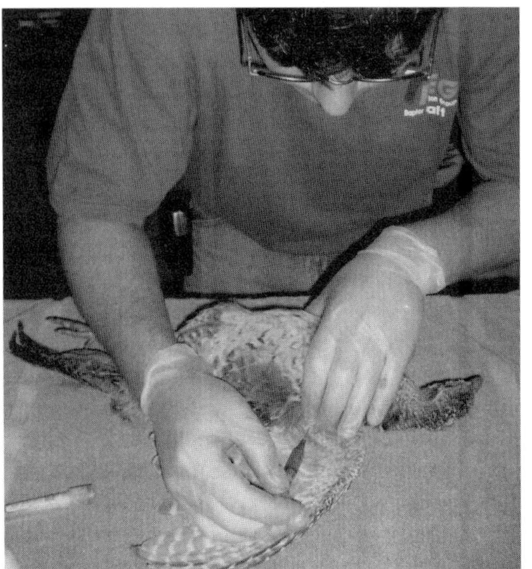

Figure 18.3. Blood collection from the cutaneous ulnar vein in a pheasant.

of similar size is introduced. Ideally, the species should be the same, but since in the world of wildlife rehabilitation that is not always possible, similar species may be used as a companion. The conundrum is that many wild species are sensitive to diseases carried naturally by another, which may not manifest itself as clinical disease in the second. This sensitivity continues through adulthood, and as a general rule birds should never be raised in mixed flocks or crowded conditions.

In the wild, even through species may share a common habitat, they usually do not have enough close contact to allow disease transference. In many species, very little is known about disease transference. Textbooks on avian medicine freely discuss the lack of information (Altman et al. 1997). New information is continually discovered. Check with an avian veterinarian experienced in game birds for specifics of diseases, species incompatibility, and drug sensitivities. Use antibiotics sparingly in wild galliformes as they may suppress the birds' immune systems. Antiprotozoals may be necessary in some species, particularly turkeys, and are often included in commercial turkey diets.

Commercial feeds, which are developed specifically for certain species, may be toxic to other galliformes. For instance, feed developed for chickens may be toxic to pheasants and partridge due to the addition of halofuginone. Commercial turkey food containing antiprotozoals can inhibit cecal flora and cause death in grouse and other sensitive species (Altman et al. 1997). For this reason natural food is best for the wild galliformes.

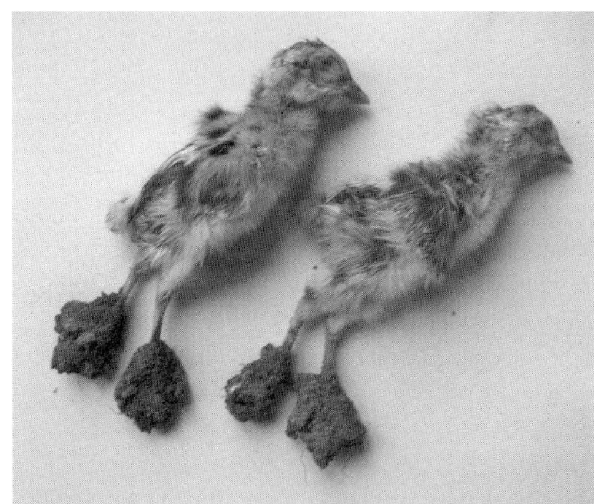

Figure 18.4. Mud-balling causes the feet to become encased in heavy, solid material and may be lethal.

Mud-balling

Mud-balling may occur with ground-dwelling birds, both in the wild and in captive care (see Figure 18.4). The problem begins when wet conditions turn soil sticky, allowing it to adhere to the feet of young birds (Welty 1982). Multiple layers build up around the feet until they are encased around a ball—thus the term *mud-balling*. This may cause death from exhaustion as the bird struggles to free itself, or inability to walk, eat, or maintain other normal behaviors. In captivity this process can occur in brooders with very young chicks, or in outdoor facilities. Wet feces mixed with any soft substrate such as wood shavings, can also cause balling. Foot deformities can result from even minor cases if not corrected quickly. The hardened material acts as a cast, retarding growth in rapidly growing young. Treatment consists of soaking the feet in warm water to soften the material. Be careful pulling it off because fractures may occur or the skin may be torn.

Splayed Legs

Splayed legs can happen when a young bird slips on unstable substrate, stretching ligaments beyond their normal range. If caught early, it can be corrected using Vetrap (3 M) or similar material to "soft-splint" the legs in a natural position. The feet should be separated by normal standing or walking distance (see Figure 12.3). The bird should be able to walk and maintain normal behavior with the splint on its legs. Standing and walking while splinted is important to maintain muscle tone and development. Depending on the severity, the legs should remain splinted for a few days to a week. Adjust the splint daily in newly hatched birds to accommodate their rapid growth (Altman et al. 1997).

Cannibalism

Cannibalism may occur in all galliformes when kept in captivity. Many theories exist on the causes of this, from nutritional deficiencies to overcrowding to poor sanitation (Woodward 1993). It is likely that multiple factors play a part in the phenomenon. Providing adequate space and good food in plentiful amounts is a proper place to start for prevention of this destructive behavior. Stress from human or domestic animals should be kept to a minimum.

While in brooders, chicks will often pick at the toes or legs of others. Check the victim for bleeding or physical abnormality, such as crooked toes, that could attract attention. Feces or bedding adhered to the vent or feet may resemble bits of food and cause picking by other chicks. All areas that are open sores should be treated with antibiotic ointment. Open wounds must be healed before reintroducing birds that have been cannibalized by cagemates.

Removing an aggressive bird for even a short time seems to break the cycle of picking, and it may be enough to solve the problem. Introducing fresh greens with roots and soil still attached may also distract the birds and resolve picking.

Birds in outdoor facilities pick feathers of others or themselves when under either physiological or environmental stress. Check all factors, including making sure there is adequate high-quality food available, no predator harassment, and a stress-free environment. Domestic animals including dogs that live on the property can be responsible for stress. The birds see domestic pets as predators and will react as such. Release may be the best option if you are unable to locate the stressor.

DIET

Wild galliformes have very specific food needs. Although some can survive on prepared commercial diets, many cannot. Unfortunately, there is no hard and fast rule to indicate which will be relatively hardy patients and which are delicate beyond expectation for even the most experienced rehabilitator.

As a generalization, species that have been raised commercially, such as pheasants and quail, are hardy and have a high success rate when raised in captivity. By contrast, wild turkeys and grouse are delicate in captive care. Wild turkeys differ in many ways from domestic varieties, including the fact that they have 35% more brain capacity than domestics.

There is often wide variation in food habits for grouse species. Complicating things, these diets change with the season. Considering there are 16 grouse species in the northern hemisphere alone, it is virtually impossible to give successful diets for each within this chapter. The best approach is for the rehabilitator to become familiar with the species found in each region and their diets. This is one reason a history and location where the bird was found is more important in galliformes than for most patients. Young patients of these sensitive species will require extra effort to successfully raise to release.

Getting youngsters to eat can be challenging. The first food of grouse chicks is ants or other tiny insects. The rapid movement of an insect attracts chicks, and they are usually stimulated to begin eating. A large-sized dog food bowl will work as a miniature habitat for a small shovel of active ants. Ants can overwhelm youngsters and bite them, so be sure to monitor them well.

Wild grasses or weeds pulled from the ground with some soil left on the root (Hayes 1992) is very interesting to chicks. Most instinctively begin scratching the roots, eating as they do. Be sure grass is safe, nontoxic, and has not been sprayed with pesticide. The act of eating will encourage chicks to eat other food offered. Kitten or puppy pellets (Hills Science Diet), soaked overnight in the refrigerator with an equal amount of water, should be offered in a shallow dish. Before serving, add tiny mealworms, bloodworms, waxworms, tubifex worms, or naturally occurring insects from the region. Some commercial game farm growers suggest crumbling a red dog treat and using it to top food. The red color is said to attract the attention of the chicks (Woodward 1993).

If a young patient still refuses to eat despite the above measures, try sprinkling dry baby cereal or dried crumbled insects on the chicks' back. During the natural preening behavior they will invariably get some food in their mouths, recognize it as food, and begin eating.

If all else fails, use a drop-by-drop method with the emaciation diet described earlier in this chapter. Tube-feeding can be used but is stressful to these delicate species.

Warm water (Hayes 1992) should be provided in shallow saucerlike dishes lined with pea gravel or sand substrate. This prevents the chick from slipping and splaying its legs. Some sand may also be eaten for grit to aid digestion. Chicks should be prevented from ingesting large amounts of sand as impacted crops can result. Commercial chick water founts are available at most farm supply stores and work well. Colorful marbles put in the drinking water prevent tiny game birds from drowning while attracting interest to the water supply (Ritchie et al. 1994; Hayes 1992; Woodward 1993).

Once the youngsters begin to eat, continue providing soaked kitten or puppy pellets topped with small mealworms, tubifex worms, and other insects as a staple diet during the first month of life. The saturated pellets must be changed several times per day to prevent souring. Add grasshoppers, crickets, and finally grain as the chicks grow and show interest in new foods. Wild natural greens cut into tiny bite-size pieces are a good addition to the diet. Romaine lettuce can also be used. Cutting the greens into small bits will help prevent large pieces from impacting in their crops. Adults perform this service for chicks in the wild.

HOUSING

Brooders

Commercial brooders used for chicken or game farms also work well for wild chicks. If the brooder has been used in the past for domestic species, clean and sterilize it well. Many wild species are highly susceptible to diseases found in domestic chickens and turkey poults. Commercial brooders are meant to brood many chicks at a time and may not be the best choice if you have only a few to rear.

If only a few chicks are in care, a smaller setup may be more practical. A clean cardboard box, $16 \times 20 \times 20$ in ($40 \times 50 \times 50$ cm), or plastic storage container is a good option. A clip-on reflector heat lamp, found in the hardware section of many stores, should be firmly secured on one side of the box. A 40–60 watt bulb is usually adequate to provide a temperature of 95–99°F (35–37.2°C). Check the temperature under the heat lamp and move the lamp either up or down to reach the correct temperature.

Single chicks rarely live. For that reason it may be helpful during the first few days of confinement to house the chick with a day-old bantam chick or older chicks to lower stress and encourage eating. However, be aware of the possibility of bacterial, viral, or other infectious diseases that can be transferred in these cases. It is recommended that any domestic fowl be from a closed flock or vaccinated for common diseases before they come into contact even briefly with a wild individual.

Mixed-age housing has advantages and disadvantages that must be weighed. Older chicks may suffocate, injure, or not allow newly hatched young to feed. Use care if this is the only option for housing. Older chicks that have begun to eat on their own may encourage and teach younger ones how to eat and drink. Observe the birds carefully for any aggression and separate immediately if it occurs. Networking with other rehabilitators is suggested and very helpful with housing multiple species or varied ages.

A windup alarm clock and mirror with a clean feather duster or cotton mop head (Ritchie et al. 1994) may be helpful to provide the youngster with a substitute parent figure. If using a feather duster, make certain no chemicals or preservatives have been used. Toxic fumes may result when chemically treated feathers become wet. Synthetic feathers may be the safest for this use. White muslin fabric placed on top of the substrate during the first week of life allows the caregiver to observe the feces and be alert to digestive problems or whether the young birds are eating. The fabric also helps prevent chicks from developing an impacted crop by ingesting large amounts of plant material or sand. Other substrates that work well for the brooder can be coarse sand, pea gravel, clean soil, or natural dry leaf litter. Firm substrate will prevent young birds' legs from slipping and splaying out. Fine sand can cause eye problems in young chicks. Wood shavings (not cedar), or natural leaf litter from the chick's natural habitat combined with pea gravel can be used as substrate as the chicks mature.

No matter what substrate is used, it must be kept clean and dry to prevent bacterial growth and disease. Some people suggest wooden boxes; although they work well, they retain moisture and are more difficult to sanitize after use (Woodward 1993).

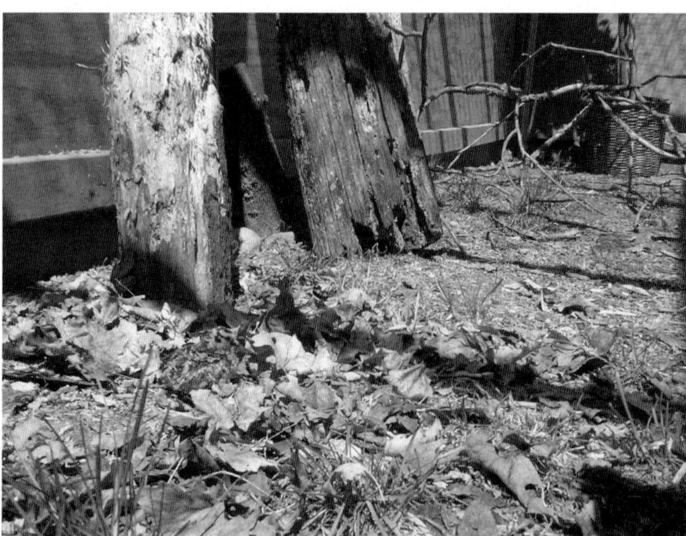

Figure 18.5. Enclosures should have natural leaf litter and soil for birds to practice foraging behaviors.

The behavior of the chicks will be the guide as to whether the temperature is too warm or cold. Chicks that are too cold will huddle under the heat lamp and hesitate to come out to eat or drink. If they are too hot they will droop their wings and stand away from the lamp. A heat lamp on one side of the box enables them to choose to stay close or move away from the heat if needed.

As chicks develop and become more active, they will require larger and taller brooder boxes and lower temperatures. Lower the temperature in 5°F (2.8°C) increments weekly or more quickly if chicks display signs of being too hot. Many galliform chicks can fly within a few days to a week of hatch. For that reason, a top for the brooder box is essential to keep the chicks inside. Chicks will need to remain under a brooder for 5–6 weeks. When they are fully feathered they may be moved to an outdoor area. A supplemental heat source and protected indoor area must remain available in cooler climates until the birds have acclimated completely.

Outdoor Facilities

Galliformes are often prey for other animals and therefore have a strong stress reaction to the sight and sound of predators. Seeking cover and hiding is their reaction to fear. Birds do not eat or drink well when forced to "hide" from predators even as their metabolism and need for calories increases with the added stress.

Pens made to raptor specifications work well, offering the birds access to natural sun and rain and protection from predators (Gibson 1996). A visual barrier installed at least 3 ft high around the perimeter of the enclosure will lower stress in captive birds by providing privacy. Galliformes destined to be released to the wild do best in enclosures planted with native plants, berries, apple trees, and other nontoxic plants to provide cover. The author uses dwarf variety fruit trees to prevent damage to the netting covering of the pen. A shelter, such as a lean-to or building, should also be provided for severe weather and shade protection if needed.

The size of the enclosure will depend on the species of the bird in care. Natural soil is the best substrate for these species. The enclosure should be freshly tilled at least once per season, or before young galliformes are introduced, to prevent parasites and disease that may be harbored in the soil left by previous inhabitants. If the substrate of the enclosure is pea gravel or other material it should be sanitized. Cover the substrate with several inches of natural litter (leaves, decaying bark, and soil) from a forest floor in the region (see Figure 18.5). Leaf litter is a natural habitat and will give young birds an opportunity to exercise normal foraging behaviors. Sand in one area of the pen is beneficial. Galliformes use sand or light soil as a grooming aid and also as grit for digestion.

The size of the prerelease enclosure will depend on the species of bird in care. The enclosure size of

30 × 30 × 10 ft (9 × 9 × 3 m) will accommodate 5–10 young grouse until release. Crowding increases stress and opportunities for disease. Natural logs, some hollow to provide shelter, are useful and will help birds become accustomed to "wild habitat" prior to release.

It is natural for galliformes to live with a parent, usually the hen, until they are fully feathered, sometimes through the fall of their first year. Some adults, such as males and juveniles approaching adult status, are often not compatible. Many species are territorial and will be aggressive to others in the group. Watch for signs of this behavior and separate those individuals that cause injury. Injured birds that are bleeding also must be removed for their safety until no fresh injury is visible.

Predator Guards for Housing and Enclosures

The first step to protecting patients from predation is to not attract predators to the area. Grain spillage should be cleaned up and no excess food left outside the pens. Solid barrier fences block visual temptation for predators. Trees bordering enclosures may allow avian predators to perch and climbing predators to access the enclosure, so they should be carefully evaluated. Digging animals such as skunks, can be discouraged with 1 × 0.5 in (2.5 × 1.25 cm) hardware cloth buried 2 ft (60 cm) straight into the ground and angled outward from the pen another 2 ft (60 cm). The use of galvanized heavy gauge wire is wise because less substantial wire may deteriorate and require costly maintenance. Some rehabilitators have success using multiple strands of electric fencing on the outside of the perimeter fencing, starting inches from the ground and placed about 1 ft (30 cm) apart to a height of approximately 5 ft (1.5 m), which is generally adequate to discourage most predators. Check with local wildlife officials for a list of predators that frequent the area and regulations for legal means to control them. Humane trapping using live traps or other methods may be needed for persistent pests. Local regulations may affect translocation of live-trapped predators. Under no circumstances should poison ever be used to control predators. The chance of poisoning nontarget species is great. For the most complete protection, the enclosure should be covered to prevent avian predation, premature release, or wild visitors that may bring parasites or other problems to the pens.

RELEASE CRITERIA

Everything about wild galliformes is unique and release is no different. Most species do not fly well nor move great distances, so dispersal is not an option for these birds as it is with most other avian species. It is therefore important for them to be released into good habitat and away from humans and domestic animals. Release should occur after the bird is fully feathered, acclimated to outdoor temperature, and experienced with natural food. Let them go in late summer, or fall and winter in areas that have moderate temperatures. Do not release birds in spring or when breeding or nesting occurs in the natural population of the same species. Wild galliformes vary greatly in this aspect but some may defend their territories vigorously.

Many galliformes are hunted. Consider the hunting season dates in timing release. For best survival, release birds after hunting season ends or a few weeks before to allow the bird to acclimate without threat. Postrelease supplemental feeding can continue, but is generally not needed.

AUTHOR'S NOTE

The rehabilitation of wild galliformes can be challenging. Wildlife rehabilitators have contact with species rarely handled, particularly as chicks. Working with these delicate species gives the wildlife rehabilitator an opportunity to be a valued partner in natural history information development and disease research. It is essential to keep good records of diet, housing, and treatment regimes. Both successes and failures with every aspect of care are important and should be shared with the wildlife community. Full necropsies of mortalities should be done to document disease processes, which may be poorly understood. Adding to the knowledge of a species is an important endeavor and one in which the rehabilitator can play an active role.

ACKNOWLEDGMENTS

I owe much to my grandmother and parents who filled my young life with galliformes both wild and domestic, infecting me with their own love of birds. Thanks to my family: my husband Don; our children, Darrell, Katrinka, and Sarah; and now grandchildren Hunter, Madalyn, and Alexander, who continue to share my life with aves.

REFERENCES

Altman, R.B., Clubb, S.L., Dorrestein, G.M., and Quesenberry, K. 1997. Avian Medicine and Surgery. W.B. Saunders Co., Philadelphia, pp. 944–959.

Anderson Brown, A.F. and Robins, G.E.S. 2002. The New Incubation Book. Hancock House Publishing Ltd. Blaine, Washington, pp. 206–213.

Atwater, S. and Schnell, J. 1989. The Wildlife Series: The Ruffed Grouse. Stackpole Books, Mechanicsburg, Pennsylvania, pp. 130–138.

Baicich, P.J. and Harrison, C.J.O. 2005. Nest, Eggs, and Nestlings of North American Birds, Second Edition. Princeton University Press, Princeton, New Jersey, 347 pp.

Bump, G., Darrow, R.W., Edminster, F.C., and Crissey, W.F. 1947. The Ruffed Grouse: Life History, Propagation and Management. New York State Conservation Department, pp. 179–226.

Delacour, J. 1978. Pheasant Breeding and Care. T.F.H. Publications Inc., pp. 18, 443–448.

Elphick, C., Dunning, Jr., J.B., and Sibley, D.A. 2001. The Sibley Guide to Bird Life and Behavior. Alfred A. Knopf, Inc., New York, pp. 73–77, 233–245.

Erickson, L. 2006. 101 Ways to Help Birds. Stackpole Books, Mechanicsburg, Pennsylvania, pp. 73–74, 76, 203.

Gibson, M. 1996. The ABC's of housing raptors. Journal of Wildlife Rehabilitation 19(3): 23–31.

———. 1997. Natural history: Square one for wildlife rehabilitation. Journal of Wildlife Rehabilitation 17(1): 3–6, 16.

———. 1998. Putting baby back. Journal of Wildlife Rehabilitation 21(2): 33–40.

Hayes, L.B. 1992. The Chinese Painted Quail, Their Breeding and Care. Leland Hayes' Gamebird Publications, 161 pp.

Johnsgard, P.A. 1988. The Quails, Partridges and Francolins of the World. Oxford University Press, pp. 202–205.

Landers, L.J. and Mueller, B.S. 1986. Bobwhite Quail Management: A Habitat Approach. Tall Timbers Research Station and Quail Unlimited, 39 pp.

Martin, L.C. 1993. The Folklore of Birds. The Globe Pequot Press, pp. 69, 153.

Ritchie, B.W., Harrison, G.J., and Harrison, L.R. 1994. Avian Medicine: Principles and Application. Wingers Publishing Inc., Lake Worth, Florida, 1384 pp.

Rogers, L.J. and Kaplan, G. 2000. Songs, Roars and Rituals, Communications in Birds, Mammals, and Other Animals. Harvard University Press, Cambridge, Massachusetts, pp. 20, 83, 90.

Rupley, A. 1997. Manual of Avian Practice. W.B. Saunders Co., Philadelphia, pp. 265–291.

Sibley, D.A. 2000. The Sibley Guide to Birds. Alfred A. Knopf, Inc., New York, pp. 134–149.

Skutch, A.F. 1976. Parent Birds and Their Young. University of Texas Press, pp. 312–315.

Welty, J.C. 1982. The Life of Birds, Third Edition. Saunders College Publishing, Philadelphia. 754 pp.

Williams, Jr., L.E. 1991. Wild Turkey Country. Northword Press, 160 pp.

Woodward, A. 1993. Commercial and Ornamental Game Bird Breeders Handbook, Hancock Wildlife Research Center, pp. 181–188, 272–290, 357–359.

HELPFUL WEBSITES

http://www.mcmurrayhatchery.com/index.html.

http://www.naga.org/.

http://www.gamebird.com/.

http://www.agmrc.org/agmrc/commodity/agritourism/gamebirds/.

http://www.lelandhayes.com/.

http://www.avianpublications.com/items/fowl/itemB15.htm.

19
Cranes

Marjorie Gibson

NATURAL HISTORY

Cranes are classed among the oldest families of birds. Of the 15 species in the Gruidae family worldwide, 9 are threatened or endangered. Cranes are tall stately birds with long necks and legs, and heavy bills. They have distinctive silhouettes with the tertial feathers drooping over the rump in a bustle. Cranes are best known for strong mate fidelity, intricate "mating dances" and the practice of siblicide.

Two species are found in North America, with another species, the Common Crane (*Grus grus*) of Eurasia, being sighted occasionally. The Sandhill Crane (*Grus Canadensis*) has six subspecies, including Canadian, Greater, Lesser, Florida, Mississippi, and Cuban. The Whooping Crane (*Grus Americana*) is endangered in North America.

Sandhill Cranes are 34–48 in (0.8–1.2 m) tall with wingspans of 73–90 in (1.8–2.3 m), with variation in size depending on the subspecies. Whooping Cranes are 52 in (1.3 m) tall with wingspans of 87 in (2.2 m). Successful captive breeding programs for Whooping Cranes have been established, and these birds are currently being reintroduced to regions within the U.S. With continued success of captive breeding and reintroduction, it may be possible to encounter wild Whooping Cranes in need of rehabilitation within the next decade.

Cranes are long-lived and monogamous. They nest in marshy areas and build simple nests of vegetation gathered from around the nest site. The gathering of nesting material plays an important role in nesting because a watery barrier must be created around the nest site. This act may contribute to the reproductive success of cranes. Both male and female incubate the two eggs, which hatch asynchronously in 28–36 days.

Young cranes are called *colts*. Crane colts can be very aggressive to each other and siblicide is common. Asynchronous hatching gives the older chick an advantage, but leaves the second egg and resulting chick as a "backup" if the first colt should perish. If both chicks survive past hatch, they are generally separated, with each adult taking one chick and acting as its primary parent. In this way the young are physically separated until tolerance is attained.

Crane colts are precocial at hatch. They are covered with thick rusty brown-colored down. They are active after hatch and can leave the nest the same day. Young cranes follow their parent, often walking underneath the abdomen of the adult as they move through the marsh. They can swim short distances. There is a wide variety of vocalizations that occur between adult cranes and their young. Sounds can change from a soft pumping noise to an aggressive trumpet when danger is near. The young vocalize a soft purring sound, almost constantly to maintain contact with the adult as they walk. Adult cranes feed the young by killing prey such as crustaceans, frogs, snakes, or mice, and thrashing it to bits for the youngster. They also teach chicks to secure their own food by turning over mud or soil in upland areas to expose insects or aquatic invertebrates. Crane colts are naturally attracted to movement and shiny objects and learn to feed themselves quickly.

Cranes in the wild eat a wide variety of plant material—insects, aquatic invertebrates, frogs, small animals, and even small birds if the opportunity presents itself. Hence, do not house them with songbirds or young ducklings. Although plant material is ingested in small amounts, most of the diet the first 6–8 weeks of life consists of insects, invertebrates, and larger vertebrates that have been killed and ripped apart by the adults.

Captive Breeding Facilities

Husbandry of captive and breeding cranes has been researched extensively by scientists at Patuxent Wildlife Research Center in Laurel, Maryland, and The International Crane Foundation in Baraboo, Wisconsin. Through these excellent sources, wildlife rehabilitators have access to a wide variety of information on the various aspects of captive crane care. One of the best reference books and a must for every rehabilitator considering cranes is *Cranes: Their Biology, Husbandry and Conservation* by David Ellis, George Gee, and Claire Mirande (1996).

Although information on long-term captive care of cranes is excellent, it must be kept in mind that the rehabilitation of cranes will have a different approach when compared to permanent captive and breeding care. Those differences focus on preparing for life in the wild in the case of a colt, or return to the wild in the adult. The captive care of birds in rehabilitation is a short period, rather than their entire life. Some of those differences will be discussed in this chapter.

CRITERIA FOR INTERVENTION

Cranes' large size, interesting behavior, and considerable folklore draw the interest of the public when nest sites are close to human activity.

Adults

Most calls received by wildlife centers concerning adult cranes will be those hit by cars, shot, or accidentally poisoned from overspray or run-off in agricultural areas. Large die-offs of cranes have been reported due to mycotoxins. These are produced by fungi that grow on crops that have been left unharvested. Cranes species may be hypersensitive to mycotoxins (Ellis et al. 1996; Altman et al. 1997). Lead poisoning and ingestion of items such as screws or staples also occur. For this reason, the crane patient with digestive problems should be x-rayed to determine whether ingested material is the source. Gruidae as a family tend to be temperature-hardy. However, individuals exposed to extreme cold without protection may suffer frostbite to the toes. Patients with frostbite are usually birds that have been unable to migrate for some reason and are forced to remain in extreme winter temperatures.

Chicks

Very young cranes may be found with hypothermia. Those chicks that are hatched during very cold temperatures have a poor chance of survival. Although able to thermoregulate to some degree, circumstances require youngsters to follow their parent through wet, marshy habitat soon after hatch. Periods of cold temperatures, particularly when prolonged, often prove to be too harsh for survival. Colts admitted in this situation will always be hypothermic, will be cold to the touch, and have delayed or minimal response to stimulation. In serious cases, they can be mistaken for being dead. Young cranes with hypothermia can be revived, even when there is lack of movement, with application of heat.

The appearance of a crane colt, with the long neck, legs, and soft coloring, is attractive to the public, and once spotted, they are often victims of kidnapping from the wild. Dogs, cats, and wild predators are also a threat. The incidence of all of these increases when nest sites border parks, agricultural, or other recreational areas. Advice to the public plays an important role in assuring normal, uninjured youngsters stay in the wild with their parents.

Questions to Ask the Public When Answering Calls

1. Is the crane standing or lying down?
2. Is blood visible?
3. Is the youngster running and active?
4. Can the youngster hear an adult crane vocalizing or see an adult in the immediate area?
5. Is the youngster in immediate danger? (If dogs or aggressive children are chasing it, for example, a chick can be temporarily captured and placed back in the area when the danger is gone.)

Young cranes, although very mobile, can be easily captured. Colts can suffer heat exhaustion, capture myopathy, or injury when chased. In most cases, parent birds are in close proximity. Adults can become aggressive in defense of their young. Initially, the adult response is to become vocal. The vocalizations increase in volume and tone to warn the youngster of approaching danger and "predator" of the adult presence. The stout and heavy beak of an adult crane can be very dangerous.

Parents occasionally abandon newly hatched cranes. This phenomenon is likely if weather at hatch is extreme and chances of the colt's survival are minimal. Siblings can injure or kill each other. Although siblicide occurs more often in captive situations, it can occur in the wild. Care must be taken when housing even very young or debilitated cranes together.

INITIAL CARE AND STABILIZATION

If the colt is cold to the touch but responsive, put it in a dark, quiet box on heat of 90–95°F (32–34°C) until the core body temperature returns to normal and is stable (104–108°F, 40–42°C). The patient should be gently massaged with a warmed towel to stimulate response. When the youngster is stable, an exam can be done.

Do not give oral fluid or diet to a colt that is non-responsive. Oral fluid can be given only when the colt is able to hold its head up for at least brief periods on its own. Oral emaciation diet should be the first food for colts coming out of hypothermia, or in critical condition (see the section "Diet," later in this chapter).

Give fluids warmed to 100.4–102.2°F (38–39°C) (Samour 2000) subcutaneously to chicks that are weak or poorly responsive or orally via gavage tube to strong chicks. The author prefers to be conservative in fluid amounts given, giving 5% of body weight (50 ml/kg) at a maximum to avoid overhydrating crane chicks. Fluid therapy is important in cases of starvation or other conditions where dehydration is present. Dehydration will almost always be an element in starvation cases and should be addressed immediately.

Handle colts as little as possible. This is important both for keeping the stress level low and in consideration of injury that may result due to handling. The body structure of members of the crane family is conducive to injury at the smallest provocation. A heightened awareness of possible injury must be built into the handling protocol of members of the Grus family. When handling is necessary, take care to protect the legs. A towel can be used to hold and gently restrain young cranes (see Figure 19.1). One hand should be under the feet at all times if the patient is a youngster. Joints and legs are very delicate in cranes and inappropriate handling can cause permanent damage to the integrity of the legs, pelvis, or joints.

If the patient is thin and has not been eating, give emaciation diet via gavage tube into the crop (after initial rehydration). Use minimal amounts at first (5 ml) to make sure the digestive system is moving before offering solid food. Once the young patient is stable, a full exam and additional medical intervention can be done (see Figure 19.2).

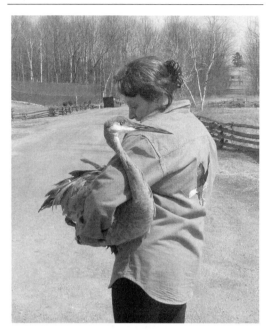

Figure 19.1. Restraining a crane involves holding the bird facing backward with the legs and feet restrained. Safety glasses are also prudent.

COMMON MEDICAL PROBLEMS

Cranes are subject to several viral diseases, fungal diseases, and a host of bacterial and parasitic conditions. Cranes in the wild have and tolerate many parasites. It is not necessary to evaluate every patient unless secondary problems are apparent. If the patient presents with or develops diarrhea, has poor weight gain, or is lethargic, a workup should be done to identify the problem. Good sanitation, pen rotation, fresh food, and clean water are the best means with which to prevent disease.

Respiratory Disease

Respiratory disease is common in crane colts. General symptoms include pale mucous membranes and lethargy in the early stages of any respiratory

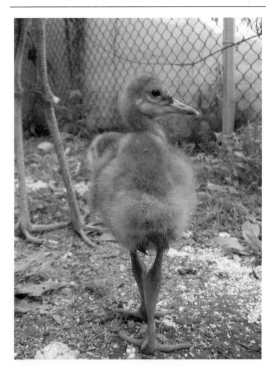

Figure 19.2. Young colt walking toward foster parent's legs.

condition. Chicks exhibiting signs of illness should be given supplemental heat (90–97°F, 32–36°C) and supportive care immediately. Raspy or open-mouthed breathing requires immediate intervention. In very young chicks, the problem is generally bacterial in nature; however, after 2 weeks of age, fungal disease including aspergillosis and coccidioidomycosis should be considered with appropriate medical care (Altman et al. 1997).

Parasites such as *Syngamus trachea* (gapeworm) occur in cranes and create respiratory symptoms. Earthworms serve as an intermediate host. This parasite should be considered in any young cranes, particularly those that have been fed or have access to earthworms early in their life. Gapeworm produces many symptoms, including head shaking, raspy sounding respirations, open mouth breathing, and coughing. In some cases, the worms are easily visible as red threadlike strands on the wall of the trachea when viewed down the glottis from inside the mouth. Eggs can be detected in the feces. This parasite can cause death in young cranes from anemia, asphyxiation from mucous production or even tracheal ulceration (Ritchie et al. 1997; Rupley 1997). Treatment once diagnosed is Ivermectin or Thiabendazole.

Heatstroke

Heatstroke can occur in cranes, particularly on hot summer days. This can be prevented with a few simple measures. Provide a shelter or shaded area in the compound. Only emergency handling should be done on hot days. If handling cannot be avoided, do it in the cooler early morning hours. Provide an adequate water supply. Be certain the crane is able to drink from the water container. The long beak requires a deep dish or pail. Cranes cannot drink from a shallow dish.

Heatstroke is demonstrated with gasping, panting, rapid breathing, staggering, and wings held away from the body of the crane or drooping. If the body temperature remains elevated death may result. If heatstroke is suspected, cool the bird immediately by placing its body or parts of its body in cool water. Cold packs may be placed under the wings to facilitate more rapid cooling. For birds that are conscious, alert, and capable, a swimming pool may be used to allow the bird to cool itself.

Injuries to Bones and Beaks

This section covers only injuries that can result in the full recovery and wild release of a crane. Many orthopedic procedures have been developed that work well for captive cranes, including leg prosthesis. Information for these procedures is available in many excellent textbooks, many of which are listed in this chapter's reference section. One of the best resources on avian medicine, which includes wild species, is Altman et al. (1997). Serious (e.g., open, comminuted, or close to a joint) fractures should be evaluated and repaired by your avian veterinarian.

Cranes often present to rehabilitation facilities with damage to the beak. Beak injury can be caused by a collision with an object or defensive maneuvers by the crane itself. In most cases, a broken tip of the beak needs little intervention unless it is bleeding or interferes with the ability of the bird to eat or drink. Some filing of the broken area, either with a hand file or Dremel tool, is recommended to create a smooth surface.

Serious fractures of the beak can be repaired with self-curing dental acrylics reinforced with Kirshner wires. Most healing takes place in 4–6 weeks with the wires being removed at that time. In young cranes, the splint must be changed frequently to accommodate the growth of the beak.

Broken wings can be successfully repaired by a variety of methods. Bandaging, splinting, and surgical repair are all valid methods of response to a wing fracture. Which technique is used will depend on how recent the fracture is, which bone is fractured, or whether it is a closed or open fracture.

Broken legs, although difficult to repair, can be attempted with the use of a sling to hold the body in a natural upright position. Due to weight-bearing exercise need of young cranes, this method is generally reserved only for adults or juveniles that have achieve full height. If a sling is used, the caregiver must be certain the vent area is uncovered and allows the bird to defecate.

Nutritional Problems

A diet too rich in protein and sulfur-containing amino acids can cause deformities of the wings and legs. Overgrowth of the primaries causes a condition commonly known as *angel wing,* with the tip of the wing turning up in an unnatural position. This occurs when feather growth exceeds muscular development. Angel wing can usually be corrected if caught early, by bandaging the wing in a natural position for 3–4 days.

Take care to check any housing for unnatural shiny objects, such as staples or pieces of wire. Cranes are attracted to shiny objects and will ingest such material, which can cause death.

Feather Problems

Quality of feathers is often underestimated in evaluating suitability for release of both captive-raised cranes and those that have been rehabilitated. Attention to feather quality (stress bars, dull or dirty, broken feathers, and defects such as barb defects) is essential. Feathers are responsible for maintaining waterproofing to prevent hypothermia, as well as for flight. Feathers directly affect the survival of a bird living in the wild. Malnutrition or other conditions can cause feather changes and indicate that the bird is not ready for release. Birds that fit this description should be retained and given supportive nutritional care. Feather damage can be so severe as to delay the release of an otherwise releasable crane until molting occurs.

Broken primaries can occur with injury, or as a result of a viral infection. Feathers can also be broken or in poor condition due to even a short time period in inadequate or inappropriate housing. Primaries can be *imped,* a process by which replacement feathers are fixed artificially into existing feather shafts, with the same methods as those used for raptors.

DIET

While in captivity, a very young crane colt can be encouraged to eat from a bowl if a red item, simulating the tip of the parent's beak, is placed into the food dish. Care should be taken that the simulated beak is sturdy and not an ingestion danger to the colt.

The diet of cranes varies with age. It is important to remember that while the adult diet includes vegetation and grain, the diet of a young crane, for the first 45–60 days, consists almost entirely of killed insects, invertebrates, and aquatic vertebrates.

Feeding live insects or animals to a very young crane is dangerous and not recommended. Young birds do not have the experience, skill, or digestive enzymes to kill and digest live prey. The parent kills all but the smallest insects for the first weeks of life, and continues to kill larger prey for several weeks.

Offer as much natural food, such as insects and aquatic invertebrates, as the colt will eat. Fresh food should be available at all times. Cranes reared in captivity but destined to go back into the wild need a natural diet. This is not only for nutritional support, but to develop their normal intestinal flora and gain experience foraging as well. Cranes grow at a rapid rate and ingest large amounts of food to provide the calories, minerals, and other nutrients to support their metabolic needs.

When augmented with natural foods, a successful basic diet can consist of Science Diet Feline or Canine Growth pellets saturated in water overnight in a refrigerator. Do not feed pellets before they are fully saturated. Care must be taken to assure the pellets remain refrigerated before use and are changed once a day at room temperature or more frequently in warm conditions. Once soaked in water do not keep pellets more than 3 days in the refrigerator before using, as they will sour and spoil with age. Allow the colt to eat as much as it wants during the day. Grain can be added once the young crane is more than 45 days old. This regime must be accompanied by substantial exercise for the growing colt.

After 30 days of age, small live crustaceans should be offered along with mayfly larva, moths, mealworms, waxworms, and other invertebrate prey. The colt may play with the new food items for several days before it successfully kills and eats them. It is important to offer a variety of items because each provides elements needed in the diet. It is best if the young crane has access to enclosed natural areas so it can graze and select a wide range of natural insects and vegetation on its own. If the nonreleasable foster parenting method of rearing is used, a nonflighted adult in or adjacent to the natural area will assure the colt does not wander. After 60 days of age crayfish, frogs, mice, and grain can be added to the colt's diet.

Commercial starter diets such as Zeigler Crane Breeder (Zeigler) diet are easily obtained and can be used to supplement a natural prey diet. It is important to note the difference in a maintenance diet used for adult birds and the starter diet used for the active growing stage of youngsters. The type of protein used in the diet of a colt is important.

Diets with a high percentage of sulphur-containing amino acids must be avoided because they contribute to developmental abnormalities such as leg and wing problems. For instance, fish should be fed in very small quantity because they contain a higher percentage of these amino acids. Breeders suggest a diet with 24% protein, 1.4% calcium, 0.90% phosphorus, 0.7% methionine and cystine, and 1.3% lysine. The kcal/kg is higher in starter or chick diets than those developed for adult birds. Maintenance diets have lower protein levels and can be used once the crane is over the age of 2 months (Ellis et al. 1996).

It is not suggested that a crane in rehabilitation be fed exclusively an artificial or commercial formula. If commercial diet is the only food offered, intake should be limited to prevent weight gain too quickly. If this occurs, the bird may become unable to support itself and deformities of the limbs may result.

Natural diet may be difficult to provide daily in quantities large enough for the captive crane patient. Most cranes will eat commercial diet once it is introduced. Sprinkling corn or insects on top of the commercial diet will encourage first-time investigation. An adult crane will do well on a commercial maintenance diet containing about 19% protein. Introduce breeder formula if an adult patient is held to early spring or breeding season. Breeding formulas offer higher protein and calcium, and they metabolizable energy. The importance of maintaining dry or pelleted commercial foods in a dry and fresh condition cannot be overemphasized.

Observe the wild rehabilitation patient from a remote location, or by a camera located within its enclosure, to make certain it is eating. If the bird is not eating, tube-feeding should be initiated within 24 hours.

Emaciation Diet for Crane Colts

The following is a recommended diet for emaciated crane colts:

- 2 oz (56 g) human baby mixed grain cereal, such as Gerber's brand
- One 2.5 oz (71 g) jar of Gerber's baby meat food (beef, chicken, turkey or veal)
- One 2.5 oz (71 g) jar water
- One 2.5 oz (71 g) jar human infant electrolyte replacer such as Pedialyte

Whip ingredients together, adding more water if needed until the diet will pass through a size 14 French red rubber feeding tube (catheter tube). Make the diet thinner for very weak patients.

Diet should be prepared fresh each feeding in the amount needed (see Figure 19.3). Start newly hatched colts with 5 ml and monitor how fast the crop empties. Increase the quantity fed as the chick successfully empties its crop. Feed the amount that fills the crop and is able to be moved out of the crop in an hour. If the chick regurgitates or fluid comes up, cut back the quantity given. Continue tube-feedings until the chick is eating on its own. Offer food items when the chick is able to stand. The diet must be warmed to 90°F (32°C) when administered but it should not be hot or crop burns will result. Microwave heating is not recommended due to uneven heating of the food particles. Feeding cold diet may well put a fragile patient into shock and result in death.

If the bird has diarrhea or is losing fluid, add extra isotonic electrolytes. In most cases of simple starvation or emaciation, the kidneys and most organs are functioning at a low level. Adding electrolytes will add sodium to already stressed kidneys and may cause shutdown.

If prepared baby meats are not available, steam pure fresh meat (no fat) until it is fully cooked. Puree the meat using a blender. The mixture may need reblending before each feeding to maintain a liquid fine enough to pass through a feeding tube.

This is not meant to be an all-inclusive balanced diet. It is used only to get a bird back on its feet so it can digest whole or natural food again. Very ema-

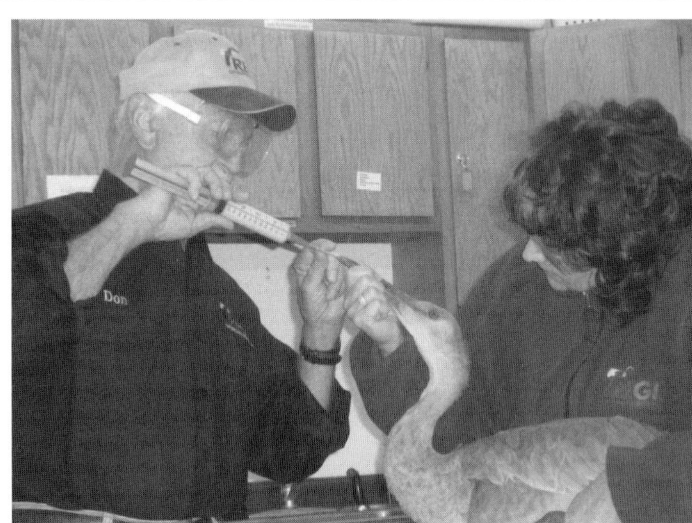

Figure 19.3. Author and husband, Don Gibson, tube-feeding a juvenile crane.

ciated birds need the process of "refeeding," which gives them a small amount of simple food to get their digestive system moving and calories coming in, but not overloading a body that is in fragile condition. Adding vitamins and other supplements may cause the patient to die.

EXPECTED WEIGHT GAIN

Sandhill Crane chicks typically grow rapidly from a tiny 6 in (15 cm) high hatchling to adult height in 56–64 days. By 3 months they should have attained adult weight, including muscle weight if able to fly. Weighing the bird frequently carries risk of habituation and damage to the delicate legs, hence monitoring each chick's attitude and appetite is a better indication of progress. Body weight of North American cranes may also vary considerably by geographic region.

HOUSING

Young Colt

Housing for a stable colt can be a simple cardboard box approximately 36 × 24 × 30 in (90 × 60 × 75 cm) with a reflector lamp. The lamp should be in one corner, safely attached, so it does not come into contact with the chick. One part of the box must be maintained at 95–99°F (35–37°C) for a hatchling. Older colts need less heat, but they require supplemental heat until they begin to feather out or have regained health. Decrease temperature in 5°F increments each week or more rapidly if the youngster shows signs of being too warm, such as moving to the opposite side of the box.

Substrate for the bottom of the box should provide firm leg placement without slipping (Ellis et al. 1996). Pea gravel, soil, or fabric can be used. Sand can be tried but may cause eye irritation with possible complications. If sand is used, the colt should be observed carefully for behaviors such as frequent rubbing of its face or head indicating eye irritation. Do not use wood shavings, kitty litter, or any material other than natural soil that can be ingested by the patient. Intestinal blockage can result. Wet shavings or grasses harbor fungus and may result in respiratory infections. Whatever material is used, keep it dry and clean. Cranes walk in their food and bring feces from the substrate into food.

Water pans for a very young crane should be a stable no-tip variety. Durable nontoxic cake pans make good water dishes for very young birds. Cranes grow quickly, and their needs for drinking receptacles change with growth. Make certain the youngster can actually drink. The long beak necessitates deeper water pans than those provided for most bird species. If the colt can walk into the pan, firm substrate such as pea gravel should line the bottom for secure foot placement.

Once a youngster can eat on its own, provide a raised bowl such as a cat or dog dish that cannot tip. Crane colts will inevitably step into anything they can. If the bowl can be tipped, it will be, and it may

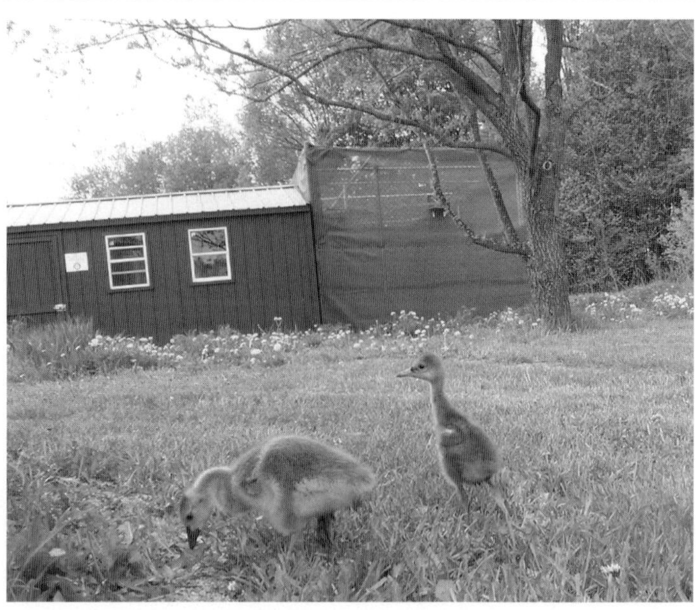

Figure 19.4. Colt with Canada gosling companion.

cause injury. Both water and food should be changed frequently to prevent bacterial growth.

In any housing, take care to check for any unnatural shiny objects, such as staples, bits of wire, or nails. As discussed previously, cranes are attracted to shiny objects, and ingestion can cause death (Ellis et al. 1996). It is good practice to use a commercial magnet attached to a pole to scan the entire ground area in the pen prior to cranes being housed. This is particularly true when using new or recently remodeled construction.

Young cranes need adequate room to exercise. Joints and ligaments grow at a rapid rate along with the rest of the body. A youngster reared without significant exercise will be unable to support itself and cannot survive. If any swelling is noted in the ankle, or the colt sits down on its hocks frequently, begin a more aggressive exercise program immediately. Swimming is an excellent means of exercise for cranes in addition to walking (Ellis et al. 1996). A camouflaged gown, matching the landscape in color and design, can be used when walking or grazing crane chicks to prevent imprinting or habituation. The author uses gowns of fabric that appear to be tall grass, matching the habitat of our exercise area.

It may be helpful during the first few days of confinement to house the colt with a young waterfowl companion, such as a Canada gosling close in age (see Figure 19.4). This may prevent stress and encourage eating. Some rehabilitators have had success using week-old baby chicks as companions. However, be aware of the possibility of infectious diseases that can be transferred in these cases. The urge to siblicide does not generally apply to other species companions of sufficient size to not appear as prey.

A windup alarm clock and mirror with a feather duster may be helpful to provide the youngster with a substitute parent figure. If you use a feather duster, make certain no chemicals or preservatives have been used. Toxic fumes may result when chemically treated feathers become wet. Synthetic feathers may be the safest for this use.

Colts over the Age of 30 Days

A large natural area fenced with 1 × 0.5 in (2.5 × 1 cm) coated wire provides the most secure pens. A rectangular pen is the most versatile shape and allows for the most natural exercise for youngsters. Weasels or rodents can access larger-diameter wire and may kill young cranes. Cranes can also injure themselves by getting their heads or beaks caught in larger-diameter fencing.

Solid or opaque material 4–6 ft (1–1.7 m) high attached to the inside of the fence is recommended. The solid barrier is necessary to prevent self-inflicted injury. Cranes may seriously injure themselves running into fencing when frightened, during escape attempts, or when reacting to sudden movement inside or outside the pen. A solid barrier is also helpful to lessen habituation by providing a visual barrier to human activity.

The natural behavior of young cranes includes jumping into the air simulating the adult mating dance. This behavior is done for various reasons, including greeting other cranes or as a stress reaction as well as the legendary mating ritual. The enclosure should be tall enough to allow this movement without causing injury to the bird or feathers. A 12–15 ft (3–3.5 m) high perimeter fence is generally considered sufficient for all age cranes.

Enclosures should have natural shade areas that allow the birds to be sheltered from heat or other weather extremes. Privacy areas, either a building or area with solid roof and fencing, should be provided.

Cranes love to bathe, and they benefit from a shallow pond with a nonslip bottom. Water must be flowing, changed often, or have a filtration system to prevent bacterial growth and algae. Until the age of 6 weeks, supplemental heat must be used if temperatures drop below 50°F (10°C).

Sandhill colts can fly at 56 days. Anticipate the first flight in advance to prevent premature release.

Predator Guards

Caging is more complex than to keep captive birds from escaping. As important as keeping the birds in, is keeping undesirables out. Birds depend on caregivers to keep them safe while in captive care. Even those that, when healthy, have the ability to protect themselves need protection from physical injury or disease transference during rehabilitation.

Predator guards are a must for all enclosures housing wildlife patients, and cranes are no exception. There are many successful fencing techniques to discourage predators. Multiple methods, including buried fencing, electric fencing, and humane trapping of persistent predators or other techniques may be required on a single enclosure in order to adequately protect wild patients. It will be necessary to customize the protection of your enclosures to the predators and type of soil native to your region. This information will be best obtained from wildlife agencies within your region.

One important approach to protecting your patients from predation is to take steps not to attract predators to your pens. This will involve not leaving excess food around and spilled grain outside the pen. Solid barrier fences will block visual attraction. Trees near or bordering enclosures may allow avian predators to perch and climbing predators to use as a launching platform to access the enclosure. Digging animals such as skunks can be discouraged with buried 1 × 0.5 in (2.5 × 1 cm) galvanized wire hardware cloth. The wire should be buried 2 ft (60 cm) straight into the ground and angled outward from the pen another 2 ft (60 cm). The use of galvanized moderately heavy-gauge wire is wise, because less substantial wire may require costly maintenance or replacement every few years. Some rehabilitators have success using multiple strands of electric fencing on the outside of the perimeter fencing. This technique will discourage climbing predators such as raccoons, mink, and fishers. Several strands of electrical fencing starting a few inches from the ground and going up approximately 5 ft from the ground is generally adequate to discourage most predators. Check with local wildlife officials for a list of predators that frequent your area and for regulations on legal means to control them. Humane trapping using live traps or other methods may be needed for persistent predators. Local regulations will also affect the translocation of live-trapped predators. Under no circumstances should poison be used. The chance of poisoning nontarget species is great, including the cranes being protected. For the most complete protection the enclosure should be covered or enclosed to prevent avian predation, wild visitors that may bring parasites, and premature release.

IMPRINTING VERSUS HABITUATION

Imprinting and habituation are very different behaviors. Imprinting is the permanent alteration of sexual identity and species orientation. Imprinted birds can be imprinted to humans, objects, or even another species when cross-fostering techniques are used. During early efforts to save the Whooping Crane from extinction, Sandhill Cranes were used to cross-foster Whooping Crane colts. The result was the young Whooping Cranes never learned the courtship behavior expected of a Whooping Crane and were rejected by them. Sandhill Cranes also rejected the young Whooping Cranes likely due to vocalization variations (Ritchie et al. 1997; Baughman 2003).

The process of imprinting begins soon after hatch and continues at least through the first month of life.

Recent evidence suggests that imprinting can occur in birds with a long life span and slow maturity postfledge. Imprinting is thought to be associated with food delivery during the first days or weeks of life. It is at this time the young bird incorporates and retains important sounds and behavior clues that become a permanent part of its identity. Imprinting prevents natural reproduction in terms of recognizing or attracting a mate. Vocalization development of imprinted birds may be retarded, with chick calls being retained for a lifetime. Aggression often occurs in imprinted birds, particularly when they reach breeding age. Imprint aggression can be extreme. Imprinted birds should be considered dangerous and unpredictable. Human-imprinted birds can pose a serious danger to humans and should never be released to the wild or used in wildlife petting zoos due to the unpredictable nature of this aggression. If they are maintained in captivity they should be handled by only the most experienced handlers.

Habituated cranes do not respond with appropriate caution or fear to humans, dogs, or situations to which they have been repeatedly exposed without consequence. Release of a habituated bird may create a variety of problematic scenarios, none of which are healthy for the crane. There are methods that can retrain a habituated crane and incorporate it into the wild population. Housing habituated cranes with normal cranes is very important to their success. Restrict contact with humans as soon as possible. Aversion techniques such as noise-making may encourage the habituated bird to reconsider the level of comfort with things that will prove dangerous to it in the wild.

Consider a crane that has been reared with contact with a family dog. Although that dog may not cause the crane harm, other dogs likely will once the bird has been released. The bird must have the correct fear response to survive. Habituation can be reversed, imprinting cannot.

Cranes are curious by nature and both imprint and habituate easily to human caretakers. There are several successful methods by which to raise wild crane colts without imprinting them to humans. Some habituation will be likely; however, prerelease time spent with other cranes will alleviate habituation. It will not alter imprinting:

- Pair each chick with a nonreleasable crane foster parent (see Figure 19.5). This is the least labor-intensive and produces the best results if an appropriate adult is located. The limiting factor is that each adult can generally rear only one colt at a time due to sibling rivalry when others are introduced. Adult cranes may be aggressive to colts. If this is a problem with a bird that is available to use as a foster, install Plexiglas or screening that will allow the adult to be in sight and hearing of the colt. This way it can still serve as a role model.
- Raise colts in visual and auditory contact with other cranes of the same species.
- Play audio recordings of wild cranes with young.
- Rear in a sheltered area with a taxidermied adult crane mounted in the head-down position if a live foster is not available.
- As a last resort if captive fostering is not an option, use costume rearing, with the human caregivers dressed as cranes or covered in material similar in color to the adult crane, and a puppet that mimics the adult crane closely in size, shape, and coloration. Sounds are important to a youngster, so human voices must be kept to a minimum. Recordings of breeding cranes should be used.

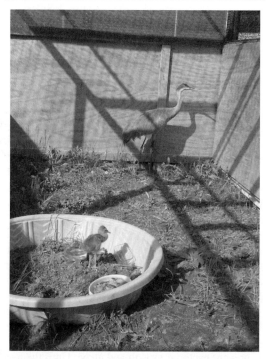

Figure 19.5. Young colt in aviary with foster parent.

PREPARATION FOR WILD RELEASE

By the time colts are several months old at the end of summer (late August in Wisconsin), they should be introduced to each other to form prerelease "family groups." Once colts are this old the urge to siblicide declines, but individuals should be monitored closely and aggressive individuals placed in visual and auditory contact with other colts only. Some colts are sociable and others are not.

RELEASE

Most crane species are migratory and migrate in flocks. During the winter months, even nonmigratory cranes gather in groups (Ellis et al. 1996).

Young cranes must be in excellent body and feather condition and comfortable with their natural diet, hunting techniques, and other cranes before they can be released into the wild. It is beneficial for young cranes to socialize with others prior to release. Captive raised orphans that range freely in a large, fenced, natural area with little human contact are the best prepared for transition into the wild. Cranes can be aggressive to their own species; however, once they become juveniles their tolerance for each other increases. By fall migration, youngsters, if allowed to socialize with others, will have formed a "family group." Releasing these juveniles in their family groups, in early fall, offers an excellent chance at survival.

Wild-reared colts may spend the first winter with their parents (Kaufman 1996). For a lone crane, release timed early in the spring after overwintering may increase survival. A *soft hack* release, where food and shelter continues to be provided after release, is the best release option for these birds. If soft hack is not an option, release in early spring with a migratory flock if possible. The release area should be natural habitat where prey is abundant, and it should not have nesting cranes in the area. Check the nesting dates in your region to assure a safe, unchallenged release.

Rehabilitated adult cranes must have flight exercise prerelease. This is particularly important if the cranes are a migratory species and are released in fall in areas other than wintering destinations.

Release of adults should occur in the area in which they were found if at all possible. Cranes are monogamous and may be aggressive to others in their territory. Adults can also be released into a migratory group. Location of staging areas for migration or migratory groups of birds can be found by maintaining good communication with state biologists, local Audubon or birding clubs, or even landowners in the area.

AUTHOR'S NOTE: A WORD ON THE IMPORTANCE OF NETWORKING

Networking with others is the most valuable tool available to wildlife rehabilitators. Networking is, in part, how we gain information concerning regional nuances of animal behavior and needs. This information can make all the difference in the welfare of your wild patient. Local agency biologists, university researchers, veterinarians, avid birders or landowners—all make great networking partners. It is only through the help and advice of others that wildlife rehabilitation can be done successfully. This is particularly true with sensitive species that have exacting requirements for success. As professional wildlife rehabilitators it is our responsibility to make certain the animal in our care has the best possible chance at recovery and survival after release.

ACKNOWLEDGMENTS

My love and gratitude to my husband for his in-house editing, and my family for their support and patience through years of field work and as thousands of wild birds made their way through our rehabilitation facility and back into the wild. Thanks to Dr. Barry Hartup for his help with this chapter. And finally, to the cranes from whom we continue to learn. Their time with us, spent in rehabilitation, is brief but invaluable in allowing us to better understand their species.

SOURCES FOR PRODUCTS MENTIONED

Zeigler crane feeds: Zeigler Bros, Inc. PO Box 95, Gardners, PA 17324, (800) 841-6800, http://zeiglerfeed.com/bird.htm.

REFERENCES

Altman, R.B., Clubb, S.L., Dorrestein, G.M., and Quesenberry, K.E. 1997. Avian Medicine and Surgery. W.B.Saunders Co., Philadelphia, 1070 pp.

Baughman, M., ed. 2003. Reference Atlas to the Birds of North America. National Geographic, pp. 136–140.

Ellis, D.H., Gee, G.F., and Mirande, C.M., eds. 1996. Cranes: Their Biology, Husbandry and Conservation. U.S. Department of the Interior, National Biological Service, Washington, D.C. and International Crane Foundation, Baraboo, Wisconsin, 308 pp. Available free online at http://www.pwrc.usgs.gov/resshow/gee/cranbook/cranebook.htm

Gibson, M. 1994. Natural history: The square one for wildlife rehabilitation. Journal of Wildlife Rehabilitation 17(1): 3–16.

——. 1996. The ABC's of housing raptors. Journal of Wildlife Rehabilitation 19(3): 23–31.

Harrison, H.H. 1975. Birds' Nests. Peterson Field Guides, Houghton Mifflin Co., pp. 54.

Kaufman, K. 1996. Lives of North American Birds, Kenn, Houghton Mifflin Co., pp. 173–175.

Ritchie, B.W., Harrison, G.J., and Harrison, L.R. 1997. Avian Medicine: Principles and Application. Wingers Publishing, Inc., Lake Worth, Florida, pp. 842–849.

Rogers, L.J., Kaplan, G. 2000. Songs, Roars and Rituals. Harvard University Press, pp. 70–89, 128–140.

Rupley, A. 1997. Manual of Avian Practice. W.B. Saunders Co., Philadelphia, pp. 265–291.

Samour, J. 2000. Avian Medicine. Harcourt Publishers Limited, pp. 102–104.

20
Pigeons and Doves

Martha Kudlacik and Nancy Eilertsen

NATURAL HISTORY

The family Columbidae (order Columbiformes) comprises 313 species worldwide. Nine species of pigeons and doves are native to North America including Band-tailed Pigeon, Mourning Dove (so called because of its mournful coo), Inca Dove, and White-winged Dove. Four species have been introduced, most notably the Rock Dove or Common Pigeon (Leahy 2004), plus three species from genus Streptopelia: the Spotted Dove, Eurasian Collared Dove, and Ringed Turtle Dove. For the purposes of this chapter, the family will be considered as a unit. Specific differences will be noted as necessary.

Columbids range in size from 6–30 in (15–75 cm). They are plump with small heads and short legs and are generally drab-colored, though some iridescent patches are common. The bills are slender with a cere or operculum at the base.

Pigeons and doves feed largely on grains, seeds, and fruit, and are often seen on the ground in groups. Features that set these birds apart from other birds are their ability to drink without raising their heads and the ability to feed their young with a secretion produced in the crop known as "crop milk."

Pair bonds are formed for life; unfortunately, the high mortality rate of these nonaggressive birds means that new pairs are formed yearly. A common city sight is a male pigeon doing a courtship "dance" of rotating in one spot and bobbing near the female. The Rock Dove chooses man-made ledges that somewhat mimic its native cliff nest sites; doves may select hanging baskets, intersecting phone wires, house gutters, or low bushes or trees. Nests are flimsy platforms of sticks, dried grass, and twigs, which usually contain two eggs ranging from white to pale blue. As their eggs are often lost to predators or gravity, these birds will often nest multiple times in a season. Hence, presentation of orphaned and injured chicks may occur nearly any time of the year.

Incubation is 14–19 days, with parents sharing incubation and feeding duties. The altricial young hatch with pink or gray skin covered in long down and eyes closed. Feet are anisodactyl with three toes forward and one toe back. Chicks grow rapidly and attain near-adult weight by 3 weeks of age (see Figure 20.1). The most common predators of columbids include Peregrine Falcon, Cooper's and Sharp-shinned Hawks, and the domestic cat. Native Band-tailed Pigeons may be differentiated from Rock Doves (feral pigeons) by legs that are yellow rather than red or pink, and bills that are yellow with a black tip.

CRITERIA FOR INTERVENTION

Doves are frequent victims of cat attacks, window strikes, and car collisions. Young are often found on the ground after storms when heavy wind or rain causes the flimsy nest to collapse. Loss of parents to predators is very common as the dove is a favorite prey for hawks. Crows and jays will attack chicks as well.

Pigeons are likely to present with pellet gun injuries, poisoning, car collision injuries, and feather damage from bird repellant substances. Their young are often orphaned due to nest removal by exterminators because the nests are frequently found on ledges and rooftops of business buildings.

Because of frequent nest damage, returning the young to the original nest is almost never possible and orphaned doves and pigeons make up a large percentage of birds presented to rehabilitation centers. However, doves are one of the easiest birds

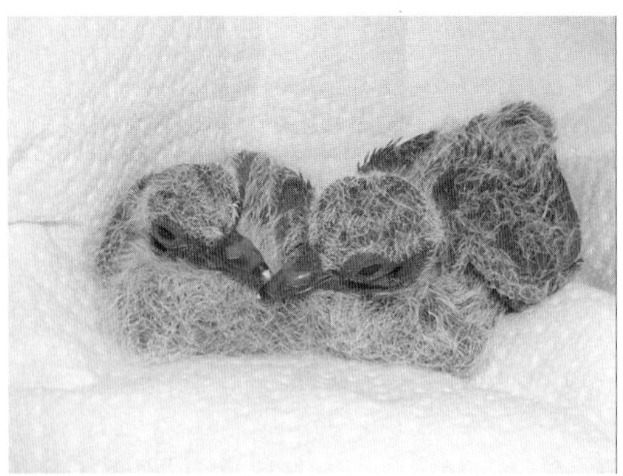

Figure 20.1. Two nestling Mourning Doves.

to re-nest under the right conditions. The parents will follow the baby's cries for food and often a parent dove will try to continue caring for a grounded baby by feeding it and brooding it as much as possible. Grounded babies will not survive on the ground, so if the chick is warm and alert and the parent birds are nearby, the re-nesting should be successful. Use a makeshift nest (small natural fiber basket lined with dried grass or the remains of the old nest) and attach it to a branch in a nearby tree. Make sure that the nest is protected from exposure, especially to afternoon sun. Observe the nest from a distance to make sure the parent birds are caring for the baby. It might take an hour or two for the parents to return.

Rehabilitators often receive banded racing pigeons that are injured or lost. Band numbers on birds registered with the American Racing Pigeon Union are in a series of letters and numbers (e.g., AU 99 ABC 1234) and can be used to locate the bird's owner (see http://www.pigeon.org/lostbirdinfo.htm).

Domestic doves or pigeons either escape or are released at public events. Some of the more popular fancy pigeons are tumblers and rollers and they are often identifiable by features not seen in wild birds: feathered feet, shortened beaks, ruffed neck feathers, very large size (up to 900 g). Proper species identification is necessary to determine whether release or captivity is suitable. Rock Doves are not protected by the Migratory Bird Treaty Act of 1918, so permits are not required to rehabilitate or keep them.

RECORD KEEPING

To comply with Federal regulations, records should be kept per the Minimum Standards for Wildlife Rehabilitation (Miller 2000); state or regional wildlife agencies should be contacted for additional requirements. As a minimum, the following information should be kept: species; date admitted; location found; approximate age; reason admitted for care; medical problems; admission weight; final disposition, including transfer, death, euthanasia, or release date and location. Contact information for the finder is useful in the event that more information is required.

A detailed medical record should also be kept with each bird detailing findings of the initial examination, medications administered, daily body weight, progress of treatment, and behavioral notes. A daily feed and care chart should be maintained throughout the birds' stay in captivity. It is particularly useful to note effect of temperature, hydration, and types of feeding on crop clearance.

Each bird should be assigned a patient number. If multiple birds are being cared for, small plastic numbered leg bands (National Band and Tag Company) available from avian and poultry suppliers should be used to track individual progress.

INITIAL CARE AND STABILIZATION

On arrival, do a quick examination to identify injuries that are life-threatening, which should be addressed immediately. Because columbids are common prey, they frequently present with feather loss, lacerations, crop tears, and bone fractures; these should be assessed for survivability to prevent wasted rehabilitation efforts. However, it can be quite amazing from what level of tissue damage these species can fully recover. Nestling and fledgling birds often arrive cold and dehydrated, so a common rule is to keep the animal "warm, dark, and quiet" for at least 15–20 minutes after arrival before doing a thorough examination. Place fully feathered birds in a covered padded container atop a heating pad on low setting. Be aware that a bird (especially an adult) that seemed lifeless on intake is likely to become active and attempt escape once it reaches normal temperature. Hatchlings should be warmed to higher temperatures (85–90°F, 29–32°C) on arrival and should never feel cold to the touch of a warm human hand.

Birds may also arrive hyperthermic due to extreme heat. Symptoms may include rapid, shallow, or open-mouthed breathing, weakness; instability; and nystagmus (rapid eye movement). This can cause irreversible organ damage and must be reversed by placing the bird in a cool area, offering cool water (if able to drink) or in severe cases, placing in a plastic bag up to the neck and immersing in cold water to quickly lower the temperature. Take care not to induce hypothermia in the process.

After the bird's body temperature has returned to normal, fluids are administered based on hydration status. A well-hydrated bird will be alert and have skin that snaps back easily, bright eyes, moist mucus membranes, and well-formed moist feces. A moderately dehydrated bird will be less than fully alert and have dry, flaky skin, dull eyes, unformed feces, and tacky mucus membranes with stringy saliva. A severely dehydrated bird will be lethargic or unconscious, with skin that "tents" when slightly pinched, and will have sunken eyes, dry or absent feces, and dry mucus membranes.

All birds are assumed to be at least mildly dehydrated on admission. Depending on the cause and percentage of dehydration, reversing this condition can take up to 24 hours. If the bird is alert, it may be rehydrated orally with warm (100°F, 38°C) lactated Ringers or pediatric electrolyte solution administered in either of two ways: by using an eye dropper to run drops of the solution along the beak, or by gavage. If the bird is not swallowing on its own or fully alert, fluids should be given subcutaneously. Give 5% of body weight (50 ml/kg) in fluids orally or subcutaneously. If a chick has a crop filled with food from its parents, hydrate the bird orally until the crop empties before commencing further feedings.

COMMON MEDICAL PROBLEMS AND SOLUTIONS

Trichomonas is a flagellated protozoan parasite transmitted through mouth-to-mouth contact between parent and chick or through the ingestion of contaminated water. Shared water sources are common sources of infection. This parasite does not have a "cyst" stage and is effectively killed by drying or exposure to many disinfecting agents. Oral lesions consisting of cheesy, foul-smelling masses cause gagging, neck stretching, difficulty swallowing or breathing, and regurgitation. When the lesions begin to block the esophagus, the bird is unable to eat and a slimy discharge is produced from the beak. Fledglings with severe cases may present emaciated with obvious masses in the throat. Definitive diagnosis is made by identifying the flagellate on a wet smear taken from the mouth. However, many experienced rehabilitators can make a presumptive diagnosis by gross exam. Treatment with carnidazole (Spartrix, Janssen Pharmaceuticals) at 20–30 mg/kg orally once is generally effective (Carpenter 2005). Metronidazole may also be used. If the esophagus is blocked such that a feeding tube cannot be inserted into the crop, especially if the bird is emaciated and neurologically abnormal, euthanasia should be considered. Special care must be taken to disinfect dishes and feeding implements because Trichomoniasis is contagious to other species of birds and can quickly kill many passerines. It is prudent to house passerines away from columbids for this reason.

There are several other potential crop problems. Failure of the crop to empty normally is termed *crop stasis* or *sour crop* and can occur in doves and pigeons of all ages. Causes include immunosuppression, crop infections, foreign bodies (such as bedding materials); inappropriate food items such as earthworms or dry rice; poor feeding technique (overfeeding, cold or indigestible formula); and, less commonly, vitamin/mineral deficiencies (vitamin B1 and copper). In severe cases, the crop may need to be emptied by a veterinarian and any underlying problems treated. Candida (yeast) infections are a common cause of crop stasis and can be avoided by providing a clean, stress-free environment with proper nutrition and limiting the use of antibiotics. Crop impaction results from feeding large quantities of dehydrated food. Tubing a small amount of warm water and massaging the crop may loosen the mass. If the crop mass fails to move after several hours, consult an avian veterinarian familiar with columbiformes. Crop burns occur when formula is too hot. A visible hole can appear over the crop and the surrounding area may become swollen and discolored with a foul odor and matted feathers. Most often these birds require euthanasia. Crop tears may be caused by predator attacks. These can be successfully sutured by isolating the individual layers of crop and overlying skin.

Pigeons often present with ectoparasites, such as feather lice and flat flies (Hippoboscidae). If these parasites are noted, spray the bird (while covering the head) with a topical antiarthropod spray such as UltraCare Mite and Lice Bird Spray (8 in 1 Pet Products). Provide adequate ventilation during and after application to prevent inhalation of vapors. Pigeons also often have several intestinal parasites, such as capillaria and coccidia. Emaciated chicks or chicks with diarrhea should have fecal testing for parasites. Capillaria may be treated with fenbendazole at 50 mg/kg orally once daily for 3–5 days.

Treatment may need to be repeated in 14 days. Coccidia may be treated with toltrazuril (Baycox, Bayer) at 20–35 mg/kg orally once (Carpenter 2005).

Avian pox is a viral disease that can affect most or all avian species. It presents as wartlike nodules on unfeathered parts of the body such as the feet and beak. Recovered birds are thought to be immune to the particular strain they survived. It is a self-limiting disease with no specific treatment other than supportive care and prevention of secondary bacterial infections. Supportive care includes careful attention to diet, housing and stress. Cleaning the lesions daily with dilute chlorhexidine or povidone iodine solutions may reduce incidence of secondary bacterial infections. Pox is contagious; it can be spread through insect bites and contact with cuts, open wounds, or scabs. It can also be passed indirectly by contact with contaminated perches, dishes, and utensils. To prevent the spread of disease to uninfected birds, keep infected birds separate from healthy birds (i.e., in another room), wash and disinfect housing and feeding items separately, and wash hands carefully before handling or feeding another bird. Always handle pox birds last when feeding, medicating, or examining. The disease can be latent and appear in a bird presented for care due to the illness/injury and stress of captivity.

Splayed legs can occur in developing birds when there is not enough support from the nest during joint development. Incorrect substrate that allows no traction (e.g., newspaper) can cause splaying in older nestlings. At first, the hock appears flattened, widened, and swollen. As the condition worsens, the tendon at the hock may slip, and the tibia and metatarsus become twisted or bowed. In early stages, supplementation with B vitamins may help. If the legs are flexible enough to be positioned correctly, the legs can be hobbled. A curled foot or toe may be caused by a fracture or vitamin B_2 (riboflavin) deficiency. A *snowshoe splint* is often successful in guiding the foot/toes into the anatomically correct position. This can be made from cardboard or thin Styrofoam cut in the normal foot shape. With the foot splayed out in the proper position, tape the foot to the splint. It may take several tries to get it fitted correctly so that it stays on and is comfortable for the bird. Remove the splint to check the foot's progress every other day and replace as needed.

Parent birds occasionally use human hair or fishing line for nest material, which may wrap around a nestling's foot or leg causing necrosis. If the damage is not severe enough to prevent future survival, the material and any necrotic tissue can be removed under anesthesia with magnification to remove tiny constricting fibers, and treated topically and systemically with antibiotics.

Fecal matter may cake around the vent area, causing blockage. This can be caused by dehydration, improper diet, or illness. Gently wash the fecal matter away with warm water on a soft cloth. The bird should defecate once the blockage is gone. Check for signs of dehydration.

One of the most common predators of both young and adult doves is the domestic cat. The cat's oral flora contains *Pasturella multocida*, a gram-negative rod that is highly infective and can kill a bird quickly if not treated. If a bird is admitted with any reported interaction with a cat, it should be put on antibiotics immediately regardless of the confirmed presence of puncture wounds. *Pasturella multocida* is usually susceptible to Clavamox (amoxicillin plus clavulanic acid) at 50–100 mg/kg twice daily for 7–10 days or Keflex (cephalexin) at 100 mg/kg twice daily for 7 days (Carpenter 2005). Continue antibiotic therapy until wounds have completely healed. Lacerations should be cleaned and closed primarily with sutures or surgical glue whenever possible. Scalp lacerations are quite common. Scalp tissue appears to be quite sensitive; if anesthesia is not available, surgical glue is the closure of choice. Hygroscopic dressings such as BioDres (DVM Pharmaceuticals) and Tegaderm (3M) are also useful options when primary closure is not an option.

DIET OR HAND-FEEDING RECIPES

The number and variety of hand-feeding diets being used in rehabilitation and captive breeding are such that they cannot all be covered in a short chapter. The underlying principle is to mimic the natural diet as much as possible. The first 2–3 days of life, columbids are fed crop milk, which is high in protein and fat. About day 3 or 4, small amounts of regurgitated seed are added to the milk; crop milk production ceases about day 7–9 and regurgitated seed is fed throughout the fledging period (Yuhas 2000).

Hatchling Diet

The following is a recommended diet for hatchlings:

- 1 jar Gerber's chicken and gravy human baby food

Table 20.1. Mourning Dove tube-feeding schedule (weights based on California population). Feed hatchling diet to chicks of weights in **bold**. Birds on the hatchling diet may not require as frequent feeding as is listed. Check the crop at the interval and feed when crop empties.

Weight (grams)	Quantity (ml)	Hours between Feeds
10	**1**	**1**
15	**1.5–2**	**1–1.5**
20	**1.5–2.5**	**2**
25	2–3	2
30	2.5–3.5	2
35	4	2
40	5	3
45	5	3
50	6	3
55	6	3
60	6–7	3
Above 65 grams, skip meal if any seed in crop.		
65	6–7	3–1/2
Newly admitted juvenile mourning doves over 70 grams will usually self-feed unless debilitated, emaciated, or otherwise compromised.		
70	8	4
80	8	4
Above 90 grams, do not tube-feed unless bird is debilitated. Healthy juveniles will almost always self-feed at 90 grams.		
90	9	3×/day
95	9–10	3×/day

- 1 Tbsp plain nonfat yogurt
- 1 ml corn oil
- 1/8 tsp Avi-Era avian vitamins (Lafeber)
- 100–150 mg elemental calcium from 250–375 mg calcium carbonate

Nestlings and Older Diet

After the fourth day of life, add 1 tsp of Exact (Kaytee) and a small amount of extra water to the Hatchling Diet recipe. As each day goes by add a little more Exact and less chicken (see Table 20.1). After the seventh day add 2 Tbsp of strained mixed vegetables human baby food. Diet should be the consistency of creamed soup. Allow the mixture to set for 5 minutes before feeding because gases are released during this time, which can cause bloating problems. The mix may also become too thick and more water may need to be added.

A good quality mix of white millet, safflower, or sunflower hearts and fine cracked corn, together with small caliber grit to facilitate grinding in the gizzard, is used for weaning and self-feeding birds. A small amount of grit per bird is adequate. Beware of giving birds large amounts of grit, as they may overeat nonnutritive material. "Pigeon mix" seed blend may be used for pigeons, but occasional fledgling pigeons will prefer smaller seed mixes more typically fed to doves. If a fledgling is difficult to wean or not self-feeding when old enough to do so, try a different seed mix.

FEEDING PROCEDURES

Just as there are a variety of diets, there are also many feeding methods, each with its advocates. Two methods will be described here.

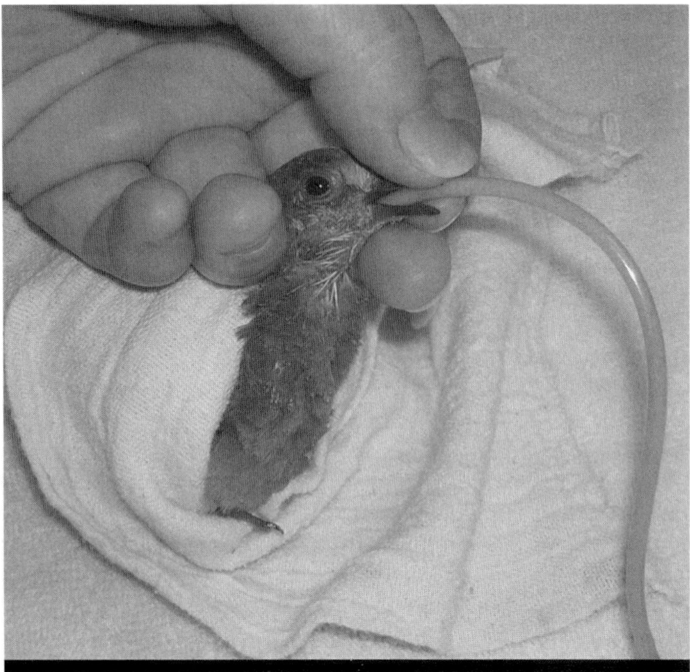

Figure 20.2. Tube-feeding a Mourning Dove. Note that using this hold on the head keeps thumb and forefinger free to manipulate beak and tube during feeding. Keep the neck extended during feeding. Wrapping snugly in towel restrains fractious birds but is not necessary for habituated chicks.

The first method simulates the natural feeding action of young doves, whereby they insert their heads into the parent's mouth and throat and eat from the crop. Warm the formula to 85–90°F (29–32°C) and draw up into a syringe barrel. Secure a cohesive bandage (Vetrap, 3M) over the wide opening and cut a slit to accommodate the bird's beak. While the container is held, allow the bird to feed from the syringe. This is considered a more natural feeding method; however, it can be messy and time-consuming, and it may be difficult to tell how much the chick has consumed. Clean any food on the feathers immediately with warm water to prevent infection or feather damage.

The second method is by gavage, or tubing. This technique takes practice but is invaluable when feeding large numbers of birds. Feeding syringes should be constructed well ahead of time. The length of tubing required is that which reaches past the glottis and into the crop. Most doves require tubing of 3–4 in (7.5–10 cm) (see Figure 20.2); pigeons may need tubing as long as 6 in (15 cm) (see Figure 20.3). Intravenous extension set tubing cut to an appropriate length makes an excellent feeding tube. This tubing is typically 1/8 in (3 mm) in diameter, which is sufficient to pass the diet. Lightly burn the cut end to avoid sharp edges and prevent internal crop lacerations. Steel feeding needles are also used by some rehabilitation centers, but are not necessary for columbiformes because there is no risk of the bird biting off the tubing. Attach the flexible tubing to a feeding syringe and fill with warmed formula. Remove any large air bubbles from the syringe and wipe the outside of the tubing clean of any formula. Moisten the end of the tubing with warm water. Wrap the bird securely in a soft cloth, and extend the neck to straighten the esophagus. Open the beak with a finger and introduce the tubing into the mouth, aiming toward the bird's right side of the back of the mouth. Advance the tube slowly until ruffling of the feathers over the crop is observed. If at any time there is resistance, stop and remove the tube. When the tube is in place, deliver the formula steadily into the crop. Make sure the tube does not slip out from the crop and that there is no formula welling up in the mouth; these can cause the bird to inhale formula (aspiration). If any food pools in the bird's mouth, pull the tube immediately and clear the bird's mouth.

Perform any treatments and give medications before feeding to avoid squeezing a full crop and causing aspiration. Young columbids will beg frantically when they are hungry, and often when they are not. To avoid crop problems, do not feed again until

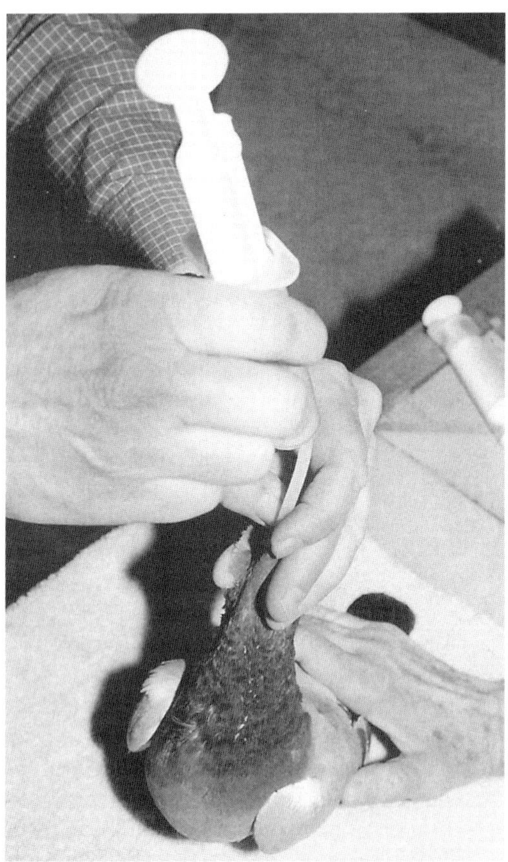

Figure 20.3. Tube-feeding a pigeon. Note neck is fully extended. Tubing must be inserted deep enough to reach the crop.

the crop has emptied. An overstretched crop can sometimes be supported with a "crop bra," a piece of Vetrap wrapped around the bird's chest so the crop does not overhang the keel bone. Crop capacity of most columbids is 10% of body weight (100 ml/kg).

EXPECTED WEIGHT GAIN

Figure 20.4 graphs the expected weight gains for both the Mourning Dove and the Rock Pigeon.

HOUSING

To maintain wildness in orphaned birds, it is crucial to raise them in pairs or small groups of similar ages and sizes. Never combine doves and Rock Pigeons together because the larger, more aggressive pigeons may kill the doves. Band-tailed Pigeon fledglings may display extreme stress responses to handling. If this occurs, wean the bird as soon as possible. A calm, nonaggressive, self-feeding role model to show the bird how to eat seed may be useful, even if the role model is of a different species.

For hatchlings and nestlings, nests can be made with a plastic bowl or berry basket covered with absorbent paper toweling and lined with facial or toilet tissues. White unscented paper products are preferred. All hard surfaces and plastic mesh must be covered with tissue; these species may injure themselves if placed in unlined berry baskets. Taper the lining at the bottom of the nest (making an inverted cone) to prevent leg splaying. Nest size will be dependent on number and size of the birds; the birds should be able to shift comfortably but remain close together. Most dove and pigeon species have two chicks at a time, so keeping birds in pairs is ideal. Most are sociable and will accept higher numbers of chicks in groups without dominance issues. The rim of the nest should be low enough to allow the birds to defecate over the edge. Line the bottom of an aquarium or incubator with paper towels and place the nest inside. Place a small jar with cotton balls and water and thermometer inside. Cover the top of the aquarium with cloth and monitor the temperature (see Figure 1.3). Optimum temperature for unfeathered birds is 85–90°F (29–32°C); humidity should be approximately 50%. Heating pads can be used for heat under a covered aquarium. Check temperature frequently when setting up new housing. Do not use heating pads with automatic shutoffs, and beware of overheating the chicks.

Doves and pigeons grow rapidly. As the birds grow, they require less heat. Monitor for signs of overheating (gasping, dehydration) or chilling (fluffed feathers). When they are fully feathered, they may be moved to the next stage of housing. A laundry basket that has been screened on the inside and lined with paper towels can be used for most birds. Cover the top with fiberglass screening or mesh and secure with clothespins. A perch can be made from a brick or similar-sized piece of wood wrapped in wax paper or plastic wrap, and then in a paper towel, taping the ends underneath. This keeps the perch from absorbing fecal matter. The perch should be high enough to keep the bird's tail from bending on the bottom of the basket; having several perch sizes will allow for growth. There should be enough room to keep feathers from touching the

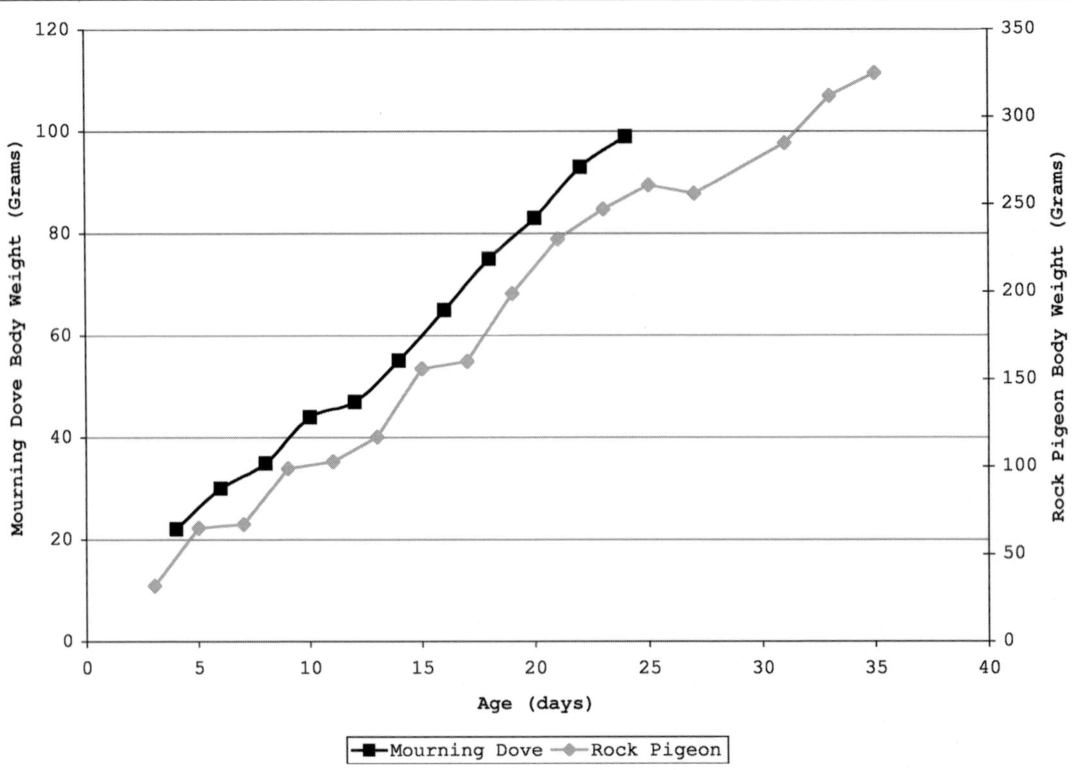

Figure 20.4. Expected weight gains of hand-reared Mourning Doves and Rock Pigeons.

walls of the basket. Clean or change perches daily or as needed to remove fecal material. Stick perches may be used but it is recommended that these be kept very close to the floor; avoid stick perches with highly stressed birds because they may damage their feathers.

Provide a small cardboard box with an opening so the younger birds can group inside for warmth and security. Using branches with leaves will also provide security plus natural enrichment. Natural-looking plastic vegetation from craft stores can also be used. Clean and sanitize with a bleach solution as needed.

Wide flat jar lids of various diameters can be used for seed. Pigeons in particular will learn to eat faster with food presented in this manner rather than in a deep crock-style food dish. Water should be provided in bowls at least as deep as the bird's beaks are long, but not so high that the bird cannot reach. For pigeons, use dishes at least 1–1.5 in (2.5–3.5 cm) deep. Place seed and water dishes at the opposite end of the basket from the perch to prevent contamination from droppings.

Whenever possible, housing may be placed in a protected outside area to provide natural sunlight. Full spectrum lighting can be purchased that provides both UVA and UVB light for times when natural light is not available.

Transfer the bird to an outside flight cage when it has been self-feeding and maintaining weight for 7 days. Never allow the bird to fly free inside a building.

WEANING

Doves and pigeons can learn to pick up seeds at an early age. Housing weaning-age birds with slightly older birds that are self-feeding will usually speed the weaning process. The older bird should be close in size to the younger and not aggressive, especially when dealing with pigeons. Adult pigeons often are not tolerant of younger birds that are not their own and can do serious damage and even kill a youngster. Some young pigeons learn to self-feed as early as 2 weeks of age or as soon as they can walk, and the majority of doves and pigeons are enthusiastic about learning to eat on their own. Monitor weight and check crops carefully and frequently. Although some birds seem to be pecking, they may not be taking in sufficient food for growth.

A crop with seed in it is usually described as feeling like a bean bag. Palpate the crop gently, rolling the skin between two fingers. A bird that is successfully feeding itself will have noticeable seed in the crop. If it does not, monitor droppings and continue to supplement the bird's diet with formula until the crop is consistently full of seed. If added feedings are necessary, make one of the feedings in the late evening to ensure the bird has enough food to last through the night.

When the bird has been self-feeding and continuing to gain weight for at least 7 days inside, it can be transferred to an outside flight cage or aviary. Minimum standards for columbiformes are dimensions of 12 × 8 × 8 ft (3.6 × 2.5 × 2.5 m) (Miller 2000). Plywood, fiberglass, or hardware (wire) cloth can be used for the sides of the cage; sand floors allow sifting and cleaning between occupants. Wire sides and the ceiling should be screened to prevent feather damage caused by panic flights. Doves may "flush" when frightened in the aviary and are at risk of lacerating their scalp on the ceiling.

PREPARATION FOR WILD RELEASE

Pigeons and doves are flock birds and therefore should be released into a flock of their own species. Prior to release, the birds should be completely self-feeding outside for at least 1 week and have heavy muscling on the breast. In addition to acclimation to outdoor conditions, time in the aviary will demonstrate the bird's stamina; do not release if the bird appears winded with short flights. Feathers should be intact, waterproof, and free of parasites. Any bird that does not appear wary of humans or other animals is not suitable for release. If a bird has spent significant time without other birds, introducing additional birds of the same species may help a human-habituated bird to "wild up." Whenever possible, never raise a bird alone if it is intended for wild release. Check weather forecasts and release only when weather will be calm and dry for 2–3 days. Early morning releases enable the bird to adjust to its surroundings before nightfall. If birds are to be released in areas that allow hunting, it is prudent to postpone release until the season is ended.

ACKNOWLEDGMENTS

Martha Kudlacik would like to thank Wildlife Rescue, Inc., in Palo Alto, California for historical data, and to Rebecca Duerr, DVM, and Kathy Tyson, DVM, for developing WRI's Mourning Dove feeding table. Nancy Eilertsen would like to thank Linda Hufford, who has been a continual source of moral support, knowledge, and sanity stabilization for many years.

SOURCES FOR PRODUCTS MENTIONED

Carnidazole (Spartrix): Janssen Animal Health, available in the U.S. through Global Pigeon Supply, 2301 Rowland Ave, Savannah, GA 31404, (800) 562-2295, www.globalpigeon.com.

Toltrazuril (Baycox): Bayer Animal Health, available in the U.S. through Global Pigeon Supply 2301 Rowland Ave, Savannah, GA 31404, (800) 562-2295, www.globalpigeon.com.

Ultracare Mite and Lice Bird Spray: 8 in 1 Pet Products, Hauppauge, NY, (800) 645-5154.

Leg bands: National Band and Tag Company, 721 York St, Newport, KY 41072-0430, (800) 261-TAGS (8247).

Vetrap and Tegaderm: 3M Corporate Headquarters, 3M Center, St. Paul, MN 55144-1000, (888) 364-3577.

BioDres: DVM Pharmaceuticals, Subsidiary of IVAX Corporation, 4400 Biscayne Blvd, Miami, FL 33137, (305) 575-6000.

Kaytee products: 521 Clay St, PO Box 230, Chilton, WI 53014, (800) KAYTEE-1.

Avi-Era Avian Vitamins: Lafeber Company, Cornell, IL 61319, (800) 842-6445, www.lafeber.com.

REFERENCES

Carpenter, J.W., ed. 2005. Exotic Animal Formulary, 3rd Edition. Elsevier Saunders, Philadelphia, pp. 135–344.

Leahy, C.W. 2004. The Birdwatcher's Companion to North American Birdlife. Princeton, New Jersey, Princeton University Press, pp. 223, 638.

Miller, E.A., ed. 2000. Minimum Standards for Wildlife Rehabilitation, 3rd Edition. National Wildlife Rehabilitation Association, St. Cloud, Minnesota, 77 pp.

Yuhas, E.M. 2000. New Approaches to Hand-rearing Mourning Dove (Zenaida macroura) squabs. Proceedings of the 2000 Symposium National Wildlife Rehabilitators Association, St. Cloud, Minnesota, pp. 25–43.

21
Parrots

Brian Speer

NATURAL HISTORY

The order Psittaciformes is represented by 80 genera and approximately 360 different species, and includes all of the parrots. Parrots are popular in aviculture, in public and private zoologic collections, and are exceedingly popular as companion animals throughout the world. There are approximately 77 genera within this order. Only one remaining species, the Thick-billed Parrot (*Rhynchopsitta terrisi*), is a native parrot to the continental United States. Approximately 90 of the species within this order are considered to be endangered, critical, or vulnerable species. The Caribbean and Latin American regions are home to 44 parrot species that are considered endangered, critical, or vulnerable. This represents nearly 31% of their total parrot species. All species in this order are altricial and hatch young that are blind and virtually naked. Altricial young require long periods of feeding before they are strong enough to fledge and leave the nest on their own. All parrots nest in holes and cavities and produce white eggs. Incubation periods for parrots range from 16–28 days, and young fledge in 30 days to 6 months. Many species of parrots continue to feed their young for many months. The social structure of parrot flocks varies among species, and the nature of socialization and learning needed by these fledglings varies considerably. Techniques of hand-rearing and postweaning for psittacine bird species being hand-reared are dependent on the individual species needs and the ultimate desired destination of the chicks. Birds designated for the pet trade will be socialized differently than those that are intended for breeding or reintroduction programs. Some parrot species, such as cockatoos, may be more predisposed to behavioral problems if socially imprinted on their human stewards and not taught ornithologically normal social interactions and daily maintenance behaviors consistent with their species and natural biology. Most often, parrots are hand-reared in captivity as a portion of a planned breeding program, in contrast with the rearing or orphaned wild birds. They may be hand-reared as a result of parental rejection; for a planned commercial or hobby avicultural endeavor; for medical reasons; as a part of a conservation program or, on occasion, as a supportive care measure for wild chicks that have been presented for assistance and support.

THE DEVELOPING EGG AND EMBRYO

The embryo is formed from a fertilized blastoderm or germinal spot on the ovum. Females carry the sex linked chromosome and are responsible for determining the sex of the avian embryo. Each ovum carries either a Z or W chromosome, whereas the male is ZZ, and his spermatozoa can contribute only a Z chromosome. Three layers of membranes protect and segregate the developing embryo. The extra embryonic membranes consist of two layers—the ectoderm and mesoderm, or endoderm and mesoderm, depending on the interface of the individual membrane. As the blastoderm matures, the amnion grows out around the developing embryo to form the sac containing the amniotic fluid. The embryo develops suspended in this amniotic fluid, which is in turn surrounded by the amniotic membrane. The second concentric membrane, the chorion, expands to line the inner shell wall. The third membrane, the allantois, develops from the hindgut of the embryo and also lines the inner shell. The combined membranes are called the chorioallantois, and this highly vascularized surface acts as both respiratory and excretory systems for the embryo. Blood vessels of the chorioallantois carry oxygen from the shell lining to the embryo and bring carbon dioxide back to the surface. This inner shell lining then acts like a large, passive lung. Metabolic wastes are deposited in part as urate crystals within the allantois. The insoluble urates are the most biologically inert form of nitrogenous waste. If birds, like mammals, excreted nitrogenous wastes as ammonia (urea), they could not reproduce by laying eggs: The ammonia within the egg would quickly prove to be toxic to the developing embryo.

THE NURSERY

Within the nursery is housed the highest concentration of avian life in a breeding facility. This population is vulnerable to the greatest amount of loss due to mechanical failure, human error, infectious disease, or combinations of these three factors. These young birds should be considered to be the most environmentally sensitive, immunologically vulnerable to infectious disease, and most time-consuming in their care. The nursery is an individual and separate entity of the closed-aviary conceptually managed facility. All principles of controlled traffic flow, as are applied in the entire aviary, apply directly within the nursery as well. The eggs and offspring located in the closed facility nursery represent the yield of financial investment, hard work, knowledge, and avicultural skills. The potential impact of either primary or secondary infectious disease processes, if not properly managed, can be both emotionally and financially devastating to the aviculturist and the well-being of the neonates within.

Records

At the time of entry to the nursery, all eggs or chicks should have an individual record initiated and assigned. Closed banding is the most popular form of permanent identification, although microchip implantation may also be used in older chicks or some precocial chicks such as the ratite species. Eggs may be identified with pencil coding on their shells. Newly hatched chicks are not banded at that age and care must be taken to maintain the identification of those chicks until they are large enough to be permanently identified.

Specific areas of value for hand-feeding psittacine bird records should potentially include:

- Identification (leg band, microchip number, or other markings)
- Species
- Parentage
- Date of hatch
- Date that hand feeding was initiated
- Formula being used
- Age in days
- Weight (daily or as appropriate to the species)
- Volume fed
- Frequency of feedings
- Comments (e.g., changes in droppings, feeding response, crop transit time, etc.)

Traffic Flow in the Nursery

In those facilities that maintain separate incubation and nursery areas, a general floor plan should be established. This floor plan should allow a specific traffic pattern to be used to promote the efficient use of time and materials and also serve as a passive barrier to waste and contamination. The so-called "spaghetti test" is a helpful aid toward establishing a fluid floor plan. By tracing the daily activity that will occur within a building for normal work tasks, the amount of overlapping and inefficiency of motion will become evident in a floor plan/entire facility analysis. If the projected foot traffic begins to resemble a "spaghetti ball," the relative risk of cross-contamination and motion/time inefficiency should dictate a change in blueprints.

A key consideration throughout the entire incubation and hand-rearing process is traffic flow. Minimized traffic, particularly in the high-risk areas such as the incubation, hatching, and nursery rooms will allow for lower infectious disease risk as well as lower stress to the eggs and chicks. Controlled and minimized introduction of potential infectious pathogens into the nursery is of key importance. Careful thought is strongly recommended regarding how people, the eggs, visitors, etc., are moving into and within the designated incubation area.

ARTIFICIAL INCUBATION

Most psittacine aviculturists will set eggs into the incubator on the same day that the egg is harvested from the nest. In part, this procedure originates from the fact that there is less knowledge about the specific date of lay, and this is a reality to a certain degree with psittacine aviculture. If the eggs have not yet been set by the parents, and incubation has

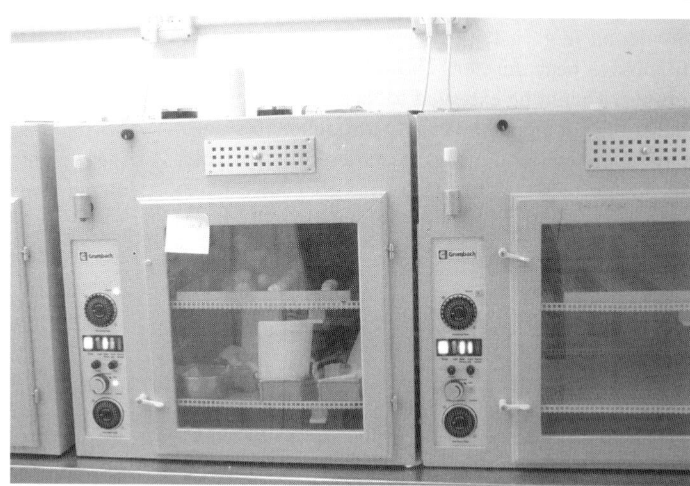

Figure 21.1. The ideal incubator provides the desired incubation parameters while resting in a temperature- and humidity-controlled room.

not started embryogenesis significantly, storage can be utilized to synchronize hatch groups. Once incubation has started either naturally or artificially, the eggs should not be cooled, because there is significant risk of embryonic mortality if the egg is warmed, cooled, and then warmed again. Should the eggs need to be stored, however, this is done ideally at a temperature of approximately 59°F (15°C) until they are set into the incubator. During the initial period of egg-cooling in storage or in the nest, the air cell develops from the separation of the inner and outer shell membranes. Minimal movement or vibrations of the eggs during both storage and incubation is important because handling during storage and the initial aspects of development can predispose to early embryonic mortality as well as malpositions. Washing psittacine eggs prior to incubation is an uncommon procedure. For identification, eggs should be marked with a #2 pencil, not ink or felt.

The three most important variables that need to be simulated in an artificial environment for incubation are temperature, humidity, and turning of the eggs. It is mandatory that all of these three factors be provided consistently by the incubator. Successful artificial incubation requires complete attention to the details of record keeping, care and monitoring of the equipment, egg handling technique, and brooder management. There are numerous testimonials available regarding specific incubator manufacturer choices, settings, and techniques used. However, many of these testimonials are exactly opposite of each other! It is very important for the operator of an incubator to listen to these testimonials and carefully try to separate fact from fiction. The same goes for their attending veterinarian or caregiver.

The ideal incubator serves as a "room within a room" (see Figure 21.1). The incubator should be capable of providing the desired incubation parameters while resting in a temperature- and humidity-controlled room that remains independent of daily climatic conditions and variations. Without this type of control, fluctuations should be expected within the incubator unit, and the potential problems that can result. Construction of this unit should be with nonporous materials for two reasons: improved temperature and humidity control and improved ability to effectively clean and sanitize or sterilize. In some situations, incubation may be successfully accomplished with psittacine eggs using brooding chickens.

Temperature

The temperature settings of the incubator generally control the developmental speed of the embryo. Individual testimonials of temperatures ranging from 99.0–99.3°F (37.2–37.4°C) have proven successful for psittacine egg incubation. The heat of the incubator should be consistent and uniformly distributed within the unit. Consistency and accuracy are attained by regularly monitoring temperature with multiple thermometers. It is not recommended that the operator "trust" any one thermometer or piece of monitoring equipment. Uniform distribution of temperature is accomplished through the air circulation (e.g., a fan) system within the unit, or by passive heat transfer. Those units with low air turnover should be expected to vary in their ability to distribute temperature evenly throughout the unit, particularly when the unit becomes progressively filled with eggs. Those incubators that have been altered for improved ventilation may actually have created an increase in temperature variability through increased heat loss.

Humidity

Relative humidity controls the rate of weight loss of the egg during the incubation process. As the eggs are incubated, weight loss through water evaporation is a normal process. "Wet chicks" is a term used to describe chicks that have demonstrated inadequate weight loss during the incubation process. "Wet" altricial chicks tend not to show the classic edema demonstrated by precocial chicks, but may simply have a weaker-than-normal hatch; increased tendency to splay the legs; and, possibly, immunosuppression-linked problems. "Dry or sticky chicks" generally refers to those birds that have lost excessive weight during the incubation process. Although wet or sticky psittacine chicks do occur, the phenomenon is less visibly apparent than what is commonly described with precocial chick hatches. Weight-loss calculations can have considerable value in the diagnosis and management of suspect humidity issues in the psittacine hatchery.

Turning of the Eggs

The frequency and specific details of rotation of the eggs is perhaps one of the most overlooked aspects of incubation. Most psittacine eggs are incubated lying in a horizontal position. Turning the eggs is mandatory to allow for uniform development of the vascular supply of the embryo throughout the embryonic membranes. Without this web of vessels, the developing embryo will become deprived of adequate oxygen exchange and can potentially die. General poultry recommendations for egg turning are a 90° turn, a minimum of four times per day. The turning mechanism of the incubator should be smooth because rough turning can be associated with an increase in early embryonic mortality. Obviously, mechanical turning as well as hand-turning of eggs potentially can be too rough, resulting in an increase in embryonic mortality. Careful evaluation of the turning processes of an incubation system is strongly advised for this reason.

Weight Loss Formula

Egg weight losses may be calculated using the following steps:

1. Calculate the grams lost per day of incubation.

$$\frac{\mathit{Starting\ Weight} - \mathit{Current\ Weight}}{\mathit{Days\ Incubated}} = \mathit{grams\ lost\ per\ day\ of\ incubation}$$

Example:

$$\frac{26.00\,gm - 24.05\,gm}{14\,days} = \frac{1.95\,gm}{14\,days} = 0.14\,gm/day$$

2. Calculate anticipated weight loss for the total incubation period for the species.
   Grams lost/day × 28 days incubation period
   Example:
   0.14 g/day × 28 days incubation period = 3.9 g
3. Calculate anticipated weight loss as a percentage of the original weight.

$$\frac{\mathit{Anticipated\ weight\ loss}}{\mathit{Starting\ weight}} \times 100 = \%\ \mathit{weight\ loss}$$

Example:

$$\frac{3.9\,gm}{26\,gm} \times 100 = 15\%\ \mathit{weight\ loss}$$

Most avian species' eggs lose in the range of 15% (13–16%) of their original weight during the incubation process, and this is also true for the order Psittaciformes. This weight loss is regular and consistent throughout the entire period, and as a result, these calculations allow for predictability of the ultimate percentage loss to be anticipated. This linear weight loss relationship is a grossly underutilized monitoring tool in psittacine egg artificial incubation at present time. As a result, weight loss deficits are often not as easily recognized or prevented.

HATCHING

Throughout the development of the embryo, the egg steadily loses water by transpiration through the

Table 21.1. Malposition classification and descriptions (domestic poultry criteria).

Malposition I	Head is between the thighs (position assumed immediately prior to hatching position).
Malposition II	Head is in the small end of the egg. Approximately 50% of the embryos can hatch from this position if they do not suffocate. Manual intervention may help reduce mortality rates associated with this position.
Malposition III	Head is toward or under the left wing instead of the right wing. This is a lethal position because the embryo tends to rotate counterclockwise to hatch, which it cannot do in this position.
Malposition IV	The embryo is rotated with the beak away from the air cell. It is impossible to successfully hatch from this position, although the chick will often pip the shell and frequently pip a vessel and cause hemorrhage from the chorioallantoic vessels.
Malposition V	Chicks have their feet over their head. This position makes rotation very difficult and the embryo usually fails to hatch. This is an uncommon malposition in psittacine birds.
Malposition VI	The beak is above the right wing. This is a nonlethal variant of normal positioning.

chorioallantoic membrane. Because of the combination of water loss and the loss of yolk fats metabolized during development, the egg is much lighter at hatching than when it was laid. The eggshell, too, is thinner than when it was laid because the chick has absorbed much of the calcium from the inner shell lining. In the imminent hatching period, the chick absorbs the remainder of the yolk sac into the abdominal cavity and also begins to swallow any remaining amniotic fluid.

Two specialized structures found only in hatchlings aid the chick in its struggle to break open the shell. A small, sharp *egg tooth* develops on the dorsal tip of the rhinotheca and is used to *pip* and cut out of the shell. A substantial enlargement of the complexus muscle (pipping muscle) in the proximal dorsal cervical region helps brace the neck and cushion the head as the chick forces the egg tooth through the shell. After hatching, most of the fluid within the complexus muscle is reabsorbed, and this muscle continues to function as an extender of the head in most adult birds. The egg tooth is lost in the first few weeks following hatching.

Immediately prior to the start of the hatching process, the air cell expands to encompass approximately 20–30% of the total internal egg volume. At the same time, the embryo shifts from a position with its head between its legs to raise its head up and underneath the right wing. These changes can be noted by candling, and are termed the *drawdown*. At the start of the hatching process, the beak of the embryo penetrates the inner shell membrane where it forms the inner wall of the air cell, and the lungs become functional by inspiring air from the air cell. An increase in plasma CO_2 is associated with the trigger for the *internal pipping* process. The *external pip* occurs when the chick cracks or cuts the outer shell membrane and shell. Again, rising CO2 in the air cell chamber serves as the trigger for the spastic neck and associated muscle contractions involved in the hatching process. In the domestic fowl, a period of about 20 hours elapses between pipping and hatching. Most parrot species normally hatch within a 24-hour period from internal pip to completed hatch.

Problems with the Hatch

The above table (see Table 21.1) is provided to furnish basic information that will allow for troubleshooting problem hatches. Keep in mind that the management actions recommended are based on overall incidences of problems, rather than isolated incidents. Recommendations to change nursery protocols based on isolated incidents could easily lead to more significant problems.

BROODERS

The function of a brooder is to provide an artificial environment for feeding and maintaining chicks immediately following hatching. Consistent and

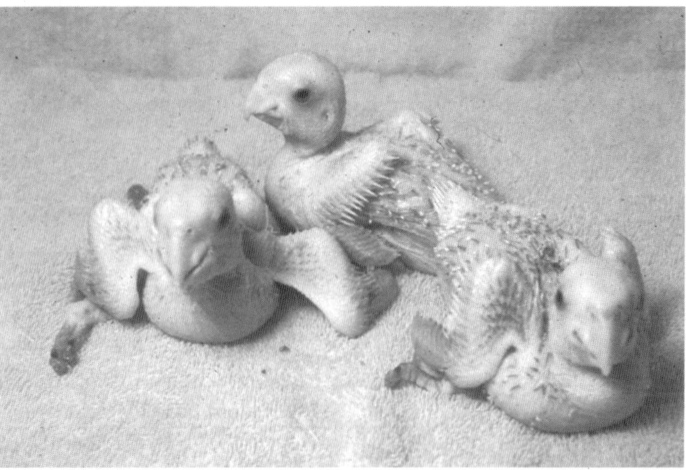

Figure 21.2. These young Golden Conures (*Aratinga guarouba*) still require considerable environmental humidity and warmth due to their naked and exposed skin, with vulnerability to heat and moisture loss.

accurate temperature and humidity control is again a key requirement for brooders, as it was with incubation. The design of these units should incorporate reliable and uniform control of temperature and humidity. In general, an air circulation system with a low rate of air exchange or a passive air flow/heat delivery system is believed to be desirable to maintain an optimal brooder environment for newly hatched psittacine chicks. A brooder that is too hot may result in dehydration, delayed gastrointestinal (GI) transit times, stunting, and other problems. Likewise, a brooder that is too cold may also cause delayed GI transit problems. Inadequate humidity is a common contributor to dehydration issues as well. As a general rule of thumb, humidity is maintained as high as possible with newly hatched chicks, and is decreased proportionately to common room conditions as natal down and contour feathers emerge, covering their naked skin (see Figure 21.2). Brooders should be nonporous, and easy to clean and disinfect. Substrate material that the chicks are maintained on should be clean. Extremely young chicks are frequently reared on toweling or fine shavings. As these chicks become older, wood shavings are used even more frequently. The ability to provide stable footing for the growing chick is an important consideration in substrate selection, and judicious concern for possible consumption of shavings by these chicks is needed. Nest materials that should be avoided include cedar shavings, soil, peat, and leaves, due to their potential to irritate the respiratory tract and to be contaminated with Aspergillus spores.

DIETS

There are a number of formulated diets designed for hand- rearing psittacine chicks. These products are easily obtained from commercial bird retail stores, or directly through online ordering sources. Commercially manufactured hand-feeding products are utilized much more frequently in psittacine aviculture than home-made diets and recipes at the present time. Commercial formulas range from 16–26% protein, 3–16% fat, and 2–10% fiber. These hand-feeding diets are mixed freshly at the time of each feeding, using water heated to a temperature of 103–105°F (40–41°C), according to manufacturer's recommendations. With day-1 newly hatched psittacine chicks, often there will be a diluted formula offered. This is empirically done. Starting with the manufacturer's recommendations, the formula may be mixed slightly thinner for the newly hatched chicks, but care needs to be taken as much as possible not to dilute the caloric density of the formula.

Excessively thin or dilute diets predispose to caloric deprivation, and excessively thick diets may predispose to delayed gastrointestinal transit time, dehydration, and secondary problems (see Table 21.2). Both of these extremes may result in stunting or delayed growth in the chicks.

Table 21.2. Common pediatric problems.

Clinical Presentation	Differential Diagnostic Considerations
Crop stasis	Dehydration Formula too hot Formula too cold Hypomotility related to stunting Malnutrition Primary or secondary infectious disease Sour crop as a secondary complication Brooder temperature too high Brooder temperature too low Brooder humidity too low Exogenous stressors (light, etc.) Foreign body obstruction of GI tract Normal variation in motility during 24-hr period Toxicoses
Regurgitation	Crop stasis Normal behavior for species and age Inadequate feeding practices Imbalanced brooder environment
Sinusitis	Inadequate brooder air quality Foreign objects in nares Primary or secondary infectious disease Inadequate feeding protocols
Splay-leg (see Figure 21.5)	Inadequate brooder substrate Wet chicks Weak chicks Inattentive nursery management
Tibiotarsal rotation	Splay-leg Traumatic injury Inattentive nursery management Malnutrition/metabolic bone disease
Anteroflexed P1/P4	Stunting Inappropriate brooder substrate Malnutrition Inattentive nursery management
Constricted toe syndrome	Specific etiology not known Genetics? Humidity? Bacterial dermatitis/hypersensitivity?
Diarrhea	Normal for age and species Bacterial imbalance/infection of GIT Enteritis Primary or secondary infections Overmedication Malnutrition Gut hypermotility Gut hypomotility Pansystemic disease Endoparasitism Polyuria?

Table 21.2. *Continued*

Clinical Presentation	Differential Diagnostic Considerations
Stunting	Malnutrition Inadequate feeding volume/day Inadequate caloric intake/day Crop stasis Inattentive nursery management Excessive brooder temperature Inadequate brooder temperature Inexperienced hand feeders Inadequate adult breeder parenting Large interval between first/last hatch Aviary disturbances Infectious parental disease Infectious disease (primary or secondary)

Some common commercial hand-feeding diet manufacturers in the United States are listed in the section "Sources for Products Mentioned" at the end of this chapter.

HAND-FEEDING TECHNIQUE

Most psittacine chicks will have a variable degree of a feeding reflex, or "pumping" reflex. The beak does not need to be held during hand-feeding in most circumstances, and there actually is risk of trauma to the immature beak tissues if inadvertent pressure or bruising occurs. The specific hand-feeding techniques that are used are oriented to support the head and neck of the bird, to solicit a feeding reflex, and to deliver formula at a rate consistent with the swallowing rate of the chick. Despite their age and difference in syringe sizes, each chick is fed basically the same way. The left hand is used to guide the head upward to facilitate easier flow of the food into the oral cavity. The beak does not need to be handled at all, or very little during hand-feeding. The hand-feeder's job is to support (not restrain) the head and neck, which is amazingly strong yet wobbly. It is important to support the chick and feeding syringe, concurrently, in a manner that prevents bruising or trauma to the pharyngeal tissues or the rictal phalanges of the developing upper mandible (see Figure 21.3). These types of traumatic or bruising injuries are a likely origin of asymmetrical beak growth, resulting in scissors beak deformities or other problems.

A common, but now recognized as outdated, requirement for hand-feeding young parrots was to allow the crop to completely empty between feedings. In reality, this predisposes to hunger, stress, decreased caloric intake for the chicks, and stunting. Parent-fed psittacine chicks are known to vocalize for parent attention and feeding prior to complete emptying of their crops. The more current hand-feeding techniques attempt to simulate parent feeding, where the crop is not allowed to empty between feedings. The volume of hand-feeding formula to be fed is dependent primarily on the crop capacity of the chick. A general rule is to feed approximately 10% of the chick's body weight with each feeding. Typically, the crop is filled to, or close to, the point of seeing formula beginning to come up the upper cervical esophagus. The cervical esophagus starts at the caudal aspect of the oral cavity and ends at the crop, down the right side of the neck. There is no specific requirement for feeding on the right side of the bird's mouth, contrary to common and popularly held belief. The frequency of hand-feeding also varies considerably between species and age, but is dictated primarily by chick crop motility and growth rates.

EXPECTED WEIGHT GAIN

It is recommendable to monitor chick weights during hand-feeding, and to compare with established normal developmental parameters for the species as a point of reference, particularly if the hand-feeder

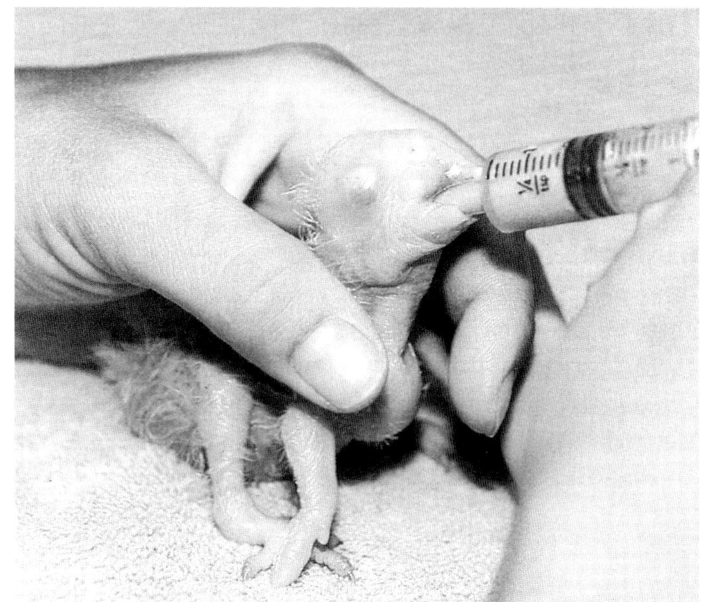

Figure 21.3. Most psittacine chicks will have a variable degree of a feeding reflex, or *pumping reflex.* This chick is rapidly pumping up and down, while the head is being gently supported by the hand-feeder. A general rule is to feed approximately 10% of the chick's body weight with each feeding.

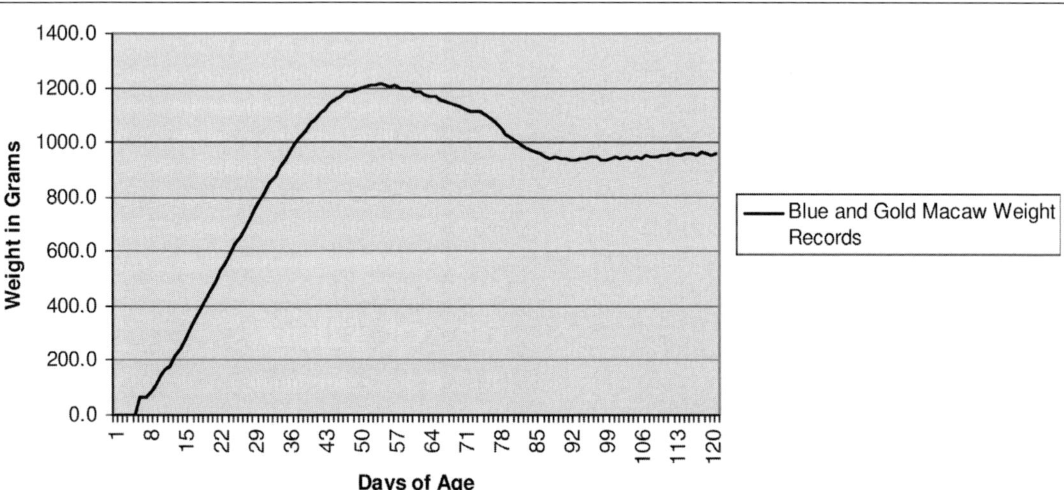

Figure 21.4. Average weight gain graph for Blue and Gold Macaw chicks (*source:* Abramson et al. 1995).

is less experienced with a particular species (see Figure 21.4). One manner of utilizing a set of normal weight gain data in monitoring chick growth is itemized in the following equation:

$$\frac{\textit{chick weight at X days of age}}{\textit{"Normal"}} \times 100 = \textit{Percentage of "normal" weight for X days of age}$$

By not only monitoring the daily gain in grams for the hand-fed chicks, but also monitoring the chick's relative percentage of normal, the hand-feeder is better positioned to detect developmental anomalies earlier. As a result, there will be more time to make management changes as needed to guide the chick's development towards normal.

HAND-FEEDING EQUIPMENT

Various sized luer-lock and catheter tip syringes (3 ml–60 ml) are commonly used for hand-feeding psittacine chicks. Red rubber catheters or other soft rubber tubing may be used for tube or gavage feeding if needed. Manufactured metal gavage tubes may be used for feeding psittacine chicks in some circumstances. These items need to be carefully cleaned and disinfected after use, to minimize transfer of infectious disease agents.

CHICK HOUSING WITHIN THE BROODER ENVIRONMENT

Many day-1 hatch chicks are initially placed individually in small cups or other plastic containers with paper towel substrates beneath them. This type of housing allows for individual attention to the chicks, and particular attention toward sanitation and cleanliness. Not all hatched chicks are placed in these types of environments, however. Some are maintained as a functional group or clutch together, and some chicks may be more comfortable if they are on shavings or other more natural substrates. Most parrot species are nest-cavity breeders, and their chicks generally are not naturally exposed to much sunlight during the early aspects of their lives. As a result, it is recommended to maintain the lighting of the nursery and brooder environment comparatively dim until the chicks become more developed and active. In addition, providing a darkened recess into which a chick can retreat is consistent with their natural biology, and recommendable.

WEANING AND FLEDGING

The age of fledging is variable among the many species of psittacine birds. In general, the larger the species of parrot, the longer the weaning and fledging period will be. As the chicks develop, their inquisitiveness, contour and flight feathers, and motor skills develop. During this time period, these birds should be offered a variety of foodstuffs to learn to eat. In general, the maintenance-type diet that is planned for these birds is the primary "weaning" foods offered. During this weaning period, birds are allowed to become more active and to socialize and interact with others of their same species, or even individuals of other species when appropriate. During this time, they are allowed to develop their foraging skills, to learn different food items, and to still have a comfortable nesting environment to retreat to. Common types of table foods that may be offered and taught to the bird include most vegetables, pastas, and fruits. These are not intended to become a daily mainstay, but can become acceptable as treats, special foraging-type items, etc., after fledging and weaning. Hand-feeding formula is still offered to these birds, but should they reject those feedings, no further efforts to forcibly feed them should be made. Ultimately, chicks will take less and less hand-feeding formula and ultimately reject hand-feeding entirely. Some of the time-honored but antiquated force-weaning techniques that are well described in the common literature can be quite stressful to parrot chicks, and can result in secondary problems. Furthermore, these force-weaning techniques often downplay the importance of socialization, physical activity, and exploration aspects of the weaning and fledging period for these birds. There is a normal drop in body weight during the fledging and weaning period for most parrots, with common estimates being up to 15% weight drop. Typically, this weight is regained over the next 6 months to 1 year of life.

PEDIATRIC PROBLEMS

Most of the current literature relating to psittacine pediatrics describes ailments and their subsequent treatment (see Figure 21.5). There is usually a mention of "secondary disease" and primary managerial problems, but less emphasis on the real roots of the problem or how to "think out" a problem starting with the diagnosis. With this in mind, the following information is provided to stimulate thought as to the underlying causes (hence, true cure potential) for several pediatric ailments. Keep in mind that psittacine pediatric medicine, in many ways, is an aspect of avicultural or flock medicine. The individual bird diagnosis leads toward potentially other thoughts and actions from the astute veterinary clinician.

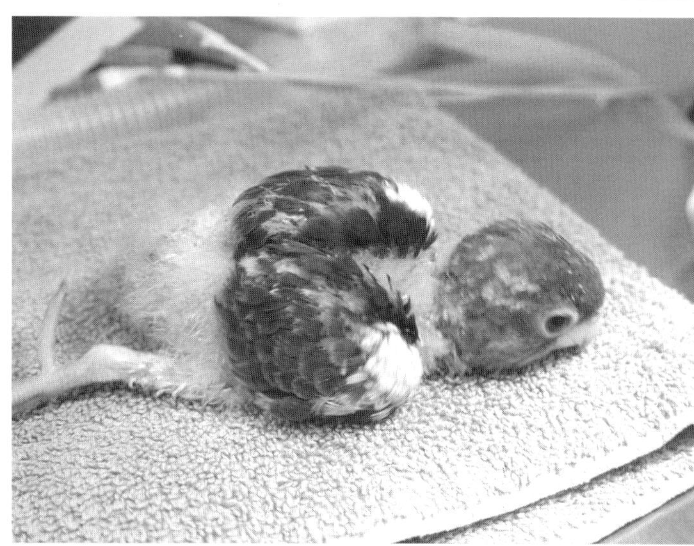

Figure 21.5. This young Meyers Parrot chick (*Poicephalus meyeri*) suffered from a combination of a splay-leg condition, tibiotarsal rotation, stunting, delayed crop motility, and metabolic bone disease. Significant orthopedic abnormalities were surgically corrected, ultimately allowing the bird to function and appear with close-to-normal posture.

Table 21.2 illustrates some of the considerations that would be appropriate for some common pediatric problems that could be encountered in the psittacine nursery.

ACKNOWLEDGMENTS

Thanks to my wife, Denise, and my family for tolerating and supporting my "bird habit" over all of these years, and special thanks to Joanne Abramson for sharing her photos and input from our book, *The Large Macaws*.

SOURCES FOR PRODUCTS

Zupreem, 10504 W. 79th St. Shawnee, KS 66214, (800) 345-4767, www.zupreem.com.

Roudybush, Box 908, Templeton, CA 93465-0908, (800) 326-1726, www.roudybush.com.

Lafeber Company, 24981 North East Road, Cornell, IL 61319, (800) 842-6445, www.lafeber.com.

Pretty Bird International, Inc., PO Box 177, Stacy, MN 55079, (800) 356-5020, www.prettypets.com.

Kaytee, 292 E. Grand, Chilton, WI 53014, (800) 669-9580, www.kaytee.com.

Hagen, 50 Hampden Rd, Mansfield, MA 02048, (800) 225-2700, www.hagen.com.

Harrison's Bird Diets, 7108 Crossroads Blvd, Suite 325, Brentwood, TN 37027, (800) 346-0269, www.harrisonsbirdfoods.com.

REFERENCES

Abramson, J. 1995. Captive breeding and conservation. In Abramson, J., Speer, B.L., and Thomsen, J.B., The Large Macaws. Raintree Publications, Fort Bragg.

Abramson, J., Speer, B.L., and Thomsen, J.B. 1995. The Large Macaws. Raintree Publications, Fort Bragg.

Balinsky, B.I. 1975. An Introduction to Embryology. W.B. Saunders, Philadelphia.

Forshaw, J.M. 1973. Parrots of the World. Lansdowne Press, Melbourne.

Johnson, A.L. 1986. Reproduction in the Female. In Sturkie, P.D., Avian Physiology. Springer-Verlag, New York, pp. 403–431.

Juniper, T. and Parr, M.L. 1998. Parrots; A Guide to Parrots of the World. Yale University Press, Hong Kong.

King, A.S. and McLelland, J. 1984a. Birds: Their Structure and Function. Bailliere Tindall, Philadelphia.

———. 1984b. Female Reproductive System. In King, A.S. and McLelland, J., Birds: Their Structure and Function. Bailliere Tindall, Philadelphia, pp. 145–165.

Low, R. 1986. Parrots, Their Care and Breeding. Blandford Press, Dorset.

———. 1998. Hancock House Encyclopedia of the Lories. Hancock House, Blaine.

Monroe, B.L. and Sibley, C.G. 1993. A World Checklist of Birds. Yale University Press, New Haven.

Perrins, C.M. and Middleton, A.L.A. 1985. The Encyclopedia of Birds. Facts on File, Inc., New York.

Sibley, D.A., Dunning, J.B., Elphick, C. 2001. The Sibley Guide to Bird Life and Behavior. Chanticleer Press, New York.

Speer, B.L. 1991. Avicultural Medical Management. In Rosskopf W.J. and Woerpel R.W., eds., Veterinary Clinics of North America, Small Animal Practice. W.B. Saunders, Philadelphia, pp. 1393–1404.

22
Lorikeets

Robyn Arnold

NATURAL HISTORY

There are 53 species of lorikeets belonging to the family Loriidae. Lories and lorikeets are small- to medium-sized "brush-tongued" parrots found in the Pacific region. Lories are unique among the parrots due to the structure of their tongues. The ends of their tongues have long papillae, which allow the lories to collect pollen and nectar. Unlike most parrots they lack a muscular gizzard, therefore requiring a soft diet. Most lorikeets are not sexually dimorphic and can be identified only by using DNA sexing, feather sexing, or surgical sexing techniques.

Captive species have bred successfully when offered the appropriate space, proper diet, and nestboxes. Sexual maturity occurs between 1 and 4 years. In the wild they breed only when trees are in blossom because they cannot leave the nest for long periods of time to feed, and are thus restricted to a small area in the vicinity of the nest. Some species can breed at any time of the year with an optimal climate. They nest in tree cavities and hatch altricial young that are blind and nearly featherless. Young are fed regurgitated adult diet of pollen and nectar.

Most species will produce a clutch of two eggs. Incubation lasts 22–27 days. The eggs may be carefully candled after a minimum of 10 days to check fertility (see Chapter 3).

The second egg may not hatch for more than 48 hours after the first chick has hatched. After 72 hours, carefully candle the egg. If there is no sign of life, the remaining egg is pulled so as not to infect the surviving chick.

CRITERIA FOR INTERVENTION

One of the most common reasons for intervention is due to a frequent problem where captive lorikeet pairs overpreen or occasionally severely pluck the feathers from their young. In these instances, the chicks are removed from the pair between 20–25 days, at about the time the feathers are emerging. One consideration for this overpreening behavior is that captive lorikeets often have smaller environments and do not need to forage for food, causing them to spend too much time in the nestbox. Enrichment such as browse; small parrot toys; food items like whole apples or grapes; or alternative items that may be shredded, such as paper or bark, may help mitigate this problem.

Lorikeets going into a public feeding aviary are often hand-reared to acclimate them to people. Generally, if the parents take good care of the chicks, hand-rearing could commence at about 5 weeks of age.

Other reasons for intervention are abandonment of the chicks, or parents and/or chicks that are ill. Improper care by the parents may require intervention and occurs more frequently during colder months.

Pulling chicks for short periods of time to feed, weigh, or warm them or to clean the nestbox generally does not pose any serious problems. The amount of time chicks are pulled from their nestbox should be kept to a minimum for each procedure. After chicks are returned to the nestbox, observe to ensure that parents are attentive and tending to the chicks properly.

MONITORING NEW HATCHLINGS

Usually a clutch consists of two eggs. The eggs usually hatch more than 24 hours apart; therefore, it is common for the first chick to be 5 or more g heavier than the second throughout the rearing process, and occasionally when there is a greater time difference between the hatching of the eggs, there may be as much as a 10 g difference in weight. The chicks will maintain their difference in weight until they approach their adult size. Chicks are visually inspected two to three times per day to ensure they are being fed by the parents. If everything is going well, the chicks may be removed every 2–3 days for acquiring weights and to change the nestbox substrate. When moving the chicks, put them into a small bowl or box filled with dust-free shavings or a smooth-textured cloth and cover with a towel or small blanket to keep them warm. As they grow, the nestbox may need to be changed more frequently. Watch carefully that parents attend to them after returning them to the box.

If parents spend too much time out of the nestbox during the colder months, the chicks will perish quickly. Note that double and triple brooding is common when chicks are pulled for hand-rearing. This is frequently seen in Trichoglossus species, and careful planning should take place to help avoid having chicks hatch in the colder months. Using dummy eggs to add time between clutches often helps but does not always work. Some pairs of birds will reject artificial or "dummy" eggs and will accept only their own eggs that have been pinned, and the contents removed. One trick to add strength to the pinned eggs is to remove all of the contents, fill them with water, and seal the hole with a tiny drop of candle wax. These eggs may decompose over time and should be checked every few days. Check the nestbox frequently because some pairs will lay their eggs on top of the dummy eggs.

If a clutch hatches during the colder months, use tarps or blankets to help insulate the enclosure as well as heat sources such as heat lamps or radiant heat panels on the inside of the enclosure. Heat lamps must be covered with protective caging to prevent contact with the birds, and they should be secured to the structure to be safe. Be prepared to hand-rear the chicks as early as a few days of age.

RECORD KEEPING

Detailed record keeping is important. Records will be useful information for future clutches or simply for communication with others who may be involved with a hand-rearing project. Once chicks have been pulled, a daily chart documenting their weights and the times they were fed will help determine proper times between feeding and will that ensure weight gain is proper. Chicks should be weighed before the first morning feed when the crop is empty. Charts should also include brooder temperatures, food temperatures, chick activity, and willingness to eat. Everything observed should be logged at each feeding. Abnormalities such as changes in fecal consistency or amount should also be noted.

INITIAL CARE

Before the chicks are pulled ensure that the brooder is set up and is maintaining at the proper temperature, generally between 80–90°F (26.7–32.2°C). Attempt to have the brooder at the same temperature as the nestbox. Nestbox temperatures will vary, and it is best to obtain the temperature reading of the nestbox by placing a thermometer in it when the parents are not present.

After placing the chicks in the brooder observe them to determine whether they are comfortable. A chick that is too warm may pant or spread out its wings to cool off. A chick that is too cold may shiver or shake. Temperatures may need to be adjusted. This can be accomplished by adjusting the thermostat (if you have one) or by adjusting a blanket or towel over the top of the container housing the chick. Do not cover the brooder completely; ensure that there is proper air flow. Some commercial brooders will also come with plexiglass or a wood top. These may be replaced with a blanket or towel if needed. Close monitoring for the first 2–3 days is important. Keep the area quiet where the chicks are housed so they may adjust to their new surroundings. The first day they are generally quiet, but that will change. Within a day or two the chicks will start vocalizing at feeding time as well as throughout the day and night. They may vocalize for several hours after feeding. This is normal.

The first feeding of chicks that have been pulled at 20–25 days of age is challenging for the birds and handlers alike. You will need to teach the neonates how to eat formula from a bent spoon (see Figure 22.1). The temperature of the formula is crucial and should be very warm but not hot enough to burn. Test on your wrist before giving the formula to the bird. Gently hold the bird's head between your thumb and forefinger. Guide the bird's head toward the bent spoon and slowly tilt the spoon until formula flows towards the beak. Once a drop or two enters the mouth, if it is the right temperature, the chick will willingly take the entire spoonful, which is about 0.5 ml. If the temperature is too cool they will not accept the formula and will show no interest in eating. For Trichoglossis, the chicks usually will swallow about 1 ml during the first feed. Monitor the level of fullness by watching the back of the neck. The crop

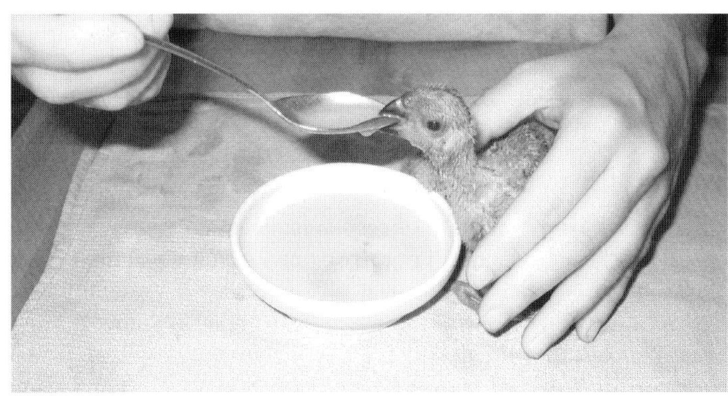

Figure 22.1. Feeding 23- and 24-day-old Rainbow Lorikeet chicks with bent spoon.

may be visualized through the thin skin extending around the back of the neck. The nectar formula may be seen filling the crop and extending into the back of the neck area. Stop feeding the chick when the formula begins filling this area. The formula may need to be reheated more than once during this time, especially if multiple chicks are being fed. Most chicks will take spoon after spoon with very little time in between. Always allow the bird to swallow completely before continuing with a new spoonful of formula. Be cautious moving the chicks back to the brooder and do not put any pressure on their crop or they will regurgitate their feed.

COMMON MEDICAL PROBLEMS

Hypothermia during the colder months is one of the more common problems seen. There are no medical problems that are specific to lorikeets; however, overpreening the chicks by the parents could lead to more serious problems. See Chapter 21 for other medical problems affecting psittacines in general.

DIET RECIPES

Chicks should be fed a nectar/baby bird feeding formula mixture (Kaytee exact) using distilled or boiled water initially. Regardless of the age they are pulled from the nest, chicks are introduced to the formula by first offering them 1/2 Tbsp (7.4 ml dry volume) nectar powder (use only the powdered product that is normally combined with water before feeding), 1 tsp (5 ml dry volume) baby parrot feeding formula (Kaytee exact), and 1/4 C (59 ml) distilled water. This recipe is appropriate for feeding two chicks.

As the chicks grow, the nectar formula is increased accordingly, and as they approach 55 days of age, other food should be introduced.

CHECKLIST FOR SUPPLIES

The following is a recommended list of supplies to keep on hand:

- Distilled water
- Psittacine baby bird feeding formula
- Nectar powder
- Feeding charts
- Scale
- Bedding (linens and/or dust free shavings)
- 1 ml syringe
- Curved spoon
- Small (shallow) feed dish or bowl
- Measuring spoons (1 tsp and 1 Tbsp)
- 1/4 C (60 ml) measuring cup
- Disinfectant
- Sponges

FEEDING PROCEDURES

Lorikeets are generally straightforward to feed. Hatchlings should be fed with a small curved spoon for 1–2 weeks, after which they quickly learn to eat from a larger bent metal spoon. They tend to consume the formula rapidly to the point of almost gorging themselves. The chicks are very sensitive to the temperature of the formula initially, regardless of the age when they are pulled from the nestbox. The first few days and up to 1 week, the formula will need to be very warm, between 102–110°F (39–43°C), for them to accept it. Always check the temperature of the formula on your wrist before feeding to ensure that it is not so hot it could damage the sensitive tissues of the mouth and esophagus of the chick.

If the formula spills onto the chick, remove it with a warm moist cloth before it dries. As the chicks mature, their eating behaviors become more sloppy and formula frequently drips from their mouth onto their feathers. Ensure that all feeding equipment is disinfected between each feed.

HATCHLINGS

Hatchlings should be checked every hour, feeding only when the crop is empty or nearly empty, which is usually every 2 hours. Always wash hands thoroughly before handling chicks or the feeding equipment. Plan to feed the chicks every 2 hours around the clock for 7 days. The time between feeds may slowly be increased, starting when the chicks are making a steady daily weight gain; this is usually between 7 and 10 days. Feed at regular intervals throughout the day and increase the time between feeds at night. A 1 ml syringe may be used for feeding newly hatched chicks of the smallest species, but most will eat from a small, bent baby spoon. Young chicks will quickly adapt to eating from a larger bent spoon. Drop the formula into the mouth from a short distance, being careful not to insert the syringe or spoon into the mouth. The chick will take it willingly. Do not force any food into the mouth or down the throat. If the chick is not interested in accepting the formula, the food may not be warm enough, and should be heated and offered again. Once the chick begins eating, administer the food in a controlled manner while the chick is actively swallowing. Give the chick enough time to completely swallow after each small increment before offering the next. As they grow, they seem to want the formula faster than they can eat it. Observe the crop as it fills with nectar. Use that as your gauge to know how much to feed. When the nectar can be seen filling the crop at the back of the neck, it is time to stop. Avoid filling the mouth completely with food, because it may compromise their breathing. Some birds will eat better if the food is given in multiple small amounts; others will take their entire meal rapidly. Note that if the formula is offered too fast it may come out the nares.

EXPECTED WEIGHT GAIN

Figures 22.2 and 22.3 graph the expected weight gains of Rainbow Lorikeets and Perfect Lorikeets, respectively.

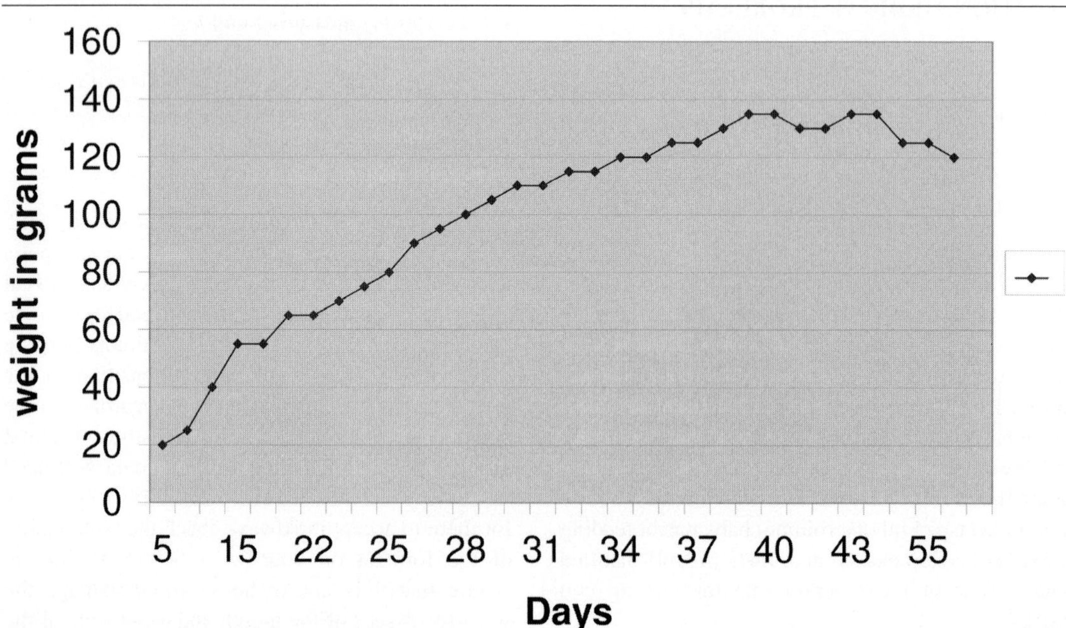

Figure 22.2. Rainbow Lorikeet weight gain chart.

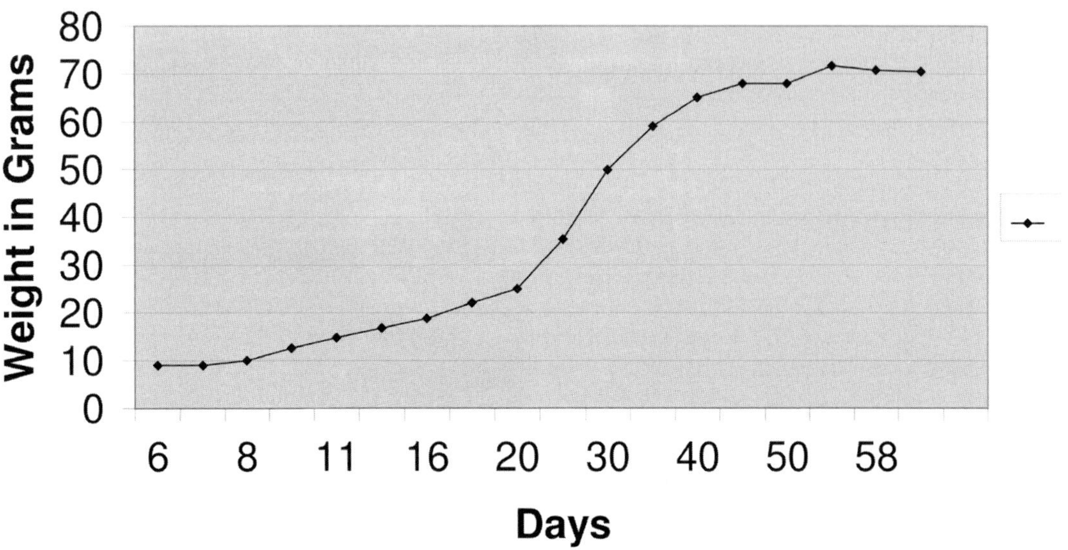

Figure 22.3. Perfect Lorikeet weight gain chart.

HOUSING

Hatchlings should be kept in a brooder at 85–90°F (29.4–32.2°C). Brooders of all kinds may be purchased through breeders, specialty pet stores, and the Internet. A home-made brooder that works well is a small plastic ice chest (Igloo) with a towel or blanket covering the top. Use a digital thermometer with the sensor close to the birds. An additional heat source, such as a heat pad, is not necessary if this brooder is kept in a warm room over 68°F. Another useful home-made brooder is made using two small plastic cat litter boxes. Put one upside down on top of the other and cut a large hole in the top box. Place a heating pad under one-half of the lower box to allow a warm zone and a cooler zone so the chicks may select their thermal comfort. Place a towel between the heating pad and the box. This arrangement is more difficult for maintaining a comfortable temperature, but use the digital thermometer and a towel or blanket on top if necessary. If the room is kept at a continuous temperature, the temperature inside the brooder will be easier to control. Hatchlings are best kept on pillowcases or a smooth towel. Towels and pillowcase should be free of holes and hanging pieces. Terrycloth towels are unacceptable. Dust-free shavings may also be used. The bedding should be changed daily and replaced with new dry bedding.

Place a washed, small, safe stuffed animal and or a new, small feather duster in the brooder with the chicks (see Figure 22.4). Both of these items should be free of small ingestible parts, and the chicks should be unable to tangle themselves in any part. The chicks utilize these items to huddle next to for warmth and for a feeling of safety and comfort.

WEANING

Throughout the feeding process, a small shallow bowl is often used to hold the formula, which is then fed to the chicks using the spoon. When the chicks are 5–6 weeks old, one or both will start to show interest in the bowl full of formula rather than the spoon. Normal chicks are always anxious to eat. Encourage the chicks to dip their heads in the bowl by gently guiding the head toward the bowl. Tapping the spoon in the bowl may be helpful to draw their

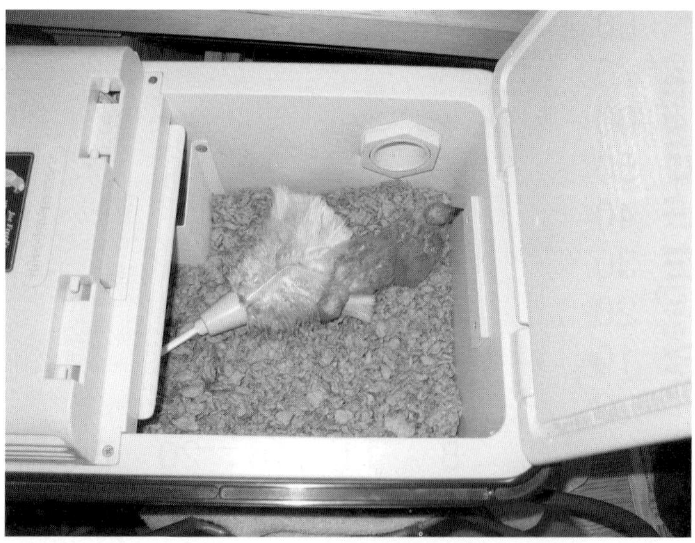

Figure 22.4. Lorikeet chicks in portable commercial brooder with a feather duster.

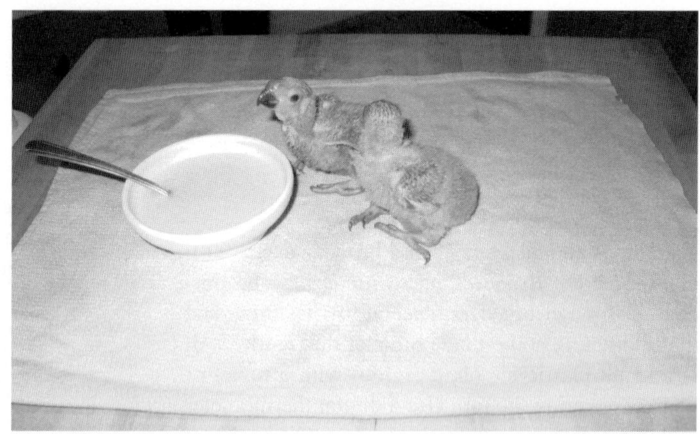

Figure 22.5. Rainbow Lorikeet chicks (23 days old and 24 days old) next to shallow feed bowl.

attention to the formula (see Figure 22.5). They will quickly learn how to eat from the bowl, but will initially take only one or two gulps of very warm food, and then the remainder will need to be fed using the spoon.

The process of weaning them to eat all of their formula from a bowl may take from 7 to as many as 20 days. At about 40 days of age introduce small amounts of pureed fruits into their nectar mixture. At this time, introduce small pieces of soft skinless fruit and vegetables (no avocado, which may be toxic) for them to play with. This is also the time to introduce a safe small toy such as a plastic chain, wood blocks, or thin cardboard. Toys with any size rope or twine attached are inappropriate. As soon as the birds start exploring, put a small low perch in one area of the brooder. A dowel or small branch may be set on the ground or slightly elevated. When they are fully feathered and start to become active, which could be a few days to a week, they are ready for a small cage with low perches and food bowls still on the ground. As they get stronger, bowls and perches should be raised to help encourage them to climb and increase their activity.

Exposing the birds to different types of foods, toys, perches, foliage, and people will help ensure a well-adjusted, friendly bird. See Table 22.1 for a recommended weaning schedule.

Table 22.1. Approximate schedule for weaning lorikeets.

Day 50–53	Reduce the baby feeding formula (Exact) by half; the nectar amount stays the same.
Day 55	Introduce fruit puree or cut-up skinless fruit pieces.
Day 60	Reduce the distilled water in the formula by half and replace it with the same water the birds get as adults.
Day 67	Discontinue baby formula (Exact).
Day 70	Discontinue all distilled water, replacing it with the same water the adult birds are offered.

The chicks are now receiving their adult diet. Overnight care may be discontinued between 54–64 days. Sometimes spoon-feeding during the day may be necessary to maintain proper growth.

Captive adult lorikeets are generally fed a commercial nectar diet and a variety of pureed or cut-up fruit. Lory life (Avico) and Nekton are available at most pet stores. Rainbow Landing is also a good diet, but it is not available in stores. Small amounts of vegetables are sometimes added to fruit mixture for extra nutrition. Lorikeet pellets are also available, but they should not be fed as a sole diet. A combination of all of the above should be fed. Lorikeets lack a muscular gizzard to process seeds or nuts; therefore, only soft foods should be fed.

PREPARATION FOR AVIARY RELEASE

After the birds have had some time to practice flying they may be taken to an introductory aviary, which is often a small aviary that is large enough for them to fly in and may house calm nonaggressive birds or other fledged chicks. This allows them to socialize with other birds. Allow them to spend 2–3 hours per day in this aviary for a few days, gradually increasing the time. This requires close supervision to ensure that the other birds are acting appropriately and that the young birds are eating. If no other birds are available for the introductory aviary, housing the young birds in an aviary adjacent to the main aviary is the next option for socialization. Weigh the chicks daily until they have maintained their weight for at least 2 weeks. The young birds are now ready to be introduced to their final aviary housing.

ACKNOWLEDGMENTS

Thanks to Bobbie Meyer, Laura Guinasso, and Dyann Kruse for their assistance with this chapter.

SOURCES FOR PRODUCTS MENTIONED

Lory life Pre-Mix Nectar Diet, Avico, Cuttlebone Plus, 810 North Twin Oaks Valley Road, #131, San Marcos, CA 92069, (760) 591-4951, (800) 747-9878, www.cuttleboneplus.com.

Nekton products, www.nekton.de.

Rainbow Landing, P.O. Box 462845, Escondido, CA 92046-2845, (800) 229-1946, lorynectar@earthlink.net.

Kaytee Exact (Baby Parrot Feeding Formula), 521 Clay St., Chilton, WI 53014, (800) Kaytee-1 or (920) 849-2321, www.kaytee.com.

REFERENCE

Low, R. 1998. Encyclopedia of the Lories. Hancock House Publishers, Blaine, Washington.

23
Roadrunners

Elizabeth Penn Elliston

NATURAL HISTORY

Geococcyx californianus, the Greater Roadrunner, is also known by many local names such as Chaparral Cock, Snake Killer, Lizard Bird, Churca, Paisano, and Correcamino. The only American cuckoo to take up permanent residence north of approximately 26°N latitude, this bird inhabits the arid environment of the American Southwest and north central Mexico. These cuckoos start nesting early and frequently choose thick evergreens or stationary farm equipment as a nesting site (see Figure 23.1). They may have as many as three broods in a season. Both male and female are exemplary parents, and pairs may produce broods of up to six young in a clutch (Ohmart 1973). Parents start incubating as soon as the first egg is laid, for an incubation period of 17–20 days. Consequently, there may be a great variation in the age and development of chicks in a nest. Chicks may leave the nest at about 2 weeks of age, but are under the supervision of their parents for another 30–40 days (Whitson 1976) as they refine their foraging skills.

Upper parts of the adult bird are streaked brown and white with some iridescent shades of green, blue-black, and purple on the wing. Tail feathers have white "thumbprint" markings on the tips typical of cuckoos. The blue/black erectile crest on the head may be raised and lowered in displays, which may also expose brightly colored apteria, which are unfeathered postorbital spaces colored bright blue close to the eye, fading and blending to bright orange distal to the eye. The eye, shaded by prominent protective lashes, has a pale yellow or grey to reddish-orange iris. The black decurved bill is about 5 cm in length. Legs are long and bluish terminating in a zygodactyl toe arrangement with toes number 2 and 3 pointing forward and 1 and 4 pointing backward. Normal adult body temperature has been reported by Calder (1968) as 104°F (40°C) and confirmed by the author. Adult weights range from 221–538 g (Dunning 1984).

Roadrunners are obligate faunivores. They hunt and eat any kind of small prey such as mice, lizards, snakes, small birds, insects, and snails. They may pick up and eat a variety of nonanimal material (chili peppers), which is usually cast out when the indigestible material builds up in the muscular stomach. Prey is prepared for swallowing whole by whacking it on a nearby rock or other hard surface.

CRITERIA FOR INTERVENTION

Roadrunners may be brought into captivity as eggs from nests displaced from machinery, as hatchlings from similarly displaced nests, as fledglings that have been kidnapped or caught by dogs or cats, or as adults that have met with some accident. Roadrunners are very dedicated parents and seemingly uninjured fledglings should have a physical exam to rule out both subtle and obvious injuries. If results are satisfactory they should be reunited with their parents.

RECORD KEEPING

See Chapter 1, "General Care," for record keeping suggestions.

INITIAL CARE AND STABILIZATION

The main rule of initial baby bird care is to provide warmth, rehydration, and feeding, in that order. Warm chicks before giving fluids, and then hydrate them until they start passing droppings. Only then is it safe to commence feedings. Feeding a cold or

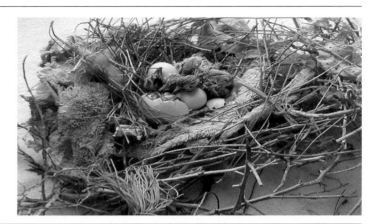

Figure 23.1. Roadrunner nest with three hatchlings and two eggs.

dehydrated baby bird before it is warm and hydrated will probably kill it.

New patients should be allowed to rest for 15–20 minutes in a warm, dark, quiet container before examination. If the bird is not able to stand, it should be placed in a soft support structure such as a rolled cloth donut or paper nest. Do not allow the bird to lie on its side or other abnormal positions. Hatchlings and nestlings should be placed in a climate-controlled incubator if available. When the animal is warm and calm, it may be hydrated orally and/or subcutaneously (SQ). Warm sterile fluids such as 2.5% dextrose in 0.45% sodium chloride or lactated Ringer's solution may be administered SQ at 5% of body weight once, although repeated administrations may be needed for extremely dehydrated birds. Gaping, active hatchlings or nestlings should be orally hydrated until they produce droppings. Give a few drops of warm oral fluids every 15–20 minutes with a small syringe or eyedropper and allow the bird to swallow completely before giving more. Once the amount the chick is able to swallow is understood, the amount may be raised to 2.5–5% of body weight in several mouthfuls. Human infant electrolyte fluids (unflavored) are excellent for oral rehydration of baby birds. Ensure that the bird is warm before administering fluids, and that the bird is both warm and well-hydrated before receiving food. Start the bird on a hand-feeding formula after it begins passing droppings.

If the bird is depressed or not swallowing well, oral rehydration must be performed very carefully, because there is a greater risk of aspiration of fluids into the respiratory system. It may be better in this circumstance to wait for the animal to absorb SQ fluids, rather than giving oral fluids too quickly. If SQ fluids are not an option, give tiny amounts of oral fluids deep into the mouth and ensure that the bird swallows everything before giving more.

COMMON MEDICAL PROBLEMS AND SOLUTIONS

Young roadrunners usually present with injuries from animal bites, or as orphans from loss of parents. Injured birds may require splints for broken bones. Dense styrofoam makes a very nice supportive but lightweight splint. For lacerations, the author prefers covering with a bio-occlusive dressing such as Op-site (Smith and Nephew) or Tegaderm (3M) to sutures or any other closure. In the author's experience, these dressings are well tolerated by most birds and do not require a decision about closure or drainage, because the material acts as a substitute skin. These dressings also serve to keep feathers out of wounds. Some brands of this type of product absorb exudate as well.

Subcutaneous emphysema (air under the skin) may occur as the result of a cat attack. This usually resolves without treatment. If the bubble is interfering with mobility or compromising breathing, it may be necessary to remove the pressure by puncturing the bubble with a sterile needle, avoiding any visible skin blood vessels. If the internal puncture into an air sac has not closed, the bubble will reinflate. A slightly elastic pressure bandage may help resolve the emphysema, but is often hard to apply and may be stressful to the bird. Consult your avian veterinarian for medical advice regarding antibiotic treatment for puncture wounds.

DIET RECIPES

Roadunners are obligate faunivores and do well on diets that are fed to raptors (see Chapter 14, "Hawks, Falcons, Kites, Osprey, and New World Vultures") for diet information). However, unlike raptors, roadrunners typically do not cast (regurgitate) bones, fur, teeth, or chitinous insect exoskeletons. In adults, the entire ingested animal is reduced to a thick, tarry, malodorous fecal dropping. In the healthy nestling, droppings are very large and encapsulated in a gelatinous envelope.

These rapidly developing youngsters evolved in the desert, and they need the proper calcium to phosphorus ratio (2:1 by weight) with adequate vitamin D3 and sun from the earliest age.

Characteristic of all cuckoos, roadrunners typically do not pick up and eat dead food unless they have learned to do so. In training young roadrunners for release, they are given an advantage if trained to pick up almost anything that could be food, live or dead, and examine it.

FEEDING PROCEDURES

Roadrunner hatchlings, after being well hydrated so that they produce large gelatinous droppings, can be fed pieces of food as large as they can swallow. The food should be lifted from a soak of fluid (water or 0.9% saline) to provide plenty of fluid and prevent dehydration. Hatchlings have bright red gapes with a fringed pattern in the mouth that includes both white spots and a black tip to the tongue. They gape vigorously and make a whining, growling sound when begging. They should be fed whenever they beg in response to stimulus. If even the slightest wrinkle appears on the abdomen, they are becoming dehydrated. This condition should be immediately corrected by hydration with isotonic fluid.

The amount of food needed each day can be calculated with the formula $(BW_{Kg})^{.75} \times 78 \times 1.5 = 24\,hr$ maintenance requirement. A young bird needs 1.5–3 times maintenance for healthy growth. See Appendix 2 for tables of these values by body weight. A good way to measure the amount fed is to weigh the day's planned food at the beginning of the day and at the end of the day after feeding has ceased. The difference is, of course, the weight of the food consumed. Each prey species will vary in caloric density, but the author's rule of thumb is to estimate faunivore prey items at 1 kcal/g.

Self-feeding roadrunners coming in to rehabilitation may have a difficult time learning to eat nonmoving food. It is often important to give them foods that they do not have to kill, so that they receive sufficient calories and variety during the healing period. Encouraging them to self-feed is important because force-feeding these birds, even only twice a day, is very stressful to them. Sometimes presenting the food with a puppet will help, sometimes dressing a piece of meat up with spare feathers or fur will be enough to let the roadrunner know that this is food. Once they learn that this unlikely looking stuff is food, they will often begin to self-feed easily.

As with raptors, roadrunners imprint when their eyes have opened and cleared. As this process is occurring, it is important to provide chicks with a conspecific imprint model. This may be a foster parent, slightly older sibling that responds to begging, or a puppet made from a roadrunner skin (Elliston 1998). Puppets may be used with feeding implements such as long hemostats or a syringe with a long rubber tube attachment for feeding liquid diets.

Hatchlings

Hatchlings, between 13–18 g, should be weighed every morning, hydrated, and fed 5 times/12–14-hour day or whenever they gape (see Figure 23.2).

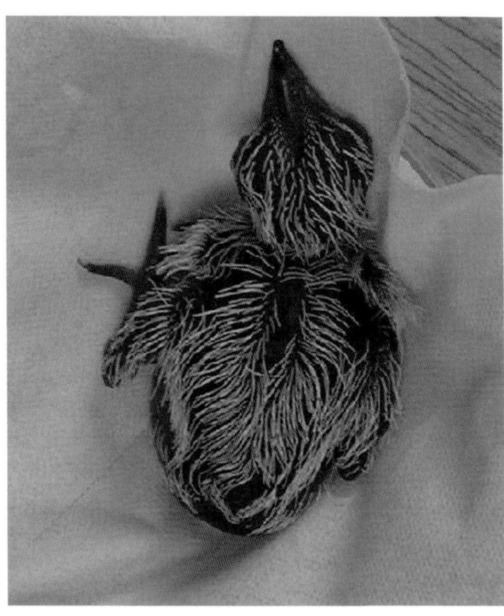

Figure 23.2. Hatchling roadrunner. Note white down on black skin.

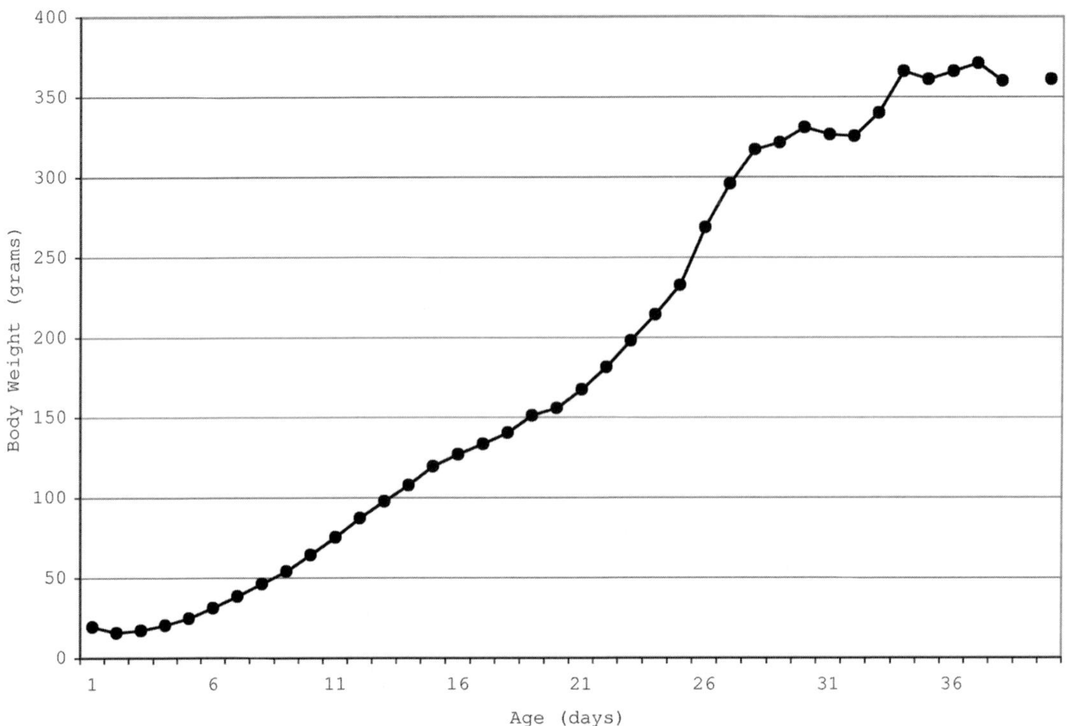

Figure 23.3. Mean weight gain of hand-reared Greater Roadrunner chicks (n = 10).

Allow the birds to get plenty of sleep between feeds and at night. The internal temperature of hatchling roadrunners is about 105°F (40.6°C) (author, unpublished data). They should feel hot to the touch and look like little black balloons with sparse white down on their feather tracts. If a bird refuses food, reevaluate the temperature, hydration status, and physical condition.

Nestlings and Fledglings

Fully and partially feathered birds should be fed 2–3 times a day when they call or beg. Roadrunners stop begging when they are full. In nature, their parents probably start to feed them when the day becomes warm and cease when they go to roost at about 1 hour before dark. They can be fed by a surrogate parent (foster sibling or adult) or blunt forceps and a puppet surrogate.

EXPECTED WEIGHT GAIN

Unlike many other species, roadrunners do not gain their full adult weight before learning to forage (see Figures 23.3, 23.4). Their exact age may be determined by the length of the central retrices, unless, of course, the bird has met with some mishap that has caused feathers to be lost or damaged.

HOUSING

Hatchlings should be kept at around 99°F (37°C) and 40–50% humidity. A variety of materials may be used to create a replacement nest. A woven basket of the right dimensions makes a perfect substitute nest for roadrunners. It can be lined with soft material when the birds are very young, and droppings can be removed with toilet paper. However, the sticks of the basket provide a perfect substrate for developing legs and feet. Young birds should sit in the nest with their legs folded underneath their heavy bodies. Legs allowed to splay may become deformed. A healthy nestling will deposit droppings over the rim of the nest, which makes maintaining cleanliness easy.

At 10–11 days when they are fully feathered and beginning to move around, the nestlings can be placed outside where they can interact with their

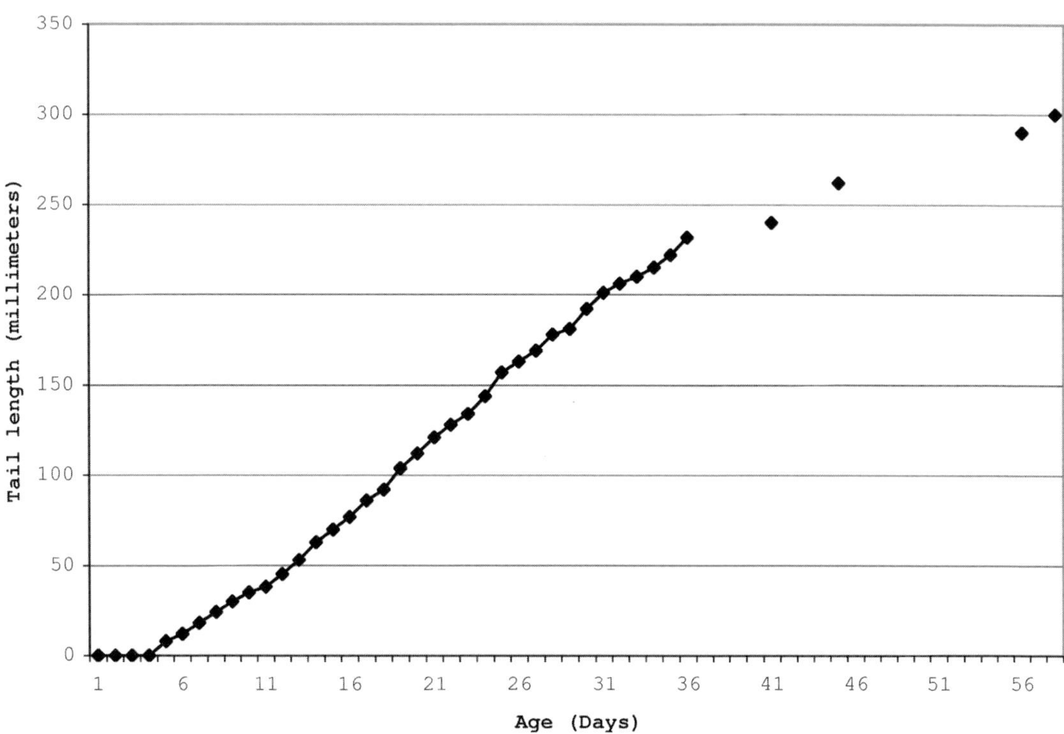

Figure 23.4. Mean tail growth of hand-reared Greater Roadrunner chicks (n = 10).

environment. The 16 × 8 × 8 ft (4.9 × 2.4 × 2.4 m) enclosure for a maximum of six birds (Miller 2000) should contain plenty of room to sun- and dust-bathe. Perches at various heights are important for exercise and night use (see Figure 23.5). A pool of water is attractive, but not necessary for these desert birds. It is wise, however, to provide drinking water at all times.

As soon as the youngsters are able to manage their heavy bodies on their legs, they begin to exhibit typical roadrunner sunning behavior. Their bodies are extended, their wings spread and their rumps exposed to the sun. In this way, since they don't need to generate their own heat, their daily caloric requirement for food may be reduced by 41–50% (Calder 1968; Ohmart 1971).

By 2 weeks of age, young birds pick up and play with objects but rarely swallow them. In the third and fourth weeks they begin to whack and eat their prey. At this time, they should be offered mealworms (*Tenebrio molitor*) and superworms (*Zoophorba moriom*) to stimulate foraging behavior (see Figure 23.6). By the end of the fourth week, they may be picking up dead mice and whacking them, soon graduating to catching and killing live mice. Not surprisingly, birds raised by a conspecific surrogate learn to hunt sooner than those raised by a puppet, and those that have had early experience opening snails are at an advantage after release. When they

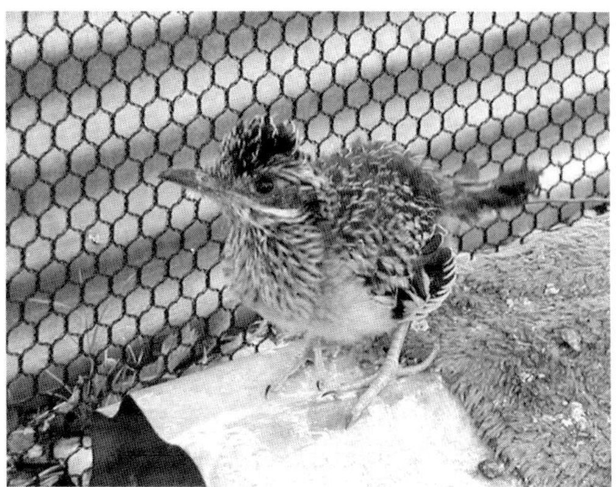

Figure 23.5. Fledgling roadrunner perching in aviary. Aviaries should have ample perching objects of varying heights.

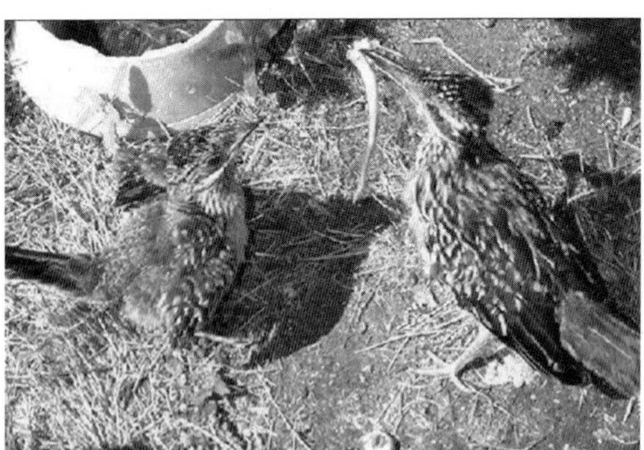

Figure 23.6. Two fledgling roadrunners in aviary learning to pick up food.

have left the nest, birds should be weighed less frequently than every day, to prevent too much habituation.

WEANING

As soon as the birds begin jumping in and out of the nest and are old enough to begin exploring their environment, desert furnishings such as hunks of bark, cactus skeletons, and other similar objects should be provided. It is important to confine the live food of these animals so that it cannot escape, but it is equally important to stimulate foraging. Leaves and detritus, as well as game bird starter, chopped fruit, and potatoes, can be placed in large pans with Tenebrio or Zoophorba larvae, which may attract other "wild" insects into the hunting area. As the birds become competent killing large superworms, they can be introduced to live mice. It may be necessary to continue to feed some nonliving meat material (chicken neck pieces, ground turkey balls supplemented with calcium) to the youngsters because live prey is costly, and also to provide variety and good nutrition in the diet. However, learning to pick up and eat nonmoving food is clearly very advantageous to the young hunter in the wild because it allows the bird to scavenge while refining its hunting skills.

It is difficult to keep captive hand-reared roadrunners for long without having them become habituated to people. Making sure that they are exposed to only one caregiver helps keep them wild, as does only one or two approaches with food per day once the birds are weaned. If birds are heard calling, it may mean that they are not being provided with adequate foods stores in which to forage. If an individual ever appears lethargic or less active than usual, it should be removed and its condition assessed.

PREPARATION FOR WILD RELEASE

To avoid habituating young roadrunners to humans, restrict human contact to one person and only when food is being presented. It may be necessary to call other rehabilitation facilities to find conspecifics for placement of single orphans.

Success at avoiding habituation should be seen by the time the birds are ready for release. They should be wary of humans rather than coming up to caretakers for food.

RELEASE

Roadrunners are not migratory and are quite territorial. It is important to release them at a time and in areas in which they can find plenty of prey and will not be harassed by domestic pets. In the season of plentiful range locusts and other prey, young birds are well tolerated by resident adults until natural dispersal occurs. Each chick should weigh at least 275 g on release and be exclusively foraging and sunning to fulfill its energy requirements. There should be no begging from the caregiver if food is present. A good way to catch up a young roadrunner for release is for the regular caregiver to approach them in the dark, pick them off their perch, and place them in a dark cardboard box. They can then be transported to the release site with as little stress as possible. The box should be opened on the ground and the birds allowed to exit at will.

ACKNOWLEDGMENTS

Thanks to Nancy Lee Olsen for sharing her extensive collection of literature and Janine Perlman for critical reading. Thanks to the Albuquerque office of the U.S. Fish and Wildlife Service and the New Mexico Department of Game and Fish (NMDGF) for permits and for bringing us displaced eggs and young of New Mexico's state bird. Thanks to the Share with Wildlife Program of the NMDGF for continued support of Wildlife Rescue Inc. of New Mexico (WRINM). Most of all, thanks to the supporters and members of WRINM who made the acquisition of this information possible through giving displaced nestling roadrunners their careful attention.

SOURCES FOR PRODUCTS MENTIONED

Op-site Flexifix dressing: Smith & Nephew, Inc., 11775 Starkey Road, P.O. Box 1970, Largo, FL 33779-1970, (800) 876-1261, http://www.opsitepostop.com/.

Tegaderm: 3M, 3M Center, St. Paul, MN 55144-1000, (800) 364-3577.

Invertebrate food supplier: Rainbow Mealworms, 126 E. Spruce St., Compton, CA 90220, (800) 777-9676, https://www.rainbowmealworms.net/home.asp.

Invertebrate food supplier: Fluker Farms, 1333 Plantation Ave., Port Allen, LA 70767-4087, (800) 735-8537, http://www.flukerfarms.com/.

REFERENCES

Calder, W.A. 1968. There really is a roadrunner. Natural History 77(4): 50–55.

Dunning, J.B., Jr. 1984. Body weights of 686 species of North American Birds. Western Bird Banding Association Monograph No. 1. 39 pp.

Elliston, E.P. 1998. MOM—Made to Order Mother. 1998. International Wildlife Rehabilitation Council Conference Proceedings, p. 138.

Miller, E.A., ed. 2000. Minimum Standards for Wildlife Rehabilitation, 3rd Edition. National Wildlife Rehabilitation Association, St. Cloud, Minnesota, 77 pp.

Ohmart, R.D. 1971. Roadrunners: Energy conservation by hypothermia and absorption of sunlight. Science 172: 67–69.

———. 1973. Observations on the breeding adaptations of the roadrunner. Condor 75: 140–149.

Whitson, M.A. 1976. Courtship behavior of the greater roadrunner. Living Bird 14: 215–255.

24
Owls

Lisa Fosco

NATURAL HISTORY

Owls make up the order Strigiformes and are divided into two distinct families based on natural history as well as anatomical differences. Barn owl species make up the family Tytonidae, which includes about 14 species. The family Strigidae, also known as the "typical" owls includes about 167 species worldwide and is further divided into two subfamilies: Striginae (long-eared and forest-adapted owls), and Buboninae (small-eared and visually hunting species.)

Owls are found on all continents except Antarctica. Most species are nocturnal and all are hunters that will scavenge only when necessary. They hunt by both sight and sound, and most species have feathers adapted for noiseless flight. In general, owls are relatively sedentary, with only the smaller and more specialized species being migratory.

The reproductive period of owls tends to be prolonged compared to other raptor species. They have a long incubation period, and the prefledging period is also comparatively long in most species. Cavity nesting species usually remain securely hidden in their nest for most of their prefledging time where they are visually isolated from their surroundings. Unlike other owls, most of these species use no visual cues in any of their food-begging behaviors.

Tree-nesting species tend to grow and develop at a faster rate. They are more physically active and mobile, climbing up and around the nest as legs develop. This behavior often results in owlets of these species leaving the nest before fledging. Unlike some other avian and raptorial species, this is considered a natural behavior and rarely impacts parental care. Also unlike other raptors, juvenile owls of most species tend to remain with the parents for relatively long periods of time after fledging while they are learning and refining their hunting skills.

CRITERIA FOR INTERVENTION

Whenever possible, healthy owlets should be returned to the nest site for familial recovery. Healthy owlets should be well-fleshed, bright-eyed, and responsive to all stimuli. Feathered nestlings are usually accepted when placed safely off the ground in the vicinity of the nesting tree or structure. If the owlet repeatedly grounds itself, is in a structurally questionable nest, or is in an urban or visible location, protective measures may be helpful. Temporary barriers surrounding the tree base at a minimum distance of 6 ft in radius may provide a protective barrier for domestic predators and human attention.

Unfortunately, owlets are commonly kidnapped due to their visibility on the ground and their proximity to people and domestic animals. Uninjured owlets should not be considered orphans unless the parent clearly rejects them. Captive rearing of the highest standards still tends to have a permanent impact on their learned abilities and skills, as well as their general behavior. These factors are crucial for long-term survival.

Many species have been known to readily accept young that have been gone for several days and even extended periods. In 2001, the author rehabilitated a nestling Great Horned Owl with a fractured ulna for 22 days and then successfully reunited it with the family group where it fledged naturally.

Young owlets that are repeatedly forced from the nest, or those that have been actively ignored by parents are often candidates for intervention. Those with large numbers of ectoparasites or those attracting flies are also candidates for rehabilitation.

If captive rearing is the only option, owlets that are to be released into the wild should never be raised alone. Every effort should be made to house nestlings with conspecifics and ideally in view of the natural habitat. Regardless of the age or condition of the bird, human interaction and all contact with people or domestic pets should be minimized whenever possible.

RECORD KEEPING

All records should include detailed information on the location where the bird was found as well as the circumstances of the rescue. Regulating wildlife agencies should be consulted for specific requirements or for local licensed wildlife rehabilitation options.

In addition to basic legal documentation, records should be kept on individual animals throughout their care. Birds should be weighed, aged as best as possible, and have a physical exam to identify or rule out any potential health concerns or injuries.

Proper development and general health status may be best assessed by closely monitoring and documenting body weight, feeding habits and behavior, digestive function, and feather condition, as compared to their wild counterparts. Physical development of most owl species has been observed, documented, and is accessible for reference with minimal research. This information is an essential resource when rearing any unfamiliar species. Special attention should be given to diet, nutritional needs, and feeding behaviors throughout development, because these factors impact bone growth and behavioral maturation.

INITIAL CARE AND STABILIZATION

New patients that appear to be stable should be assessed for thermal needs and then should be left alone to settle down and de-stress. Covering the box or cage with a dark towel and moving it to a quiet room for a few minutes is often sufficient.

Once the animal is warm and calm, it should be weighed, rehydrated, and given an initial physical exam. Record its initial body weight in grams or in the smallest and most accurate unit available (see Figure 24.1). Check the bird's keel and pectoral muscle to assess overall state of health. Keel should not be "sharp" or remarkably prominent in owlets of any age. It is normal for owls to have asymmetrically placed ears for triangulation of prey location by sound. Severely malnourished or emaciated birds should be fed a few pieces of organ meat as soon as the bird is warm and hydrated. A little food goes a long way when stabilizing a weak or starving baby.

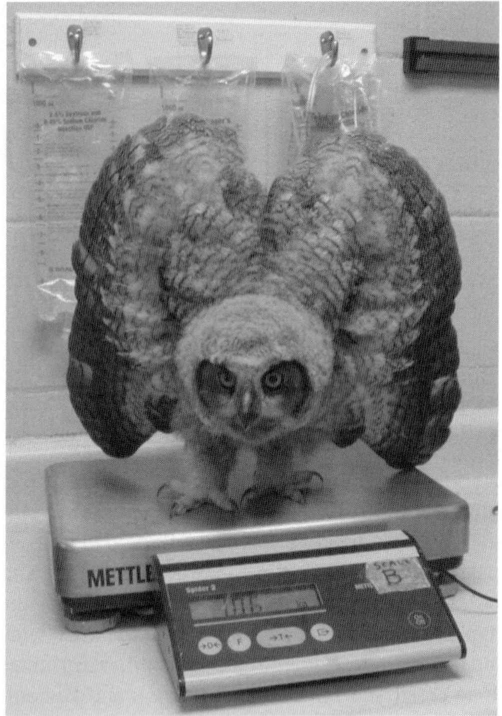

Figure 24.1. Fledgling Great Horned Owl standing on scale.

All new birds should be hydrated. Rehydration volume should be based on approximate level of dehydration. Healthy, hydrated birds should receive a bolus volume of 5% of their body weight in grams (50 ml/kg), those that are severely dehydrated (mucoid or tacky mouth, sunken eyes, wrinkled skin and eyelids) should receive up to 15% (see Figure 24.2). Consult or enlist an avian veterinarian if necessary. Warm, sterile, isotonic fluids such as lactated Ringer's solution or 0.9% sodium chloride should be administered subcutaneously or, in critical cases, intravenously. Large liquid volumes should not be given orally unless that is the only option. Owls are anatomically designed to eat and digest solid prey items only. They may easily aspirate liquids while swallowing or in any body position where the head is not elevated above the body. Small volumes or sips of liquids can be given orally to those requiring additional gastrointestinal hydration or those not capable of processing whole foods.

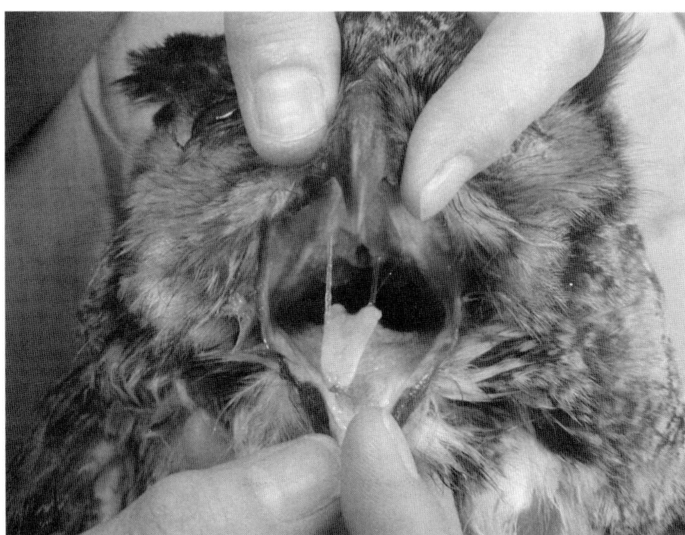

Figure 24.2. Dehydration may result in stringy or mucousy saliva.

Once the bird is warm and hydrated, a physical examination should be performed, and any injuries or remarkable conditions should be recorded and treated. The approximate age should be established based on physical development and feeding initiated. Ideally, the bird should be fed relatively soon after being admitted. It is best to feed after handling because stress can increase the likelihood of regurgitation and therefore the risk of aspiration. For malnourished, very weak, or unstable birds, all handling and treatment should be as quick as possible. In these circumstances, check weight, hydrate quickly, and if warm enough, feed one or two pieces of organ meats. Then leave the bird alone on heat in a dark quiet area. An hour or two later, the bird is likely to be at least a little stronger.

Well-fleshed, healthy owlets should be encouraged to reach for and take their own food as soon as they are capable of holding up their heads. Size and presentation of food items should be based on digestive abilities of that stage of development. Never force-feed a young owl unless absolutely necessary. It is not unusual for a new chick to ravenously accept food on intake, and then, after a forcible and negative feeding experience, to avoid eating on its own or even to actively refuse food when offered. Carefully assess dietary needs and make a feeding plan before feeding a new patient.

It should be noted that well-fleshed animals with no apparent injuries should be kept in captivity only when there is no other option. It is after this initial exam that plans should be made to return any potential candidates to their family.

COMMON MEDICAL PROBLEMS AND SOLUTIONS

Traumatic injuries in owls should be treated as they would be in other avian species. Due to the anatomical absence of a protective brow bone, eye injuries are common in owls and unfortunately, are rarely documented. A thorough eye exam should be performed in all owls with any suspicion of trauma because these injuries may result in functional limitations that may affect flight as well as hunting ability. All cases with a history of ocular trauma should be considered for release based on a well-evaluated ability to hunt live prey in optimal light conditions for that species.

Injuries to the cornea should be confirmed by the positive uptake of fluoroscein stain on the corneal surface. Treatment with nonsteroidal ophthalmic agents may be helpful. Do not use steroids if there is corneal damage with positive fluorescein stain uptake. Corneal scars and opacities in the outer areas of the cornea may or may not affect visual function depending on their density and location. Visible blood in the anterior chamber (hyphema) may be a common result of traumatic injuries. Treatment with topical corticosteroids may be helpful, although blood is often reabsorbed without treatment. Age-

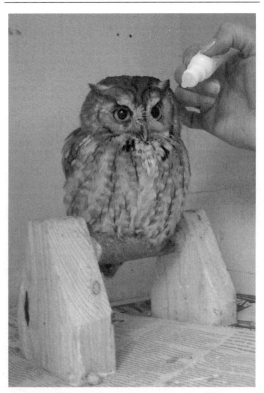

Figure 24.3. Eastern Screech Owl with traumatic anisocoria having eye medication applied without restraint.

related retinal degeneration in owls has been documented (Redig 1993).

Based on the natural behaviors of the larger-bodied owls, they can often be given topical eye medications without necessitating restraint (see Figure 24.3). Often, if the protected hand holding the medication is brought in from the side of the bird, the owl will remain focused on the individual and not respond to the hand or the administration of the medication.

Parasites

Wildlife species are common hosts to many species of parasites. Like other opportunistic pathogens, they may become a significant strain on compromised individuals and should be treated in compromised or recovering patients. Gastrointestinal parasites should be diagnosed by fecal analysis and treated accordingly.

Blood Parasites

Several blood parasites are commonly identified in owl species, including Plasmodium, Leucocytozoan, and Haemoproteus. Routine bloodwork should include analysis of a blood smear in these species. Plasmodium species are the causative agent of malaria in birds as well as humans. Vectors include three genera of mosquitoes. The primary vector of Leucocytozoan is black flies in the genus Simulium. Haemoproteus species are commonly transmitted by hippoboscid or flat flies. Infections are often subclinical. Consult an avian veterinarian for treatment options.

Ectoparasites

Feather mites, lice, and hippoboscids (flat flies) may be found all over the body. Due to the prevalence of vector-borne diseases, these parasites should be eliminated in clinical or group settings. The bird can generally be safely and thoroughly de-parasitized with a light dusting of Sevin Dust (diethylcarbamazine, GardenTech). Lightly rub powder through feather layers down to the skin. Avoid the facial area in those birds with respiratory concerns. One good dusting on intake will not only benefit the host, but will reduce the transfer of parasites to other patients or resident birds. It is prudent to wear gloves when applying pesticides to patients. See Chapter 1, "General Care," for information on caregiver exposure to pesticides.

Maggots and fly eggs should be manually removed as soon as possible. Sites that allow penetration or are easily penetrated, such as wounds and bodily orifices, should be cleared immediately. Although some species of flies target only compromised tissue, the larva of most common fly species are much less selective and are just as likely to feed on healthy structures. Once the eggs hatch, they can burrow through healthy tissues and often result in damage worse than the original trauma. The use of Capstar (Nytenpyram, Novartis) is often administered orally to weaken and reduce the number of deeper and less-accessible active larvae. Birds should be closely monitored for continued hatching as well as for any resilient live maggots and treated twice daily until all larvae are eliminated.

DIET

Owls are studied and even admired for their efficient breakdown of whole food. Only the most digestible and nutritious parts (organ meat, muscle, fat) are utilized, and the remaining less-digestible parts (bones, hair, feathers) are efficiently collected and formed into a pellet or casting that is ejected or spit out. Owl pellets are often used in educational programs.

As in other areas of captive wildlife management, the optimal and most healthy diet is one that most closely resembles the wild diet of that species. Although adult birds may tolerate modified diets, growing juveniles with developing bones may be permanently and irreversibly affected by incomplete or unbalanced diets. Ideally, owlets that are physically capable of digesting whole food should be fed a complete and fully balanced diet. Calcium, phosphorus, and fat content should be optimal in selected food sources. Whole adult prey items are always preferred.

In situations where food quality and availability are limited, care should be taken to supplement the necessary vitamins, minerals, and deficient components as needed for each meal. It must be emphasized that supplementation should be calculated carefully based on analysis of the food source as well as nutritional requirements for that species. As with other growing birds, calcium and phosphorus must be balanced at a 2 : 1 ratio by weight to avoid development of metabolic bone disease. Feeding whole adult prey animals avoids this problem. As a general rule, if whole adult prey items are not fed, calcium must be supplemented at a level that provides twice as many milligrams of elemental calcium as phosphorus in the deficient food. Bone meal is not an appropriate calcium supplement because it also contains phosphorus at a fixed ratio to calcium. Powdered calcium carbonate is the calcium supplement of choice.

FEEDING PROCEDURES

Frequency of feeding should be based on the digestion and clearance time of meals. Since owls lack a true crop, the gizzard is often used as an indicator. An empty, flaccid, or ill-defined lower abdomen represents a presumably empty gastrointestinal tract. When full, the gizzard is easily palpated as an obvious, dense, round mass in the lower abdomen. Body weight should be monitored daily and should begin to show a consistent daily increase within no more than 48 hours after intake.

Careful consideration should be used when formulating a feeding plan for growing owls. Hatchlings and young unfeathered nestlings do not have fully developed digestive systems. In most species, the male provides the food and the female stays with the young as a source of heat, protection, and feeding. She will tear food into edible pieces depending on the age of the chick. When cutting food into bite-size pieces, the size of the mouth and throat should be considered. The following sections on feeding considerations are based on the natural history and development of growing owls. Captive recommendations should ideally replicate general natural behaviors.

Hatchlings

The digestive system of newly hatched owls may take as long as 36 hours to be functional in most species. Hatchlings may be hydrated orally with a few drops of water once vocalizations become persistent. Solid food should not be offered to most species for the first 24 hours; the chick's vocalizations at this age are believed to stimulate specific hormonal responses in the parents, not to actually acquire solid food yet. Digestive function in unfeathered hatchlings can be confirmed by the passage and elimination of droppings.

Young hatchlings of most owl species are usually fed every few hours, with 4–5 feedings daily. At this young age, food should be torn into small pieces of easily digestible parts, such as organ meat, muscle, and skin. These bite-size pieces are gently rubbed on the edge of the beak. Food should not be colder than room temperature and should be fresh. Although easily digested parts are preferred, parents do not debone or carefully eviscerate prey. Fragments of bone, skin, fur, and stomach contents are included in the natural diet at all ages. Using this as a reference, a small fragment of bone should be included in the diet of healthy hatchlings, because they require calcium even at this young age (see Figure 24.4). Be sure to remove any sharp edges that may irritate or injure their sensitive esophageal tissue. Tenderizing pieces with a mortar and pestle may be helpful when necessary.

Owlets should be bright eyed and active before feeding and may sleep soundly after a satisfying meal. Weak, slow babies with dull eyes should be evaluated for problems as quickly as possible. Often, hydration and adjustment of supplemental heat can make a significant difference. Compromised individuals of any age should be fed small amounts often and should be given highly digestible and

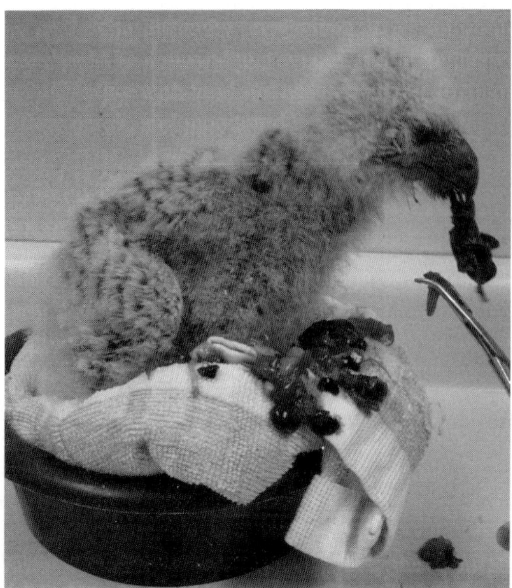

Figure 24.4. Owlet eating offered pieces of rodent prey.

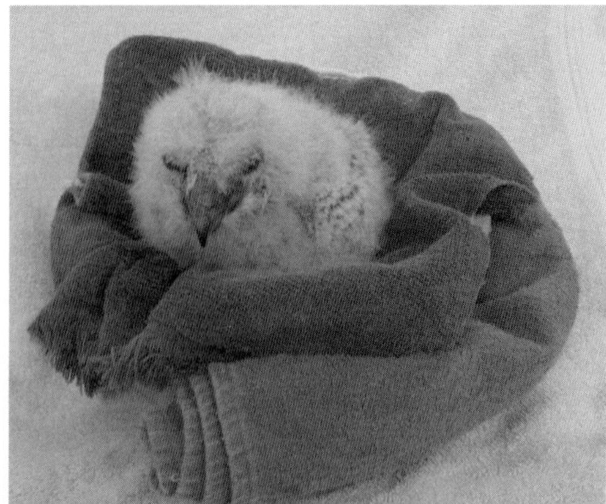

Figure 24.5. Owlet in appropriately sized cloth nest.

balanced foods until they are digesting and processing food correctly. Body weight, digestive function, and general behavior should be monitored throughout growth.

Nestlings and Fledglings

Size and quality of food pieces should be increased as the baby grows and develops. Skin, fur, and feathers should be gradually added and pellet formation monitored and recorded. Digestibility of bones is also evident in pellet appearance. Healthy birds that are gaining weight, eating well, digesting food efficiently, and producing normal-looking pellets should be offered increasingly complete meals until food can be presented in its whole form. Healthy babies that are old enough to physically process whole food should never be offered anything less. Tree-nesting species learn to tear whole food at an early age. Exceptions should be made only when necessary in individual cases.

HOUSING

Hatchlings and Nestlings

At this young age, the mother's body provides a constant source of heat. Owlets will huddle against or burrow underneath her for warmth or may move or lean away to cool off. The nest floor should be placed safely on a protected heating pad set on the lowest setting and should be positioned with up to 80% of the floor on heat to create a heat gradient. Owlets should seek or use heat as they would a warm-bodied parent. Any individual actively and continually moving off or away from heat should be watched closely because this is often the first observable behavior of dying chicks. If noted, consult an avian veterinarian immediately.

Artificial nests should be designed with respect to each species' nesting style and should be placed in the back corner of the cage or incubator. Cavity-nesters should be offered a nest box large enough to allow movement, with solid walls for natural security as well as for a physical boundary (see Figure 24.5). These species tend to huddle and lean in corners and will likely fall over the rim of conventional open nests. Tree-nesters should be offered bowl-shaped nests with edges high enough to crouch behind and lean against but low enough to reach heads out over the rim. Heavy crocks and dog bowls padded and covered with fabric can be used as a nest structure for larger bodied clutches and smaller heavy bowls may be ideal for smaller species. Many owl species will sleep with neck limp and head hanging over edge.

Whatever style of housing is used, the front of the cage should be adequately covered to provide the nest with a visual barrier to human activity but should also allow partial exposure to light.

Thermoregulatory abilities develop as feathers grow, and supplemental heat can be gradually removed once the bird is adequately insulated.

Owlets may be housed in heavy, dark plastic kennels. The nest should be placed in a back corner with adjacent holes covered. Natural perches of the appropriate size for these birds should be provided to ease the first step out of the nest. The size of the kennel should be at least as wide as the length of the wingspan and should be enlarged as the birds grow.

As vision improves with age, the young nestlings become increasingly aware of their surroundings. It is presently believed that programmed identification and recognition behaviors develop during this period (McKeever 1987). Social development and permanent associations are consistently linked to this stage of cognitive development. Owlets that remain in their natural environment through this stage usually exhibit much wilder and more aggressive behaviors. They actively respond to human presence and seem to recognize natural threats. Those that were captive or in a modified environment during this stage may still recognize and avoid handling and human activity in general, but they are usually less aggressive and behave more passively in comparison.

It is imperative that conspecific companions be provided. Ideally, surrogate or foster owl parents should be present or at least visible at all times, and human presence should be reduced or, if possible, eliminated. As soon as each owlet is reliably self-feeding, growing, and able to maintain body temperature, the cage should be set up outside for increasing lengths of time until the bird is acclimated to ambient outdoor temperatures. If extreme weather and drastic temperature changes necessitate indoor shelter for these young babies, they should still be placed near a window for visual stimuli. Protected structures with open doors or windows (porches, garages, sheds) may help acclimation in questionable climates. If the temperature drops more than 15°F (8°C), a supplemental heat source should be offered as an option to all ages.

Fledglings

Owlets quickly become more physically active and mobile. They start to stand and will begin to branch or climb on and around the nest edge and beyond. In many tree nesting species, family groups, including the mother bird as well as siblings of varying sizes, may be easily observed throughout the tree. As active and mature as these adolescents may appear, their flight feathers have a long way to go. Fledglings raised in captivity should be housed outdoors as early as possible. They spend much of their time watching their new world from the comfort of their perch.

Aviaries for small owls have a recommended minimum size of 8 × 8 × 8 ft (2.4 × 2.4 × 2.4 m). Medium-sized species such as Barn Owls should have aviaries of at least 10 × 30 × 12 ft (3 × 9 × 3.6 m). Large owls such as Great Horned Owls require large flight cages of minimum dimensions 10 × 50 × 12 ft (3 × 15 × 3.6 m) (Miller 2000). Development of flight agility can be enhanced by designing the aviary in a *L* shape or by placing movable baffles extending from the side walls that birds must bank and turn to fly past. Live prey arenas must be included for all species. These can be as simple as a large metal tub in which live rodents are placed, or an arena that may be set into the floor of the enclosure. Prevention of prey escape is an important factor. As birds become more adept at catching prey, the rodents should be allowed more hiding places within the arena.

RELEASE CONSIDERATIONS

Flighted juveniles of most owl species remain in the nesting territory for a considerably long period of time. Parents continue to provide food as owlets leisurely practice their flight and hunting skills. Owls seem to require more overall support during their training than other species of raptors. Young owls should be restricted to hunting of live prey for at least 3 weeks before release. Late-season captive-reared birds that were not exposed to what seems to be necessary training are less likely to survive their first winter. Many facilities overwinter fall owlets to allow extra time for practice and overall maturation. First-year owls that are released in the fall should be soft-released and provided with a feeding station. It is not uncommon for Great Horned Owls to return to a recognized feeding spot several times over the course of the winter. Nature would not provide this extra time and amount of assistance unless it was necessary for survival.

ACKNOWLEDGMENTS

I would like to gratefully acknowledge and dedicate this writing to my family.

SOURCES FOR PRODUCTS MENTIONED

Sevin Dust: GardenTech, PO Box 24830, Lexington, KY 40524-4830, (800) 969-7200.

Capstar (Nitenpyram): Novartis Animal Health, (800) 637-0281.

REFERENCES

Bent, A.C. 1938. Life Histories of North American Birds of Prey. Dover Publications, New York.

Engelmann, M. and Marcum, P. 1993. Raptor Rehabilitation. Carolina Raptor Center.

Fosco, L. 1997. Great Horned Owls: Natural history and its role in wildlife rehabilitation. Proceedings of the International Wildlife Rehabilitation Council Annual Conference. Concord, California, pp. 173–177.

Johnsgard, P.A. 1988. North American Owls: Biology and Natural History. Smithsonian Institution Press, Washington, D.C., 295 pp.

Long, K. 1998. Owls, A Wildlife Handbook. Johnson Publishing Company, Chicago, 181 pp.

Macleod, A. and Perlman, J. 2003. Wildlife Feeding and Nutrition. International Wildlife Rehabilitation Council, 73 pp.

McKeever, K. 1987. Care and Rehabilitation of Injured Owls. W.F. Rannie Publishing, Lincoln, Ontario, Canada, 128 pp.

Miller, E.A., ed. 2000. Minimum Standards for Wildlife Rehabilitation, 3rd Edition. National Wildlife Rehabilitation Association, St. Cloud, Minnesota, 77 pp.

Redig, P.T. 1993. Medical Management of Birds of Prey. The Raptor Center at the University of Minnesota.

Tyler, H.A. and Phillips, D. 1978. Owls by Day and Night. Naturegraph Publishers, Inc., Happy Camp, California. 208 pp.

Walker, L.W. 1993. The Book of Owls. University of Texas Press, Austin, 255 pp.

25
Goatsuckers

Linda Hufford

NATURAL HISTORY

The goatsuckers are classified within the order Caprimulgiformes, which consists of five diverse but fascinating families with many unusual metabolic and lifestyle adaptations. The most current taxonomy places order Caprimulgiformes near the owl (Strigiformes) order by DNA-DNA hybridization (Sibley and Ahlquist 1990). The goatsuckers, family Caprimulgidae, nighthawks and nightjars, will be discussed in this chapter in detail as representatives of their order. Other Caprimulgids include the owlet-nightjars (Aegothelidae), sometimes referred to as *moth owls* in their native Australasia. These tiny long-tailed birds with an upright posture are capable of torpor during cold days. Also Australasian natives, the Frogmouths (Podargidae) are named quite descriptively for their wide cavernous mouths as well as their booming night sound. Prey consists of mostly insects, some of which are enticed within range by an odor exuded from the mouth of the bird. Frogmouths are kept in many zoological institutions because unlike many birds in this order, they can adapt to eating out of dishes. Potoos (Nyctibiidae) are South American birds that have a unique feature of the eyelids: two small slits that allow the bird to see even with the eyes closed. Perched on a tree with their beaks upraised, these long-clawed birds look like broken branches. Among the most interesting and unique of all birds, the Oilbirds (Steatornithidae) of South America are so named because the young are fed rich, oily fruits until at about 30 days of age when they are 150% the weight of the adults. At one time, the chicks were rendered to make torch oil. These cave-dwelling frugivores are thought to be unique in that they use echolocation in near-total darkness.

The term *Goatsucker* (family Caprimulgidae) is a common inclusive name that includes subfamilies of the New World nighthawks (Chordeilinae) and the typical nightjars (Caprimulginae). In North America, the birds known by the common names of Chuck Will's Widow, Common Pauraque, Whip-poor-will, Common Poorwill, and Buff-collared Nightjars are considered nightjars. Those known as Common Nighthawks, Antillean Nighthawks, and Lesser Nighthawks are usually referred to as nighthawks.

Both subfamilies have common general physical traits. Their large flat heads blend into the rounded body to give the appearance of the birds having no necks. A tiny weak bill with prominent nares (the nostrils of which are flexible tubes) conceals a cavernous mouth that is shockingly large when opened. Also owl-like is the lack of development of a true crop.

Short, tiny, weak legs seem to disappear when the bird is perched. Caprimulgids have an anisodactyl toe arrangement with three toes forward and one toe back, and there is partial webbing between the front-facing toes. Located on the inner claw of the middle toe of some species is a pectinated claw, also known as a *feathercomb.*

Virtually silent flight is accomplished as it is in owls, with softened leading edges of the primaries. Camouflage coloring, combined with a unique horizontal perching position, make these birds virtually disappear when resting on a branch or in leaf litter (see Figure 25.1). The feathers are cryptically colored with penciling, blotching, and mottling. The fragile, loose feathers are colored brown, tan, gray, or rust, and the hues blend well with the natural background of their chosen environments. Generally, those in higher altitudes are lighter in color, as are those found in desert areas.

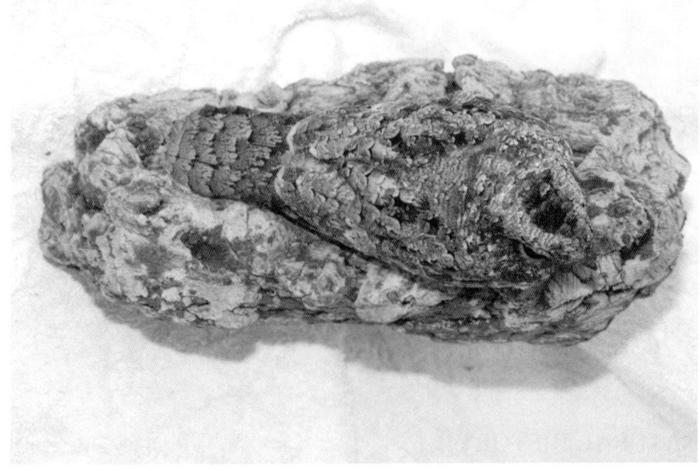

Figure 25.1. Goatsuckers have cryptic plumage that allows them to blend into their environment (photo courtesy of Peter Butler).

All species engage in dust-bathing to condition their delicate feathers. Adult birds may also indulge in aerial bathing when relaxed. Because the oil gland in goatsuckers is atrophied, preening consists of distributing fat from the feathers of the breast with the use of the bill and the pectinated claw. Some species have a strong, earthy smell.

Goatsucker wings are designed for maneuverability and swiftness to pursue the variety of insects that compose the majority of their diet (see Figure 25.2). Even the eyes of the goatsuckers are designed for their nocturnal or crepuscular hunting habits; the large dark eyes have a tapetum that reflects unabsorbed light, resulting in a distinctive red or red-orange eye-shine. The eyes are situated laterally, offering a wide view during flight. One feature unique to goatsuckers is the ability to control their upper eyelids.

Generally, nightjars have rounded wings with no white feathering. They are nocturnal feeders and have obvious rictal feathering. The wingtips do not extend past the tail, and they have feathered tarsi. Nighthawks, on the other hand, have pointed wings with white covert feathers that are visible when they are sitting. There may be white patches on the wings, the specific markings of which vary by species. The wings cross over the back and extend beyond the tail. Rictal feathering is obscure or does not exist in these crepuscular and nocturnal birds. The long forked tail is also distinct. Although most goatsucker chicks are raised in a similar manner, it becomes essential near release time to identify the proper

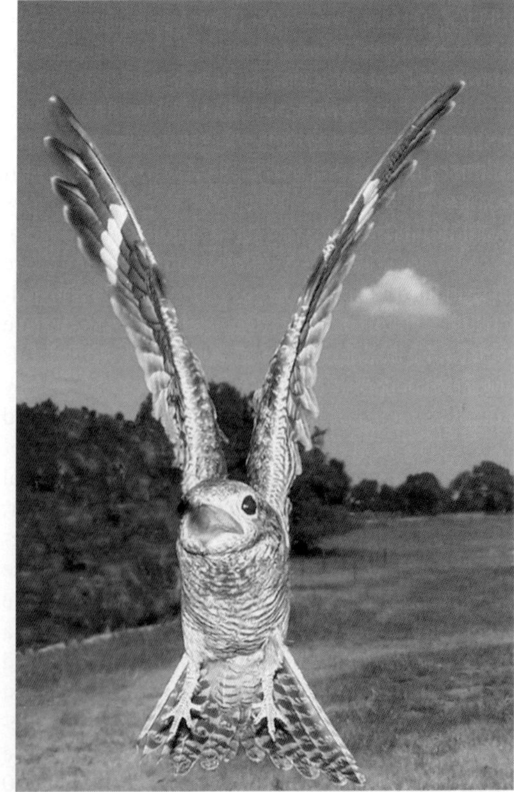

Figure 25.2. Goatsuckers are extremely agile fliers and must have full flight dexterity to qualify for release.

Table 25.1. Characteristics of six species of N.A. goatsuckers.

Common Name	Chick Down	Bill Color	Legs/Feet Color	Adult Weight
Common Nighthawk	Gray, buff w/mottled dark-brown upper parts	Dark blue-black	Drab brown	58–91 g
Lesser Nighthawk	Buff with mottled brown upperparts	Black	Gray, brownish	34–55 g
Chuck Will's Widow	Golden brown or yellowish ochre	Dusky, pinkish beige, black tip	Dull buff	94–137 g
Whip-poor-will	Cinnamon, pale buff, brown, fades to yellow tan	Dark brown, black	Purple-gray or brown	49–68 g
Common Poorwill	Pale buff, gray-buff, tinged purple	Brown or black	Pinkish-brown	31–58 g
Common Pauraque	Brown, pinkish buff	Black	Gray	43–66 g

release criteria and to recognize the signs of physical maturity of each species. The use of a good field guide may help identify specific species or subspecies of goatsuckers; weights and territorial ranges may also be helpful (see Table 25.1). Particularly in the northern parts of the U.S. and Canada, most species can be ruled out by location. This is not always possible in the southern U.S. or northern Mexico during migration.

Migration is achieved for some species in flocks during daylight hours. Nonmigratory species, primarily the Common Poorwill, enter torpor, a state resulting in a lowered heart rate, breathing rate, and metabolism with reduced response to external stimulation.

Reproduction

After an aerial courtship, during which the male often "booms" and tail-flashes, the pair bond and breed. Generally, two eggs (rarely up to four) are laid on consecutive days on the ground, on broken tree stumps, or on flat roofs with little or no nesting materials.

Incubation is 17–21 days, with either the male or the female being the primary daytime caregiver, species-specifically. Also species-dependent is whether the eggs hatch together or on consecutive days. When necessary, the adult will move the eggs out of direct sunlight or dangerous circumstances by pushing the eggs with feet or breast.

With weak feet and a tiny bill, goatsuckers are basically defenseless against predators; camouflage is one of the few defenses available for the adults and the young. The nest is made of natural earth-tone materials, the eggs are patterned to be obscure, and the still chicks' down blends well with the surrounding area. Adults on a nest use techniques to change their body profiles by flattening the upper feathers to the body, lowering the head to the ground, and changing the posture of the body to engulf the nest. The bird then closes its eyes and maintains complete stillness. If this camouflage attempt does not work, the adult will aggressively defend the nest by flaring its feathers to appear larger and will launch an intimidating but harmless open-mouth attack while hissing.

If threats are not effective, attempts to lure and confuse will follow. The female may feign a broken wing in an attempt to lure the predator away from the nest while the males may circle and dive on the intruder while wing-clapping.

Development of Chicks

The chicks begin peeping before hatching. The eggs pip, and then open in perfect halves. The semiprecocial chicks are capable of movement within the nest on the day of hatch. For species where hatch weights are published (Cink 2002; Poulin et al. 1996), the chicks weigh 5–6 g and have a very sparse covering of soft down. Pinfeathers emerge along the wing and scapular tracts by day 10. When the nest is disturbed, chicks will rapidly scatter, with each chick going in a different direction away from the nest as an effort to confuse the predator. By day 16 for nightjars, and day 18 for nighthawks, the primaries are unsheathed and chicks respond to parental warning cries by hopping or flying short distances. Chicks become thermally independent between days 20–23, depending upon species. They are no longer brooded, but continue to be fed by the parents. At about 25 days of age, chicks are capable of catching their own food, although parents may still furnish backup feedings. By day 30, the chicks of all species are feeding independently and flying well. They leave their nest permanently. Migratory species will join a flock in preparation for their long journey at about 7 weeks of age.

CRITERIA FOR INTERVENTION

Chicks may come into care for a variety of reasons: they may be found when remodeling or repairing a flat roof, recovered from construction sites where nests are accidentally disturbed, and even from the backs of delivery trucks, where the parents may have chosen an unfortunate nesting site. Re-nesting recently discovered uninjured chicks is the best resolution, but if that is not possible they can be raised with care relatively easily.

INITIAL CARE AND STABILIZATION

As with any young bird, warming first is essential. Place the bird in a padded container on a heating pad set on low for 15–20 minutes until it is relaxed and warm. Please see Chapter 1, "General Care," for stabilization of newly admitted birds.

Goatsucker feathers are extremely delicate, and extreme measures must be taken to ensure that damage is not sustained in captivity. Use a silk or polyester material (such as a scarf) to protect the feathers during handling. If it is an emergency situation and such material cannot be located immediately, thoroughly wash and rinse the examination area and the examiner's hands with soap and water to remove any oils that could contaminate the feathers. Be aware that even young chicks will probably hiss and gape in a very threatening manner; this is a harmless but startling tactic. Do not hold the bird by the legs, as is common when examining raptors. Many goatsuckers will remain still at approach, and then suddenly flush. To avoid injuries to the bird, one hand should be placed above the bird, while the second hand does a slow approach from the side. Uninjured chicks may be quite adept at evasive running maneuvers and may leap unexpectedly off the examination table.

The eyes should be clear and liquid-looking, and the eyelids rather loose-fitting. During daylight or under bright lights, the eyelids may appear to be half-opened. This is normal. Hold the bird with the feathers laying in proper alignment and the wings folded against the body. To check wing alignment, hold an index and third finger on either side of the neck, pinning the bird down. A detailed palpation of the wings can be achieved by holding one folded wing against the body while examining the other. To check the mouth, brush or blow softly on the rictal feathering. This may trigger a snapping motion, so be prepared with a halved tongue depressor or a large paper clip to enter from the side of the mouth. Once in place, these can then be slowly turned sideways to open the mouth enough for viewing, without risking injury to the jaws. Examine the remainder of the body as you would any species of bird. Common Poorwills found during cold weather should be evaluated for torpor. Torpid birds should be slowly warmed before examination in order to fully evaluate their condition. Torpor is an energy-conserving reduction of the heart, respiratory, and metabolic rates. The torpor of a Common Poorwill studied in 1994 recorded body temperatures of less than 41°F (5°C), which constitutes the lowest body temperature ever recorded for any species of wild bird. One experiment kept a poor-will in torpor at 50°F (10°C) for 100 days, with a resulting weight loss of only 10 g of stored fat (Howell and Bartholomew 1959). Torpor can be induced by either a 20% weight loss or by cold weather. Even poor-will chicks have been found in torpor.

COMMON MEDICAL PROBLEMS

Little is known about the medical disorders of these species; most chicks are brought into care through unnecessary seizures. Adult goatsuckers commonly arrive with injuries from vehicles. The birds are attracted to insects, which are, in turn, attracted to car headlights. Many times this collision results in a compound fracture or semiamputated wing. Most rehabilitators consider nighthawks with serious wing fractures to be candidates for euthanasia, due to the need for perfect flight maneuverability. Well-aligned, midshaft fractures of the radius, ulna, or metacarpal

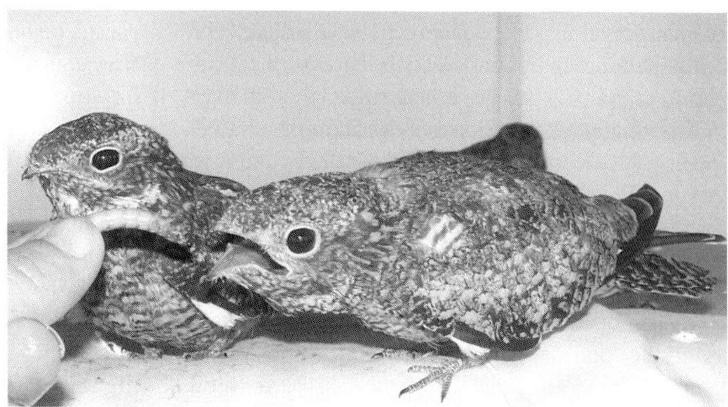

Figure 25.3. Chicks being hand-fed will lunge forward with mouths open to accept food. Note the extremely small feet typical of goatsuckers.

bones with minimal soft tissue damage may have a better prognosis, but should be evaluated on a case-by-case basis. All wing injuries must be considered extremely serious; a nighthawk or nightjar without viable flight is a nonreleasable bird. Goatsuckers may present with skin lacerations from predator attacks. Keep any feather removals from wound cleaning to an absolute minimum, and any tape applied in the course of wing wraps or other bandaging must take feather condition into account. See Chapter, 1 "General Care," for suggestions of antibiotic therapy for birds with open wounds.

FEEDING PROCEDURES

In captivity, all goatsuckers must be hand-fed. Neither the adults nor juveniles will self-feed in captivity, although they will often learn to accept foods flung or dropped for them, and they may fly to insects held aloft. The technique used while feeding is important. Perhaps because of the lateral eyes, goatsuckers appear not to recognize a still body as food. When hand-feeding, use a "zooming" motion with the food held in blunt forceps or hemostats, lightly brushing or tickling the rictus feathers. In the wild, parents feed chicks regurgitated insects two or three times each dusk and dawn. In captivity they are fed three or four times a day on a diet of primarily commercially available insects such as mealworms, waxworms, superworms, and crickets dipped in an insectivore formula (see Chapter 34 "Passerines: Hand-Feeding Diets"). As wide a variety of insects should be used as possible. The insects most often found in stomach contents of smaller goatsuckers are beetles, moths, flies, mosquitoes, grasshoppers, plant lice, locusts, horseflies,

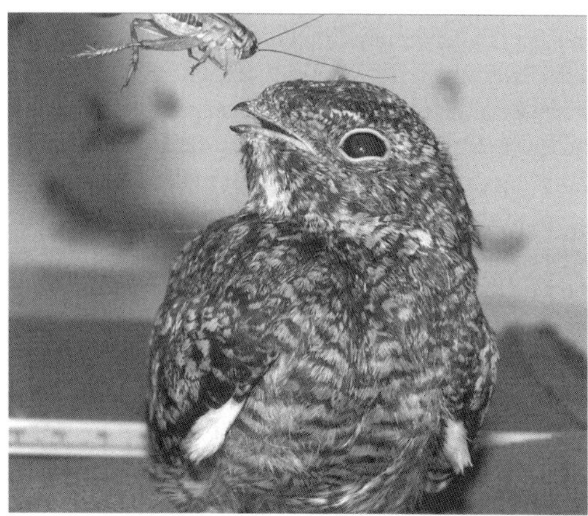

Figure 25.4. Insect prey may be offered with forceps. A zooming motion with the offered food may stimulate the chick to eat.

winged ants, wasps, bees, chinch bugs, and caterpillars. The much larger Chuck Will's Widow has even been found to have consumed whole small birds and small mice. Chicks will adapt easily to hand-feeding, and will come to the realization that food is imminent when the caretaker nears the cage. Caution should be used because the chicks will lunge toward the feeder with wings outspread and mouths wide open, often with a frantic-sounding peep. Chicks should be fed as much and often as demanded (see Figures 25.3, 25.4). A short rest during the feeding period, followed by an offer of additional food, works well.

Adults, on the other hand, are notorious for being difficult to feed in captivity. The normal heavy feeding times of most species are during the 45-minute period just after dawn and before dusk. The birds will be more cooperative during this time period while in care. To reduce stress, first attempt to use the zooming motion mentioned in the general feeding section. Many adults will quickly adapt to this method. For the less cooperative, gently open the jaws and insert the food toward the back of the mouth. Hold the head up slightly with one fingertip beneath the jaw after the feeding because it is common for the adults to shake their heads to dislodge the food or they may hold and dispose of it later without swallowing. Check the substrate several minutes after each feeding for signs of regurgitation. Adults may eat only at the periods of time of their normal feeding in the wild. If repeated feeding attempts during these times fail and the bird is in danger of starvation, force-feeding may be necessary. Hold the bird's body wrapped with a scarf in the left hand (for right-handed caregivers), and use the right hand to come beneath the body with the thumb and fourth finger on either side of the bird's temporal-mandibular joint (the intersection of the upper and lower jaws). Very gently pry open the joint with both sides receiving equal pressure. As soon as there is gape, insert a paper clip from the side of the mouth to the opposing side. The index and second finger can be used to hold the food, and when the jaws are open the food can be pushed to the back of the mouth, using care to place the food on top of the tongue.

An insectivore hand-feeding formula (see Chapter 34) can be used with a Catac ST1 nipple (Catac Products Limited) at the end of a syringe using the same approach. Goatsuckers are difficult to feed by gavage. Great care must be taken when forcing the mouth open, because the mandibles are very easily broken. However, if necessary, a 6 in (15 cm) section of cut-off IV extension set or other narrow flexible tubing may be used to tube-feed. Burn the cut end of the tube to avoid sharp edges and attach the female fitting of the tubing to an appropriately sized syringe. Open the mouth as described previously while restraining the bird on a table, and then visualize the opening to the esophagus within the mouth. Spiral the tubing down this opening such that the tube curves around to follow the esophagus as deep as the end of the bird's ribcage. When inserting the tube it may feel as though the bird has a 90° bend in the esophagus from straight down toward the table and then abruptly curving to be parallel to the table. Adults have been successfully maintained for several weeks during care in captivity using this method. Again, beware of causing any damage to the delicate feathers during handling. Feed 5% of body weight in volume of hand-feeding formula (50 ml/kg) 4–6 times a day: for example, 2 ml formula 4–6 times a day for a 40 g bird (R. Duerr personal communication). Weigh the bird daily at the same time each day to track gains, because the metabolism of the individuals may vary. After feeding, all birds should be wiped carefully with a damp cotton swab or ball to remove any residual food or fluids from the rictal and facial feathers and nares. When old enough for flight, place the bird in a large flight cage and introduce into the cage flying insects such as dragonflies, beetles, moths, butterflies, and bees. Each bird should be weighed daily to assure no weight loss, and backup hand-feeding should be continued until the birds are released. Some goatsuckers, primarily Chuck Will's Widows and Lesser Nighthawks, have been observed in the wild picking up small pieces of rocks and swallowing them. This may be due to a need for supplemental minerals, or it may be as an aid in digestion. While in care, crushed eggshells or oyster shell calcium can be made available by sprinkling on the substrate surface.

EXPECTED WEIGHT GAIN

Chicks should gain weight daily and should reach or exceed adult weight by the time they are 4 weeks of age. See Table 25.1 for adult weights of several goatsucker species.

HOUSING

Wire cages should be avoided at all times. Most rehabilitators use solid-sided caging for young birds or injured adults during recovery. Plastic port-a-kennels or airline kennels for dogs are a good choice if the front grates are covered with insect screening. A light stitching with heavy thread through the weave of the screening will hold it in place. Avoid using duct tape or any other type of adhesive that may come loose and cause feather damage. In an emergency, a draped cardboard box may be used.

Substrate

Clean sand is recommended as a substrate, and it provides the additional benefit of heating evenly. The sand can be sculptured to provide indentations and raised areas. An added benefit to sand is that the birds may use it for dust-bathing, which will help with feather conditioning.

Egg-crate foam, actual egg cartons, or even shredded newspapers piled irregularly can be laid across the bottom of the cage to provide contoured flooring. This substrate can then be covered with fleece. Fleece is washable, inexpensive, and has the additional benefit of being available in various patterns. If given a choice, choose a dark variegated pattern. Fleece will not catch the tiny toes of the bird, as will a looped towel, nor does it have feather-damaging oils, as newspapers do. Insecticide-free dry leaf litter may also be placed on the bottom of the cage in uneven piles if replaced regularly to avoid mold. Darker colors or camouflage patterns seem to provide comfort to the birds, even the youngest chicks will generally choose to sit or lie on the colors with which they best blend (see Figure 25.5).

Cleanliness is of extreme importance, whatever substrate material is chosen. The substrate must be maintained meticulously to avoid feces or spilled formula from contacting and damaging the delicate feathers. Occasionally, a casting may be found, which will contain undigested insect parts; this should also be disposed of during cleaning.

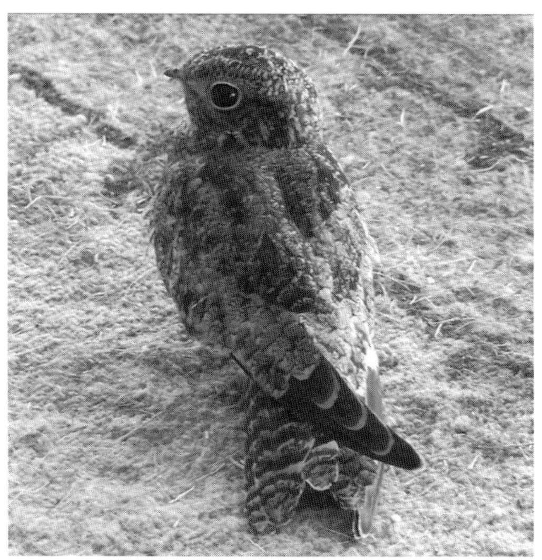

Figure 25.5. Goatsuckers may be more relaxed on substrate that allows them to blend in. Use dark or mottled substrate whenever possible. Dark carpeting is shown.

Perches

Typical songbird perches are not utilized by goatsuckers. They will perch either on the ground, or laterally and horizontally on a wide branch or rock. While in care, an elevated area may be provided through the use of a contoured substrate, a large branch or small log, or a large rough rock. Rocks and sand will retain heat better than woods, and both rocks and woods can be elevated enough to keep the delicate feathers away from feces.

Providing Water

Some rehabilitators have noticed that the birds will defecate in water dishes, but none have reported goatsuckers actually drinking water while in care. In the wild, some goatsuckers have been observed drinking by skimming still water with their lower jaws while flying, or rarely while sitting at the edge of a still-water pond. Moisture is presumed to be primarily provided by the fluid content of insects, many of which are comprised of 70% fluids. Young chicks or injured adults may drown or become chilled, so water should be made available only to healthy adults in prerelease housing.

Providing Supplemental Heat

There are two important considerations when artificially heating. Temperatures that are too cool may induce torpor in some species, too hot may induce gular fluttering. When chilled, the metabolism is slowed. Gular fluttering uses metabolic energy to cool the body. Neither of these conditions is conducive to the bird's well being.

Heat should be furnished for any chick less than 3 weeks of age, or for a traumatized adult. Heat can be provided in the form of a heating pad placed under the cage, through the use of an overhead heat lamp, or with reptile ceramic radiant heaters. Heaters have the advantage of producing heat without producing light, which is a consideration for nocturnal species. Full-spectrum lighting can be provided with the use of heat lamps. Generally, the ambient air should be approximately 90°F (32.2°C) for older chicks or injured adults, slightly higher for younger chicks. Whichever method is chosen, be certain the heat source is placed to avoid overheating the enclosure. Overhead heat lamps should be encased to prevent contact that may cause singed feathers or legs.

Observation is essential. Watch the movements of the bird; if it prefers to lay far away from the heat source, consider reducing the temperature. If laying directly beneath or above the heat source, consider increasing temperatures by small increments and continue to observe. Although studies have shown that Common Poorwills efficiently tolerate the extreme heat of their desert and prairie environments by using gular fluttering to facilitate a heat exchange, this fluttering may be an important sign of overheating when you are using an artificial heat source. If you observe this behavior, immediately remove the heat source until the ambient air has cooled, and watch carefully as you slowly reintroduce heat.

WEANING

Because most species will not eat from a dish, an approximation of weaning occurs when the bird proves that it is capable of feeding itself by catching free-flying insects. Once the flight feathers have fully emerged, move the chicks to an outdoor aviary. A lightbulb (enclosed in a wire basket to prevent close contact) placed in the cage and away from the birds should invite native flying insects at the appropriate feeding times. If necessary, insects can also be netted and put into the cage for testing purposes. Miller (2000) recommends an aviary size of 8 × 16 × 8 ft (2.4 × 4.9 × 2.4 m) to contain a maximum of six birds. Prior to release, a complete physical examination is important. Feathers should be checked carefully for any signs of distress that may hinder flight maneuverability, any previous fractures checked for alignment, and eyes examined. If there is no obvious reason not to release, the bird should be flight-tested and exercised in the largest flight cage available to build up muscle strength.

Maneuverability must be exceptional. A flight cage with obstructions, such as hanging branches or even sheets of canvas, should be utilized for observations of banking and swerving capabilities. Keep in mind the hunting practices used by the individual species; these will range from sustained flight, as in nighthawks, to short sallies by many other species. All members must have the ability to corner, bank, dive, swerve, and gain altitude quickly.

RELEASE

It may be important for sedentary birds to be released into the area where originally found; however, during migration the bird may not have a local home territory, so release should be in an area that is safe, provides the proper foods, and allows the bird a high likelihood of survival. When planning a release, keep in mind that goatsuckers are crepuscular or nocturnal birds. After a full feeding, release right at dusk or just before dawn. Choose a safe area away from traffic, raptors, and, if possible, where the recent use of insecticides is unlikely. This provides the birds with an opportunity to begin their freedom safely. Whenever possible, time releases according to weather and moon phases. A clear forecast and a full moon will enhance foraging. Goatsuckers that are not physically capable of catching sufficient numbers of insects should never be released. Very few nonreleasable birds are placeable because they do not learn to self-feed, and few care facilities are willing to maintain a feeding regimen for the life of the bird.

ACKNOWLEDGMENTS

The author wishes to acknowledge and thank many fellow rehabilitators who generously contributed their experiences, among these particularly Gloria Halesworth, Sigrid Ueblacker, Rebecca Duerr, and Nancy Eilertsen.

SOURCES FOR PRODUCTS MENTIONED

Catac nipples: Catac Products Limited, Catac House, 1 Newnham Street, Bedford Mk40 3jr England, Tel: +44 (0) 1234 360116, Fax: +44 (0) 1234 346406, http://www.catac.co.uk.
Also available from Chris's Squirrels and More, LLC, P.O. Box 365, Somers CT 06071, (860) 749-1129, http://www.thesquirrelstore.com

REFERENCES

Bent, A.C. 1962. Life histories of North American Cuckoos, Goatsuckers, Hummingbirds, and Their Allies. Dover Press, New York, 506 pp.

Cink, C.L. 2002. Whip-poor-will (*Caprimulgus vociferus*). In The Birds of North America, No. 620 (Poole, A. and Gill, F., eds. The Birds of North America, Inc., Philadelphia.

Cleere, N. 1998. Nightjars: A Guide to Nightjars and Related Nightbirds. Yale University Press, New Haven, Connecticut, 317 pp.

Forbush, E. and May, J. 1939. Natural History of American Birds of Eastern and Central North

America. Houghton Mifflin Company, Boston, 553 pp.

Howell, T.R. and Bartholomew, G.A. 1959. Further experiments on torpidity in the poor-will. Condor 61(3): 180–185.

Ligon, J.D. 1970. Still more responses of the poor-will to low temperatures. Condor 72(4): 496–498.

Miller, E.A., ed. 2000. Minimum Standards for Wildlife Rehabilitation, 3rd Edition. National Wildlife Rehabilitation Association, St. Cloud, Minnesota, 77 pp. http://www.nwrawildlife.org/documents/Standards3rdEdition.pdf.

Perrins, C. 1979. Birds: Their Life, Their Ways, Their World. Reader's Digest Association, Pleasantville, New York, 411 pp.

Poulin, R.G., Grindal, S.D., and Brigham, R.M. 1996. Common nighthawk (*Chordeiles minor*). In The Birds of North America, No. 213 (Poole, A. and Gill, F., eds. The Academy of Natural Sciences, Philadelphia, and The American Ornithologists' Union, Washington, D.C.

Sibley, C.G. and Ahlquist, J.E. 1990. Phylogeny and Classification of Birds: A Study in Molecular Evolution. Yale University Press, New Haven, Connecticut, 976 pp.

Terres, J. 1991. The Audubon Society Encyclopedia of North American Birds, Wings Books New Jersey, 1053 pp.

26
Turacos

Kateri J. Davis

NATURAL HISTORY

The turacos of order Musophagiformes, are found solely in Africa south of the Sahara. There are 23 species of turacos in five genera, with several subspecies identified. Common names are many, including *plantain-eater, go-away bird, loury,* and *touraco,* although *turaco* is currently the most popular.

All species are about the size of a chicken with long tails, short rounded wings, zygodactyl toe arrangement, and strong legs for running along and bounding off branches. They have smooth plumage and crests, which most can erect at will. A unique characteristic is that turacos possess two actual copper-based feather pigments: turacoverdin (green) and turacin (red).

Although there are five genera, turacos can be grouped into four basic categories: the greens (genus Tauraco), purples (genus Musophaga), greys (genera Corythaixoides and Crinifer), and the blue (one species, the Great Blue Turaco, *Corythaeola cristata*). The purples tend to be called plantain-eaters and the greys tend to be called go-away birds. There is variation in habitat, diet, and behavior between the green/purple and grey groups.

Most species of turacos are found in pairs or small groups in the mid-canopy section of evergreen and rain forest environments, with the exception of the grey group, which inhabits the drier savanna areas. Fruit is the main diet of most species, with the grey species taking more leafy fare. Occasional animal protein in the form of grubs or other insects is sometimes taken.

Turacos are monogamous and make a flat, insubstantial stick nest, much like a pigeon. They are semideterminate layers of 2–3 white eggs. The young are fed by regurgitation. All species, except the White-bellied Go-away Bird, *Criniferoides leucogaster*, are sexually monomorphic.

CRITERIA FOR INTERVENTION

Because of their color and other display qualities, turacos are some of the more commonly kept softbill private avicultural subjects in the United States and Europe, as well as being popular in many zoological institutions. The Houston Zoo in Texas, U.S. has been a leader in turaco husbandry for years. The green turacos are the most commonly kept turacos in the U.S., followed by the purples and then the greys. The Great Blue Turaco is extremely rare in captivity in the U.S. The Houston Zoo has had success with raising this species, but none are in private hands.

Hand-rearing of turacos is done usually to increase productivity of a pair, for the safety of the chick, or to have a tame adult.

RECORD KEEPING

See Chapter 29, "Mousebirds."

INCUBATION OF EGGS

In addition to cases of rescuing eggs that would be destroyed, turaco eggs are sometimes removed and artificially incubated to induce a pair of birds to lay again within a couple of weeks. It is much better for the parents to be able to raise the chicks on their own, but in certain cases, such as rare species, this is a valid technique as long as it is not overused and the female's health put at risk from excessive egg production.

Turaco eggs can be artificially incubated at a temperature of 99–100°F (37.2–37.8°C) and 45% relative humidity in a standard incubator unit. They should be turned 180° in opposite directions every 1–5 hours. Evidence of fertility can be seen by candling methods around days 7–10. See Chapter 3, "Incubation of Eggs," for greater detail.

Incubation times vary between species and even individuals. Green turacos hatch in 19–23 days, and Great Blues take 31 days. Purple and grey turacos fall between these values. Hatching can take up to 48 hours.

INITIAL CARE AND STABILIZATION

Turaco chicks are semiprecocial, opening their eyes soon after hatching (see Figure 26.4), and are very alert to their environment. Chicks in the nest will hiss, threaten an intruder with an open mouth, and defecate when handled. When incubator hatched, they will imprint on the human caregiver and typically not show these reactions unless frightened.

The newly hatched chick can stay in the incubator for a few hours until it is dry (see Figure 26.1). No food should be given the first 12–24 hours so that the yolk sac can be absorbed. The umbilicus may be swabbed with an iodine solution to help prevent infections. Watch behavior for insight into the comfort of the chick because turaco chicks will pant when too hot and will not gape or feed when too cold.

COMMON MEDICAL PROBLEMS AND SOLUTIONS

Turacos, especially the greens, are hardy and typically have few health problems. They are a group that can be affected by iron storage disease, or hemachromatosis, which is a fatal dietary condition wherein the liver stores too much iron. Although they are not as prone to this as toucans and starlings, attention should be paid to a turaco's diet, thus avoiding animal-based iron foodstuffs and citrus fruits. Low-iron softbill pellets, such as Kaytee Exact Mynah, Mazuri Softbill, or ZuPreem Softbill, should be chosen.

The most common problem seen in hand-raised turacos is splay-leg due to improper substrate. From day 1 turacos must be kept on a substrate that can be gripped easily, such as wire/plastic mesh and fibrous grass or hay. If the chick is on a surface that is too slick, the legs may be permanently damaged. In mild cases of splay-leg, the legs may be taped in position and allowed to heal for a few days. If applying tape in this manner, be sure not to cover the bird's vent with tape. Placing the chick in a small bowl to force his legs to stay under his body in proper position may sometimes be effective.

HAND-FEEDING DIET

The different groups of turacos require different diets. The greens and purples are the most com-

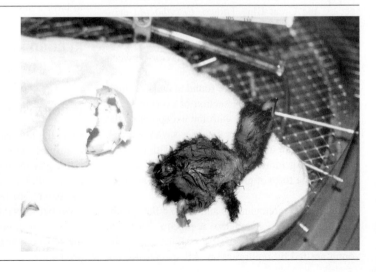

Figure 26.1. Freshly hatched Livingston Turaco in incubator drying off.

monly and successfully hand-raised, and they are more frugivorous. The greys and the Great Blue Turaco are more herbivorous as adults. Not as much is known about the nutritional needs of their chicks so rearing them is more problematic, although some people have been successful hand-raising them. There is currently much variation in hand-rearing diets used.

Feedings should start about 6:00 a.m. and continue until 10–11:00 p.m. Feeding throughout the night is unnecessary. The regularity, appearance, and amount of feces should be recorded at each feeding time to ensure that the chick is not having problems. Turaco feces are soft, brownish, somewhat formed, and sometimes have a mucous layer. If the stools are too runny, it may indicate a yeast or bacterial problem. If the stools are too dry, add a little more water to the formula. If the chick is not defecating or is straining, stimulate the vent with a warm moist swab. If the chick is not gaping and the temperature is fine, it may mean that it is constipated or dehydrated and may require fluid therapy.

Hand-Feeding Diet for Green and Purple Turacos

The following is a recommended diet for hand-feeding green and purple turacos:

- 2 parts commercial hand-feeding formula for parrots, such as Kaytee Exact Hand-feeding Formula (Kaytee Products, Inc.), mixed with warm water to reconstitute as directed on package.
- 1 part strained fruit human baby food, such as Gerber's pear, apple, papaya, or banana (Gerber Products Company).

Formula should be warm, but not hot, and should be made fresh for each meal. As the chick develops, the formula should be made with less water for a thicker pancake-batter consistency. Mashed water-soaked softbill pellets, such as Kaytee Exact Mynah, can be substituted for the hand-feeding formula in emergencies. As the chick grows, small chunks of fruit and water-soaked pellets should be fed and the amount of formula decreased.

Suggested Feeding Schedule

Larger species such as Lady Ross can take slightly larger feedings (see Table 26.1). Feeding size gradually increases throughout the day; for example, the day 2 first feeding may be 0.3 ml but by the last feeding it is 0.5 ml. Weight gain will tell the hand-feeder whether the meals are the right size.

Table 26.1. Turaco feeding schedule.

Age (days)	Meal Size (ml)	Frequency (min)
2	0.3–0.5	30
3	0.6–0.8	30–60
4	1.0–1.2	60
5–6	1.3–2.5 with pieces of fruit, such as pear, papaya, melon, apple, and soaked pellets	75

Table 26.2. Alternate turaco diet feeding schedule.

Age (Days)	Diet
0–10	Gruel mixture: fed with plastic pipette or spoon
10–18	Whole pieces of fruit and parrot pellets mixed in with gruel, offered from forceps; gradually reduce gruel
18–20	Whole foods offered from spoon or forceps
22–25	Adult turaco diet—tray left with chicks

Increase the amount of fruit and pellet pieces while reducing the amount of formula so that by day 10 or 11 the chick is eating only solid food.

Alternate Hand-Feeding Diet

The following list summarizes an alternate hand-feeding diet (See Table 26.2 for feeding schedute):

- 2 parts soaked Mazuri Parrot Breeder Pellets
- 1 part fruit: applesauce, papaya, or both
- 1 part greens: kale or endive

Add enough Pedialyte to moisten to a consistency that is from runny oatmeal to chunky peanut butter.

The solid foods offered first are usually grape, papaya, banana, or soaked parrot pellets (see Table 26.1). For Great Blue Turacos, the Houston Zoo includes additional vegetable or fruit baby food in the above gruel and increases the amount of greens in the mixture. For grey species, Mazuri Leaf-eater Primate Pellets and Mazuri Parrot pellets are included. Chicks may seem insatiable, and no problems have been seen with allowing them to eat larger amounts than other turaco species. These diets are constantly under revision, because the ideal diets for these species have not as yet been developed. Many Great Blue and grey chicks require medication for gastrointestinal upset at some point during growth. Consult an avian veterinarian for medication information.

FEEDING PROCEDURES

Turacos tend to be easy to hand-feed. They readily gape at the feeder, although older chicks that have been recently pulled from the nest take longer to adjust. Like mousebirds, they do not have a crop but have an expandable esophagus, so a swelling on the right side of the neck is normal when feeding.

Care must be taken not to overfeed to avoid aspiration. Most chicks will stop gaping when they are full but some will continue to beg even when food can be visualized in the throat. It is best to feed slowly, allowing time for the chick to swallow and not fill the esophagus to the point where food can be seen. Place the syringe on the right side of the beak while feeding to lessen the chance of aspiration. Start with a 1 ml syringe with a regular tip, and use larger syringe sizes as the chick requires more food. Some individuals will get frantic at feeding time, and the head may need to be gently corralled and held steady.

Wipe the beak and any other soiled areas of the body with a warm moist swab after each feeding to reduce the chance of infection from spoiled food. Do not allow spilled food to dry on developing feathers or get into the bird's eyes.

Some turaco species, such as Lady Ross (*Musophaga rossae*), have very prominent claws on their wrist joints resembling the Hoatzin (*Opisthocomus hoazin*). These claws disappear as the chick gets older. Also some species will use their wings like arms, to bring their body forward and push themselves upright while begging.

EXPECTED WEIGHT GAIN

Turaco chicks grow quickly. Chicks should be weighed daily before the first feeding so that weight trends can be tracked. A 5–14% increase in weight daily, depending on species, is typical, although there can be some normal fluctuation (see Figure 26.3). After day 18 or weaning, turaco chicks do not gain as much daily weight. A lack of weight gain or weight loss could mean problems, especially if it is consistent for 2 or more days. Consult your avian veterinarian if a chick becomes ill or is not progressing.

Different species of adult turacos and their chicks vary in size and weight slightly. The average hatchling weight of the green turaco species is 18–20 g.

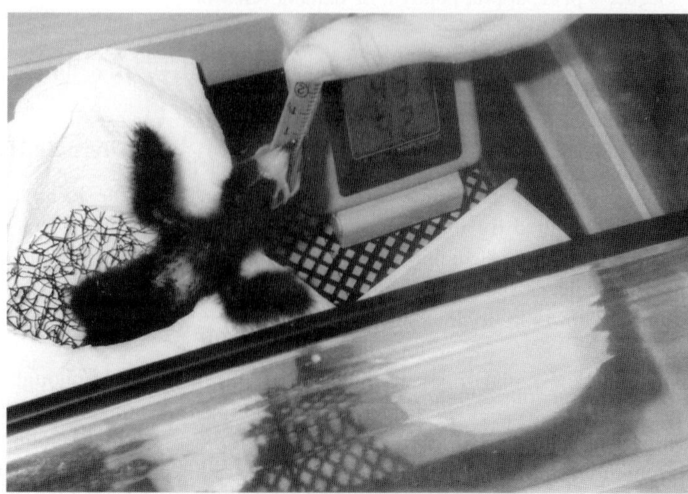

Figure 26.2. One-week-old Lady Ross Turaco in brooder. Notice how it is using its wings like arms to push itself toward the feeder.

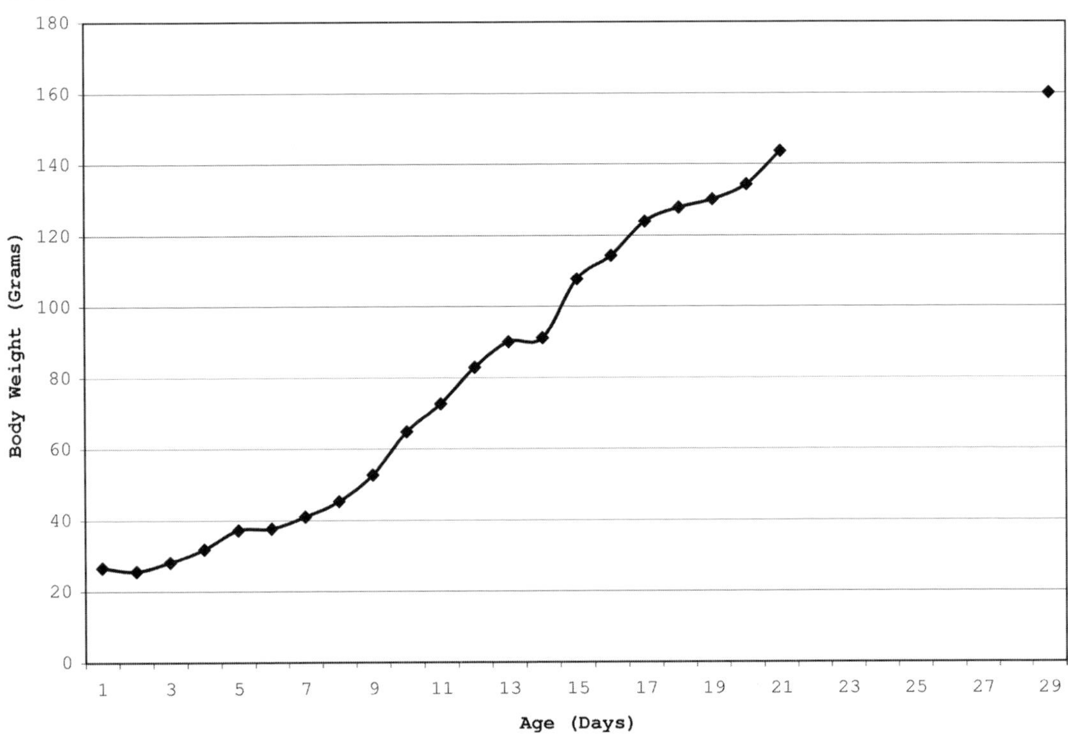

Figure 26.3. Lady Ross Turaco Growth Chart.

HOUSING

After about 12 hours in the incubator, a hatchling can be moved to a brooder (see Figure 26.2). The brooder can be a professional one or as simple as a clear plastic critter container with an adjustable heat and humidity source. Place the chick in a small bowl with a substrate that can be gripped easily and will not move aside as the chick wiggles. Keep the chick and its area clean of feces and uneaten food. A clean tissue or lightweight cloth can be draped over the bowl to simulate being brooded by a parent. As the chick grows, it will become more active, and the bowl may need to be larger so as not to tip when the chick begs. Around day 11–14, the chick will jump out of the bowl and start moving around the brooder.

Brooder temperature at day 1 should be at 96°F (35.5°C), and it should be lowered gradually, about a degree a day. Although not as crucial as temperature, humidity can be kept at 50–60% and can be gradually lowered to room humidity in the same way as the chick grows. By day 16–18, the chick can be moved to a cage without supplemental heat unless the room is colder than average room temperature of 74–80°F (23–27°C). The cage should be supplied with heavy perches on which the chick can run and bounce off. It is normal for turacos to suddenly have

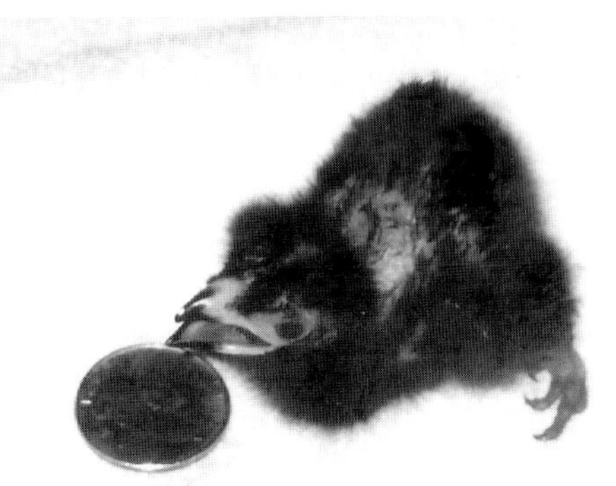

Figure 26.4. Three-day-old Livingston Turaco with quarter for size comparison.

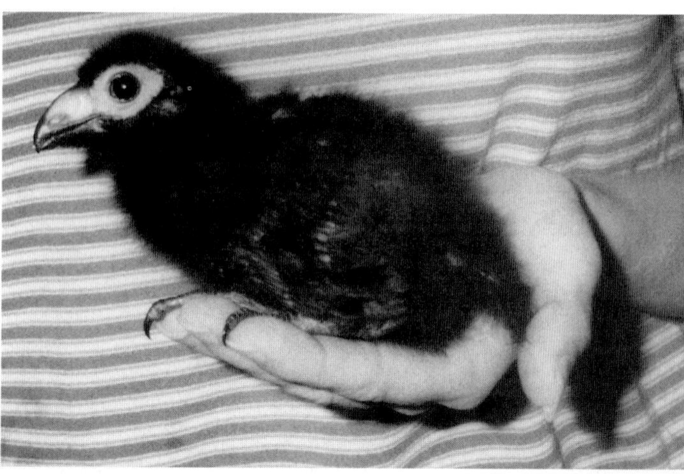

Figure 26.5. Three-week-old Lady Ross Turaco.

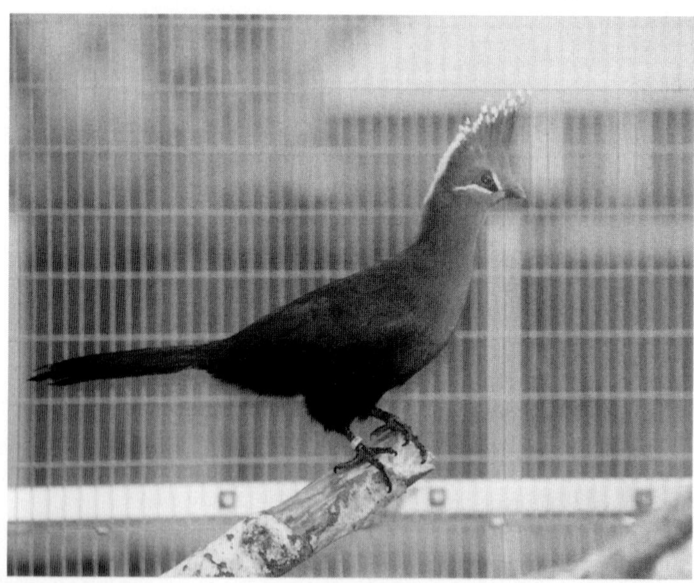

Figure 26.6. Livingston Turaco in aviary.

periods of intense excitement where the chick will be very active, flapping, and running. Flight will occur at approximately 1 month of age.

WEANING

Turaco chicks start to wean at day 18 and generally are completely weaned by day 30 or earlier (see Figure 26.5). Shallow bowls of adult food and water should be offered at day 18, and the chicks usually investigate and wean themselves. Some weight fluctuations normally occur at this time. The chicks will also start to bathe in their drinking water so frequent changes may be needed. Young green turacos' plumage is dull, and it takes several months to acquire the adult sheen and color.

INTRODUCTION TO CAPTIVE FLOCK

Young turacos, even of mixed species, can be housed together safely for awhile if they are all similar ages. Mature turacos tend to be aggressive toward each other, and it is recommended that they be housed separately or in bonded pairs. Species should be kept separately. Mate aggression and fatalities in all species are common, even after years of being together, and it can happen quickly with little or no warning. Hiding places on the ground, such as appropriately sized hollow pipes, should always be available in turaco enclosures. Use of the "howdy cage" technique described in the Chapter 29 is recommended when introducing turacos to one another. Turacos of all ages are generally safe to house with other birds, even small finches, although they may start chasing other birds when in breeding condition.

BEHAVIORAL TRAINING FOR PET TURACOS

Turacos are not birds recommended as house pets because they require large amounts of space and are very active. However, tame birds, even in large aviaries (see Figure 26.6), can be quite endearing because they will interact with people even after mature. But beware, tame birds, especially when in breeding condition, have no fear of people and can be dangerously aggressive, pecking at and jumping on faces and on heads.

Typically, turacos cannot be trained out of this behavior, so it is generally best to modify the keeper's behavior by learning to read the bird's mood and when necessary avoid direct eye contact (which is considered a challenge), keep interaction to a minimum, and wear protective headgear and glasses. Turacos will usually warn the person of these moods by approaching and displaying with open wings, head bowed, and loud calling or growling. Novice turaco owners and observers tend to be thrilled at this interaction by the bird and may feel inclined to display back by mimicking the bird's calls and actions. This just increases the bird's excitement and makes it more prone to attack.

AUTHOR'S NOTE

Although the author is working on one, there are no formal books published strictly on turacos in aviculture at this time, but a wealth of information has been published in magazines and journals. A great resource is The International Turaco Society, founded in Great Britain in the early 1990s.

The author owns Davis Lund Aviaries, which specializes in softbilled birds, and more pictures and information about turacos and other softbill birds can be found on the author's website, http://members.aol.com/DLAviaries. She would like to make contact with other people that are working with turacos and can be reached at 541–895–5149 or DLAviaries@aol.com.

ACKNOWLEDGMENTS

I would like to thank all the softbill aviculturists, past and present, who have so generously shared their experiences throughout the years. Many thanks to Hannah Bailey from Houston Zoo for sharing turaco protocols and diets. Thanks also to Pat Witman for assistance with diet information.

SOURCES FOR PRODUCTS MENTIONED

Kaytee Exact Hand Feeding Formula and Mynah Diet: Kaytee Products, Inc., 521 Clay St, P.O. Box 230, Chilton, WI 53014, (800) KAYTEE-1.

Mazuri ZuLiFe Soft-bill Diet: Mazuri Products, PMI Nutrition International, (800) 227–8941, www.mazuri.com.

ZuPreem Low-Iron Softbill Diet: ZuPreem, Premium Nutritional Products, Inc., (800) 345–4767, www.zupreem.com.

Gerber human baby food: Gerber Products Company, 445 Sate St, Fremont, MI, 49413–0001, (800) 4-GERBER.

REFERENCES

Milne, L. 1994. Touracos. AFA Watchbird. 21(6): 40–43.

Peat, L. 2000. Touracos galore. International Turaco Society Magazine 13: 8–14.

Plasse, R. and Todd, W. 1994. Turaco husbandry at the Houston Zoo. AFA Watchbird 21(6): 34–39.

Todd, W. 1998. Turaco TAG Husbandry Manual. Houston Zoological Gardens. Houston, 30 pp.

Vince, M. 1996. Softbills, Care, Breeding and Conservation. Hancock House Publishers LTD., Blaine, Washington, 278 pp.

27
Hummingbirds

Elizabeth Penn Elliston

NATURAL HISTORY

"Of all the numerous groups into which the birds are divided there is none other so numerous in species, so varied in form, so brilliant in plumage, and so different from all others in their mode of life" were the words used to describe hummingbirds by American ornithologist Robert Ridgway a century ago (Johnsgard 1983). Existing only in the western hemisphere, over 300 species of the family Trochilidae have been described, most of which occur in South America. There are several southern species that occasionally stray north into the U.S. At least 23 species in five genera occur regularly in North America, from the southern states to Alaska (Johnsgard 1983).

Hummingbirds are perching birds in the order Apodiformes. They typically fly anywhere they desire to go, using their feet only for perching. Wing use is unique to the family Trochilidae in that the shoulder structure allows a rotational or sculling motion of the wings. This enables the bird to hover for long periods and even fly backward, an ability possessed by no other type of bird.

Hummingbirds eat nectar found in a wide variety of flowers and feeders provided by humans. For over a century it has been known that they also consume large numbers of tiny insects and spiders (Baltosser and Scott 1996; Baltosser and Russell 2000; Bent 1940; Bendire 1895; Calder and Calder 1992; Calder 1993; Robinson et al. 1996; Scheithauer 1967). A bird may perch to gather nectar or hover while feeding. Nectar is drawn by capillary action up into the tongue and squeezed into the crop. Insects are obtained by hawking, and reportedly also by gleaning, though this author has rarely observed gleaning in captive black-chinned hummingbirds. Scheithauer (1966) described a "hazing" behavior of some captive hummingbirds, which flushes the insect into the air before catching it. Gleaning appears uncommon at best, and caregivers should not assume that the species they are housing will glean enough unflighted insects to fulfill dietary requirements.

These birds typically nest in feltlike cups made of plant fibers, down, fur, and cotton and are lined on the outside with lichen, bark, paint chips, or other similar material. Females lay two eggs about a day apart but begin incubating immediately, which results in an asynchronous hatch. Incubation may last from 12–19 days, most commonly about 2 weeks, and it is probably influenced by the weather during this period. The young are altricial, eyes closed with naked black skin decorated by a few filamentous white or yellowish feathers on the head and along the back feather tracts. They typically fledge at about 21 days but remain dependent on their mother for as long as 2 weeks after leaving the nest. Males do not participate in family life beyond copulation.

CRITERIA FOR INTERVENTION

Hummingbirds brought into captivity fall into three major categories. First, adults with wing or other injuries caused by collisions with windows, interaction with cats, or some other trauma that has rendered them nonflighted, are commonly found during summer months in North America. These may or may not recover flight with little treatment other than a safe place to rest and recuperate.

The second category is that of uninjured orphaned fledglings. These are birds that have left the nest and have not yet become independent. Overzealous people concerned about their well-being may kidnap them, or they may be true orphans whose mothers have met with some mishap. These birds are typically capable of flight, but their bills have not grown to full length. In addition, these birds may be making the high frequency "peep" call used by their mothers to locate them (Elliston and Baltosser 1995). These birds can easily be brought to release stage with proper nutritional support and foraging practice.

Populating the third group of displaced hummingbirds are nestlings, which have come to the attention of people and are brought into care. These birds are rarely "kidnapped" because people attentively watch the developing family and tend to remove them from the wild only when it is apparent that something has gone wrong. Indications of imminent nest failure are the failure of the parent to return to feed the young every hour or so, failure to cover naked birds at night, and the young calling from the nest. Not infrequently young are found on the ground and calling, seemingly unable to fly. These are usually nestlings that have fallen from the nest, probably due to agitation as a result of food deprivation (Elliston 1995).

RECORD KEEPING

Detailed information on the location and date where the bird was found should be recorded. A record of location will serve as a guide to suitable habitat for release and also will place the bird back where its genetic pool already occurs. Date found may be of interest should the bird become a museum specimen, or for breeding records of the species.

No matter how confident one may be that one will never forget the details of a particular bird, memory fails. Pertinent data should be recorded as it is observed. For unflighted juvenile hummingbirds, this may include daily body weights, length of bill (exposed culmen) in mm, progress of treatments, record of food given, and notes on behavior.

Wildlife regulatory agencies have minimum standards for record keeping that require tracking of individual animals undergoing rehabilitation. Check with your regulating agencies for further information. See Appendix 1, "Important Contacts," for a list of North American resources for locating permitted wildlife rehabilitators and regulatory agencies. At a minimum, the following information should be kept: date and location found, species (when known), age (when determined), reason brought into captivity, initial condition assessment, final disposition, and release location. There is often confusion between reason for acquisition and initial condition. *Reasons* can include such things as apparently abandoned (in hummingbirds, calling from nest, or parent not seen for ~12 hours), found on ground, rescued from predator, or "kidnapped." *Condition* includes such things as dehydration, out of nest, cold, starving, etc. Every attempt should be made to keep these categories distinct.

A detailed medical record should be kept on each animal, with results of the initial examination recorded and any updated information added as it happens. It is helpful when large numbers of diverse species are being raised en masse with different volunteer caregivers, to have a "Feeding Instructions" sheet that tells the next caregiver what to feed and any tips for food delivery. A chart, on which is recorded the actual time of each feeding and how much was fed, can be valuable.

INITIAL CARE AND STABILIZATION

Like any other baby bird, the main rule of initial care is warmth, rehydration, and feeding, in that order. If hummingbirds are in pinfeathers (~2 weeks of age), feathered, or perching and too old to display gaping behavior, they are probably able to regulate their own temperature and need only temporary warming until their behavior indicates that they are normothermic. Then they must be persuaded to drink an isotonic rehydrating solution before offering hypertonic nutrition. Five percent dextrose will suffice for the initial stages of rehydration while providing a tiny bit of nutrition. This fluid is isotonic and tastes acceptable to the bird. If the fluid does not taste good, the bird will refuse to drink. Although gavage for hummingbirds is possible, it is highly undesirable. Persuasion is the best route. When the bird passes some fluid droppings, feedings can commence.

If the baby hummingbird is naked, or in early pinfeathers, it is extremely important to provide adequate heat. Newly hatched hummingbirds can weigh as little as 250 mg, so heat loss is rapid. Also as a result of the birds' tiny size, hot and cool spots in incubators dictate how much heat the bird is actually receiving. Measuring heat with an indoor-outdoor wire probe-style thermometer (available at many home and garden stores) in the nest and under the bird is an effective way of monitoring the temperature of the bird. Placing the nestling in its natural nest in an incubator at 100°F (37.7°C) and covering with a small piece of flannel may provide adequate heat for all but the most tiny of chicks (see Figure 27.1). If a bird heated to that temperature fails to

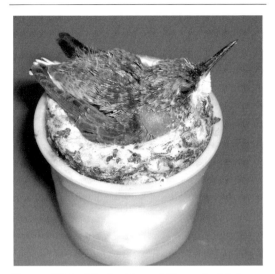

Figure 27.1. Black-chinned Hummingbird nestling. Note the full crop visible at the neck plus many feathers still in quills. Hummingbirds do well when kept in their original nest inside another container.

gape, the heat can be increased to register as high as 104°F on the probe under the bird. At that temperature, the nestling usually kicks off the covering blanket. Under all these conditions of high heat, it is important to monitor humidity in the chamber. A wide-mouth jar containing water and a cotton wick should keep the air adequately moist. Warm hydrating fluid can be introduced into the gaping bird with any tiny plastic catheter placed on the end of a 1 ml syringe. The response of a healthy vigorous nestling will be to "climb" the catheter with the pulsing pumping motion observable in parent-fed birds. Depending on the size of the bird, amounts of fluid from 0.05–0.5 ml can be given at each feeding. Observation of the crop, easily visible around the neck, can aid in determining what volume to give. Though hummingbirds manage their liquid food very well, it is better to underfill than overfill a tiny crop. Because these birds are gaping and won't taste the food, they can immediately be given a hydrating solution containing electrolytes, such as lactated Ringer's solution (LRS) or a mixture of LRS and 5% dextrose. When they look plump and start passing wet droppings, they can be fed insects and a nutritious fluid diet.

COMMON MEDICAL PROBLEMS AND SOLUTIONS

A common problem on presentation of an orphaned or injured hummingbird is that it is covered with sugar-water from finders' attempts to feed it. Nestlings may often be stuck to the nest, which can interfere with their movement or even excretory functions. It's important to free them with warm water as soon as they have been stabilized, and to clean their feathers and vent. Then, be aware that the vent must be kept clean until the caregiver is confident that the bird is regularly lifting its behind and defecating out of the nest.

Young hummingbirds rarely present with medical conditions. There have been occasional anecdotal reports of cases of trichomonas in flighted birds and outbreaks of microsporidia in nestlings in care. These can be treated with one of the nitroimidazoles, when detected (Diane Waters, personal communication). Fungal spores and *E. coli* are not uncommonly seen in examination of fecal smears, but unless some symptoms are evident the best treatment is probably good nutrition and supportive care. If a self-feeding bird seems to be holding its tongue out continually, a drop of Nystatin (Bristol-Meyers Squibb) in 3 cc liquid food often seems to address the condition (Janine Perlman personal communication).

Feather mites are a common parasite in the nests of hummingbirds. They usually appear late in the season and can be treated by removing the nestlings from the nest, treating the nest with a miticide such as Kelthane (Dow Agrosciences), and returning the birds to the nest. Residual mite poison in the nest usually takes care of any mites remaining on the birds, and, as this poison is very specific for mites, it is unlikely to harm the birds. If the parasites seem to be excessive in numbers on a feathered bird, gently wiping a cotton-tipped swab dampened in miticide over the outer feathers, especially at the top of the head, will often take care of the ectoparasites.

Another kind of mite (Ascidae), first described by Baker and Yunker in 1964, and of which about 60 species have now been described, is sometimes found on nestling hummingbirds. These little mites are seen clustered around the nares and when the bird opens its mouth the mites run up to the tip. When the bird's mouth closes the mites all run back to the top of the bill. These mites are often colored yellow, pink, or brownish and are actually flower mites. They eat nectar and pollen of particular flowers and hitch a ride from flower to flower via the visiting hummingbirds. But when they get off on a nestling bird, they have reached a dead end. These little animals can only live a few days without their flowers, and the birds need no treatment other than time or perhaps a damp cotton swab to remove them.

DIET RECIPES

Refrigerate all liquid diets between feedings, or keep the day's food in a thermos filled with ice. Begin each day with fresh diet. Whey is available in several consistencies and individual measuring spoons may vary considerably. It's important to weigh the powders until the relationship of volume to weight has been established for each individual's equipment.

Fledglings and Adults

Fledgling and adult food contains 20 mg/ml of protein (see Table 27.1). Eating 5 ml/day will provide the approximate amount needed to sustain an adult's protein requirements. If a bird is given a choice of this mix, nectar (1 part sugar to 4 parts water), and plain water, it will be able to choose the proportions of each that it needs. It has been observed that the older the bird is, the more personal the preference may be for sweetness. Adjustments for taste may be needed with small additions of sugar to coax the bird into readily drinking the above diet.

Liquid food can be offered in 3 ml syringes. The Vital HN/Whey/Sugar mix is more susceptible to bacterial and fungal growth than water or sugar alone, and it should be monitored carefully for signs of spoilage. Dripping is a sign of gas formation and fermentation. The birds will not eat something that tastes at all sour. They will starve first.

A culture of flying fruit flies should be made available to flighted birds so that they will learn through practice how to catch small insects. As they become proficient at foraging and consume more flies, intake of the protein-rich liquid food will diminish, and plain nectar or water consumption may rise.

Table 27.1. Vital HN/whey/sugar recipe for fledglings and unflighted adults (based on Elliston and Perlman 2002).

Ingredient	Amount
Water	75 ml
Vital HN powder	4 g
Granulated table sugar	25 g
Whey, powdered 100% concentrate	1.8 g
Mix the above and freeze as ice cubes.	
Thaw enough for each day and add per 10 ml:	
Yogurt, plain live-culture	0.5 ml (~10 drops)
5 : 1 cod liver oil, vitamin E oil, mixed	1 drop
B complex plus C tablet, crushed	Small pinch, to turn solution light lemon-yellow color
Add the below to the diet of any growing or skeletal injury bird:	
Calcium glubionate (23 mg/ml)	0.25 ml

Hatchlings and Nestlings

"Bloodworms," which are actually midge larvae (blood, red, or black), may be either live or frozen, and should be drained on a paper towel before weighing. Crush the worms with a mortar and pestle. Grind ingredients together, mixing well, and draw into a 1 ml syringe. Freeze stock and keep amount in use very cold. A very small container in an ice-filled thermos is an excellent way to keep this food very cold between feedings (see Tables 27.2–27.5 for recipes and ingredients).

Table 27.2. Hatchling and nestling recipe Mix 1: Fortified Vital HN.

Ingredient	Amount
Water	33 ml
Vital HN powder (no extra sugar)	8 g
B complex plus C tablet, crushed	1/20 tablet, to turn solution light lemon-yellow color
Supplemented oil (see Table 27.4)	0.025 ml
Yogurt, plain live culture	0.05 ml per ml diet fed

Table 27.3. Hatchling and nestling recipe Mix 2: Insect slurry.

Ingredient	Amount
"Bloodworms" and mosquito larvae	2 g
Supplemented calcium glubionate (see Table 27.5)	0.60 ml
Yogurt, plain live culture	Toothpick-tip–sized amount per ml fed

Table 27.4. Supplemented oil.

Ingredient	Amount
Fish body oil (omega 3)	7 drops
Cod liver oil	2 drops
Vitamin E	1 drop

Table 27.5. Supplemented calcium glubionate.

Ingredient	Amount
Calcium glubionate (23 mg/ml)	10 ml
B complex plus C tablet	Sand-grain–sized piece, to turn solution light lemon-yellow color
Supplemented oil	1 tiniest drop

Any form of calcium supplementation may be used that can be measured precisely enough to add the elemental calcium required. Calcium glubionate comes in a convenient pediatric suspension that provides 23 mg/ml.

Both these mixes will pass through the very tiniest of catheters. As the bird grows, and larger catheters can be used, tiny insects that may have a greater particulate component than ground insect larvae can be added to the slurry or to the fluid mix. As with all baby birds, diverse foods are always beneficial. "White" mosquito larvae, fruit flies, dried versions of these—all are good foods. Frozen tropical fish dealers have a variety of such foods to choose from. The innards of mealworms are not recommended because they seem to make the birds logy and unresponsive. It is beneficial to add some recently live insects to the mixture to provide certain enzymes and microbes that may not be present in the dried or preserved foods.

Tiny arthropods such as fruit flies, midges, leaf hoppers, or even brine shrimp can be fed whole with forceps to gaping birds. The chitinous coverings of any of these little animals all break down into tiny plates that can be digested without problems by baby hummingbirds.

Development of an optimal diet for the youngest of hummingbirds is an ongoing effort. Although a number of details regarding the components of suggested diets are clear, there have always been problems collecting adequate growth data to discriminate between recipes. Either people who keep meticulous data get too few birds to compare results, people who get numerous birds are too busy raising them to collect the necessary data, or others who do have data don't make them available to others. In any case, the work goes on, and those raising baby hummingbirds should make every effort to communicate with others regarding new findings.

The first priority of a newly hatched bird is to build the skeleton and organs required. Concurrently, the feathers that will cover and insulate the body and provide the tools for flight must be developed. Poor feathers in a hummingbird is a life-threatening condition; if the bird cannot fly it cannot catch the flying insects required, nor can it travel to gather the nectar needed to fuel its engines. Inadequate plumage has been the most apparent problem for rehabilitators raising very small hatchlings. As early as 1890, Ridgway observed that the mother hummingbird almost exclusively fed small arthropods to hatchlings (Johnsgard 1983).

Rather than calculate what the protein requirements might be each day based on weight, the best way to approach meeting these needs may be to just do what the mother hummingbird does: Stuff the little crops with insects at every opportunity. If one is starting with a 250 mg chick, however, it is unlikely that human implements can introduce many of even the smallest of insects into the crop. It would be difficult to deliver the 0.77 kilocalories (kcal) per day in insects necessary to provide adequate nutrition to this growing bird (see Appendix 2, "Energy Requirements for Growing Birds"). Vital HN, slightly more dilute than its standard strength, containing 0.7 kcal/ml, can, however, be fed with the use of a tiny intravenous catheter or as an effective substitute for the mother's bill. Vital HN contains a caloric distribution of protein (16.7%), fat (9.5%), and carbohydrate (73.8%). This fluid, containing only the carbohydrates present in the powder (no extra sugar) and insect slurry can be introduced into the crop and will suffice to get the bird started.

As the caregiver and the bird become accustomed to the feeding techniques, feeding becomes easier to accomplish. Packing the crop first with insect and arthropod slurry until the bird ceases to gape, and adding vitamin-enriched liquid Vital HN if the bird will accept it every 30–60 minutes or as the crop empties, becomes an easy routine. Insects and slurry are digested more slowly than fluid nutrients. As the day progresses, the bird may accept less insect material and more liquid Vital HN at a feed. If the crop slows and fails to empty, feed water and Vital HN until the crop is moving well again.

It should be understood that the use of Vital HN is to ensure that sufficient calories are actually delivered to a *very* small bird. The major food component should be invertebrates (insects, other arthropods) in quantities as great can be achieved. It is protein that will enable the bird to grow its essential strong feathers. A hummingbird without strong feathers will not survive in the wild.

Caregivers may find sticking forceps' "bites" of insects into a hummingbird throat a daunting prospect. Blending or grinding the insect component in the liquid component may produce the same results. However, under these circumstances one must remember that Vital HN is hypertonic (386 mosm/L) when made as directed on the package, and dehydration may become a risk. This is rectified by adding more water, as shown in the Fortified Vital HN mix in Table 27.2. The author finds the most reliable way to assess and maintain adequate hydration in hummingbirds is close attention to an absence of wrinkles on naked skin, and vigorous feeding behavior.

Various other diets have been reported as successfully used for raising young hummingbirds. It is the author's opinion, however, that unless the foods contain large amounts of animal protein with the amino acid profile required for a growing insectivore, successful feather development cannot be achieved (MacLeod and Perlman 2001). Indeed, personal communication with numerous rehabilitators has revealed poor outcomes using commercial diets based on soy protein in both hummingbirds and passerines (Elliston and Perlman 2002). The author strongly recommends against using any commercial hummingbird diets that contain significant amounts of soy protein. These diets have been known to cause gastrointestinal stasis in young hummingbirds and do not provide adequate types or quantities of protein for growing birds (Elliston and Perlman 2002). Although these products may be more convenient to make, the probability of birds growing substandard feathering or suffering greater mortality rates is higher, the younger the bird in question is started on these inadequate diets. Nektar-Plus (Nekton Products) is meant for adult birds and is inappropriate for growing chicks. As hummingbirds have evolved eating insects there is little reason to believe that they are able to utilize the vegetable protein provided by soybeans.

FEEDING PROCEDURES

If young hummingbirds are received fully feathered and perching, they are unlikely to gape for anyone but their mother. They can quickly be taught to self-feed with the presentation of a 3 ml syringe containing the Vital/Whey/Sugar mixture. Though they will readily accept a proven food source, it may be helpful to initially present the tip of the syringe with some kind of color. The tip of the syringe can be painted red, a bright piece of yarn can be tied around the tip, or a bright piece of cellophane can be stuck on the syringe. Since young birds have fairly short fat bills, slicing the tip of a luer syringe to about 1/4 its length, or boring out the hole in the syringe provides better access to the food. Another syringe containing plain water should also be placed within reach.

Mother hummingbirds regurgitate the contents of their crop into their young. Healthy young hummingbirds can be observed to open their bills at the approach of their mother and make vigorous "pumping" movements in accepting their mother's bills. As with many baby birds, the key to getting them to gape is to find the appropriate stimulus. Blowing on them prior to feeding seems to be the trick. As the mother hummingbird approaches, the movement of her wings agitates the filoplumes on the smallest of birds, which stimulates gaping. When the bird is gaping and reaching up, a "pinch" of insects in the tip of a pair of blunt-eye forceps can be plunged down the throat into the crop. Slightly release the grip on the insects and allow the motion of the feeding bird to dislodge them from the forceps. Remove and repeat until the bird ceases to gape. The author has found that the best posture for this kind

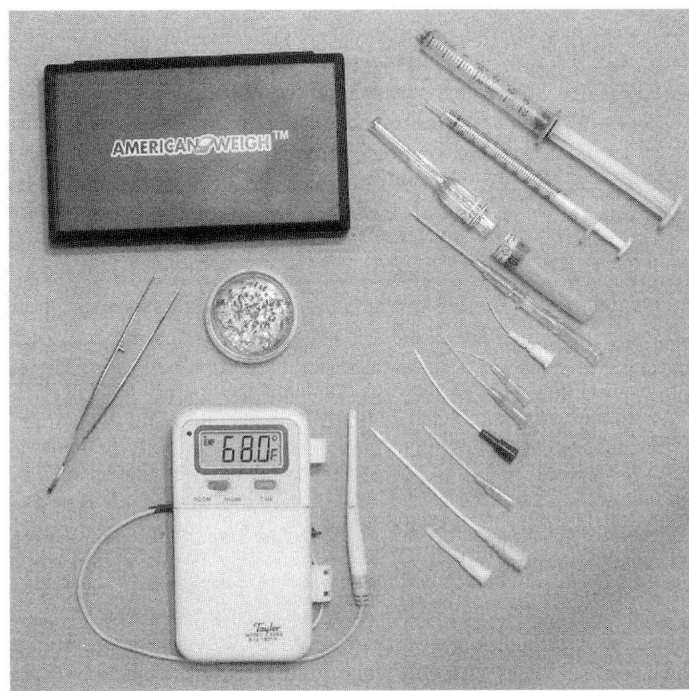

Figure 27.2. Clockwise from top left. American Weigh scale, 3 cc syringe with tip shortened and colored with red nail polish, a 1 cc O-ring syringe, a variety of intravenous catheters to be used as feeding implements (shown are 18–24 gauge), white plastic irrigation cannula, digital thermometer with probe, feeding forceps with small dish of tiny insects.

of feeding is to brace the forearm on a flat surface adjacent to the bird in its nest such that the arm can act as a lever over the bird. Holding the forceps or syringe directly over the bird, bring it down ready to plunge into the gape. Then, blow on the bird. A syringe tipped with a catheter of appropriate size can be used in the same way and is, initially, easier to manipulate.

Some rehabilitators have adopted the technique of putting insects in the fluid to deliver by syringe (Van Epps 1999). This author prefers using catheters that are too small to pass whole insects (except daphnia, the water flea) and to feed whole insects with forceps, because some birds may regurgitate when fed insects mixed into their liquid diet. Accurate assessment of the birds' tolerance for solids in the crop, and maintenance of hydration, are possible by feeding solids and fluid separately. However, a slurry may also be created by grinding insects and adding an appropriate amount of calcium to balance the phosphorus content of the insects (0.03 ml 23 mg/ml calcium glubionate per 100 mg insects fed). There may be fewer problems if the slurry and Vital mix are fed alternately as the crop empties.

Hatchlings

Hatchlings should be fed every 20–30 minutes for 12–14 hours a day, when they gape. Chicks should never be overstimulated or forced. A 1 ml syringe with an IV catheter tip, 18 gauge or smaller (see Figure 27.2), makes an excellent feeding implement for fluid food or slurry. Attach the tip securely to avoid the possibility of it disconnecting and making a mess on the bird. Administer the food in a controlled manner while the bird is actively accepting the food. Watch the crop increase in size, and stop delivery before it becomes too full. Occasionally, fluid may well up into the mouth and be swallowed again. This is not a matter of concern because healthy young hummingbirds can control fluid intake very successfully. It is better to give both solid and fluid food in small increments until the bird refuses to gape than to overfill in one application, which may cause some distress or, worse, aspiration.

If a bird with an empty crop refuses food, reevaluate the temperature, hydration status, and physical condition. Check the vent to ensure that it is clean and not stuck to the nest.

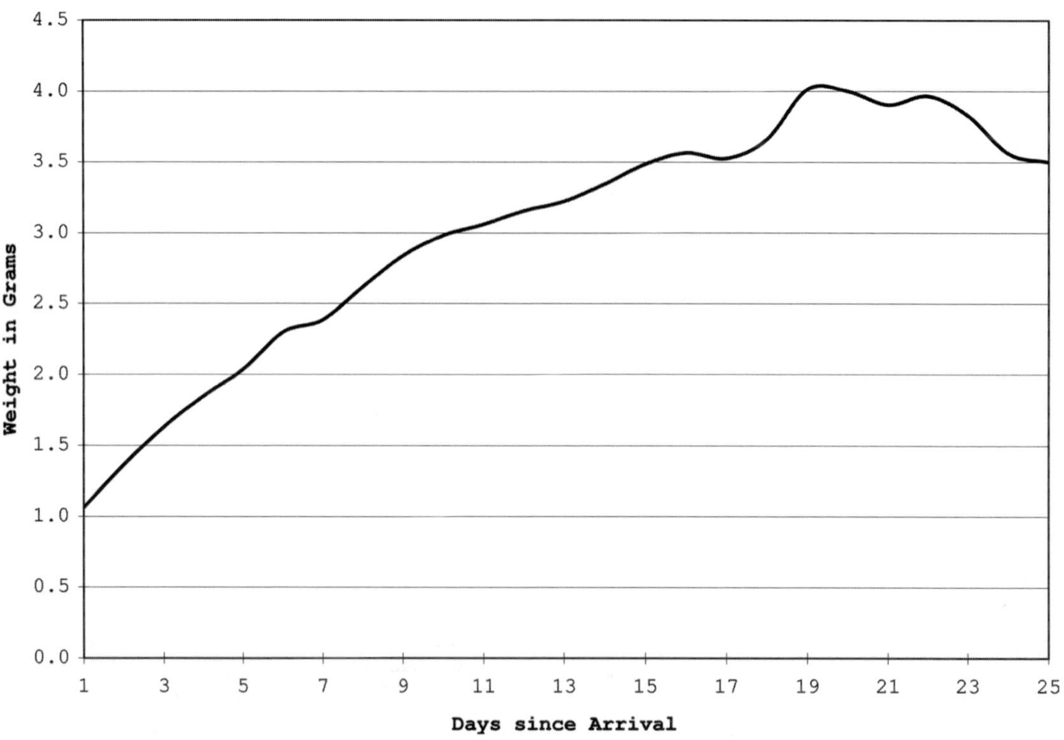

Figure 27.3. Weight gains of Black-chinned Hummingbirds for which Vital HN and insects were fed separately (n = 9).

Nestlings and Fledglings

Fully and partially feathered birds should be fed every hour or when they gape, for 12–14 hours a day. When the bird is large enough, bite sizes of about five fruit flies stuck together with water can be delivered this way with blunt-tipped eye dressing forceps. Care must be taken to get the tip of the forceps far down past the glottis, because the tongue rarely helps in swallowing insects. If the solid material is not placed far enough into the crop, the tongue will bring the particle out and wipe it off. Birds with open eyes will learn to distinguish between the forceps with solid food and the catheter with fluid food. Typically, they will open their mouths for insects until they have received enough, but will gape again when offered fluid food. The fluid food can be used to fill up the crop when insects or slurry are rejected. When whole insects are fed, calcium, in the levels noted above, should also be included in the liquid component of the daily diet (0.03 ml of 23 mg/ml calcium glubionate for every 100 mg insects).

Hummingbirds have very wet droppings that they typically eject over the edge of the nest. Fecal boli should appear very black and bulky with a spot of white urates on top. The bolus is ejected in copious amounts of urine. Try to keep the nest and surroundings clean and dry.

EXPECTED WEIGHT GAIN

Because hummingbirds may start life outside the egg at a weight of well under 1 g, a triple beam or "gram scale" balance will not be accurate enough to measure growth reliably. An electronic balance that weighs a maximum capacity of 100 g in gradations of 0.01 g can be obtained from American Weigh™, among other places, for a price in the neighborhood of $50.00 in 2006. A standard analytic pan balance can also be used. Because a bird may grow in increments of 100–900 mg a day, depending on age, this will provide an appropriate level of accuracy.

The growth curves in Figures 27.3 and 27.4 were gathered using a diet developed in the 1990s, also

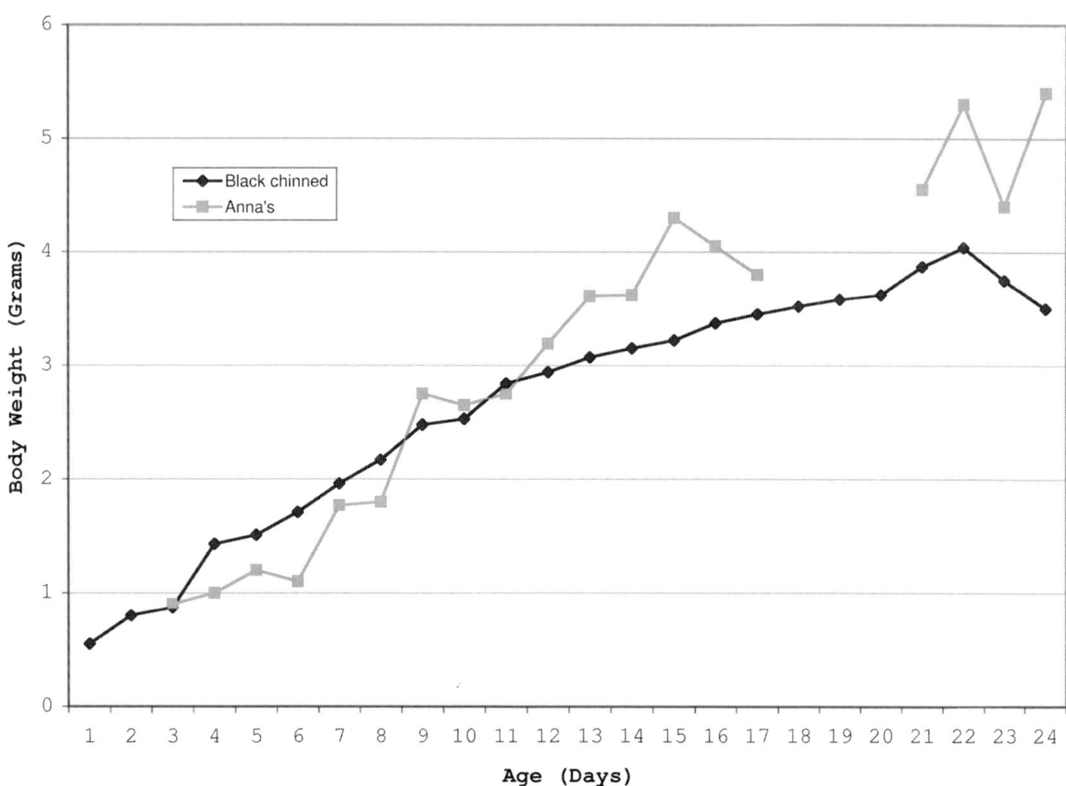

Figure 27.4. Average growth of Black-chinned Hummingbirds (n = 7) and the average growth of four Anna's Hummingbirds (n = 4) in which insects were added to standard strength Vital HN (Van Epps 1999).

composed of standard-strength Vital HN and insects. However, these diets have been subsequently been revised. The author's currently recommended diets are above.

Though the data are not as robust for the larger Annas, comparison of the two curves in Figures 27.3 and 27.4 indicates that good growth results can be obtained by feeding the Fortified Vital HN from Table 27.2 and insects separately or adding insects to the liquid mix. The limiting factor is only the size of the feeding implement, which can be mitigated by grinding the insects prior to adding them to the mix as recommended above or by blending in the liquid diet.

Weights must be taken before the first feeding in the morning because the crop can contain a significant proportion of the bird's weight. Defecation in a bird of this size can also reduce a weight as much as 30–50%. Hummingbirds should gain weight daily and reach or exceed the adult weight for the species at about 14 days of age. This may be as little as 3 g. By 10–12 days of age the young will be covered with pinfeathers and, in nature, the parent ceases to sit on them at night. By 2 weeks of age, the weight reaches a plateau. If a bird is not gaining weight, or is calling from the nest persistently, there is something seriously wrong and the feeding and housing regimen should be evaluated.

HOUSING

Hatchlings should be kept at 90–95°F (32.2–35°C) or somewhat higher (see the section "Initial Care and Stabilization," above) and 40–50% humidity. Nestling hummingbirds are very intimately associated with their nests. These are the only species for which it may be desirable to keep, or replace them into, a natural nest. If the nest is infested with ectoparasites, the birds can be removed (peeled out), the nest treated as mentioned in the section "Common

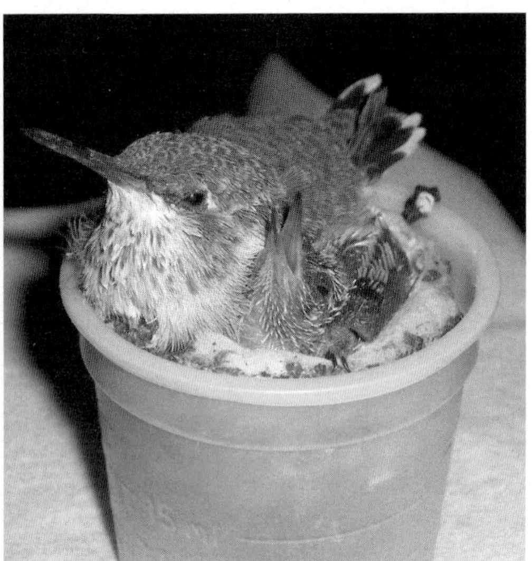

Figure 27.5. A very young Black-chinned Hummingbird chick with a chick nearing weaning age.

Medical Problems," above, and the birds returned. When daily weights are taken, it is preferable to allow the bird or birds to remain in the nest, weighing the whole thing. After the birds fledge, a tare weight can be obtained. This method may result in a slight variance in actual growth record, but it is unlikely to be more than a few milligrams; and a good visual assessment of growth can be obtained during the nestling phase.

Alternatively, a liner of a scrap of single-ply toilet paper can be used to line the nest. The bird can be removed by lifting the liner like a hammock, liner plus bird weighed, and the bird rolled back into the nest containing a clean replacement liner. This method tends to result in more accuracy of weight for a very small bird (250–1500 mg) because an accurate tare weight can be obtained each time.

Hummingbirds become able to control their body temperature between 10–14 days of age (see Figure 27.5). At this point, the parent stops covering them at night, and young can be removed from an incubator. Safety is still a major concern for these tiny young. For example, rodents that may be patrolling the care facilities at night can easily eat them.

At 19–20 days of age the birds in their nests should be placed in a secure enclosure, so that when they fledge they will be safely confined. When a nestling hummingbird takes its first flight, it starts by buzzing its wings while hanging on to the edge of the nest. At some point it lets go of the nest and shoots off in an uncontrolled direction. If it is unconfined, this is the time it lands behind the refrigerator, entertainment center, filing cabinet, or in the toilet. In any case, it will vanish. There the bird may sit for several days, or it may experiment again within hours. At this stage the bird has little control of flight and is completely dependent on its parent for food. It is at this stage of increased mobility that, under optimal circumstances in nature, the bird begins to "peep" to call its mother. In these first few days out of the nest it is important that food be placed in locations easy to reach from a perch on which the bird is located. As the birds become more competent in managing their flight capabilities, food can be placed where they must hover to reach it. In addition, a flying fruit fly culture should be introduced.

The enclosure can start at a relatively small size and be increased as the birds acquire flight proficiency. Unlimited activity aviaries should be at least $2 \times 4 \times 6$ ft ($0.6 \times 1.2 \times 1.8$ m) or provide an equivalent flight volume (Miller 2000). Over the next 2 weeks the birds will learn to be proficient flyers, to hover as they feed, to feed from a variety of sources, and to catch insects. Their housing should be enlarged as they learn and become skilled, resulting in release from a final large outdoor aviary.

If more than one fledgling is housed together, they will sit shoulder to shoulder at night. As they age, become more successful at foraging, and hormones begin to flow, males may become more antagonistic toward other residents of the enclosure. Sufficient syringes of food should be placed to ensure adequate intake by all birds.

WEANING

At about 19–20 days the birds can be trained to self-feed (see Figure 27.6). In order to persuade them to drink the food, sugar must be added. At this stage the birds can be offered the Vital HN/Whey/Sugar formula.

Hummingbirds are not as difficult to wean to self-feeding as many other species. They will, in fact, self-feed from the nest. However, they need to be given adequate time to learn to catch insects efficiently, and to bathe and perform other independent behaviors, but acquiring these skills is rarely a concern to the caregivers.

When the birds are in an outdoor aviary, presentation of an adequate number of insects to forage can be challenging (see Figure 27.7). The most reliable technique is to contain a healthy fruit fly culture in a jar, with the mouth of the jar covered with fiberglass netting. This will allow the flies to move in and out of the jar without risking the bird falling in. A collection of decaying fruit covered with hardware cloth can also be placed in the enclosure to attract other insects, such that the birds can approach and perch on dry nonsticky surfaces and haze the flies attracted to the food into the air. It is important to anticipate and prevent ways that the birds can get into trouble by getting caught in crevices or cobwebs, or covered with sugar water or fruit juice. A small, very shallow pan of water, or a small fountain of cascading water over rocks should be made available for bathing. Water for drinking should also be available in hanging tubes or feeders. The prerelease enclosure of the author is made predator-proof with 0.5 × 0.5 in (1 × 1 cm) hardware cloth through which a 3 ml syringe hangs very nicely. This makes it easy to place syringes of water and Vital HN/Whey/Sugar solution in a variety of changing locations from which the birds will feed ad lib. It is wise to have some Vital HN/Whey/Sugar solution located within reach of a perch so that birds that, for any reason, have difficulty hovering can reach nutritious food. The skill of the birds can be assessed by whether these tubes empty more rapidly than those that require hovering.

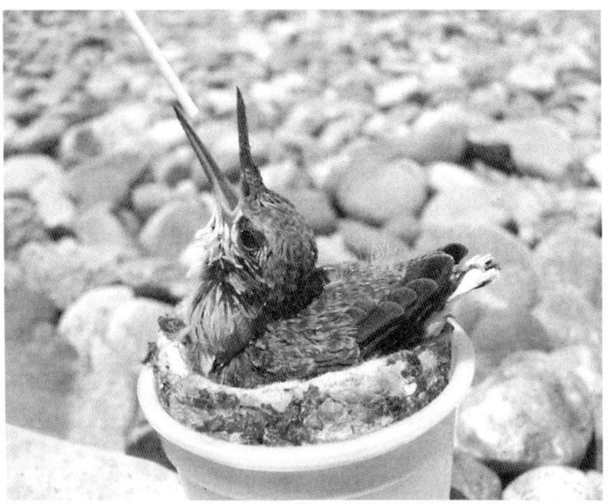

Figure 27.6. A Black-chinned Hummingbird chick gaping for a meal. Note size of feeding catheter in relation to the chick's bill (photo courtesy of Mark Gruber).

Feeders containing nectar (1 part sugar: 4 parts water) of a variety of designs, such as those that the birds reach down into (satellite), and those that offer a tubelike delivery, should be offered to optimize the bird's chances for success after release.

If the birds make any "peep" calls, check to see that all the food is available and fresh and that bathwater is clean. Any bird that peeps is not ready for release, and the reason for its distress should be addressed. Flighted birds should not be frequently weighed. Their health and condition can be assessed by their flying and feeding behavior, with less stress

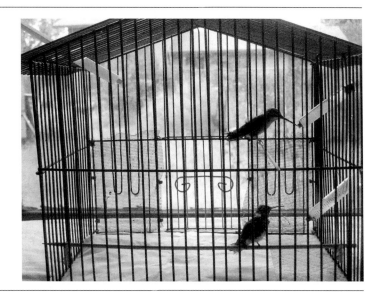

Figure 27.7. Two fledglings in indoor housing. Note ample feeding syringes placed throughout cage, some reachable by perching, some by hovering.

on the birds. If birds are found in torpor during the day or having difficulty awakening in the morning they should be removed to a smaller, more intensive care enclosure with food and water available to them as they perch, and monitored carefully.

PREPARATION FOR RELEASE TO THE WILD

Approximately 2 weeks after fledging, the birds are ready to be assessed for release. Black-chinned Hummingbirds have a bill length of 13 mm when they fledge at 21 days. Their bills reach adult length 2 weeks later (Elliston and Baltosser 1995).

A characteristic of hummingbirds is that they are fearless. Their lack of apparent fear at the approach of people may be interpreted as habituation. However, after a certain age, with only a modicum of isolation in prerelease life, it is unlikely that it would be possible to walk up to a newly released hummingbird and capture it. This is not to suggest that simply offering some attractive nutrient cannot lure a purely wild hummingbird. Lack of fear, and plentiful curiosity, can be real hazards to a hummingbird's well-being.

RELEASE

Birds should spend a couple of weeks in the aviary prior to release, with feeders hung within view outside the housing. They can observe the behavior of wild birds at those feeders, listen to the ambient sounds, and locate possible sources of nectar. Release is accomplished by opening the door of the aviary and allowing the birds to leave when they are ready. If no "peep" calls are heard after release, the process should be considered successful.

Hummingbirds are migratory in most of America north of Mexico. However, some vagrants remain in warmer climates after the others have left. If they are normally migratory within the release area, they should be released within the normal migration time, or wintered over. Young hummingbirds leave the natal area after the departure of adults, so the release window is relatively flexible. If there is doubt about late-season release, local birding organizations and 10-day weather forecasts can be consulted.

ACKNOWLEDGMENTS

Many thanks to Denise Coil and Janine Perlman Ph.D., for editorial assistance and suggestions on content for this chapter. Thanks to the Albuquerque office of the U.S. Fish and Wildlife Service and the New Mexico Department of Game and Fish (NMDGF) for permits. Thanks to the Share with Wildlife Program of the NMDGF for continued support of Wildlife Rescue Inc. of New Mexico (WRINM). Most of all, thanks to the supporters and members of WRINM who made the acquisition of this information possible through giving displaced nestling hummingbirds their careful attention.

SOURCES FOR PRODUCTS MENTIONED

Vital HN: Ross Products, (800) 258-7677, a division of Abbott Laboratories, Abbott Park, IL. Vital HN may be obtained in single packages from The Squirrel Store, (866) 907-7757, or by fax at (205) 664-1386, http://www.thesquirrelstore.com/category.cfm?Category=29.

Scale: American Weigh Scales Inc., 1836 Ashley River Rd, Suite 320, Charleston, SC 29407, (866) 643-3444.

Nystatin: Bristol-Meyers Squibb, Princeton, NJ 08543.

Kelthane miticide: Dow AgroSciences LLC, 9330 Zionsville Rd, Indianapolis, IN 46268, (317) 337-3000.

REFERENCES

Baker, E.W. and Yunker, C.E. 1964. New Blattisociid mites (Acarina: Mesostigmata) recovered from neotropical flowers and hummingbirds' nares. Annals of the Entomological Society of America 57:103–126.

Baltosser, W.H. and Russell, S.M. 2000. Black-chinned Hummingbird (*Archilochus alexandri*). In The Birds of North America, No. 495. Poole, A. and Gill, F. eds. The Birds of North America, Inc., Philadelphia.

Baltosser, W.H. and Scott, P.E. 1996. Costa's Hummingbird (*Calypte costae*). In The Birds of North America, No. 251. Poole, A. and Gill, F. eds. Philadelphia: The Academy of Natural Sciences; Washington, D.C.: The American Ornithologists' Union.

Bendire, C.E. 1895. Life Histories of North American Birds, United States National Museum, Special Bulletin 3.

Bent, A.C. 1940. Life Histories of North American Cuckoos, Goatsuckers, Hummingbirds and Their

Allies, Part II. Smithsonian Institution, United States National Museum, Bulletin 176, United States Printing Office., Washington, D.C.

Calder, W.A. 1993. Rufous Hummingbird (*Selasphorus rufus*). In The Birds of North America, No. 53. Poole, A. and Gill, F. eds. Philadelphia: The Academy of Natural Sciences; Washington, D.C.: The American Ornithologists' Union.

Calder, W.A. and Calder, L.L. 1992. Broad-tailed Hummingbird. In The Birds of North America, No. 16. Poole, A. and Gill, F., eds. Philadelphia: The Academy of Natural Sciences; Washington, DC: The American Ornithologists' Union.

Elliston, E.P. 1995. Security behavior in Black-chinned Hummingbird mothers and nestlings. Journal of Wildlife Rehabilitation 18 2:3–4.

Elliston, E.P. and Baltosser, W.H. 1995. Sex ratios and bill growth in nesting Black-chinned Hummingbirds. Western Birds 26: 76–81.

Elliston, E.P. and Perlman, J. 2002. Meeting the protein requirements of adult hummingbirds in captivity. Journal of Wildlife Rehabilitation 25(2):14–19.

Johnsgard, P.A. 1983. The Hummingbirds of North America, Smithsonian Institution Press, Washington D.C., pp. 11, 24.

MacLeod, A. and Perlman, J. 2001. Food for thought. Journal of Wildlife Rehabilitation 24(2):30–31.

Miller, E.A., ed. 2000. Minimum Standards for Wildlife Rehabilitation, 3rd Edition. National Wildlife Rehabilitation Association, St. Cloud, Minnesota, p. 37. http://www.nwrawildlife.org/documents/Standards3rdEdition.pdf.

Robinson, T.R., Sargent, R.R., and Sargent, M.B. 1996. Ruby-throated Hummingbird (*Archilochus colubris*). In The Birds of North America, No. 204. Poole A. and F. Gill, eds. Philadelphia: The Academy of Natural Sciences; Washington, D.C.: The American Ornithologists' Union.

Scheithauer, W. 1967. Hummingbirds. Thomas Y. Corwell, New York, p. 48.

Van Epps, L. 1999. Care and Feeding of the Newborn Hummingbird. International Wildlife Rehabilitation Council 22nd Annual Conference Proceedings, Tucson, Arizona, p. 72.

28
Swifts

Paul and Georgean Kyle

NATURAL HISTORY

There are 96 species of swifts and tree swifts. Four species in the suborder Apodidae occur regularly in North America. All four species produce altricial, naked, blind, and helpless young. White-throated (*Aeronautes saxatalis*) and Black Swifts (*Cypseloides niger*) nest in crevices on cliffs, with Black Swifts selecting sites near waterfalls. White-throated Swifts occasionally nest in large empty buildings such as aircraft hangers and under highway overpasses. Chimney (*Chaetura pelagica*) and Vaux's Swifts (*Chaetura vauxii*) roost and nest on vertical surfaces inside cavities such as hollow trees or chimneys. Because of the inaccessibility of the nests of White-throated and Black Swifts, little is known of the incubation and fledging periods. Chimney and Vaux's Swifts incubate 4–5 eggs for 18 to 20 days and chicks fledge at 28 to 30 days.

White-throated Swifts' feet are pamprodactyl (four toes forward) and their legs are feathered to the toes. These swifts are able to "walk about" and will burrow into crevices. Chimney and Vaux's Swifts are anisodactyl (three toes forward, one back) but are able to turn the hallux (back toe) forward. Individuals of the genus Chaetura roost by clinging to rough vertical walls and are virtually helpless on horizontal surfaces (see Figure 28.1). Their legs are covered with delicate skin rather than the scales common to passerines.

Swifts are insectivorous, and their insect prey is typically collected in flight. An expandable throat pouch is used to store insects to feed nestlings.

The authors' extensive experience with displaced Chimney Swifts is the foundation for this chapter. Although the substitute diet recommendations of this paper would be appropriate for most swift species, housing and release criteria may require adaptation based on the individual species' natural history. Input from West Coast rehabilitators has indicated that Vaux's Swifts respond well to this diet and these techniques. More extensive information on the life history and conservation of Chimney Swifts can be found in *Chimney Swifts, America's Mysterious Birds above the Fireplace* (Kyle and Kyle 2005a).

CRITERIA FOR INTERVENTION

A rehabilitator who is knowledgeable about the breeding biology and migratory habits of Chimney Swifts can often prevent the need for intervention, allowing the swifts to complete their seasonal nesting cycle in an undisturbed site. The following basic facts have been helpful in dealing with the public:

- Chimney Swifts migrate to North America from Peru and the Amazon River Basin (Coffee 1944) in the spring and are protected by federal law under the Migratory Bird Treaty Act.
- Unlike most birds, Chimney Swifts are unable to perch or stand upright and must have chimneys or similar structures in which to roost vertically and raise their families.
- The loud noises often heard by homeowners are made by baby swifts when they beg for food from their parents. The young make the most noise from about 2 weeks of age until they leave for their first flight, so most callers will have 2 weeks or less before their chimney is relatively quiet. Their nests are small and pose no safety or health hazards when the chimney is properly maintained.
- Chimney Swifts eat, and feed their young, thousands of flying insects, including

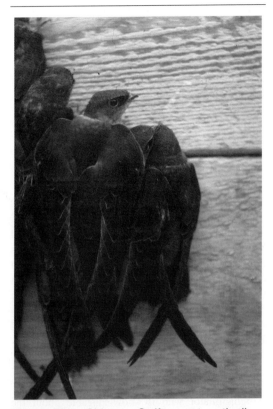

Figure 28.1. Chimney Swifts roost vertically and cuddle in closely packed groups in the wild. This behavior is also common in healthy hand-reared birds.

mosquitoes, flies, midges, winged ants and termites.

- Chimney Swifts are in North America only during the warmest part of the year and migrate back to South America by fall.

Once callers understand that it is normal for swifts to be in chimneys, that their presence is only seasonal, and that the loud sounds are the feeding calls of baby birds, most will be content to let the swifts stay the few weeks needed to raise their families.

Making sure the damper and fire doors are closed can diminish the noise and prevent birds from falling into the fireplace or flying into the house. In older fireplaces that have no dampers or in those in which the dampers are inoperable, a large piece of foam rubber can be wedged into the lower part of the flue.

Most Chimney Swift acquisitions occur when babies, juveniles, or adults fall past the damper into the fireplace. Adults become confused, fly around the house and often collide with windows. Adult birds can be caught by hand and, if uninjured, replaced on the inside wall of the chimney above the damper. Hold the bird to the wall with your hand cupped over its back until it has a firm grip on the vertical surface. Juveniles that are completely feathered, have their eyes wide open, and have been down for less than 24 hours can also be returned to the chimney in this manner. However, their ability to cling to a rough surface should be tested before replacing them. This can be done by gently holding the birds against the brick on the fireplace wall. If they are able to cling well with both feet, replacement can proceed. Placed on the inside wall above the damper and smoke shelf, they will climb up to their siblings and continue to be fed by the adults.

Nestlings are usually acquired when an entire nest with babies clinging tightly breaks loose and falls from the chimney wall. Whenever a nest or babies are found down, the smoke shelf, fireplace, screen, and surrounding area should be thoroughly searched so that all the babies are recovered.

Because the designs of fireplaces and chimneys are so diverse, there is no single solution to a fallen nest. At the very least, the nest must be replaced above the damper in the lower section of the chimney. One option is to place the nest in a shallow wicker basket and place it on the smoke shelf just above the damper. It must be either weighted or wedged in such a way that when the parents land on it to feed their young it does not tip over. Another method is to tape the nest to a broom and wedge the broom in a corner of the chimney above the damper.

Some callers may have been advised to place young Chimney Swifts outside in a basket on their roof or they may have placed juveniles on a tree in the hope that the parents would come and feed them. Although this may be sound advice in the case of some species of passerines, it will be fatal to swifts. Any Chimney Swifts that have been left outside for any length of time should be taken in for rehabilitation.

It is always important to explore every appropriate alternative before agreeing to remove a bird from the wild and accept it for rehabilitation. Once it has been determined that a Chimney Swift requires care, it should be transported in a small, cloth-lined, covered box. Terry cloth is inappropriate because the loops might entangle a bird's claws and cause injuries. A tee shirt works well, but any tightly woven cloth is fine. The cloth will provide a surface to which the birds can comfortably cling, and the darkness will keep them calm. Callers should be discouraged from attempting to give food or water to swifts. Giving no care at all can be better than causing the bird to aspirate fluids or eat inappropriate food.

Due to the inaccessible nature of the nests of other species of swift, returning a fallen chick to the nest is usually impossible. Any juvenile swift found on the ground should be admitted for rehabilitation.

INITIAL CARE AND STABILIZATION

Chilled birds should be warmed before administering fluids. Fluid therapy is essential prior to feeding the birds any solid food (Kyle and Kyle 1995, 2004). Because Chimney Swifts lack a true crop, oral rehydration can be just as effective (and safer) than either tube-feeding or injections. A combination of three products has proven to be reliable and predictable in results when used for oral rehydration: Gatorade, Nutri-cal, and STAT high-calorie liquid diet. Use only lemon-lime or other light-colored flavors. Using flavors with dark colors will make evaluation of stool more difficult.

A warmed 85°F (30°C) mix of 10 : 1 Gatorade to Nutri-cal is an excellent initial treatment. The Gatorade provides carbohydrates and electrolytes, and Nutri-cal provides readily available calories without overloading the digestive system. STAT has similar properties as the 10 : 1 Gatorade to Nutri-cal mix, but it is more concentrated. It should be used only after the bird's digestive system has begun to respond to the initial treatment.

Monitoring the consistency of a bird's stool is an effective way of determining its condition. The following protocol will insure that a swift's digestive system is fully functional:

1. Until the first stool: administer 3–4 drops of 10 : 1 Gatorade to Nutri-cal mix from a curved-tip irrigating syringe every 15 minutes.
2. After the first stool: administer 3–4 drops of 10 : 1 Gatorade to Nutri-cal mix every 15 minutes and 2 drops of STAT every 30 minutes.
3. After the second stool: Feed 1 small mealworm every hour; 3–4 drops of 10 : 1 Gatorade to Nutri-cal mix and 2 drops of STAT every 30 minutes.
4. Continue step 3 throughout the first 2 days of acquisition. As the stool improves, the number of mealworms should be gradually increased. The amount of solid food should be decreased if the quality of the stool deteriorates.

The first stool may not be a true indication of a bird's condition. Even if its parents have not fed a bird for an extended period, the first stool can be quite wet and normal in appearance. In many altricial avian species, nestlings will retain moisture by not defecating until fed. A normal Chimney Swift stool has two major parts: dark, solid material (exoskeletons and other hard, indigestible parts) and white uric acid. As volume repletion begins to occur, the accumulation of fecal material can be observed through the skin in the cloaca. If several hours have passed, no stool has been expelled, and there is a substantial accumulation of fecal material, the bird may need assistance. Swifts may be stimulated to defecate by assisting them to back over the edge of the artificial nest while still holding on with their claws. This assistance may be especially helpful for individuals with leg injuries. When expelled, the white portion of the stool should be considerably smaller than the dark portion and concentrated on the end of the stool. Any time the entire stool has a white coating, the bird is still volume depleted and fluid therapy should continue.

There is sufficient nutritional value in the rehydrating solutions alone to sustain a bird for up to 24 hours. Swifts that are volume-depleted and emaciated may be "jumpy" or hyperactive, or they may keep their eyes closed even if they are old enough to normally have them open. If any of this behavior continues for more than 24 hours, or if the stool does not normalize within that period, the swift may be suffering from an infection or injury.

COMMON MEDICAL PROBLEMS AND SOLUTIONS

Injuries

Chimney Swifts are subject to several injuries simply because of the location of their nests and their vocalizations. Fires intended to expel the unwanted animals from the chimney cause poisoning from toxic fumes, singed feathers, and burns. A veterinarian should immediately treat the inevitable respiratory problems with oxygen therapy. Burns should be flooded with sterile isotonic saline several times daily until new tissue begins to grow. Eyes should be checked for corneal damage and kept moist with an artificial tears solution.

When a swift accidentally ends up inside a house, it is often caught by the family cat or dog, or collides with windows or skylights. If puncture wounds are found or suspected, the bird should be started on an oral broad-spectrum antibiotic. Head trauma should be treated with an anti-inflammatory drug. A veterinarian should always be consulted before administering any medication.

If a leg is fractured, it must be immobilized. Because swifts' legs are relatively short, splinting is nearly impossible. A method that has worked quite well is using stretch gauze to gently bind the injured leg to the body. Do not apply tape directly to the skin of nestlings. Be sure to adjust the wrap if it becomes too tight or too loose, and be careful to not cover the bird's vent.

One-legged Chimney Swifts will be at a disadvantage, but they have been observed feeding young in the wild (Dexter 1967). However, swifts without the use of either foot will not be able to survive in the wild and should be euthanized.

A swift with a broken wing is usually a case for euthanasia. Although attempts to rehabilitate wing fractures are not discouraged, the prognosis is usually poor.

Chimney Swifts molt their feathers once each year. The molt begins in the spring and continues into the fall. In most cases, swifts with damaged or deformed feathers will not self-molt. Broken or poorly developed flight feathers of a swift in rehabilitation should not be plucked because of the danger of damage to the follicle.

Overwintering is discouraged. The muscle tone and condition of feathers in Chimney Swifts is highly dependent on flight. Chimney Swifts may survive a winter in captivity, but the chances that they will be able to fly and survive in the wild are negligible.

Illness

Whether bacterial, viral, or fungal, opportunistic organisms can easily infect a bird weakened by stress. Several recurring conditions have been observed frequently enough in hand-reared Chimney Swifts that certain symptoms can now reliably suggest impending illness (Kyle and Kyle 2004). Once these warning signs are observed, prompt action is essential because infections can quickly cause morbidity or mortality:

- Failure to respond with the feeding call within 24 hours
- Skin or mouth is dark red or white rather than pink
- Difficulty in swallowing or excessive mucus in mouth and throat
- Regurgitation of food
- Swelling, air or fluid pockets on any part of the body, but especially the face or head
- Loss of voice: mouth moves normally but bird is mute
- Poor equilibrium
- "Jumpiness" or hyperactivity after extended fluid therapy
- Abnormal stool: foul odor, gas bubbles, grainy texture of solid material, dark green or black in color, stringy in consistency

Any of these symptoms may indicate a bacterial infection. The only way to know for certain how to effectively treat the condition is to have your veterinarian or a microbiology lab perform a culture and sensitivity test. During any season, the common pathogens may change, as may the organisms' sensitivity to any particular antibiotic.

The culture will identify the organism(s) responsible, and the sensitivity test will indicate which antibiotics will best treat the infection. A throat culture taken with a sterile minitipped culturette in transport medium prior to administration of any antibiotics is usually sufficient for a diagnosis. Your veterinarian will have access to these, and it is wise to keep several on hand at all times.

Cultures generally take a minimum of 24 hours to grow and be interpreted, so it is essential to collect the sample and get it to the lab as soon as a problem is suspected. In that amount of time an infection can cause considerable morbidity. Your veterinarian may recommend a suitable broad-spectrum antibiotic to be used in the interim. In most cases, oral administration of drugs is preferable to injections.

Yeast infections are most commonly seen in juveniles and adults. This is usually indicated by a mustard-colored stool and steady weight loss in spite of good appetite or sufficient force-feeding. A veterinarian can confirm a yeast infection by microscopic examination of a fresh fecal sample. Although yeast infections left untreated are usually fatal, they can be successfully treated with Nystatin (Bristol-Meyers Squibb) at 300,000 IU/kg twice daily for 7–14 days (Carpenter 2005).

Swifts that are fed an inappropriate diet or have not received a beneficial bacteria supplement (*Lactobacillus acidophilus*) to aid in their digestion will often develop a white mucuslike material in the throat. This material may also form a hardened layer around the edges of the gape. Birds that are fed the hand-feeding diet described in this chapter usually recover from the condition within 24 hours. Failure to provide an appropriate diet will allow the condition to continue, resulting in improper development, bacterial or yeast infections, and ultimately the death of affected birds (Kyle and Kyle 2004).

HAND-FEEDING DIET

The aerial plankton that comprises the natural diet of swifts has been shown to be low in calcium. This is evident in the extremely thin-shelled nature of swifts' eggs that wither and shrivel after hatching (George Candelin, George Oxford Swift Project, personal communication 2005). Swifts do not typically have problems with metabolic bone disease. Consequently there should be no concern about this substitute diet being lower in calcium than those that are used with other avian species. This diet was specifically designed for Chimney Swifts with the assistance of nutritionists and the veterinarians of the Texas A & M University Avian Diagnostic Laboratory. Success of the diet may be measured in the high survival and release rates of birds raised on the diet as well as extensive postrelease, breeding success, and postmigration data on many hand-reared individuals studied over a 20-year period. It is important to note that many commercial avian diets typically contain grain products. Because swifts are unable to digest many of these plant-based products, these diets should not be used for swifts.

Chimney Swifts are obligate insectivores. Small and medium mealworms (*Tenebrio molitor*), if properly fed and housed, provide most of the nutritional requirements of avian insectivores (Kyle and Kyle 2004, Petrak 1982).

Mealworms, being extremely sensitive to heat, must be kept cool and dry during shipping and transport. Even if they are promptly and properly shipped, they will be dehydrated upon arrival. As soon as they arrive from the supplier they must be separated from the newsprint in which they are shipped and placed in a rigid plastic container with an ample amount of 3:2 wheat bran to cornmeal mix. About one cup of mixture is adequate for 1,000 mealworms. Moisture is provided by a white potato, sliced in half and placed sliced side down on top of the mix. The colony should be left at room temperature overnight to feed. By the next morning, the shed skins and dead mealworms will have been pushed to the top of the colony where they can be easily removed. After cleaning, the colony can be stored in a refrigerator, uncovered to prevent condensation. This will slow the activity of the colony and keep them small enough to feed to birds for a longer period of time. The colony should be taken out once each week to clean out skins and dead mealworms and allow them to feed at a normal rate. If any condensation occurs, the mealworms must immediately be sifted out and placed in a dry mix. The potato should be replaced as it is eaten by the mealworms. Small amounts of lettuce and other salad greens can also be fed to the colony.

Small birds may have difficulty digesting the skin of larger, tougher mealworms. Therefore, only the smaller ones should be used. It is inappropriate to feed cold mealworms to any bird. A small working colony should be kept at room temperature during the entire nesting season for ready use.

Some important minerals and essential amino acids must be added to the mealworms to make the diet complete. If all of the following ingredients are used, Chimney Swifts will not experience nutrition-related problems. However if even one ingredient is omitted or substituted, it will be a different diet with possibly inferior results (Kyle and Kyle 1986, 1990).

Diet Ingredients

- Small and medium mealworms (not "Jumbo")
- Avimin liquid mineral supplement
- Avi-Con powdered vitamin supplement
- SuperRich Yeast or other nutritional (not "brewers") yeast
- Nutri-cal
- Plain, active-culture yogurt (*L. acidophilus*)
- Distilled water

Utensils

- Blunt, narrow-tipped stamp tongs or forceps
- 1 saltshaker
- 8 curved-tip irrigating syringes
- 1 500 ml (pint) jar with lid
- 1 120–240 ml (4–8 oz) wide-mouthed glass jar or bowl

- 1 large-mesh tea strainer
- 1 small plastic plate

Diet Preparation

1. In the pint jar, dissolve 200 mg (0.5 tsp) Avi-con in 250 ml (8 oz) distilled water and 15 ml (1 Tbsp) Avimin. This mix can be refrigerated and small amounts warmed as needed. It will be used to drown the mealworms before feeding them to the swifts.
2. Mix equal parts of active culture yogurt and Nutri-cal (approximately 1 ml or 0.25 tsp each) into a smooth consistency and place in a curved-tip irrigating syringe. This mix should be made fresh every 2–3 hours to prevent spoilage. A larger amount of the mix may be divided among several syringes (six for 1 day) and refrigerated. Be sure to take out a syringe early enough for it to warm to room temperature before use. Do not attempt to warm the mixture with heat or in a microwave as the active culture in the yogurt may be killed.
3. Fill the saltshaker with nutritional yeast.
4. Fill a curved-tip irrigating syringe with distilled water.
5. Place a small amount of room temperature drowning mix in the small bowl 15 to 30 minutes prior to feeding time. Using the strainer, sift out an appropriate number of mealworms and place them in the drowning mix. The mealworms will absorb the vitamins and minerals in the mix.
6. At feeding time, remove the mealworms from the drowning mix with the stamp tongs (a plastic fork works well when using larger numbers of mealworms) and place them on the plastic plate. For naked birds, tenderize the mealworms by pinching all along the body of each mealworm with the tongs.
7. Sprinkle the mealworms with a small amount of SuperRich Yeast.
8. Squirt a small amount of the Nutri-cal/yogurt mix on all of the mealworms to be fed to the birds with their eyes still closed and on at least one mealworm to be fed to each fully feathered bird.
9. Feed the birds with the tongs. The segments on the bodies of mealworms overlap from front to rear (see Figure 28.2). For this reason, mealworms should always be fed "head first" to make them easier for the birds to swallow.

Feeding Procedures

Solid food should *never* be fed to any bird until it has been properly rehydrated (see the section "Initial Care and Stabilization," earlier in this chapter).

Chimney Swifts' feeding responses can be triggered by tapping the basket or by gently brushing

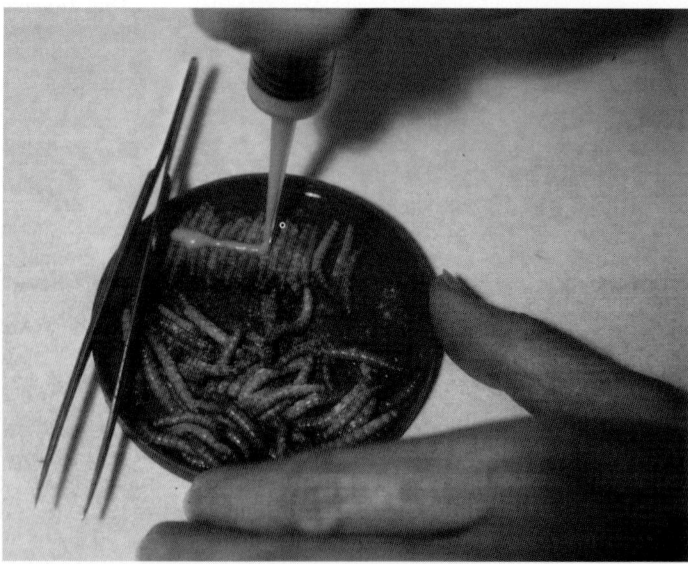

Figure 28.2. Mealworms must be specially prepared and supplemented to provide a sufficient diet for Chimney Swifts.

their faces with a facial tissue to simulate the parents' wings (Terres 1980). They respond by bobbing their heads down or throwing their heads back, chattering loudly and gulping at anything close. If a swift is allowed to bite the caregiver's finger, its mouth can easily be held open long enough to insert a mealworm with tongs. With a little practice, they will soon learn to gulp the mealworms directly from the tongs.

Each bird should be given as many mealworms as it will eat (prepared as described in the "Hand-Feeding Diet" section, earlier in the chapter) every 30 minutes, 12–13 hours per day until 10 days old. At this time, the birds will usually begin to be less responsive on the half-hour. One method of gradually extending the feeding schedule is to begin omitting one feeding during the afternoon when the birds are typically less active. Omit additional afternoon feedings on succeeding days until the birds are on an hourly schedule. The hourly schedule must be continued until release. Chimney Swifts adapt quickly to regular feedings, and maintaining a regular schedule is important in keeping stress levels as low as possible.

Older fledglings may have to be force-fed six to eight mealworms every hour until they learn to accept food from the tongs. Juveniles and adults may never learn to take food and may have to be force-fed until the time of release. Because swifts feed on the wing and are unable to perch, they never self-feed in captivity.

One or two drops of distilled water from a curved-tip irrigating syringe should follow each feeding. Place the drops on the bird's bill, not in its throat.

Because of the frantic nature of their feeding response, special care must be taken to keep the birds' faces clean. A swift's nostrils are very far forward. Be careful not to get food in them because it will harden and be difficult to remove. Each bird's face must be gently cleaned with a damp tissue whenever necessary and after the last feeding of the day.

Saliva Transfer

When Chimney Swifts hatch, their digestive tracts are sterile. They become inoculated with normal gastrointestinal flora and establish their immune competence by the transfer of saliva from the parents during the numerous mouth-to-mouth feedings. Chimney Swifts that are acquired for rehabilitation at less than 7 days old may not have fully inoculated digestive tracts and their immune competence may be substandard. These very young birds will be susceptible to potentially fatal infections from common pathogens. Although the active cultures in the yogurt provide some useful flora and aid in digestion, there is currently no substitute for the constituents of the adults' saliva.

If older nestlings, fledglings, or recovering adults are available, they may be used as saliva donors. A young swift can be inoculated by feeding it a tong-held mealworm that has been swabbed in the throat of an older swift. The process is in addition to the normal feeding schedule and should be repeated three times each day until the bird is 10 days old. The donor swifts may be those that are injured but not ill and must be receiving no medication at the time of transfer.

During a 1985 study, this procedure reversed a previous 100% mortality rate in swifts less than 7 days old. Ninety-four percent of the youngest uninjured birds inoculated that year were successfully raised to release (Kyle and Kyle 1990a, 2004). Under no circumstances should saliva from another species or the dried saliva from a Chimney Swift nest be used.

EXPECTED WEIGHT GAIN

Weighing birds daily can be extremely helpful in monitoring their development. The average growth rate for hand-reared Chimney Swifts should be 1–2 g per day for the first 3 weeks (see Figure 28.3). A weight gain of less than one-half g may indicate a metabolic problem often related to a systemic infection. A fluctuation in weight after a bird reaches 20 g is normal.

HOUSING

Nestlings

Birds less than 14 days old are nestlings incapable of effectively regulating their body temperature. They must be housed in an enclosure that maintains constant temperature and humidity, such as a human infant incubator. A suitable alternative to an incubator is a "Hospital Box": a ventilated enclosure made of wood with a glass or clear plastic front door (Petrak 1982). Heat is provided from above with the top half of a still-air poultry incubator/brooder (Kyle and Kyle 1990b). These have a built-in thermostat that is accurate to within a few degrees. Humidity

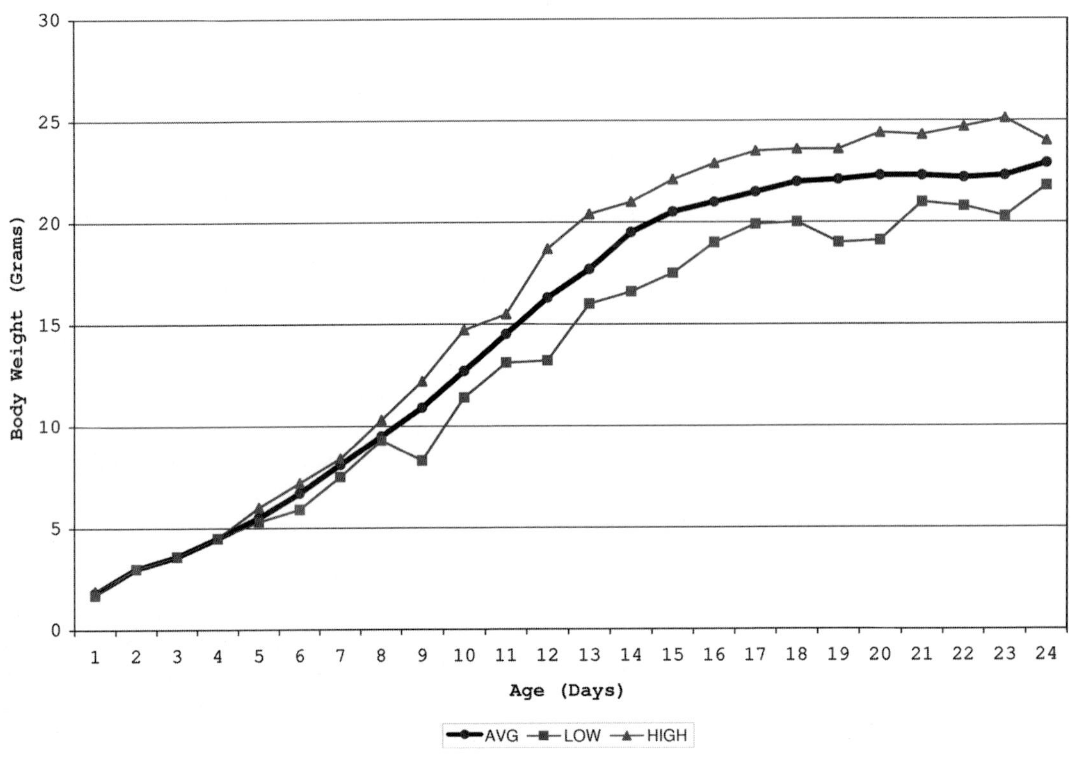

Figure 28.3. Growth rate of hand-reared Chimney Swifts (n = 12).

must be provided by a container of water with a screened top. For specific information on the construction of a hospital box, see Kyle and Kyle (1990). Incubators or hospital boxes should maintain a controlled temperature of 86°F (30°C) and a relative humidity of 50–60%.

To construct an artificial nest for nestlings within the enclosure, fold a piece of muslin cloth into a 6 in (15 cm) square (see Figure 28.4). Place this in a polystyrene supermarket mushroom container that has been thoroughly cleaned and sterilized with a mild bleach solution or other suitable disinfectant. Pressing the center of the cloth slightly into the polystyrene container will produce a shallow, dish-shaped structure that is elevated above the floor of the incubator. The nestlings will cling to the fabric and hang their heads over the edge when resting or being fed. Very young or weak swifts will defecate in the nest. A supply of clean nesting cloths should be kept available on a heating pad for quick replacement of a soiled nest. When they are a little older, they can easily back over the edge to defecate just as they would in a natural nest. Paper towels placed around the nest will aid in the removal of droppings. Some individuals will dismount the nest and roam blindly around the enclosure. This possibility should be carefully considered when setting up the enclosure.

Nestmates from the same brood should be kept together throughout the entire rehabilitation process. One brood per nest is the best arrangement. Single birds can and should be placed with others of the same age, and small broods of two or three birds can be combined.

Swifts must cling with their claws to feel secure. They have a tenacious grip even when only 1 day old. Special care must be used when handling swifts to avoid injuring their feet. When they are moved from one nest to another, their claws must be carefully worked free from the nesting material. This is most easily done by placing one hand in front of the bird and working the fingers of the other hand behind the bird's feet. The swift will usually reach forward for security when one of its feet is worked free of the cloth and will grip the hand in front of it.

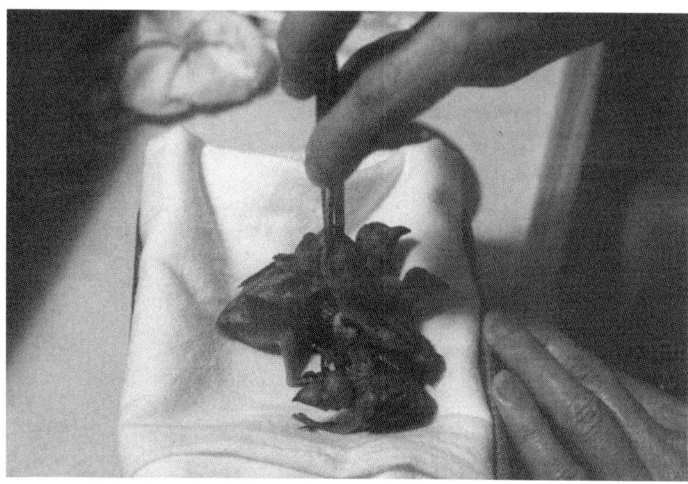

Figure 28.4. An artificial cloth-lined Chimney Swift nest will provide enough texture for the birds to be able to cling and feel secure as they would in the wild.

Fledglings

In the wild, fledglings Chimney Swifts spend their days clinging to the inside of chimneys, hollow trees, or other similar habitats. They do not actually leave the safety of the shaft until 28 to 30 days after hatching (Fischer 1958, Whittemore 1981, Kyle and Kyle 2005a,b).

Until the swifts are completely feathered and their eyes are open, they will be content on the shallow artificial nest described in the section "Housing/ Nestlings," earlier in the chapter. When their eyes are open and the body feathers are unfurled, but their heads are still covered with pinfeathers (giving the young swifts a silver or "frosty-faced" appearance), their entire nest should be placed in the bottom of a small, open-topped 12 in (30 cm) square box that has the sides lined with muslin. Lining the bottom first with a sheet of waxed paper and then with paper toweling facilitates cleaning. The toweling should be replaced at least twice during the day and once again before the birds are put to bed for the night. The cloth is draped over the sides to cover both the inside and outside of the "chimney box." The outside bottom edge of the cloth must be taped to the bottom of the box so the weight of the clinging swifts will not dislodge it.

The nest should be placed in a corner so it is in contact with two walls. The muslin will provide a textured, vertical surface for the swifts to cling to when they leave the nest. Usually, within a few hours, they will climb off the nest and onto the vertical walls (just as they would in a chimney). After a few days, when all of the swifts are off the nest, it should be removed. It is recommended that the entire chimney box be kept inside a small fiberglass-screened enclosure. At some point, the swifts will begin to exercise their wings by clinging tightly to the cloth and flapping furiously. When the swifts actually begin flying out of the small chimney box, they must be moved to an aviary.

In spite of their small size, fledgling swifts require a minimum area measuring 10 × 15 × 8 ft tall (3.5 × 4.5 × 2.5 m) once they begin to fly (Kyle and Kyle 2004, Miller 2000). Even in an aviary this large they will not be able to fly at full speed. Intermittent access to a large area several times each day is not adequate. Swifts must be allowed to fly at will if their physical and psychological development is not to be impaired (Kyle and Kyle 1990b, 2004). Details on constructing a specialized Chimney Swift flight aviary may be found in *Rehabilitation and Conservation of Chimney Swifts* (Kyle and Kyle 2004).

In lieu of a specialized flight aviary a large, empty room can be converted to accommodate Chimney Swifts. Any windows must be covered with a translucent material or fiberglass window screening spaced away from the glass panes. At least two opposite walls should be covered with a textured material such as burlap, cork, or rough-textured wood.

The aviary should be completely unfurnished except for an artificial chimney constructed of rough-textured plywood siding in the center of the

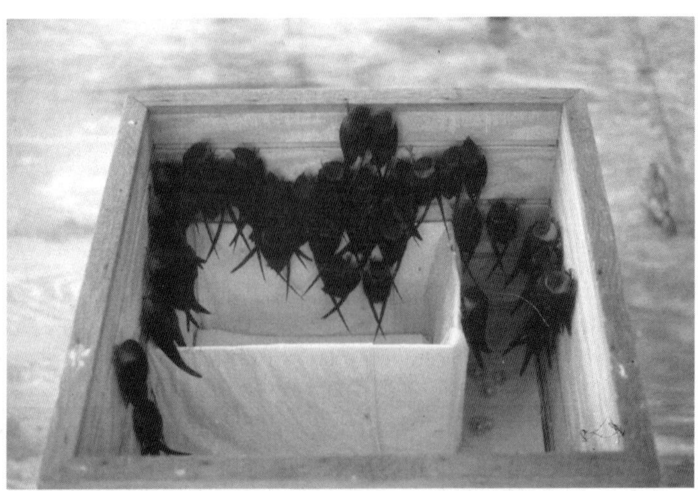

Figure 28.5. A cloth-lined "chimney box" is an excellent intermediate housing for young Chimney Swifts. They will be able to cling to the side as they would cling to the chimney wall in the wild after leaving the nest. The chimney box in this photo has been placed in the bottom of an artificial chimney inside a large flight. Once the birds have moved to the wall of the chimney, the box should be removed.

flight to serve as a roost and feeding station for the swifts. The chimney should measure about 20 in (50 cm) square, and the top should be slightly more than waist-high to the caregiver. A false bottom installed 18–20 in (45–50 cm) from the top will provide easy access to the birds. The bottom of the chimney should be covered with several layers of newsprint covered by paper toweling to facilitate cleaning.

When Chimney Swifts are introduced to the outside aviary, it is best to move the entire group, small chimney box and all, into a bottom corner of the artificial chimney just as the nest was originally moved into the first chimney box (see Figure 28.5).

The first flight is usually a stressful event for a young swift in captivity. It will go from the chimney directly to one of the walls and cling tightly. If the swifts are rounded up and returned to the chimney at each feeding, they will soon learn to return to it on their own. As the birds become more proficient, they will fly freely in and out of the chimney, fly loops around the flight, and play "tag" with one another (see Figure 28.6). Flying in and out of the chimney is excellent practice for the young birds, and a skill they will need when released.

During the heat of the summer afternoon, fledgling Chimney Swifts benefit from being gently sprayed with distilled water from a plant mister. One misting each afternoon not only cools the birds, but also encourages additional preening and helps condition feathers.

Young Chimney Swifts are extremely social creatures and seldom seem to exhibit any aggressiveness. A small chimney box will accommodate a dozen or so individuals, and the aviary described will house as many as fifty swifts at any one time. They will cuddle together with their wings overlapping each other like shingles. Keeping Chimney Swifts together in large groups seems to eliminate much of the stress of captivity and they will be able to interact with one another very much as they would in the wild.

PREPARING FOR WILD RELEASE

Classic imprinting does not seem to be a problem with Chimney Swifts. Birds that have been recaptured after release demonstrate no affection for their former benefactors.

Chimney Swifts in the wild leave the safety of the roost about 4 weeks after hatching (Fischer 1958, Kyle and Kyle 2005a,b). Hand-reared birds will not have the advantage of watchful parents when released. Additional practice in the aviary can help to compensate for this disadvantage. The extra time will improve their stamina and skill.

After 2 weeks of practice flying (when the birds are approximately 5 weeks old) release should be considered. The primary flight feathers should be completely developed, with no remaining trace of the translucent sheath that encases growing feathers. The tips of the wings should cross by at least 1 in (2.5 cm) when the bird is at rest. Release weight for

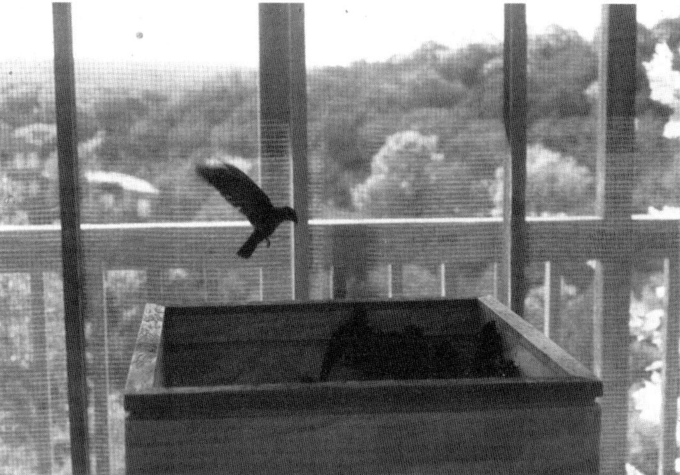

Figure 28.6. An artificial chimney provides a place for the young swifts to roost and be fed. Encouraging the swifts to return to the chimney to be fed also provides them with the practice they will need to enter and exit a chimney or similar structure when released.

hand-reared Chimney Swifts should be approximately 20 g, and the wing chord (measured from the epaulet to the tip of the longest primary) should be approximately 5 in (13 cm).

In order to survive in the wild, Chimney Swifts must be perfect fliers. They should be able to fly tirelessly in the aviary, negotiate the artificial chimney with ease, and be restless and difficult to catch to be ready for release. A swift that is reluctant to fly probably has some physical disability or is too young to release. It is important to evaluate each individual separately, and not the group as a whole.

Chimney Swifts should be released in groups 2–3 hours before sunset after the heat of the day has passed, and at a site where other swifts are feeding. They can be transported in a small chimney box with a porous covered top.

It is best to release them from a high point such as a rooftop. The chimney box should be placed at the release site and the swifts allowed to settle down from the transport. After a few minutes, when other swifts are overhead, the cover should be gently removed from the chimney box. Care must be taken not to injure birds that may be clinging to the underside of the cover. Some individuals will leave immediately, and others may hesitate. Each bird should be allowed to leave at its own pace.

Newly released Chimney Swifts will flap wildly the first few moments after leaving the chimney box. Very quickly they will begin to glide and soar between spurts of flapping. After only several minutes they will execute the rapid, jerky changes in direction that are typical of their natural feeding behavior. A release will usually attract wild swifts that will readily accept the newcomers into their group.

FURTHER STUDY

Chimney Swifts were once so common that fall roosts were likened to "smoke going back into a chimney." However, by 2004 their numbers had declined by more than 40% due to loss of habitat: first large, hollow trees and now open masonry chimneys. In the northern part of their range in Canada, they are being considered for listing on the endangered species list. More information about Chimney Swifts and conservation efforts on their behalf is available online at www.chimneyswifts.org.

ACKNOWLEDGMENTS

Two of the pioneers in Chimney Swift research were Dr. Ralph W. Dexter and Dr. Richard B. Fischer. We are honored to have had the benefit of their considerable knowledge, their encouragement, and most importantly their friendship during the twilight of their lives. Others who assisted us in developing a successful regimen for hand-rearing Chimney Swifts include Dr. Katherine Van Winkle, Betty Schuessler, Dale Zoch-Hardelik, the staff of the Avian Diagnostic Laboratory of Texas A&M University, and the Driftwood Wildlife Association.

SOURCES FOR PRODUCTS MENTIONED

Mealworms: Rainbow Mealworms, 16 E. Spruce St, Compton, CA 90224, (800) 777-9676.

Avimin: Lambert-Kay, Cranbury, NJ 08512 (available in many pet stores).

Avi-Con: Lloyd, Inc., P.O. Box 130, Shenandoah, IA 51601, (800) 831-0004.

SuperRich Yeast (not "brewers yeast"): Twin Laboratories, 150 Motor Parkway, Suite 210, Hauppauge, NY 11788.

Nutri-cal: Vetoquinol USA/Evsco Pharmaceuticals, 101 Lincoln Ave, Buena NJ 08310, (800) 267-5707.

STAT high-calorie liquid diet: PRN Pharmacal, Inc., Pensacola, FL 32504.

REFERENCES

Carpenter, J.W. 2005. Exotic Animal Formulary. 3rd Edition. Elsevier Saunders, St. Louis, pp. 172–173.

Coffey, B.B., Jr. 1944. Winter home of Chimney Swifts discovered in northeastern Peru. The Migrant 15(3): 37–38.

Dexter, R.W. 1967. Nesting behavior of a crippled Chimney Swift. Bird Banding 38(2): 147–149.

Fischer, R.B. 1958. The Breeding Biology of the Chimney Swift *Chaetura pelagica (Linnaeus)*. New York State Museum and Science Service Bulletin 368. University of the State of New York, Albany, New York.

Kyle, G.Z. 1985. An Introduction to the Role of Vitamin, Mineral and Amino acid Supplements in the Avian Diet. Driftwood Wildlife Association, Driftwood, Texas.

Kyle, P.D. and Kyle, G.Z. 1986. Hand-rearing Chimney Swifts (*Chaetura pelagica*). Wildlife Rehabilitation 5: 103–113.

———. 1990a. An evaluation of the role of microbial flora in the saliva transfer technique of hand-rearing Chimney Swifts (*Chaetura pelagica).* Wildlife Rehabilitation 8: 65–72.

———. 1990b. Housing Avian Insectivores During Rehabilitation (second edition). Driftwood Wildlife Association, Driftwood, Texas.

———. 1995. Hand-rearing Chimney Swifts (*Chaetura pelagica*): A 12-year retrospective. Wildlife Rehabilitation 13: 95–121.

———. 2004. Rehabilitation and Conservation of Chimney Swifts (*Chaetura pelagica*) (fourth edition). Driftwood Wildlife Association, Driftwood, Texas. 53 pp.

———. 2005a. Chimney Swifts: America's Mysterious Birds above the Fireplace. Texas A & M University Press, College Station, Texas. 152 pp.

———. 2005b. Chimney Swift Towers: New Habitat for America's Mysterious Birds. Texas A & M University Press, College Station, Texas. 96 pp.

Miller, E.A., ed.) 2000. Minimum Standards for Wildlife Rehabilitation, 3rd Edition. National Wildlife Rehabilitation Association, St. Cloud, Minnesota, 77 pp.

Petrak, M.L. 1982. Diseases of Cage and Aviary Birds (second edition). Lea and Febiger, Philadelphia, pp. 238, 252.

Terres, J.K. 1980. The Audubon Society Encyclopedia of North American Birds. Alfred A. Knopf, Inc., New York, pp. 868–871.

Whittemore, M. 1981. Chimney Swifts and Their Relatives. Nature Book Publishers, Jackson, Mississippi.

29
Mousebirds

Kateri J. Davis

NATURAL HISTORY

Mousebirds, or colies, are truly unique birds with six closely related species in two genera comprising the entire order of Coliiformes. Coliiformes is the only modern avian order to be entirely endemic to the continent of Africa. Mousebirds have no close relatives although they share some characteristics with turacos and parrots. All mousebird species have similar anatomy, habits, and voice, thus sharing the same avicultural care and housing requirements. Speckled, Blue-naped, Red-faced, and White-backed are the species seen in aviculture.

Mousebirds have unusual thermal physiology and are some of the very few avian species that employ torpor. They also employ sunning, clustering, and sociability techniques to help ensure their survival in an environment where food is relatively low in energy and often unpredictable in availability.

Mousebirds do not perch in typical avian fashion but rather rest their bellies on the perch (see Figure 29.1). Their legs are widely spaced and appear splay-legged to the mousebird novice. Mousebirds also hang with their feet above their heads and tail pointing down, even sleeping in this position.

Mousebirds are small gregarious birds, so named because their scampering movements through bushes combined with their gray coloring and long, skinny tails are quite mouselike. They can be found throughout most of Africa except for the northern and far western regions, inhabiting trees and bushes of dry scrubland forests and savannas as well as cultivated zones. They avoid desert and rainforest areas.

Mousebirds are mainly herbivores, eating ripe and unripe fruit as well as leaves, buds, and flowers. Insects, such as grubs, are taken on occasion.

Mousebirds are all sexually monomorphic. They are generally monogamous and live in small flocks breeding cooperatively. They help each other build loosely formed open-cup nests out of small twigs, leaves, and similar material. The young are fed by regurgitation.

CRITERIA FOR INTERVENTION

In the United States and Europe, mousebirds are slowly gaining popularity as pet birds; thus hand-rearing is becoming more common. Although parent-raised or adult imported birds can be tamed, generally hand-reared birds make the best human companions. A hand-raised mousebird can rival any species of hand-raised parrot in terms of suitability as a pet bird in a human home.

Hand-raising mousebirds is not difficult, and mousebirds are probably the easiest of the softbill chicks with which to work. Mousebird chicks that are to be hand-raised for pet quality are usually removed from the nest at 7–9 days of age. Aviculturists often use the term *pulled* for this. At this time the chick is feathered, although flightless, and very alert. It can grip well with its extra large feet, and can hang and climb within days.

In their native environment and in some avicultural settings, young and adult mousebirds sometime need rescuing, especially in stormy weather when the birds may become drenched. Rehabilitation, including hand-feeding, is sometimes needed.

RECORD KEEPING

At this time, no federal permits are required to keep and raise mousebirds. However, state laws vary and should be checked before attaining mousebirds.

Record keeping varies with each aviculturist but should include the basics, such as date hatched,

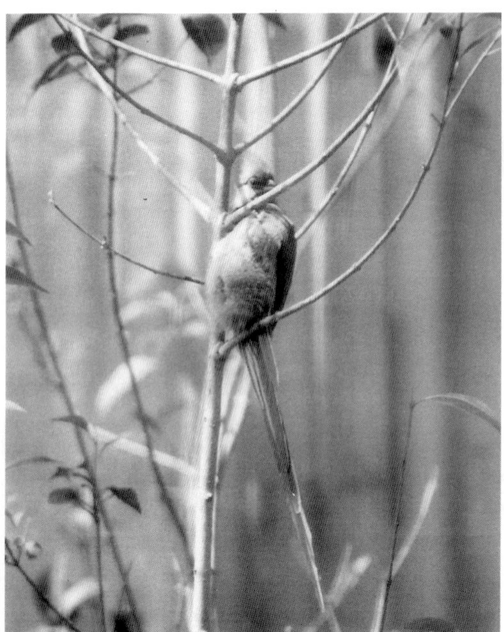

Figure 29.1. Adult Speckled Mousebird showing the unique mousebird "hang."

parents and bloodline, sexing information, and any medical issues. Leg bands or microchipping is recommended to identify and track individuals. Traditionally in aviculture, the gender of sexed birds can be visually marked by bands placed on the right leg for a male and left for a female. Tattoos are used on the appropriately sided wingweb.

INCUBATION OF EGGS

There is little reason to incubate mousebird eggs artificially. In avicultural settings, mousebirds are usually very prolific reproductively, so it is not a necessity to save every egg. Dealing with a rare species or a special case of emergency rescue would be the only instances where artificial incubation would be needed.

Mousebird eggs can be incubated at a temperature of 99–100°F (37.2–37.8°C) and 45% humidity in a standard incubator unit. They should be turned 180° in opposite directions every 1–5 hours. Evidence of fertility can be seen by candling methods around day 5 to 7.

Incubation usually lasts 12 days. Once the chick pips, it will generally hatch within the day. It is quite noisy making short calls throughout the process.

INITIAL CARE AND STABILIZATION

Heat must be given immediately to young, sick, or otherwise compromised mousebirds. When a mousebird becomes chilled, especially a youngster, whether due to environmental conditions or health problems, it can cause the bird to go into a torpid state in which the bird's bodily functions slow down, and the bird may even appear dead. Compromised mousebirds have a difficult time successfully coming out of a torpid state.

COMMON MEDICAL PROBLEMS AND SOLUTIONS

Mousebirds are relatively hardy creatures and typically have few health problems. Iron storage disease, which is common in some softbilled birds, is not documented in mousebirds.

Because of the soft nature and copious quantity of a chick's feces, the brooder and cage environments need to be religiously cleaned. If not, mold and bacteria will quickly grow, putting the chick's health at risk for aspergillosis and other infections. Unfortunately, juvenile and adult mousebirds are poor self-groomers, are oblivious of contact with their feces and food, and will soil their plumage even to the point where it impacts the feathers' ability to insulate the bird properly.

HAND-FEEDING DIET

The following sections cover recommended diets for hand-feeding mousebirds.

Days 1–6

- 2 parts commercial hand-feeding formula for parrots, such as Kaytee Exact brand Hand-feeding Formula, mixed with warm water to reconstitute as directed on package.
- 1 part strained fruit human baby food, such as Gerber's pear, apple, papaya, or banana.

Formula should be fed warm but not hot, and should be made fresh. As the chick develops, the formula should be made with less water for a thicker pancake-batter consistency. Mashed water-soaked softbill pellets can be substituted for the hand-feeding formula in emergencies.

Probiotics can be used but are not necessary; indeed, they are premixed into some commercial diets such as Kaytee Exact. Some aviculturists mix a small amount of the parents' fecal matter into the first few days' formula to promote beneficial bacteria and antibodies in the chick, but there is the possibility of introducing pathogenic bacteria and parasites.

Day 6 to Weaning

- Very small chunks of fruit, such as apples, melons, pears, papaya, and others. Avoid citrus fruits and tomatoes because of the high acid content.
- Small softbill pellets, soaked in water
- Large pellets, such as Kaytee Exact Mynah, can be soaked and then broken into small pieces.
- Water should be offered in a shallow dish.

A variety of fruits should be fed, not only to ensure nutritional variety but also to keep the bird from becoming a picky eater as an adult. Formula can be used to supplement feedings at this age, but the mixture should be made thicker every day and the majority of the diet should be the fruit mix.

FEEDING PROCEDURES

Hatchlings

Hatchlings do not have to be fed for the first 20–24 hours, getting their nutrition from the absorption of the yolk sac. The first feedings should be every 15–30 minutes, starting with only a drop or two of formula. The feeding schedule should start at about 6:00 a.m. to 11:00.p.m., with a few extra nighttime feedings for the first few days.

Mousebirds do not have crops. Their esophagus expands when fed, so a bulge can be seen on the right side of the chick's neck as he feeds. Clean the beak area after each feeding with a clean, damp swab to reduce the chance of spoiled food causing a health problem.

As the chick ages, feeding frequency can be expanded to every 1–2 hours, and amounts of formula can be gradually increased. By day 6, the chick can take 1 to 1.5 cc of formula per feeding. See Table 29.1 for adult weights of mousebird species.

After the chick realizes the feeding procedure, he will readily gape at the feeder. Chicks will signal their hunger by buzzing sounds, half-opened wings, and spastic-type movements. Speckled Mousebirds have especially pronounced movements that resemble seizures when begging. Mousebird chicks will make pumping motions while being fed and may continue to beg, even when full, and food can be visualized in the esophagus from the mouth. Beware of overfeeding, which may lead to aspiration. Smaller more frequent meals are better than larger less frequent meals.

Table 29.1. Adult mousebird weights.

Species	Weight (g)
Blue-naped	50–60
Red-faced	65–75
Speckled	50–80
Red-backed	50–75
White-backed	50–55
White-headed	35–45

Mousebird chicks will need to be stimulated to defecate after each feeding. Use a soft tissue touched to or gently rubbed on the cloaca. Feces are not in a fecal sac and are quite voluminous and soft. As the chick ages, it will defecate more and more on its own, but it is recommended that the caregiver stimulate defecation at every feeding to help keep the brooder clean.

Nestlings

Young mousebirds aged 6 days and older should be kept well fed with feedings every 1–2 hours from approximately 6:00 a.m. to 11:00 p.m. An extra feeding or two during the night is recommended the first night or two of pulling a chick.

Recently pulled mousebird chicks can be difficult to hand-feed in the beginning, and some are downright stubborn. Chicks tend to tuck their heads down and refuse to gape at the hand-feeder initially. The edge of a fingernail can be used to very gently wedge the beak open to insert the food item or syringe tip. The food should be placed just inside the beak. Care must be taken that the bird does not aspirate the food, especially with formula, and that the handler does not damage the young beak. Once the food is in the chick's mouth, it should swallow on its own.

EXPECTED WEIGHT GAIN

Mousebird chicks grow very quickly and should gain weight every day. Healthy chicks should not have a sharp keel, and, although they are generally thinner than adults, there should be muscle mass on

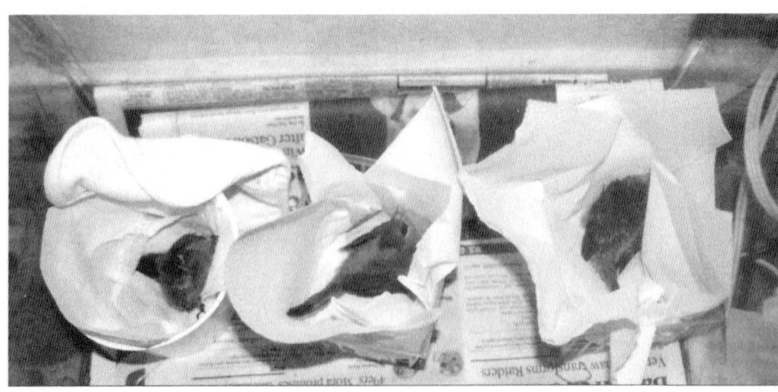

Figure 29.2. Brooder set-up with 2-week-old chicks: one Speckled Mousebird and two Blue-naped Mousebirds.

both sides of the breast. Mousebirds do not achieve their adult weight until approximately 3 months of age. Speckled Mousebirds are the heaviest of the species at between 50–80 g.

HOUSING

For the first day, hatchlings can be kept in the incubator in a small plastic bowl with a terry-cloth liner. Make a small depression in the lining to simulate a nest. The substrate enables the chick to grip with its feet as it grows. A lightweight cloth or tissue is draped loosely over the bowl so that the chick feels like it is being brooded by parents.

After the chick and its replacement nest is moved to a brooder enclosure, the temperature can be gradually lowered to 90°F (32.2°C) during the next few days. Crumpled tissues can be used over the cloth substrate for ease of cleaning, but make sure that the nest material is able to be gripped by the chick or leg problems may occur (see Figure 29.2). Mousebird chicks are very messy. Do not allow them to become soiled or damp.

By day 6, the chick will be hanging on the edge of the bowl and may hop out at feeding time. The bowl substrate can be switched to crumpled paper towels to aid in clean up.

By day 8–10, the chick is out of the nest more of the time, and it is time to provide perches and/or toys for him to start hanging on. He will soon want to hang at night instead of using the nest, and he may be moved to a more typical cage situation at this time as long as supplemental heat such as a heat lamp is given. Temperature may be gradually lowered every day until it is at room temperature by about day 14. Watch temperature and behavior closely because the chick may become torpid if the temperature goes down too quickly. If multiple chicks are being raised together, watch for aggression.

Chicks that are being raised for pet quality can be placed in separate enclosures around day 10 to ensure that they will bond closely with humans, and they must be handled daily to become successfully socialized. Mousebirds are so social that keeping a mousebird of any age by itself with no human or bird contact is cruel.

WEANING

Mousebirds wean quickly and easily. By day 11, a shallow bowl of small fruit chunks (75%) and soaked pellets (25%) can be placed in the enclosure for the chick to start investigating on its own. This proportion may be continued into adulthood. At each feeding, place the bowl in front of the begging chick and move the pieces around with a finger (see Figure 29.3). This will encourage the chick to put its beak in the bowl while gaping, thus touching the food. Feed him at an angle as close to the bowl as possible. Some birds will catch on in 1 day, but others may take a week more. Blue-naped Mousebirds tend to take longer weaning than Speckled or White-backed.

Do not discontinue the hand-feeding until the bird is about 16 days old and eating everything completely on its own. Monitor weight gain and keel muscle mass carefully. A mousebird chick is not ready for an aviary or new home release until he is a month old, eating well, and has not had supplemental heat for at least 2 weeks. At this time, he should also be able to fly, although not expertly. Adult birds will learn to eat dry pellets if pellets are gradually offered in a more dry condition during weaning.

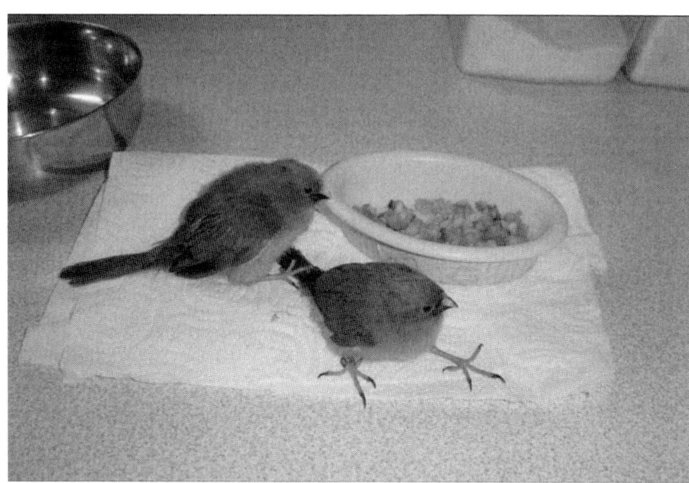

Figure 29.3. Two-week-old White-backed Mousebirds being weaned. Note small food tray with chopped fruit and soaked pellets.

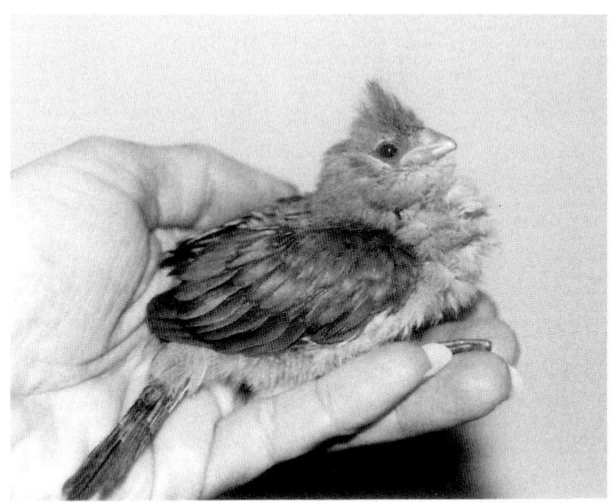

Figure 29.4. Blue-naped Mousebird, 3.5 weeks old, after a feeding. Note the distended esophageal pouch causing the neck feathers to stand up.

Make sure that young mousebirds, generally up to 3 months of age, have food available to them at all times (see Figure 29.4). They have tremendous appetites and, if they are allowed to go hungry too often, they lose weight very quickly and may go torpid.

A well-raised, hand-fed mousebird is a cuddly and loving bird that requires no extra training before entering a pet home. Because most pet bird owners are used to only parrot species, the new owner must be thoroughly educated on the unique attributes and different diet of mousebirds so that proper care will be given.

INTRODUCTION TO CAPTIVE FLOCK

Care must be taken when introducing mousebirds to each other, especially to established individuals or flocks. Intraspecific aggression is common and often fatal. Mixing species is not recommended for novices because it can be even trickier to establish harmony. Chicks can even be aggressive with each other once fledged. Typically juveniles are accepted into flocks easier than adults.

The best method is to release all the mousebirds into a new environment at the same time. If that cannot be done, then use a "howdy cage" technique, in which either the new bird or the established birds are placed in a smaller cage inside the enclosure. Because mousebirds hang on the wire, a cage within a cage in the enclosure is even better; otherwise, the birds will bite each other's toes and feet. This "howdy cage" arrangement allows the newcomer a chance to introduce himself to the other birds safely.

Once released, continue to monitor closely for signs of aggression, which include bloody toes, face, and rump area. Loss of tail feathers or a bird hiding on the ground signals problems.

AUTHOR'S NOTE

Previously little has been documented about this fascinating order of birds in captivity or in the wild.

After years of working with mousebirds herself, and compiling experiences and studies from zoological institutes and other aviculturists, the author wrote *Mousebirds in Aviculture*, the only book written on the subject. The book covers mousebirds' natural history and all aspects of the care, diet, housing, and breeding of all species of mousebirds. See http://members.aol.com/birdhousebooks for information on ordering a copy.

The author owns Davis Lund Aviaries, which specializes in softbilled birds, and more pictures and information about mousebirds and other softbill birds can be found on the author's website, http://members.aol.com/DLAviaries. She would like to make contact with other people that are working with mousebirds and can be reached at (541) 895-5149 or DLAviaries@aol.com.

ACKNOWLEDGMENTS

Thank you to all the softbill aviculturists who have shared their experiences throughout the years.

SOURCE FOR PRODUCTS MENTIONED

Kaytee products: 521 Clay St, PO Box 230, Chilton, WI 53014, (800) KAYTEE-1.

REFERENCE

Davis, K.J. 2001. Mousebirds in Aviculture. Birdhouse Publications, Sacramento, California, 140 pp.

30
Hornbills, Kingfishers, Hoopoes, and Bee-eaters

Patricia Witman

INTRODUCTION

Both facilities of the Zoological Society of San Diego, the San Diego Zoo and the Wild Animal Park, have a long history of caring for and breeding a variety of members of the order Coraciiformes. Eighteen species have been hand-reared from six of the ten families: Alcedinidae (kingfishers), Meropidae (bee-eaters), Coracidae (rollers), Upupidae (hoopoes), Phoeniculidae (woodhoopoes), and Bucerotidae (hornbills) (see Table 30.1).

NATURAL HISTORY

There are 91 species of kingfishers in the family Alcedinidae with a worldwide distribution. There are 54 species of hornbills in the family Bucerotidae, with 23 species found in tropical Africa and 31 species found in Asia to the Solomon Islands. The 25 species of bee-eaters in the family Meropidae and the 11 species of rollers in the family Coracidae are all found in the Old World. The eight species of woodhoopoe in the family Phoeniculidae are found in sub-Saharan Africa, and the single species of hoopoe in the family Upupidae is found in the Palearctic, Afrotropical, and Oriental regions (see Table 30.1).

The members of the order Coraciiformes are typically described as large-headed, short-necked, and short-legged. Most have large or long bills and have short toes on relatively weak feet, with the third and fourth toes fused at the base pointing forward. Plumage may be iridescent or green and blue pigment colors, although hornbills are black and white with some gray, brown, and cream. All are hole-nesters, whether in tree cavities, termite mounds, mud holes in banks, or some in excavated rock outcroppings. Most unusual are the hornbill species that "mud up" the nest cavity opening with mud, food, or feces, thus sealing the female and subsequent chicks inside. The female and chicks are then solely dependent on the male or helpers for food. All have white eggs that hatch into altricial chicks (Fry et al. 1992; Kemp 1995; del Hoyo, et al. 2001).

Some species nest cooperatively, but most pair up monogamously. There is a wide range in size of different species, from the pygmy kingfishers to the largest hornbills. Likewise there is a wide range of incubation periods, clutch sizes, and nestling periods (see Table 30.2).

A wide variety of insects, other invertebrates, small mammals, small reptiles, amphibians, bird eggs, and nestlings make up the bulk of the diets of the kingfishers, bee-eaters, rollers, woodhoopoes, hoopoes, and ground hornbills. Kingfishers prefer beating their prey items against a branch prior to eating. Bee-eaters mostly hunt in flight, eating bees, wasps, and related stinging species, manipulating the items until the stingers fall out. Most rollers go to the ground to feed, except the Dollarbirds that mainly take their prey in flight. Hoopoes probe for food in the ground with their long narrow bills. Although most other insectivorous birds cast a pellet made up of the indigestible chitin of the exoskeletons, hoopoes excrete it in their feces. The woodhoopoes use their long narrow beaks to probe behind bark eating, among other things, lots of caterpillars.

Although most hornbills are omnivorous, there are species that are mainly carnivorous or mainly frugivorous. When the frugivorous species are breeding, there are often many animal prey items included in the diet. The carnivorous species tend to live in the savanna and are semiterrestrial. Most of

Table 30.1. Order Coraciiformes family distribution.

Family	Common Name	# Species	Distribution
Alcedinidae	Kingfishers	91	Worldwide
Bucerotidae	Hornbills	54	Afrotropical and Oriental; marginal in Australasian
Meropidae	Bee-eaters	25	Old World
Coraciidae	Rollers	11	Old World
Upupidae	Hoopoes	1	Palearctic, Afrotropical, and Oriental
Todidae	Todies	5	Greater Antilles
Brachypteraciidae	Ground rollers	5	Madagascar
Leptosomatidae	Cuckoo-rollers	1	Madagascar and Comoro Is.
Momotidae	Motmots	10	Neotropical

Table 30.2. Incubation period, clutch size, and nestling period[a].

Species	Incubation Period (Days)	Clutch Size	Nestling Period (Days)[a]
Southern Laughing Kookaburra (*Dacelo novaeguineae*)	21–26	3	32–44
Micronesian Kingfisher (Todiramphus *cinnamonmina*)	20–23	1–3	?
White-breasted Kingfisher (*Halcyon smyrnensis*)	18–25	4–7	26–27
White-throated Bee-eater (*Merops albicollis*)	19–20	4–7	~30
White-fronted Bee-eater (*Merops bullockoides*)	19–20	2–5	~30
Blue-bellied Roller (*Coracias cyanogaster*)	18–21	2–4	25–30
Purple Roller (*Coracias naevius*)	17–23	2–4	25–30
Dollarbird (*Eurystomus orientalis*)	18–22	3–5	~23
Common Hoopoe (*Upupa epops*)	16–18	5–8	24–28
Green Woodhoopoe (*Phoeniculus purpureus*)	17–18	2–5	28–30
Abyssinian Ground Hornbill (*Bucorvus abyssinicus*)	37–41	2	80–90
Southern Ground Hornbill (*Bucorvus leadbeateri*)	37–43	1–3	86
Black Hornbill (*Anthracoceros malayanus*)	30	2–3	50
Great Hornbill (*Buceros bicornis*)	33–40	1–4	72–96
Tarictic Hornbill (*Penelopides exahatus*)	28–30	2–4	50–60
Red-knobbed Hornbill (*Aceros cassidix*)	32–35	2–3	~100
Wrinkled Hornbill (*Aceros corrugatus*)	29	2–3	65–73
Writhed Hornbill (*Aceros leucocephalus*)	29	2	?

[a] del Hoyo et al. (2001), merged with ZSSD data.

the frugivorous species live in the forest and are arboreal. Most hornbills do not drink water and rely on food as a source of hydration.

CRITERIA FOR INTERVENTION

Although parent-reared birds are preferred at both facilities, chicks may be brought in for hand-rearing as a result of parental neglect or a history of failures due to a variety of causes. Most chicks that are hand-reared are hatched using artificial incubation. This eliminates, for the most part, any chance of exposing them to parasites or infectious diseases. Chicks removed from parental care are isolated from others until the veterinary staff can evaluate their health via fecal gram stains and culture results. If parent-hatched chicks are healthy and well-hydrated (see Figure 30.1), they may be relatively easy to hand-rear when removed from the nest prior to fledging. However, it may be extremely time consuming to

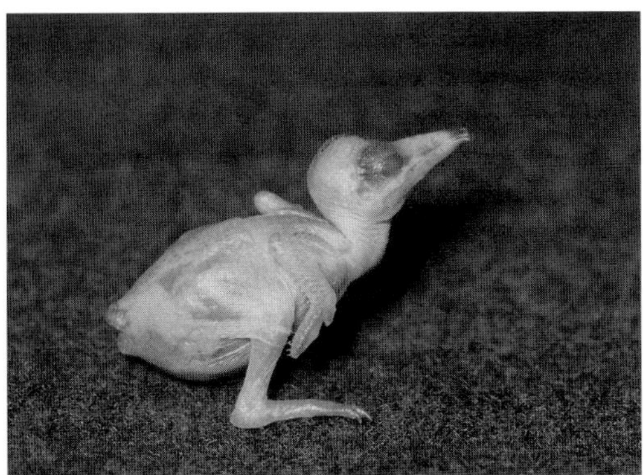

Figure 30.1. Well-hydrated White-fronted Bee-eater during first week. (Copyright Zoological Society of San Diego.)

successfully hand-rear a chick whose health has been compromised by less-than-adequate parental care.

RECORD KEEPING

Detailed hand-rearing records are kept to ensure the ability to repeat successes, share data, or track changes that lead to success. Specific information about their location, parents' identification, age, reason for removal, and condition of chick at time of removal is recorded. Care is taken to either place a band or mark with nontoxic colored felt pens all chicks for identification purposes. Detailed feed and weight records are kept (see Table 30.3). Target amounts to feed are entered along with the frequency of feedings. These are determined from past successes. The actual amounts fed are recorded, tallied, and compared to the target. Chicks are weighed every morning before their first feeding. Decisions related to target amounts to feed are based on whether weight gains or losses are in the normal range (see Figures 30.2a–d).

INCUBATION OF EGGS

Artificial incubation is used if the parents have a history of failure to hatch eggs or if there are conditions within their enclosures that would make it difficult to rear young. Incubation parameters have been determined based on past successes of closely related species. Incubation periods have been difficult to establish in cavity nesters, as it disturbs the parents to have someone investigate the nest and there are very few that have been set up with cameras for monitoring.

All of the successfully reared hornbill species and the Kookaburra were artificially incubated at 99.0°F (37.2°C) at 56–62% relative humidity (RH). The smaller eggs of the other kingfisher species, all the rollers, and bee-eaters were incubated at 99.5°F (37.5°C) at 50–66% RH. These relative humidity settings are the starting point for incubation, but percentage of egg weight loss is monitored for most eggs and the humidity was adjusted accordingly. If eggs were not losing enough weight, the humidity would be lowered, and conversely if they were losing too much weight, the humidity would be raised. The earlier these changes are made, the more effective they will be. Several small adjustments early in incubation are safer to the developing embryo than one drastic one later in incubation. Decreasing or increasing the surface area of water within the incubator will change the humidity. For example, if an egg loses only 9%, water pans with less surface area would replace the original pans in an attempt to lower the RH by 6–7%. Relative humidity should not be raised or lowered drastically, less than 10% each week.

Eggs are weighed twice a week during incubation. One method used to calculate egg weight loss is the following formula:

$$\left\{\frac{\left(\frac{S-E}{D}\times I\right)}{S}\right\}$$

where S = set weight, E = end weight, D = # days incubated since set weight, and I = incubation period. *Set weight* is the weight of the egg when it is pulled from the nest. *End weight* is the weight of the egg on any given day of artificial incubation. This formula allows the egg loss weight to be calculated even if the fresh egg weight was not obtained, and may be used at any point during incubation to determine the trend of the egg weight loss. For example, if an egg is removed from the parents after 5 days of parental incubation, the egg weighs 26 g, the incubation period is 30 days and after 7 days of artificial incubation, the egg weighs 25 g, the formula would look like this:

$$\left\{\frac{\left(\frac{26-25}{7}\times 30\right)}{26}\right\}=16.5\%$$

Table 30.3. Sample hand-rearing feed chart.

Time				0630	700	730	800	830	900	930	1000
Date	Age in days/ Body Wt/ % Change	Ca	Vit B	Meds	% of BW (Total Solids Consumed /bw)	Daily % Intake	Feeding Freq.	Target Amount to Feed/Day (bw × Daily % Intake)	Target Amount to Feed/ Feeding	Actual Solids Intake (g)	Actual Fluid Intake (ml)
24-May-06	0				23.0%	25%	7	1.25	0.18	1.07 (add all solids fed)	0.00
Amount solids fed (g)	5.00					0.18	0.19	0.17	0.20	0.18	0.15
Oral fluids											
Supplements											
Response (G, F, P, NFR)											GFR
Feces											NF
25-May-06	1				44.9%	30%	7	1.65	0.24	2.47	0.00
Amount solids fed (g)	5.50			0.32				0.32			0.31

Oral fluids	10% (Current wt – previous wt)/previous wt										
Supplements		0.01	0.02								B
Response (G, F, P, NFR)				GFR				GFR			GFR
Feces				F				F			F
26-May-06	2				36.8%	35%	7	2.39	0.34	2.51	0.00
Amount aolids fed (g)	6.82				0.33			0.32			
Oral fluids	24%										
Supplements		0.02	0.05								
Response (G, F, P, NFR)					GFR			GFR			
Feces					F			F			

Feeding response (FR): G = good, F = fair, P = poor, NFR = no feeding response.
Sample of Micronesian Kingfisher feed chart with shading indicating cells with formulas used to calculate date, age, percent body weight change, target amounts to feed, sum of amounts actually fed, and amounts of supplements. All amounts are in grams. Chart has been truncated to fit page.

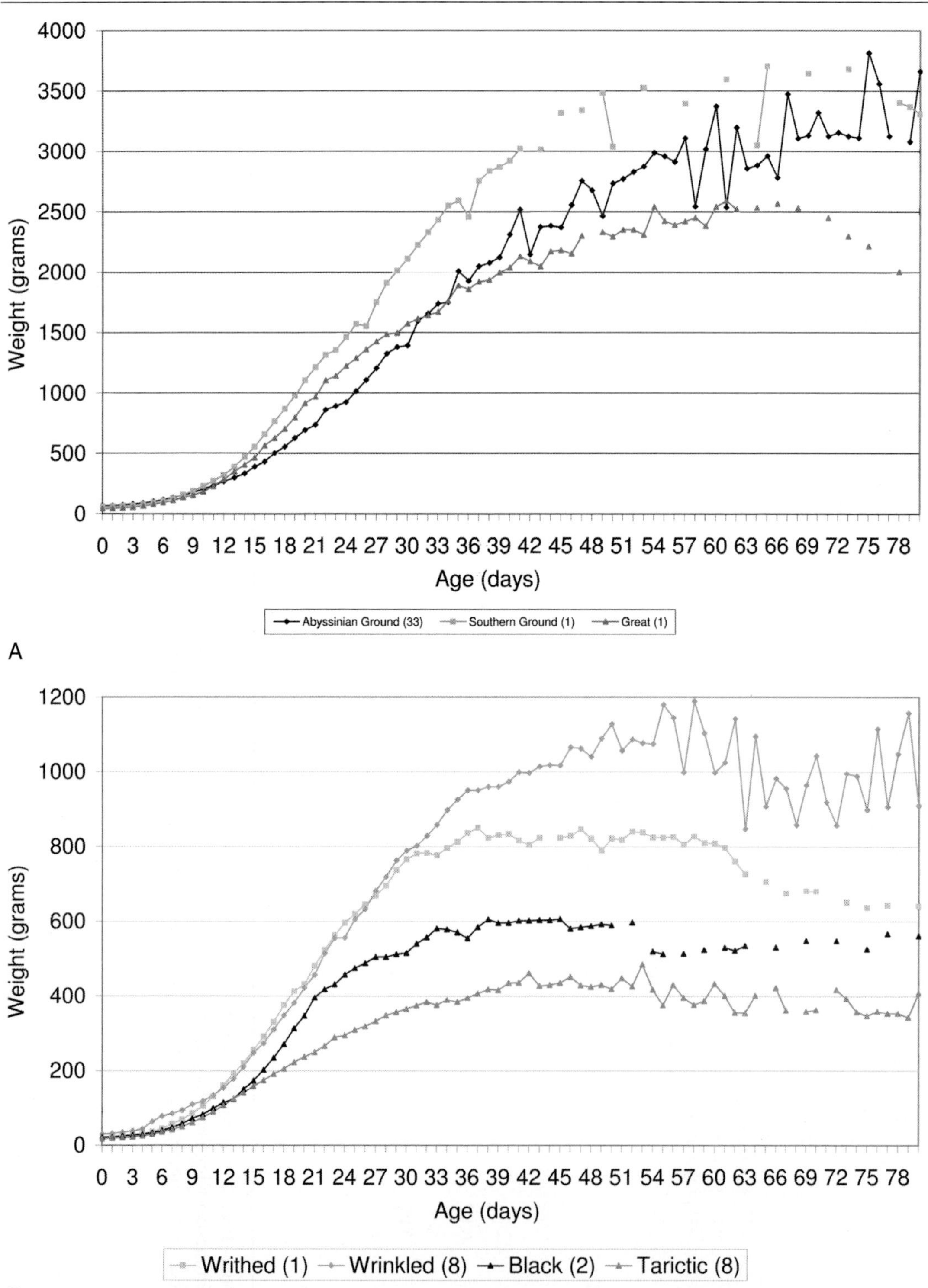

Figure 30.2. (a) Average chick growth curve for three species of hornbills. (b) Average chick growth curve for four species of hornbills. (c) Roller chick growth curve. (d) Micronesian Kingfisher chick growth curve.

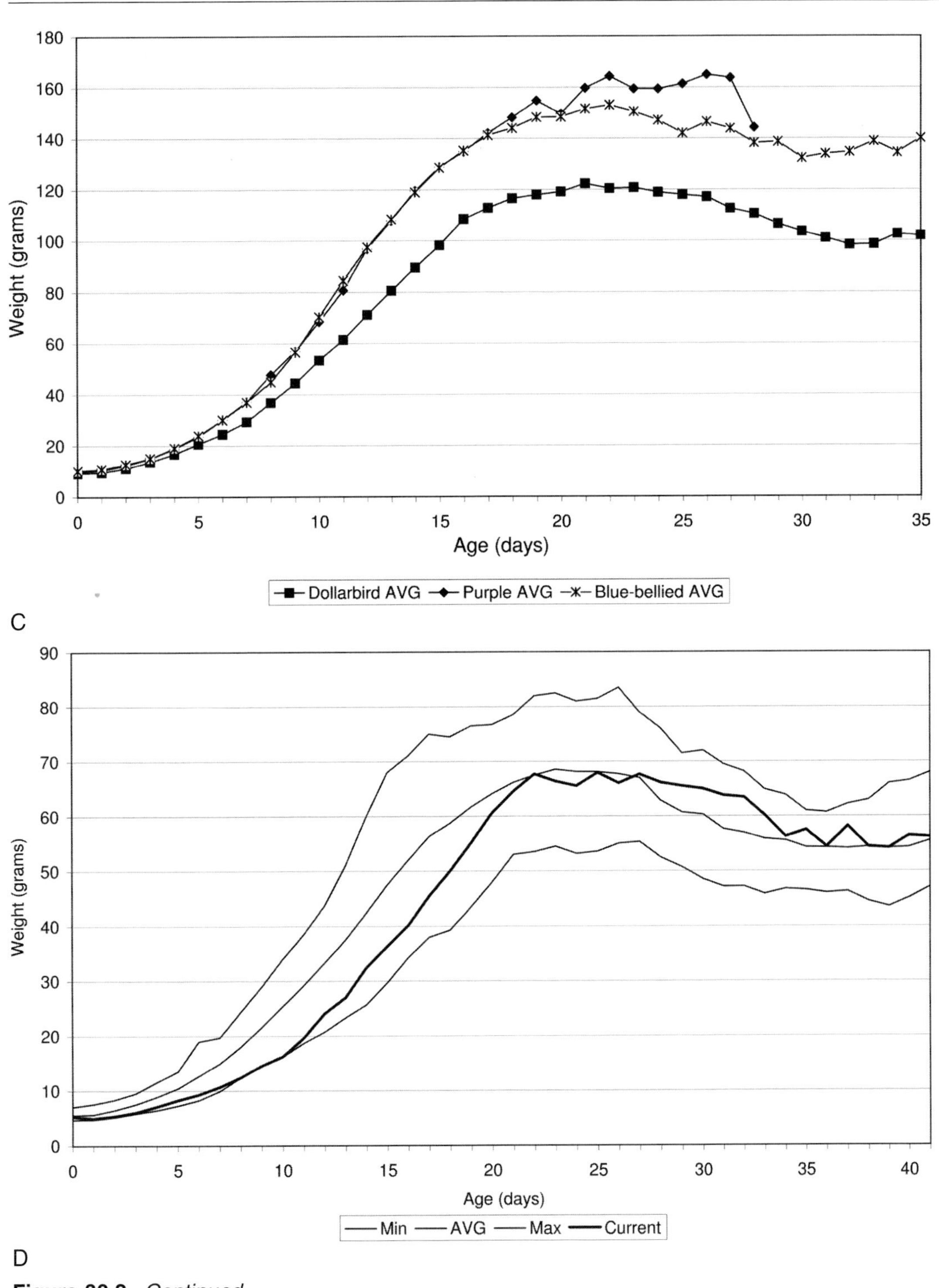

Figure 30.2. *Continued*

Table 30.4. Micronesian Kingfisher egg weight loss sample.

Egg #	Actual I	Date of 1st Wt.	Date of 2nd Wt.	D	S	E	I	I	MKF @20 Day I % Wt. Loss	MKF @23 Day I % Wt. Loss
5	20	27-Jun-95	16-Jul-95	19	7.89	7.00	20	23	12%	14%
6	21	20-Dec-97	6-Jan-98	17	7.98	7.23	20	23	11%	13%
231	21	9-Apr-98	17-Apr-98	8	7.58	7.25	20	23	11%	13%
197	21	28-Apr-99	30-Apr-99	2	7.10	7.03	20	23	10%	11%
222	21	24-Apr-00	30-Apr-00	6	6.08	5.88	20	23	11%	13%
209	23	19-Mar-04	5-Apr-04	17	7.81	7.14	20	23	10%	12%

S = set weight; E = current or end weight; D = # days artificially incubated; I = incubation period, where incubation period could be 20–23 days.

and the egg weight loss would be 16.5%. That would be within normal limits if this were a chicken egg. However, if this were a species such as the White-fronted Bee-eater and all of the successfully hand-reared chicks had hatched artificially from eggs with weight losses averaging 11.2%, the decision would be made to increase the humidity in the incubator in an attempt to slow the rate of weight loss of the egg (see Table 30.4).

Another method is to use the following formula:

$$\left\{\frac{F-P}{F}\right\}\times 100$$

where F = fresh weight and P = pip weight. This can be used at any time during incubation even if the fresh weight was not obtained and prior to pip if these values are extrapolated mathematically. The actual egg weights can be plotted on a graph along with these extrapolated values. It is then possible to determine whether the weights are in the expected range (see Figure 30.3).

The percent weight loss was 10–14% in the kingfishers, bee-eaters, rollers, and hornbills that were artificially incubated. Some of these eggs were collected as freshly laid and artificially incubated for the entire incubation period; others were collected after varying amounts of parental incubation. Eggs were transferred to hatchers approximately 3 days prior to hatching, where the temperatures were lowered by 0.5–1°F and the humidity settings were raised to 63–73% RH.

There are routine sanitation protocols that apply to incubators and hatchers to help assure that chicks hatch with minimum exposure to bacterial or viral contamination. Once a year, the incubation and hatching rooms are disinfected with a liquid disinfectant (Roccal-D, Pharmacia and UpJohn) from floor to ceiling, including all incubators, hatchers, and related equipment. On a weekly basis, the outside of all machines are wiped down with a liquid disinfectant and a UV sterilizer (Canrad-Hanovia Inc.) is used within both rooms, covering windows to protect both humans and eggs. Egg trays within all machines are disinfected between clutches. Floors are disinfected at least twice weekly with foot baths at the entrance. Traffic within the facility is limited. An ozone generator has been used routinely in the incubators recently as another means of maintaining a clean environment for eggs. The water source for humidity within all machines comes from a reverse osmosis system with a UV sterilization component. Hands are washed with an antibacterial soap before and after handling eggs. Employees wear clean uniforms every day and are expected to arrive with clean hair that is short or tied back.

INITIAL CARE AND STABILIZATION

Most neonates come to the facility via the hatchery where they've been artificially incubated. Once the chick has dried off in the hatcher, it is brought into the brooder room. The temperature of the appropriate brooder is adjusted and stable prior to the expected hatch date. Avian neonates are fed at the first sign of feeding response or within 12 hours of hatching. All food items are dipped in an electrolyte solution to moisten and provide fluids.

If a chick has been removed after hatching with the parents, its condition is evaluated and recorded.

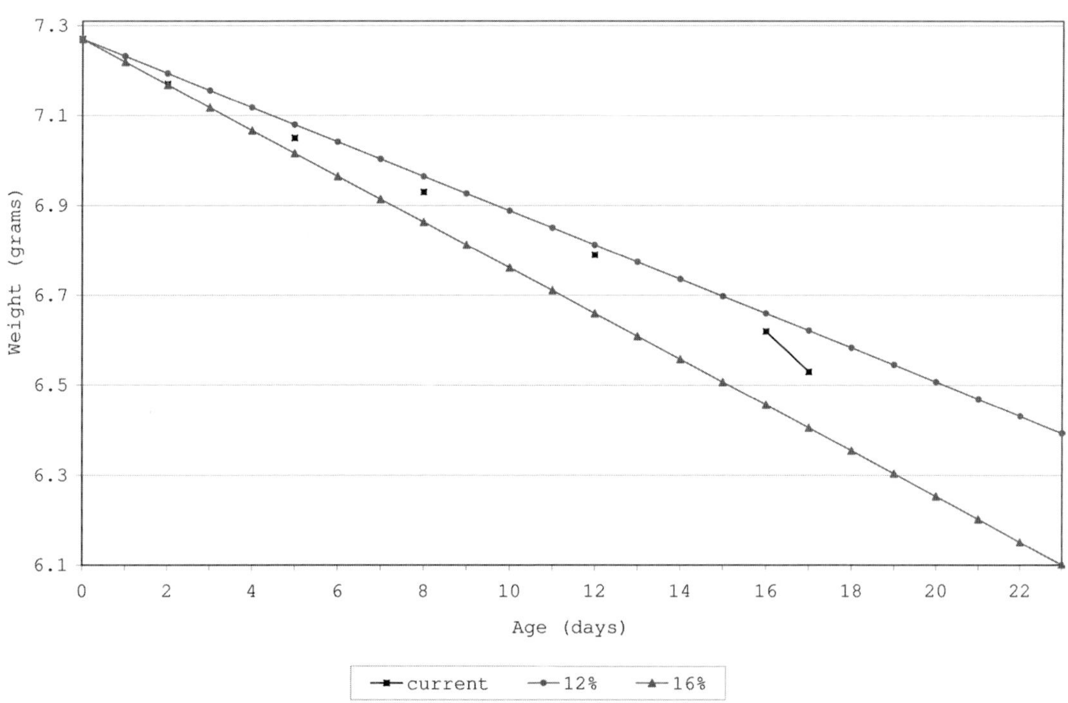

Figure 30.3. Micronesian Kingfisher egg weight loss graph.

If it is determined by "tented" skin, sunken eyes, lack of feeding response, that a chick is dehydrated, it receives 5–10% of its body weight in subcutaneous fluids (lactated Ringer's solution). If a chick has injuries, it receives treatment by a staff veterinarian. A latex glove filled with warm water is sometimes used to warm up small cold neonates by placing it among the fingers of the glove.

COMMON MEDICAL PROBLEMS

As with any species of avian neonate, bacterial infections are the most common problem encountered. A well-nourished chick reared in sanitary conditions is the least susceptible to infections. Observations about feeding responses, feces, skin, and feather condition are recorded as changes occur. Any changes that are outside the normal range are addressed as either developmental or medical abnormalities. Developmental abnormalities can occur as a result of improper nutrition, improper quantities fed or improper feeding techniques.

All of the species discussed in this chapter have been observed casting a pellet of indigestible materials (insect chitin or rodent fur) with the exceptions of the Common Hoopoe, which excretes this material, and the frugivorous hornbills that are not fed as many of the prey items as the more insectivorous or carnivorous species. In the mid-1980s when not many of this group of birds had been hand-reared, there were occasions when a chick's lack of feeding response may have been misdiagnosed as a medical issue as opposed to the normal pause some chicks need prior to casting a pellet.

Intestinal impactions associated with feeding too much chitin or fur were problems with the ground hornbills when first reared in the mid-1980s. As ground hornbills also impacted on sand, it was determined that their rearing enclosures had to be free of foreign objects that were small enough to swallow. In general, it is safer to rear chicks in relatively bare enclosures until they are old enough to be moved in with cohorts that may distract them from picking at everything around them or until they are big enough for some foreign objects to pass harmlessly through their digestive systems.

White-fronted Bee-eaters' first primaries were shorter than normal, but they grew in normal length after their first molt. At least one parent-reared chick was also observed to have abnormal tail feathers. Speculation was about a possible nutritional imbalance, but no cause was determined.

Stargazing was observed in one Abyssinian Ground Hornbill and one Micronesian Kingfisher at day 11 and day 8, respectively. Both birds received injections of B-complex vitamins, and the hornbill's condition improved within 5 days. The kingfisher did not improve for 30 days with repeated injections. It wasn't until the chick was placed in a plastic cup with a screen lid shut, holding the head in the normal position, that it did improve and was completely normal 5 days later.

DIET RECIPES

Most of the species discussed are insectivorous or carnivorous species, with the exception of some of the hornbills that tend to be more frugivorous. Regardless of the adult requirements, all chicks need protein to grow and develop normally. The most readily available commercial sources of protein are mice, insects, soaked cat or dog pet food, and supplemented meat products. Well-hydrated, plump, and juicy naked neonate mice are a source of protein that is efficient to use for many of these species. Many insects have a lot of indigestible chitin that can cause impactions in the digestive tracts of avian neonates. By using 3-week-old crickets, white molted mealworms, and waxworms during the first 7 to 10 days impactions may be avoided. Ground meat products supplemented with vitamins and minerals are available as another source of protein.

Converting an avian neonate from an easily digestible diet to an adult diet is done with a series of transitions. For species such as the ground hornbills and kookaburras, which have adult mice in their adult diets, juvenile mice from approximately 7 to 10 days provide a small amount of fur for those gradual changes. Removing the head, legs, and wings of crickets may be used as a transitional step from the soft-bodied 3-week-old crickets prior to adding adult crickets with chitin to the diet.

Some food items that are found in the captive adult diet may not be needed for hand-rearing, but adding them prior to weaning may increase the likelihood that the bird will consume a well-balanced diet as an adult. It is far easier to introduce new items to a dependent chick that is being hand-fed versus one that is already weaned. Soaked dry dog or cat food and processed meat products are two such items. Anoles are added to the diet of Micronesian Kingfishers because they are an item that is usually available, and the male uses them in courtship feeding the female.

Because none of these adult diets have a significant amount of a commercial avian pellet as a nutritionally balanced component, all of the diets used for hand-rearing are supplemented with calcium carbonate (1% of the amount of food fed the previous day) and a children's liquid B-complex high potency vitamin (Apetate Liquid). This product contains 5 mg Vitamin B_1 (Thiamine), 0.5 mg B_6 (pyridoxine), and 25 mcg B_{12} (cyanocobalamin) (1 ml/50 g of the amount of food fed the previous day). For instance, if 50 g of food was fed the previous day, the calcium supplement would be 0.5 g of calcium carbonate and the vitamin supplement would be 1.0 ml of Apetate Liquid for the following day. Crickets and mealworms are gut-loaded with a commercial calcium-based feed for 3 days prior to being fed.

The frugivorous hornbill neonates are fed approximately 70% high-protein items (neonate mice and insects) with 30% fruit for the first 10 days. The proportions gradually shift to 75% fruit and 25% protein items by approximately day 28. Papaya has traditionally been used in this facility as a source of hydration in some high-protein hand-rearing diets. By 30 days of age there is a change to a fruit mix composed of melon, apple, and other fruits as seasonally available.

The carnivorous ground hornbill chicks are fed 100% protein items. A ground meat product is introduced gradually at about 2 weeks, as is fur from adult mice (see Table 30.5).

Determining when to make these changes was initially determined by trial and error. Once success was achieved, that became the starting point for other closely related species. This underscores the importance of keeping careful records. Actual intake may vary from the target as the response of the chick and the rate of growth are taken into consideration (see Figure 30.4).

FEEDING PROCEDURE

There are three basic concerns to be addressed when hand-feeding chicks: when to feed (frequency), how

Table 30.5. San Diego Zoo Avian Propagation Center Hand-Rearing Protocol.

Common Name: Abyssinian Ground Hornbill
Species Name: *Bucorvis abyssinicus*

DAY	BROODER/TEMP.	FREQ.	DIET (by weight)	INTAKE	MISC.
1	AICU/95°F, drop 1 degree/day. Nest cup lined with paper towel/tissue.		Give Pedialyte, but wait 12–24 hrs posthatch to feed.		
2		2 hrs (7×)	100% chopped pinkies dipped in Pedialyte.	20%	Supplement w/ calcium carbonate and Apetate.
3				25%	Begin sunning.
4		3 hrs (5×)	Change to whole pinkies.	30%	
5				35%	
8	Add Nomad mat to nest.	4 hrs (4×)			May increase intake to 45% to get 15–20% wt gains.
12		5 hrs (3×)	Change to fuzzies.		Change from $CaCO_3$ to dicalcium phosphate.
13			Add 25% carnivore meat (75% fuzzie).		
14			50% carnivore meat, 50% fuzzie.		
15			Gradually change to mouse torso with no fur.		Eyes open.
17			Add small amount of fur (1 in square) and gradually increase.		Pinfeathers.
21		6 hrs (2×)			May cast pellet.
24	Move to 1/2 floor with heat, in a tub.				
30				Ad lib	
33	No heat inside.				~Day 40, self-feeding begins; leave dish between feedings.
52	Outside at night with heat.				
53					May be out of tub.
56	Outside w/out heat.				May be able to fly.
63		1 ×			Weaned.

Weight gains should be maintained at 15–20% per day.
Hornbill chicks will impact on fur, feathers, dirt, sand, and rocks.

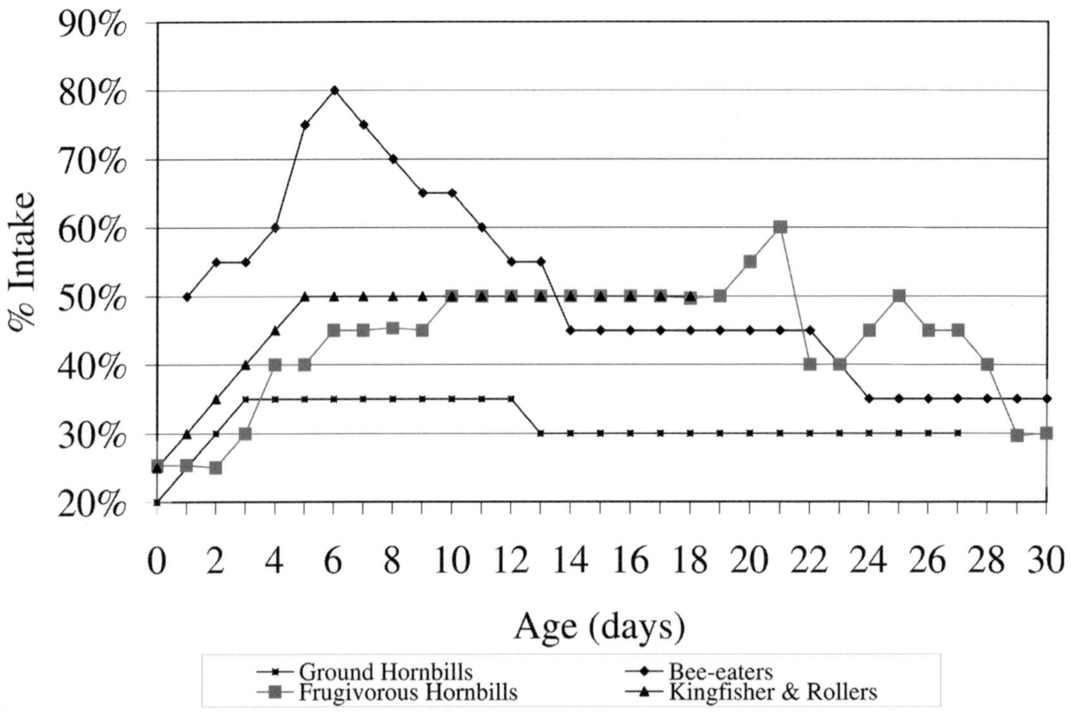

Figure 30.4. Intake targets for Hornbills, Bee-eaters, Kingfishers, and Rollers.

much to feed (quantity), and how to feed (technique). Each of these factors changes during the rearing of a chick. These transitions are what make hand-feeding such a dynamic process.

Changes in frequency of feedings occur related to each species' capacity for larger quantities of food and the greater periods of time they can go without food. As greater quantities are fed, chicks will stop eating and make it clear that it is time to reduce the frequency again. Healthy chicks are never fed by force. Keepers learn to "read" a chick's behavior and modify what they are doing to get a strong feeding response. The small bee-eaters were started at 13 times a day (every hour); all the others were started at 7 times a day (every 2 hours). Feedings occur between 6:30 a.m. and 6:30 p.m.

Forceps or curved spoons are used to feed chopped fruit or prey items (see Figure 30.5). Diet items are cut into small bite-sized pieces and are gradually cut larger as chicks grow and can easily swallow larger bites. Using blunt-tipped forceps, the food is dipped in oral electrolyte solution and placed far back into the mouth. By feeding in this manner, chicks are less apt to spit the food item back out. Chicks may regurgitate all or part of a feeding if they are fed too much, too fast, or if either they or the food items are too cold. Curved spoons have been used for hornbill chicks as they get older, and a teaspoon that was modified with the sides bent up was more efficient for delivering larger quantities.

The quantity fed has been determined differently over the years. At times, chicks have been fed to satiation or ad lib, but more often a percentage of the body weight has been used to determine the amount to be fed. This amount typically starts off at 20% of body weight and gradually increases to 35–50% in the hornbill species and 50–75% in the other smaller species during the first week. It may be held at that highest level until the chick starts regulating the amount eaten or it may be reduced gradually. The goal is to wean the chick at the same age as a parent-reared chick.

Hatchlings, nestlings, and fledglings respond to feeding in different ways. Avian hatchlings' neck

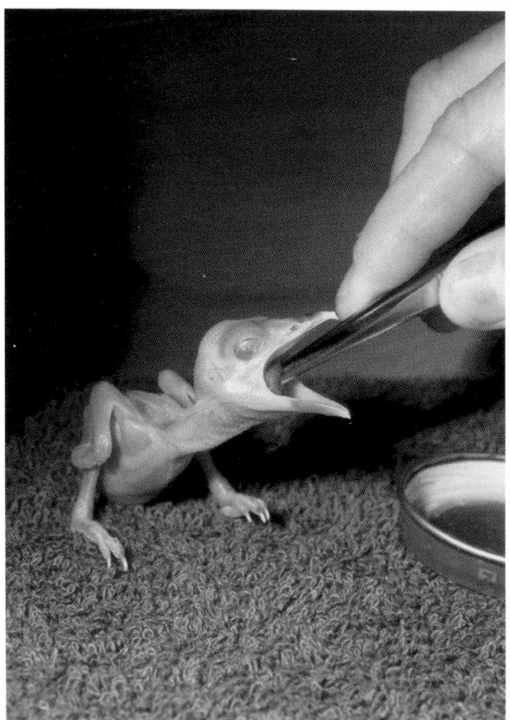

Figure 30.5. Micronesian Kingfisher during first week being fed with forceps in back of throat. (Copyright Zoological Society of San Diego.)

muscles are relatively weak and may cause their heads to sway as they reach up with beaks open for feeding. Care and attention are needed to avoid injuring the mouth with the feeding forceps. Missing the target may result in a dirty chick. Cleaning the chick with a warm damp cloth may prevent bacterial infections in the eyes and keep the feather follicles free of debris that could hinder normal feather development. Nestlings are stronger and may fall out of a nest cup in their enthusiasm to feed. It is important to ensure the safety of the nestling by never leaving it unattended while outside the brooder and to use nest cups that are deep enough to prevent a nestling from falling out. Nestlings that are close to fledgling, on the other hand, must be in a cup that they can get out of as they become more mobile.

The goal is to allow the chick to fledge at the same age as a parent-reared chick (see Table 30.2). Feeding responses often decrease near fledging. It is a difficult decision to make between allowing the chick to refuse feedings and getting enough food into it to meet its energy requirements. Using a growth curve of normal surviving chicks as a guide may make those decisions easier (see Figure 30.2).

Nowhere is it more important to have good sanitation habits than in the area of food preparation. Food is prepared indoors on stainless steel counters using separate cutting boards and knives for fruit and meat items to minimize bacterial contamination. Keepers wash their hands regularly during the preparations. All perishable food items are kept refrigerated and are not allowed to sit out in the sun after being delivered. Live forage items, such as crickets, mealworms, anoles, and mice are housed for 3 to 4 days prior to being fed to chicks. The housing, food, and water containers for these items are cleaned regularly. The sources where prey items are obtained are inspected to ensure that the product is high quality.

EXPECTED WEIGHT GAIN

Chicks are weighed daily prior to feeding until fledged and less frequently thereafter. Weights are recorded and added to a growth curve to be compared with weights of previously reared normal chicks (see Figure 30.2). Amounts of food fed are recorded, along with a rating of feeding response and the presence of feces. Feed charts are computer spreadsheets with formulas to calculate percent weight changes in chicks and to tally amounts fed of solids and fluids. On a daily basis, keepers enter the chick weight; intake target, based on a percent of body weight; and frequency of feedings, as prompted from a protocol. The target amount to be fed for the day and for each feeding is automatically calculated on the spreadsheet. For instance, if a chick weighs 10 g, the desired intake is 35% and the frequency of feedings is 7 times a day; then one multiplies 10 times 0.35 and divides by 7 to determine that the chick will be fed 0.5 g per feeding. Comparisons are then easily made between the goals for the day and what was actually ingested. Quantities of supplements given are also calculated based on the amount fed the previous day.

Observations of growth and development milestones, such as eyes opening and fledging are documented during the rearing process (see Figure 30.6). If chicks survive and have developed at the same rate as parent-reared chicks, one wants to use those same milestones as a measure for the next chicks reared (see Table 30.6).

Table 30.6. Developmental milestones.

Developmental milestones (approx. in days)	a	b	c	d	e	f	g	h
Casting pellet	6	11	20		10		20	
Eyes open	12	12	12		12	15	15	
Mobile/active	14	14	14	14	30	30	50	55
Fed ad lib	20	30	20	30	30	30	30	30
Self-feeding begins	20	17	30	26	30	40	40	40
Weaned	25	30	35	35	50	60	60	65
Flying	30	30	30	30	40	65	>55	75

[a] Kingfishers.
[b] Bee-eaters.
[c] Rollers.
[d] Woodhoopoe.
[e] Tarictic Hornbill.
[f] Wrinkled Hornbill.
[g] Ground Hornbill.
[h] Great Hornbill.

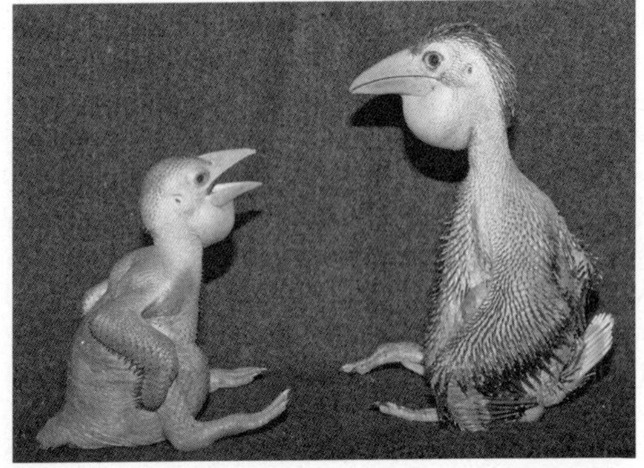

Figure 30.6. Wrinkled Hornbill chicks at day 23 and 28. (Copyright Zoological Society of San Diego.)

HOUSING

Neonates are housed in electronic acrylic brooders with a starting temperature of 94.0–96.0°F (34.4–35.6°C). Temperature is reduced by approximately 0.5–1°F (0.3–0.6°C) each day depending on the chick's reaction. Observations are made of the chick's behavior, noting whether there is shivering, panting, legs and wings splayed out, moving away from clutchmates, or huddling together. Feeding responses and fecal output may both decrease if temperature and humidity are not optimal. For the first 10 days, water pans, which are disinfected daily, are placed in the brooders to provide humidity starting at approximately 50–59% RH. This may prevent dehydration and reduce flaking skin (see Figure 30.7). Brooders are covered to simulate nest cavities and to reduce contact with keepers. Brooders are disinfected between clutches or more frequently as needed.

Chicks are placed in plastic bowls lined with paper towels and tissue paper. Looped vinyl matting (Nomad matting) is used in the bottom of the bowls to keep the chicks from sitting in their feces and to give toes something to grip. Paper is changed after each feeding, and bowls and matting are disinfected daily.

When pinfeathers open, chicks are moved into heated box brooders, wire cages, or rubber tubs on the floor. When chicks are fully feathered and perching, they are allowed access to an outside run with perches and access to a heat lamp. After a few transition days, birds are left outside day and night. Heat lamps are removed within approximately 3 days or when the ambient temperature does not drop below 50°F (10°C).

WEANING

Weaning begins when a chick can physically pick up food unaided and continues until the chick refuses

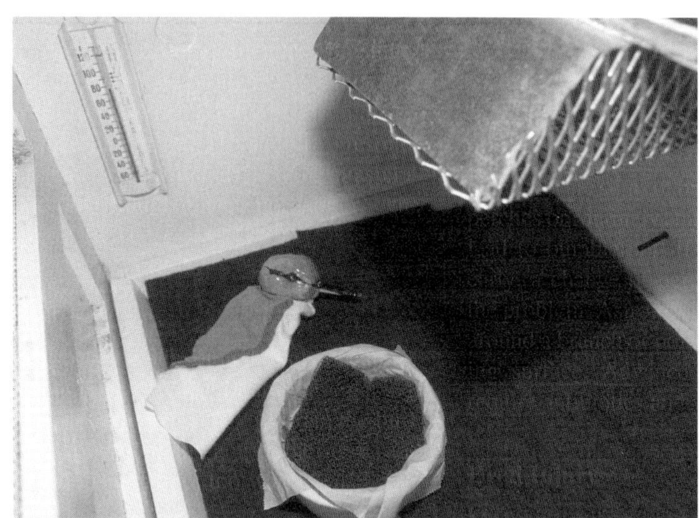

Figure 30.7. Micronesian Kingfisher puppet in box brooder. (Copyright Zoological Society of San Diego.)

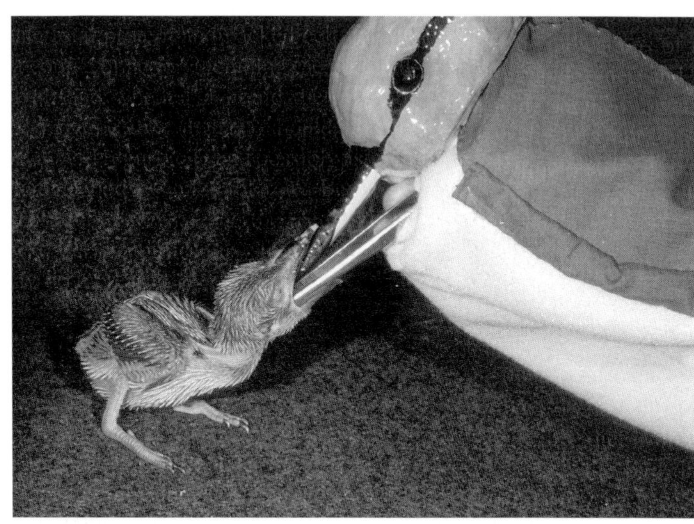

Figure 30.8. Micronesian Kingfisher at ~30 days being hand-fed with puppet. (Copyright Zoological Society of San Diego.)

to be hand-fed. Food is left with the chick between feedings when it becomes mobile. The first feeding will be omitted shortly after the chick is observed picking up food on its own. Prompting occurs at feeding time until the chick refuses all attempts to hand-feed and growth is determined to be normal.

PREPARATION FOR INTRODUCTION TO CAPTIVE FLOCK

If there is more than one chick in a clutch, they are raised in the same brooder, but in a separate nest cup to avoid siblicide. They would be permitted to fledge together and would continue to be housed together after that. Chicks that hatch without siblings may be housed either next door to older chicks of the same species or a closely related species if available.

A hand puppet has been used to rear the Micronesian Kingfisher as a precaution against imprinting on humans (see Figure 30.8). "Ghost-rearing" may be used in the absence of a puppet, where the keepers cover their body with a sheet and wear a sock over their hand while feeding. These species have not seemed to be especially susceptible to maladjusted behaviors associated with imprinting.

Table 30.7. Results of hand-rearing.

Species	# Hand-Reared	# Survived (30 days)	% Survivability
Laughing Kookaburra	4	4	100%
Micronesian Kingfisher	32	29	91%
White-breasted Kingfisher	6	6	100%
White-throated Bee-eater	2	2	100%
White-fronted Bee-eater	4	4	100%
Blue-bellied Roller	6	6	100%
Purple Roller	2	2	100%
Dollarbird	5	5	100%
Common Hoopoe	1	1	100%
Green Woodhoopoe	1	1	100%
Abyssinian Ground Hornbill	42	34	81%
Southern Ground Hornbill	1	1	100%
Black Hornbill	2	1	50%
Great Hornbill	1	1	100%
Tarictic Hornbill	13	9	69%
Red-knobbed Hornbill	1	1	100%
Wrinkled Hornbill	10	8	80%
Writhed Hornbill	2	1	50%
Totals:	135	116	86%

RESULTS

Hand-rearing protocols evolve over time as challenges are overcome and success is achieved. Changes occur related to housing, feeding frequency, diet items, and quantities to feed. Learning from past observations is the key to making changes that result in greater successes (see Table 30.7).

ACKNOWLEDGMENTS

The author acknowledges the tremendous efforts of all the bird keepers at the San Diego Zoo's Avian Propagation Center and Wild Animal Park for the care of eggs and chicks, for collecting data during artificial incubation and hand-rearing and for reviewing this for accuracy; thanks to the curators, David Rimlinger and Michael Mace, for their continued support in these endeavors.

SOURCES FOR PRODUCTS MENTIONED

Forced air incubator: Humidaire Model 20, manufactured by Humidaire Incubator Co., 217 W. Wayne St., PO Box 9, New Madison, OH 45346 (out of business).

Forced air incubator: Petersime Model 1 Incubator: Petersime Incubator Company, 300 North Bridge Street, Gettysburg, OH 45328 (out of business).

Forced air hatcher: AB Newlife Hatcher, manufactured by A.B. Incubator Ltd., PO Box 215, Moline, IL 61265.

ROCCAL-D Plus Disinfectant, Pharmacia & Upjohn Co., 7171 Portage Rd., Kalamazoo, MI 49001-0199 (616) 833-5122, FAX: (616) 833-7555.

UV sterilizer: Canrad-Hanovia Inc./Hanovia Lamp Division, 100 Chestnut St., Newark, NJ 07105, (201) 589-4300.

Acrylic brooder: Animal Intensive Care Unit (AICU), manufactured by Lyon Technologies, Inc. (formerly known as Lyon Electric Co. Inc.), 2765-A Main Street, PO Box 3307, Chula Vista, CA 92011, http://www.lyonelectric.com/index.htm, (888) 596-6872, info@lyonelectric.com.

Looped vinyl matting: Nomad Matting, manufactured by 3M Product Information Center, 3M Center, Building 042-6E-37, St.

Paul, MN 55144-1000, (866) 364-3577, http://solutions.3m.com/en_US/.

Antiseptic povidone iodine solution: Betadine solution, Purdue Pharmaceutical Products L.P., One Stamford Forum, 201 Tresser Boulevard, Stamford, CT 06901-3431, (800) 877-5666, www.pharma.com.

Candler: Hi-intensity candler, manufactured by Lyon Technologies, Inc. (formerly known as Lyon Electric Co. Inc.), 2765-A Main Street, PO Box 3307, Chula Vista, CA 92011, http://www.lyonelectric.com/index.htm, (888) 596-6872, fax (619) 216-3434, info@lyonelectric.com.

Scale: Ohaus scale, manufactured by Ohaus Corporation, P.O. Box 900, 19A Chapin Road, Pine Brook, NJ 07058, (973) 377-9000, fax (973) 944-7177, http://www.ohaus.com.

Electrolyte solution: Pedialyte, manufactured by Products Division Abbott Laboratories, Columbus, OH 43215-1724, http://www.abbott.com.

Liquid B-complex vitamin: Apatate, manufactured by Bradley Pharmaceuticals Incorporated, Fairfield, NJ 07004-2402, http://www.bradpharm.com.

Commercial avian pellet: Marion Jungle Pellets, manufactured by Marion Zoological, 2003 E. Center Circle Plymouth, MN 55441, (800) 327-7974, http://www.marionzoological.com. Outside the United States (763) 559-3305, fax (763) 559-0789, soniag@marionzoological.com.

Dog food: Iams Less Active For Dogs, manufactured by Iams Company, 7250 Powe Avenue, Dayton, OH 45414, (800) 675-3849, http://www.iams.com.

Meat products used until 1999: Nebraska Bird of Prey Diet, manufactured by Central Nebraska Packing, Inc., PO Box 550, North Platte, NE 69103-0550, (308) 532-1250, (877)900-3003, (800)445-2881, fax (308)532-2744, http://www.nebraskabrand.com, info@nebraskabrand.com.

Meat products used since 2000: Natural Balance® Meat-eating Bird Diet, processed by Dick Van Patten's Natural Balance Pet Foods, Inc., 12924 Pierce Street, Pacoima, CA 91331, (800) 829-4493, http://www.naturalbalanceinc.com.

Insect calcium feed: High Calcium Cricket Diet manufactured by Marion Zoological, 2003 E. Center Circle, Plymouth, MN 55441, (800) 327-7974, http://www.marionzoological.com. Outside the United States (763) 559-3305, fax (763) 559-0789, soniag@marionzoological.com.

REFERENCES

del Hoyo, J., Elliott, A., and Saragatal, J. eds. 2001. Handbook of the Birds of the World. Vol 6. Mousebirds to Hornbills. Lynx Edicions, Barcelona.

Fry, C.H., Fry, K., and Harris, A. 1992. Kingfishers, Bee-eaters & Rollers. Princeton University Press, Princeton, New Jersey.

Kemp, A. 1995. The Hornbills. Oxford University Press Inc., New York.

31
Woodpeckers

Rebecca Duerr

NATURAL HISTORY

There are 215 species of woodpeckers, sapsuckers, and flickers in the suborder Picidae of order Piciformes, and 22 of these species are found in North America. All species in this order nest in holes and cavities and hatch altricial, naked, blind, and helpless young. Some woodpeckers nest cooperatively and may produce broods of up to 12 young from two females. Incubation lasts 11–14 days and young fledge in 21–30 days, although some species such as the Gila Woodpecker continue to feed their young for many months (Reed 2001).

Most woodpeckers have a zygodactyl toe arrangement with two toes pointing forward and two pointing backward, and this assists in differentiating very young woodpeckers from similar-appearing passerine hatchlings. A few species such as the Three-toed and Black-backed Woodpeckers have only three toes: two forward, one back. Passerines in comparison have anisodactyl feet, with three toes forward and one back (see Figure 31.1). Hatchlings are typically pink-skinned and bald with no down at all. The neck may appear longer than a similar-sized passerine chick.

Adult diets change seasonally, with different species relying on typical food items, such as insects and other invertebrates, nuts, acorns, seeds, sap, berries, and fruit to different extents. During the breeding season, many species feed primarily on insects. Young are fed regurgitated adult diet. Some species store food seasonally, such as Acorn and Lewis's Woodpeckers. Caregivers should make every effort to become informed about the natural history and behavioral specializations of the species in their care, since the social structures of some species such as acorn woodpeckers complicate the release of captive-reared young.

CRITERIA FOR INTERVENTION

Most woodpeckers brought into captivity as hatchlings or nestlings are the result of untimely tree removal. Because nests are located inside cavities, they are usually not discovered until the tree (or cactus) has been removed and someone has noticed the young vocalizing from inside a log. By this time it is typically too late for the nest to be left undisturbed or replaced.

Fledglings are often brought into captivity after encounters with domestic pets or other mishaps such as collisions with windows. Fledglings found on the ground often have problems that require medical attention, but they may occasionally be captured by overzealous rescuers. Any seemingly uninjured fledgling that is a candidate for reunion with its parents should have a physical exam and flight test to rule out both subtle and obvious injuries.

RECORD KEEPING

See Chapter 1, "General Care."

INITIAL CARE AND STABILIZATION

The main rule of initial baby bird care is warmth, rehydration, and feeding, in that order. Warm chicks before giving fluids, and then hydrate them until they start passing droppings. Only then is it safe to commence feedings. Feeding a cold or dehydrated baby bird before it is warm and hydrated will probably kill it.

New patients should be allowed to rest for 15–20 minutes in a warm, dark, quiet container before examination. If the bird is not able to stand, it should be placed in a soft support structure such as a rolled cloth donut or paper nest. Do not allow the bird to

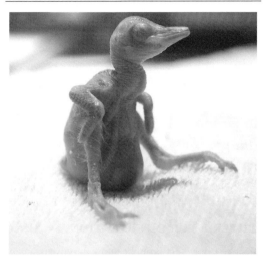

Figure 31.1. Nuttall's Woodpecker hatchling. Note zygodactyl toe arrangement (photo courtesy of Roger Parker).

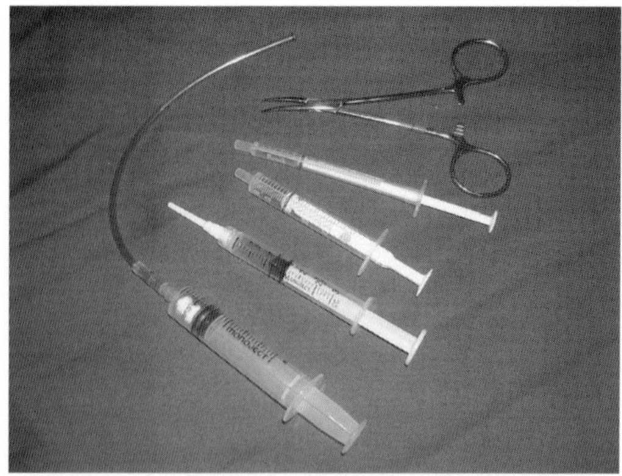

Figure 31.2. Feeding tools from top: hemostats, 1 ml O-ring syringe, 3 ml O-ring syringe, 3 ml luer-lock syringe with securely attached plastic cannula tip (Jorgenson Labs), 6 ml syringe with cut section of IV extension set tubing (note: end of tube is lightly burned to round edges).

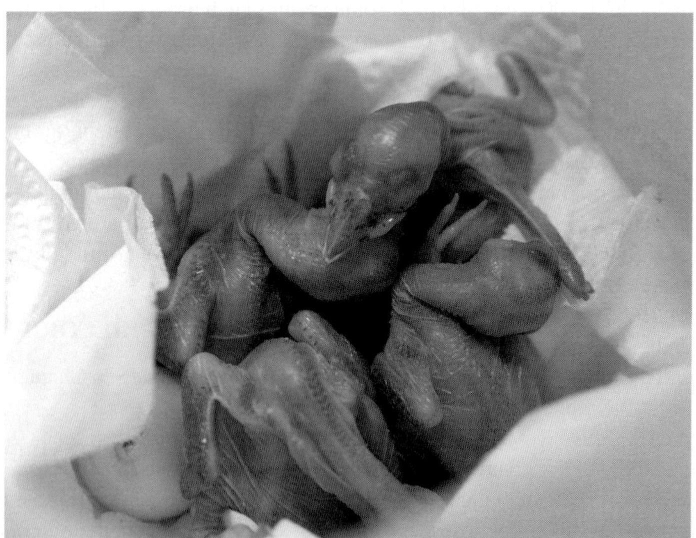

Figure 31.3. Nest of Nuttall's Woodpecker hatchlings (photo courtesy of Roger Parker).

lie on its side or other abnormal positions. Hatchlings and nestlings should be placed in a climate-controlled incubator if available (see Figures 31.2–31.4). When the animal is warm and calm, it may be hydrated orally or subcutaneously (SQ). Warm sterile fluids, such as 2.5% dextrose in 0.45% sodium chloride or lactated Ringer's solution, may be administered SQ at 5% of body weight once, although repeated administrations may be needed for extremely dehydrated birds. Gaping, active hatchlings or nestlings should be orally hydrated until they produce droppings. Give a few drops of warm oral fluids every 15–20 minutes with a small syringe or eye dropper and allow the bird to swallow

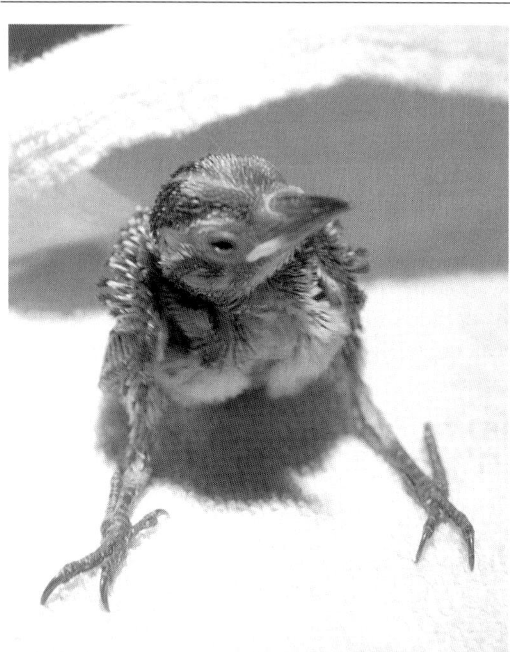

Figure 31.4. Nestling Nuttall's Woodpecker (photo courtesy of Roger Parker).

completely before giving more. Once you are comfortable with the amount the chick is able to swallow, the amount may be raised to 2.5–5% of body weight in several mouthfuls. Human infant electrolyte fluids (unflavored) are excellent for oral rehydration of baby birds. Ensure the bird is warm before administering fluids, and that the bird is both warm and well-hydrated before receiving food. Start the bird on a hand feeding formula after it begins passing droppings.

If the bird is depressed or not swallowing well, oral rehydration must be done very carefully because there is a greater risk of aspiration of fluids into the respiratory system. It may be better in this circumstance to wait for the animal to absorb SQ fluids, rather than giving oral fluids too quickly. If SQ fluids are not an option, give tiny amounts of oral fluids deep into the mouth and ensure that the bird swallows everything before giving more.

If an altricial bird does not begin passing droppings within 1 hour of giving the fluids, begin feeding the appropriate diet. However, keep the diet very dilute and the meal size small until droppings are seen.

COMMON MEDICAL PROBLEMS AND SOLUTIONS

Young woodpeckers may present with injuries from animal bites, falls, or collisions with windows. Injured birds may require splints for broken bones. Wild birds may become depressed if encumbered by heavy or confining splints, and wraps may damage growing feathers. Hence, minimally restrictive wraps and lightweight splints are recommended. For lacerations, the author prefers sutures or tissue glue, such as Nexaband (Abbott), or hygroscopic dressings, such as Biodres (DVM Pharmaceuticals), for wounds that are not able to be sutured or glued. See Chapter 1, "General Care," for more information.

Due to the structure of the woodpecker tongue, which wraps around the outside of the skull, birds with head injuries may have an impaired ability to swallow because swelling may impede the motion of the tongue. These birds may require tube-feeding to provide nutrition. Intravenous (IV) extension sets that have been cut to an appropriate length past the female end of the set make excellent small bird feeding tubes. Burn the cut-off tubing end to round off the sharp edges (see Figure 31.2). To tube-feed a woodpecker, restrain the bird with the neck extended. Measure from the mouth to the caudal end of the rib cage (where the stomach is) to determine how deep the tube should go. Gently open the beak without flexing it sideways and insert the tube along the right side of the mouth, avoiding the glottis. If the tube is correctly placed, it should easily slide down the right side of the bird's neck. When tube-feeding a bird with an impaired ability to swallow, keep the quantity small until reasonably confident the bird is not likely to regurgitate and the bird is passing normal droppings. It is uncommon for woodpeckers to present with pathologic parasitic infestations, but performing routine fecal smears and flotation is recommended. Possible parasites include coccidia, intestinal worms, mites, and feather lice.

DIET RECIPES

Woodpeckers do well when fed the same high animal protein hand-feeding diets as passerine birds. See Chapter 34, "Passerines: Hand-Feeding Diets," for recipes.

FEEDING PROCEDURES

Woodpeckers make a vigorous pecking motion that makes it a challenge to get food into their mouth rather than all over their body. Feather condition is extremely important, especially tail feathers on species that will need to use their tail as a stiff support when climbing trees. Do not allow any stray food or droppings to dry on growing feathers. If this occurs, feather loss and skin or eye infections are a possible consequence.

As with many altricial young birds, woodpeckers may eat approximately 5% of their body weight per meal (e.g., 1.5 ml for a 30 g bird). Some may tolerate higher amounts, and the very large woodpeckers may require somewhat lower amounts. Watch the droppings to gauge how much should be fed. Droppings should be moist and well formed. Loose, runny stools may indicate overfeeding, especially if the droppings look like undigested diet. A lack of droppings often indicates dehydration. Each bird should produce roughly the same amount of droppings in volume as the amount of food being fed. Any bird that has stopped producing droppings should be orally hydrated until the food currently in the digestive tract has passed. At that point, restart feedings with smaller quantities of moister food to alleviate further dehydration. Woodpeckers grow very quickly and feeding amounts may need to be adjusted daily.

Hatchlings

Hatchlings should be fed every 20–30 minutes for 12–14 hours a day. A 1 ml syringe with a disposable plastic cannula tip (Jorgensen) makes an excellent feeding implement (see Figure 31.2), although a plain 1 ml syringe may also be acceptable depending on the size of the bird's mouth. Attach the tip securely to avoid the possibility of it disconnecting and being accidentally swallowed. Do not use small detachable tips on older chicks at risk for swallowing the tip. Use a luer-lock syringe to firmly attach the cannula in older birds. Administer the food in a controlled manner while the bird is actively swallowing. Be prepared to stop instantly if the food begins to back up into the bird's mouth. If this occurs, pull the feeding implement out and allow the hatchling a moment to swallow before continuing. If the bird is not swallowing the food, clear the mouth quickly with a cotton swab. Birds cannot breathe when their mouth is full of food. Some birds will eat more comfortably if the food is given in multiple small bites; others will take their entire meal very rapidly. Avoid squirting food out of the syringe too fast as it may soil the feathers with food.

Woodpeckers don't gape like many other altricial birds, and are stimulated to eat when their beak is touched by the feeding implement. They also may be stimulated to eat even before the eyes are open by a brief period of darkness, as when a parent would block the light coming into a nest cavity. New birds that will not take offered food may need to have their beaks gently opened and a small amount of food placed at the back of the mouth to stimulate swallowing. Be careful not to bend the bird's beak to one side when opening the mouth, or the growing beak or jaw may be damaged. If a bird refuses food, reevaluate the temperature, hydration status, and its physical condition, and correct any problems found.

Nestlings and Fledglings

Fully and partially feathered birds should be fed every 45 minutes for 12–14 hours a day. The author prefers to use a 1 ml syringe for birds up to 40 g in weight. The small syringe is a good substitute for the long thin bill of the parent and fits well in the mouth. Refilling the syringe during the meal allows the bird a moment to thoroughly swallow the previous mouthful. Larger birds may feed well from a larger syringe such as a 3 ml size, with or without a cannula tip securely attached on a luer-lock syringe (see Figure 31.2). Nestlings and fledglings may appear to vigorously impale themselves on the feeding syringe, however this is normal. There is little risk of the bird being hurt as long as there are no sharp edges on the feeding implements and any tubing or catheters are securely attached to the syringe. Blunt forceps or hemostats may be used to feed insects and chunky diet recipes. Uncooperative nestlings and fledglings may require tube-feeding if unwilling to accept food from syringe or forceps.

EXPECTED WEIGHT GAIN

After a day of rehydration and adjustment to their new diet, woodpeckers should gain weight daily and quickly reach or exceed the adult weight for the species. Each bird should reach adult weight by the time it is 2 to 3 weeks old. Even the larger woodpeckers have relatively short times from hatching to fledging. If a bird is not gaining weight, the feeding regime should be critically evaluated. Older nestlings and fledglings may be difficult to feed, especially by novices, and the bird may not be getting enough calories per day. The chick should be examined again for any potential medical problems. Weight gain in sick or injured birds may be delayed while healing occurs. Birds should be at or above adult weight before beginning the weaning process.

Fledgling woodpeckers placed together in small containers for weighing or during cage-cleaning may injure one other by vigorously pecking each other in the face. Separate containers may be required.

Caregivers may be able to judge a body weight to be normal even if it varies from published accounts. For example, *The Sibley Guide to Birds* lists Nuttall's woodpeckers at 38 g, although well-muscled, acutely injured adults of that species treated at one wildlife rescue center in Northern California have typically been 32–34 g. There, fledglings were considered to be in excellent condition at 33 g when fully weaned. It is important to chart weights over time to determine optimal body weights for each species in a region.

HOUSING

Hatchlings should be kept at 90–95°F (32.2–35°C) and 40–50% humidity. Different materials may be used to create a replacement nest: berry baskets, rolled newspaper, and plastic or ceramic dishes have been used. Nests in solid dishes tend to become wet and have poor ventilation (see Figure 31.3), although some people like to use them because once warm, they hold heat well. All areas of the nest structure must be covered with tissue or paper toweling, which will allow for easy cleaning throughout the day. Cover newspaper with tissue to avoid having the birds' skin in contact with ink. Change the tissues as necessary, and do not allow the chicks' feathers or skin to become soiled. Young birds should sit in the nest with their legs folded underneath their bodies. Do not allow the legs to splay out to the sides or malformed legs or hips may result. A paper nest inside a small cardboard box cut to simulate a tree cavity may be effective as a woodpecker nest substitute, although ensure enough visibility to allow for efficient and mess-free feedings. This box may be arranged to fit within an incubator.

When the birds are fully feathered, move the nest box into a larger container. While they are still very young, additional heat may be provided by placing a heating pad set at the lowest setting beneath their container. When they fledge, they will begin to venture outside their nest (see Figure 31.4). Smaller-bodied woodpeckers do well in large laundry baskets with window screening lining, although these baskets do not provide very much vertical climbing space. Window screening also makes an excellent roof for the basket, and fledglings will spend much time climbing upside down on it. Reptariums (Dallas Manufacturing) are another option, and they may be arranged to provide vertical climbing space. Larger-bodied woodpeckers should be placed in window screening–lined wire caging of sufficient size to allow for exercise, but not so large as to impede hand feedings. Suggested cage size might be 2 ft × 3 ft × 3 ft (0.6 × 1 × 1 m). Wire cages without the screen lining may cause feather damage. Screening may need periodic repair because the birds will probably start pecking at it. Caging should be cleaned thoroughly at least once a day, wiped down with a disinfectant such as dilute chlorhexidine, and papers changed as necessary to maintain a hygienic environment. Reptariums may be laundered as needed.

WEANING

As soon as the birds are old enough to begin exploring their environment, additional furnishings such as logs, hunks of bark, large pine cones, cactus skeletons, and other similar objects should be provided. Presentation of food items to encourage self-feeding should begin at this time. Ideally, the birds should be weaned onto the identical natural food items they will be eating when they are released, although substitution for easily available items is often necessary.

Exposing the birds to the types of food items (i.e., live insects, nuts, sap, berries, etc.) they will be eating when released is essential. Presenting the birds with a variety of foraging opportunities will increase their ability to acquire food in the wild. A simple dish on the floor with food in it is not sufficient because most woodpeckers do not often forage on the ground (flickers and some others do). Creativity in developing ways of presenting food to the birds to both wean them off of hand-feeding and also to teach them food-finding skills is required. Examples of food presentation that have been found to be effective are as follows.

Worm Pillow

Cut out a 1 ft square or circle of gauze cloth. Place a handful of mealworms in the center and lay a few slices of apple on top. Bundle up the four corners and snug the worms up into a twisted-off pillow of worms. Secure the pillow with tape or string. Cut several small slits in the fabric to help catch the birds' attention, but don't make them large enough to allow the worms to escape. The apple serves to keep the worms hydrated and less interested in escape. Suspend the pillow(s) in an obvious spot. Evidence of the birds pecking at the pillow will be seen when the holes become frayed and stained with worm juices. Replace or refill as necessary. The worm pillow is also useful for nuthatches and other passerine species that glean insects from the bark of trees.

Pinecone

Place a large pinecone in a steep-sided crock or pan. Drizzle mealworms and waxworms over the pinecone periodically. Smaller mealworms are optimal as the larger ones fall off the cone too quickly. The steep-sided dish helps prevent worm escapes. This method is also useful for bushtits and other small insectivorous passerines.

Cactus Skeleton

Stuff the inside of the skeleton with a mixture of moistened ground high-quality dry cat kibble, peanut butter crumble (see Chapter 36, "Thrushes," for recipe), and mealworms. Fruit, berries, and other food items may also be wedged into the skeleton. Place the skeleton in a tray in the cage. Skeletons may also be mounted vertically on a flat stand inside the tray or placed in a corner. This method may be messy, but it provides interesting foraging.

Routered Log

Drill numerous holes and depressions in various-sized stumps and logs that fit in the caging. Fill the depressions with nuts, acorns, kibble, killed fresh or thawed frozen crickets, mealworms, or other insects. Careful application of peanut butter may assist in holding food items in holes, although this may be difficult to clean. Routered holes may also be filled with diluted maple syrup (1 part syrup to 9 parts water) to create a sap well for sapsuckers. Garnish the well with live or crushed insects. When using sticky food items, be careful not to create a feather-contamination hazard.

Stump-Mounted Dishes

Standard plastic wall-mounted pet bird dishes may be adapted to hang on the side of a vertical stump. Insert appropriately sized eye screws into the wood to allow the wire hook variety of dish to be placed. This type of dish may also be hung at the top of a stump by wedging the wire hangers between the bark and wood. Nails may be used to attach a plastic dish anywhere on a piece of wood, although if the dish is hard plastic a hole needs to be drilled first to avoid cracking the dish. Remember when mounting such dishes that the birds may peck at them very aggressively, and the mounting needs to be secure to avoid it being quickly dislodged.

Commercial Woodpecker Feeders

These feeders provide a variety of food items, usually various nutmeats. These are a good option for birds that may be released late in the season and may be partially dependent on feeders during the winter after a soft release.

Fruit Feeder

Poke indentations into an apple half. Fill the cavities with a mix of hand-feeding diet plus a small amount of maple syrup, crushed kitten kibble, chopped fruit, and live or crushed insects.

When the birds are consistently at or above adult weight, have fully grown-out feathers, and are showing an interest in the food choices offered, it is time to begin weaning them. Use forceps or hemostats to feed the birds meals of more adult food items instead of hand-feeding formula. Clean and stock the cage in the morning with a fresh assortment of food choices.

There are many possible regimens for reducing and then eliminating the birds' dependence on human caregivers for meals. Some rehabilitators cut back on the morning feeds first in order to encourage hungry interest; others make the intervals between feedings longer.

From the former feeding interval of 45 minutes, extend it first to 1 hour for 2–3 days, and then 2 hours for 2–3 days. If the birds are holding their weight at 2-hour feeds and their droppings have ample solids, continue cutting back feeds to 3-hour intervals for a few days and finally discontinue feedings entirely. If the birds were above adult weight when weaning began, it is normal for them to drop up to 10% of their body weight while weaning. If uncertain about the bird's weight status or unable to weigh birds daily, monitor the plumpness of the breast muscling closely. If any bird has dropped significant amounts of weight during the process, lost breast muscle mass, or has sparse lime-green or urates-only droppings, return the bird to 45-minute feeds and reexamine the animal for any medical problems. Try again after the bird has fattened up and reevaluate food presentation.

Once the birds are eating consistently in their small cage and maintaining weight without any supplemental hand-feedings, they are ready for an aviary. If the outdoor climate is significantly different from indoor temperature, the birds should be acclimated by gradual exposure over the course of 24–48 hours before being put in the aviary. Acclimation may be accomplished at the same time as the final stages of weaning. If acclimation is skipped, birds may die if they are suddenly subject to extremely hot or cold temperatures.

Aviaries should be at least 4 × 8 × 8 ft (1.2 × 2.5 × 2.5 m) for small-bodied woodpeckers and 8 × 16 × 8 ft (2.5 × 5 × 2.5 m) for large-bodied woodpeckers (Miller 2000). Aviaries should be constructed of window screening–lined wire mesh on a metal frame, because wooden aviaries may be quickly destroyed by woodpeckers just being themselves (see Figure 31.5). Ample logs must be provided, and fresh clean water should be available at all times. Avoid areas of bare wire mesh because it can damage the birds' tail feathers. At least half the aviary should be shaded for protection from the elements, and the log furnishings should provide a wide variety of perching and climbing opportunities. Food should be presented off the ground on shelves and logs as described in the section "Weaning" above.

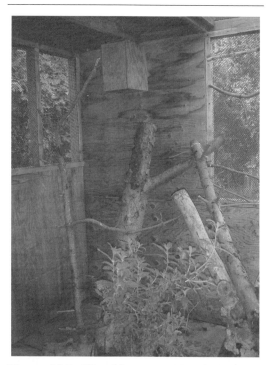

Figure 31.5. Wood-frame woodpecker aviary with ample logs, climbing surfaces, and nest box (photo courtesy of Veronica Bowers).

PREPARATION FOR WILD RELEASE

To avoid habituating the birds to humans, interact with them only at mealtime and avoid raising solitary birds. It may be necessary to call other facilities to match up single birds. Hatchling and nestling woodpeckers may also be mixed with similar-sized passerines, but they may need to be separated at fledgling age. If housing a woodpecker with another species, monitor closely for problems with aggression. Birds that are fighting or are frightened of each other may be too preoccupied to learn to self-feed. Siblings may also require separation due to aggression. Watch for small bloody wounds around the bill or between the eyes.

Dim lighting is fine for hatchlings and nestlings because they would be in a dark cavity in the wild. However, once birds are feathered, use light-colored sheeting as visual barriers to block views of human activity without blocking the light.

Success at avoiding habituation should be seen by the time the birds are in the aviary. They should be wary of humans rather than coming up to caretakers for food. Usually, woodpeckers that are admitted as older nestlings or fledglings do not readily habituate to humans.

RELEASE

Birds should spend 7–14 days gaining flight experience in the aviary prior to release, and should be able to fly short-duration flights lasting for 5–10 minutes of continuous flight at ambient temperatures without panting. Birds should shed water when misted and should weigh as much as a normal adult. Whenever possible, release birds in their home neighborhood. Choose the release day to avoid weather extremes.

Release in the morning, because woodpeckers are diurnal.

Most woodpeckers are not migratory, although some move to lower elevations in winter (Reed 2001). Many species cache food for winter consumption. If birds are released late in the year it may be advisable to do a soft release where an affiliated person can provide supplemental food until spring.

Some species, such as Acorn Woodpeckers, are not likely to accept unfamiliar fledglings into an established territory, although the family should recognize missing members if they are returned within a few weeks. It is preferable for Acorn Woodpeckers to minimize aviary time in order to get the bird back to its home territory quickly.

Anecdotal success has been achieved by consolidating young Acorn Woodpeckers from different rehabilitation groups into a new social group in the aviary, and then releasing the group into a suburban neighborhood that lacks an acorn colony, but has ample mature oak and pine trees (Sue Kelly, personal communication). More research is needed to establish the best possible ways to release orphaned birds of species with complex social systems. Placement into permanent captivity may be necessary in certain cases.

ACKNOWLEDGMENTS

Thanks to Guthrum Purdin and Susie Brain for editorial assistance and suggestions on content, and to Casey Levitt, Courtenay Dawson-Roberts, and Juanita Heinemann for teaching me about raising woodpeckers.

SOURCES FOR PRODUCTS MENTIONED

Nexaband: Abbott Animal Health, North Chicago, IL, 60064, (888) 299-7416.

Biodres: DVM Pharmaceuticals, Subsidiary of IVAX Corporation, 4400 Biscayne Blvd, Miami, FL 33137, (305) 575-6000.

Cannula (J-12 teat infusion): Jorgensen Laboratories, Inc., Loveland, CO.

Reptarium: Dallas Manufacturing Company Inc., 4215 McEwen Road, Dallas, TX 75244, (800) 256-8669.

REFERENCES

Ehrlich, P.R., Dobkin, D.S., and Wheye, D. 1988. The Birder's Handbook: A Field Guide to the Natural History of North American Birds. Simon and Schuster Inc., New York, 785 pp.

Miller, E.A., ed. 2000. Minimum Standards for Wildlife Rehabilitation, 3rd Edition. National Wildlife Rehabilitation Association, St. Cloud, Minnesota, 77 pp.

Reed, J.M. 2001. Woodpeckers and allies. In Elphick, C., Dunning, J.B., Jr., Sibley, D.A., eds. The Sibley Guide to Bird Life and Behavior. Knopf, New York. pp 373–383.

32
Toucans

Martin Vince

INTRODUCTION

The Toucan family—Ramphastidae—comprises a total of 35 species of toucans, toucanets, and aracaris. *Ramphastids,* as they are generally known, are in the Order Piciformes along with their close relatives the woodpeckers and barbets. Toucans nest in tree cavities that are either abandoned parrot nests or cavities excavated by the birds themselves within the trunks and boughs of rotting trees. Aracaris and toucanets are the smallest members of the family; their nest cavities are approximately 7 in (17 cm) in diameter and extend to 12 in (30 cm) below the entrance hole. The large toucans, genus Ramphastos, require cavities of approximately 9 in (22 cm) in diameter that extend to 16 in (38 cm) or more below the entrance hole. The ideal nest site may be a semirotten palm log approximating these dimensions that can be modified by the birds themselves. Toucans have fairly strong beaks and are capable of excavating a nest chamber in soft wood. In captivity, nestboxes may also be used. However, they are poorly accepted by members of the genus Ramphastos, which are generally much harder to breed than the aracaris and toucanets.

The reader will be familiar with the famous lightweight, honeycomb structure of a toucan's bill. For the chick, however, the structure becomes increasingly unwieldy; and the only way the bird can remain upright is to sit in a backward-leaning position with feet up in the air. Indeed, young toucans have a patch of boney ridges on the back of each leg that acts as a shoe while the feet themselves are elevated for the first couple of weeks. The boney "shoes" disappear at fledging as they are no longer needed. This apparently comical situation is important for the caregiver to realize because older chicks will fall forward if left unaided on a countertop.

All toucans are omnivores, using their serrated bills to eat small animals, as well as an array of vegetation and fruits. The sexes are alike in nearly all species. Two to four plain white eggs are laid directly on the floor of the nest chamber, with no materials added. Both sexes incubate the eggs. Aracaris and toucanets incubate for about 16 days; the large toucans incubate for about 18 days. Chicks fledge at 6–7 weeks of age, and can feed themselves reliably at 10–12 weeks of age.

CRITERIA FOR INTERVENTION

Most toucans are hand-reared by design, either from incubator-hatched eggs, or as older chicks taken from the nest for taming. Some, however, will be found abandoned on the aviary floor or may be retrieved from a nest because they are sick or abandoned or the parents are incapable of rearing them. All require immediate care, and the proactive aviculturist will be prepared with an incubator or brooder that has been operating at the correct temperature for some days.

RECORD KEEPING

Although hand-rearing a chick is a memorable experience, inevitably memories fade, making detailed record-keeping essential if successes are to be repeated and failures avoided. The ability to hand-rear toucanets and aracaris is a rare skill, and the ability to hand-rear large species of the genus *Ramphastos* is even more uncommon. It is important, therefore, that all hand-rearing information is carefully recorded to ensure the probability of future successes with these species.

Computerized records are strongly favored over paper ones. Hand-feeding notes may be recorded in a table, which eliminates illegible handwriting, makes email consultations simple, and facilitates graphing and other statistical operations. Miniature photographs of the chick are also easily inserted into a table, providing perfect benchmarks for future chicks.

INITIAL CARE AND STABILIZATION

A chick found on the aviary floor will usually be hypothermic and should be cupped in warm hands and carried to an incubator or brooder. If the chick is uninjured, vigorous movement will usually be detected as its body temperature begins to rise. Toucan chicks are robust and, depending on age and injuries, have moderately good prospects of surviving such an event.

COMMON MEDICAL PROBLEMS

Misaligned Beak

Toucans have extremely malleable beaks until about 3 weeks of age. The tip of a toucan's bill (1/8 in, 3 mm) may become misaligned for various reasons, including syringe pressure during feeding. The defect is relatively easy to rectify by applying gentle pressure to the tip of the bill in the direction that opposes the curvature. Gently bend the tip of the mandible 20–30 degrees beyond center, repeating the procedure 3 or 4 times per day, or as often as recommended by your veterinarian.

Candida Overgrowth

Some aviculturists use the antifungal drug Nystatin (Bristol Myers Squibb) orally as a prophylaxis treatment in the hand-rearing of toucans. The use of Nystatin for the first 2–3 weeks seems to do no harm and should help reduce the risk of *Candida*. There is enough anecdotal information to suggest that the use of Nystatin is helpful. However, it is also the case that toucans may be hand-reared without using Nystatin. Ultimately, the decision is made by the aviculturist and the avian veterinarian.

Impaction from Organic Material

When young chicks are taken from the nest, be aware that they may have been fed inappropriate items such as wood chips, sticks, cable ties, or other small nonfood items by their parents. The chick itself may also have eaten bark and soil from the cavity floor. Watch for poor weight gains or the appearance of soil in feces for clues as to whether the chick could be impacted. As a routine precautionary measure, a chick may be given a small amount of mineral oil (between 0.1 and 0.2 ml depending on the size of the chick) as a laxative after being removed from the nest.

DIET RECIPES

When fed by their parents, toucans receive a high-protein diet for the first several days, beginning with large insects and progressing to small animals such as baby birds, mice, and small reptiles. Even though fruit is the mainstay of the adult diet, it is only when the chicks are 4–7 days old, depending on the species, that they receive fruit from their parents. This seemingly unusual initial diet is normal for fruit-eating birds and should be taken into account when hand-rearing their chicks.

Toucan chicks may be successfully reared using a small amount of pureed fruit (apple or papaya for example), "pinkie" (newborn) mice and a proprietary hand-rearing formula developed for parrots, such as Kaytee exact (Kaytee). The precise recipe is probably not critical, but an approximate mix by weight of 20% pureed apple and/or papaya and 80% Kaytee exact original formula made to the appropriate ratio of water:Kaytee exact powder (see Table 32.1) seems to be satisfactory. In addition to this mixture, and in keeping with the natural feeding pattern, the author recommends dribbling the innards of pinkie mice into the chick's mouth or pureeing pinkies for syringe feeding. It is recommended that a calcium supplement (calcium carbonate) be used daily until fledging. Chicks are fed approximately 0.5 g of pharmaceutical grade calcium carbonate per day from 1–10 days of age, gradually increasing to 1.5 g per day for chicks 10 days and older.

The above-mentioned foods produce very satisfactory results. It must be said, however, that the ingredients are intended to cover all the nutritional "bases" because the rearing of toucans is still a rare event, which lacks scientific study. The success of this diet belies the fact that it still needs improvement. The fruit component is arguably questionable at a life stage that does not receive fruit in nature (i.e., during the period 1–7 days of age). Future work may explore the benefits of reducing or eliminating the fruit component from diets fed to chicks aged 1–7 days old. The feeding of pinkie mice may also cause concern due to the well-known risk of iron storage disease. The risk is certainly real. However, in the initial days of life, a chick has an especially high nutritional requirement and the heme-iron of meat is less likely to give rise to iron storage disease than at any other time of life. On average, withholding small amounts of pinkie mice, at least during the first several days, appears to be more problematic than not, producing sluggish or negative weight gains.

FEEDING PROCEDURES

As with many species, toucan chicks may be hard to rouse in the morning. Gently tapping on the countertop may be needed to stimulate activity because the vibration and sound equate to an adult landing on the tree trunk; making whistling or chirping sounds may also be helpful.

A toucan chick has poor control of its head, which tends to flail about during feeding. One's fingers can be ringed around the head, providing a stable feeding target and making accidents less likely.

Toucans lack a crop, and they may become temporarily full after receiving only a small part of the diet. Once the portion of food has been swallowed, however, the chick will again appear hungry and demand more. Once a chick reaches 10 days of age, it is normal for a feeding to take at least 15 minutes, as the bird goes through multiple full-empty cycles. Finally, however, the head flops completely backward as the bird truly becomes full. Feeding a toucan chick properly, therefore, takes considerably longer than other species the reader may be familiar with, such as parrots. An expert may feed a parrot chick in less than a minute, but no amount of practice can speed the feeding of a toucan.

After each feed, the author recommends cleaning food residue from inside and outside the chick's mouth using a moistened cloth or cotton-tipped swab.

Days 1–6

To promote yolk sac absorption, wait several hours before giving the first feed. The initial feed should be mostly liquid [distilled water or an oral electrolyte such as Pedialyte (Abbott Labs)], with only a minimal amount of Kaytee exact. For subsequent feeds, the Kaytee formula should be progressively

Table 32.1. Feeding chart for young chicks.

Age	Water	Kaytee exact original hand-rearing powdered formula
Day 1	6 parts	1 part
Day 2	5 parts	1 part
Day 3	4 parts	1 part
Day 4	3 parts	1 part
Day 5	3 parts	1 part
Day 6	3 parts	1 part with the introduction of small pieces of pellets and fruit

thickened according to this approximate schedule (see Table 32.1).

Hatchlings should be fed every 60–90 minutes for 14 hours. Initial feeds on day 1 should be approximately 2–3% of body weight, increasing to 3–4% of bodyweight by the afternoon of day 1 (e.g., 2% of a 9 g bird: $0.02 \times 9 = 0.18$ ml per feed.) It is a good idea to deliver the food in amounts as small as 0.05 ml until greater confidence is achieved, rather than giving a single food delivery as one might with a parrot, for example.

For at least the first 4 days, the chick should be fed using a 1 ml syringe. Depending on personal preference, the syringe may be fitted with a feeding tip, such as a plastic teat infusion cannula tip. A plain 1 ml syringe may be equally preferred, especially in the case of large species (genus *Ramphastos*). Accidental food aspiration is a significant cause of mortality in hatchlings at this stage. Within the first week, therefore, consideration should be given to transitioning onto small food pieces. This approach creates a more natural presentation for the chick and carries a lower risk of aspiration than syringe feeding. From 6 days of age, the toucan chick is able to eat small pieces of pellet that are thoroughly soaked in water. The caregiver should use the same brand of pellet that is intended for the bird's adult diet. Low iron pellets are recommended such as those manufactured by Kaytee, Mazuri, and ZuPreem.

Day 7 Onward

At approximately 7 days of age, it is relatively easy to feed pieces of the adult diet either from forceps

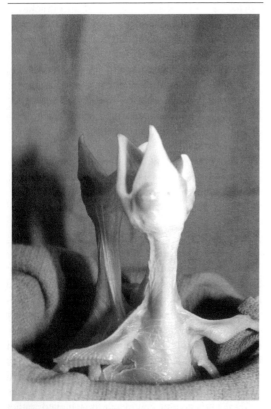

Figure 32.1. Nine-day-old toucans responding to stimulus.

or one's fingers. This may be possible as early as 4 or 5 days of age in the case of large chicks. Delivering food directly into the mouth tends to be easier with a pair of forceps, but fingers are safer for older chicks because they are far more active (see Figure 32.1). At 7 days of age, feeding frequency may be reduced to 6 or 7 times per day over 12 hours. At 2 weeks of age, 5 feeds per day are sufficient, and by 5 weeks of age 3–4 feeds per day are sufficient.

At about 3 weeks of age, toucans become fussy eaters and routinely spit out their food. One's index finger may be used to push food into the bird's mouth to encourage swallowing. Otherwise, food will sit unnoticed in the mouth and create a choking hazard when the bird slouches.

Toucans are very light-sensitive at this age, perhaps instinctively knowing that a change in lighting signals the arrival of a parent at the nest hole. Be careful not to cast a shadow over the brooder when checking the chick unless you plan to feed it at that moment. Even before the eyes are open, the bird will know you are there; and certainly do not turn the room light on or off unless you are prepared to disturb the chick. This is most awkward at the end of the day when the room lights have to be turned off. In the case of incandescent bulbs, a dimmer switch will greatly alleviate the problem because the lights may be gradually dimmed.

EXPECTED WEIGHT GAIN

Weigh the chick at the same time every 24 hours on scales designed for the purpose. Digital scales are ideal since they are quick and easy to read, minimizing the disturbance to the chick. An acceptable daily weight gain can fall within a range as wide as 5–15%, although the average (mean) daily weight gain should be about 10%. If the weight gain is outside the range of 5%–15%, either adjust the amount per feed or the time interval between feeds.

Poor Weight Gains

Example: if a chick is fed every 75 minutes but only experiences a 2% weight gain, the feeding frequency may be increased to every 60 minutes. Changes should be gradual. Normally, either the feeding frequency *or* the amount per feed will need to be changed to achieve the desired weight increase. Weigh the chick after 12 hours to help predict the 24-hour weight. If the 12-hour weight suggests that action is needed before waiting until tomorrow, one has the option of giving additional late feeds to better support the chick through the night. It is easiest to preempt tomorrow morning's poor weight by taking action tonight. If the weight does not improve the following day, consider these possibilities:

- Dehydration may be the problem, especially if the chick has recently suffered parental neglect. Provide liquid feeds approximately half the amount of a normal feed 2–4 times during the day.
- The brooder temperature may be too low. Consider a 1–2° increase, and look for changes in feeding response/attitude.
- Add pinkie mice to fortify the diet for chicks aged 1–7 days, as described in the section "Diet Recipes," earlier in this chapter.
- Weight gains will fall to near zero at 4 weeks of age because nutrition is used for feather production—not physical growth.

In general, the caregiver must carefully calculate daily weight changes using an array of tools to correct the course according to the individual chick's performance. If extraordinary weight gains are achieved (such as 40–50% in 24 hours), check for a mathematical error or fluid retention, both of which are possible. Do not panic if 1 day produces a low or negative weight gain, especially if the previous days saw large increases. Add pinkie mice if weight gains are sluggish; monitor the chick and look for panting or lethargy that may be suggestive of overheating or being cold, respectively. Overall, the chick should be as comfortable and as unstressed as possible to maximize weight gains and promote well-being.

HOUSING

If more than one chick is being hand-reared, experience has shown that chicks are best kept together for the first couple of days. The long neck of each bird drapes over a sibling, with the arrangement appearing to be comfortable and self-supporting; perhaps the touch is even stress-reducing (see Figure 32.2).

Likewise, a single chick appears to be more restful when supported by a suitable surface such as a cloth-covered golf ball. Chicks may be contained in a small bowl lined with a towel. The towel provides important traction for the bird's feet, as well as a soft rim over which the chicks will drape their heads (see Figure 32.3). After only a few days they will prefer the edge of the bowl for neck support. By this time their flailing heads will become a hazard to each other, and separating the birds into individual bowls is recommended.

Thus, at about 3 weeks of age it is advisable to separate the chicks into their own brooders, or at a minimum they should be protected from each other by cardboard barriers. Feeding two or three toucans in a single container may be hectic, and birds' faces will get whacked by wildly competitive siblings if each is not protected from the others. At about this age, the chicks are large enough to be removed from the bowls. Toweling on the floor of the brooder is the ideal substrate, providing traction and cushioning, as well as being removable for easy cleaning. A lot of work is created by using towels because they have to be changed at every feed, but they are excellent for the purpose.

FLEDGING

At about 6 weeks of age, the most precarious part of the rearing process begins. Parrots may be content to languish in the brooder for a prolonged period of time, calm and tame after having been hand-reared. Toucans, on the other hand, have a powerful urge to fledge and will bounce and crash about in their brooder if that urge is forestalled. Fledging will happen, whether one is ready or not. Watch for signs of fledging, such as a readiness to fly from the brooder. When the time is right, move the brooder into a small aviary or enclosure. The bird may fly immediately into the new surroundings, or more likely will observe them cautiously for a few more days before "fledging" at its leisure.

Do not clutter the aviary with too many perches. Select straight tree branches of about 2 in (4.8 cm)

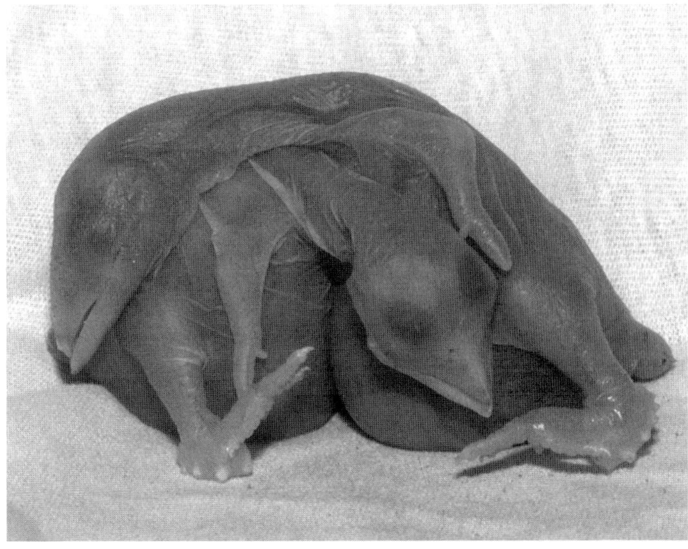

Figure 32.2. Toucan chicks draped over one another appears to be comfortable, self-supporting, and perhaps stress-reducing.

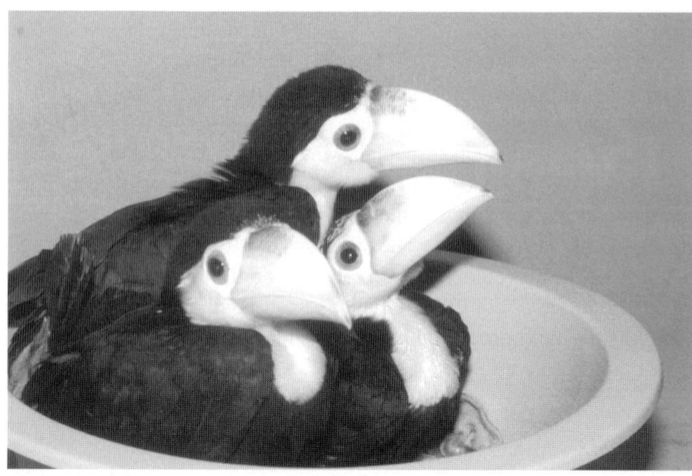

Figure 32.3. Five-week-old toucan chicks contained in a plastic bowl with a soft rim.

in diameter with rough bark that the birds can use to clean their bills. Fledgling toucans can fly only about 4 ft (1.2 m). However, after just a few days, young birds will fly greater distances and will need perching to accommodate that growing ability. Three perches, spaced 4 ft (1.2 m) apart, are ideal because they provide both a short distance and longer distance of 8 ft (2.4 m) for when the bird is ready. If possible, provide at least one high perch for roosting, with the main perches being about 5 ft (1.5 m) above the ground.

Toucans are inquisitive. They are constantly exploring their environment and thus have the frightening capacity to locate and swallow loose nails, screws, and the like if given the opportunity. Constantly check the fledgling's environment for dangerous foreign objects. Add leafy branches to the enclosure, as well as vines, logs, or other natural items that might occupy the birds. Change these items frequently to maintain interest.

Expect the birds to begin feeding themselves at about 8 weeks of age, becoming completely self-feeding at 9–10 weeks of age. If possible, attach the food pan at perch level to make feeding easier for them.

ACKNOWLEDGMENTS

Thanks to all of the staff of the Riverbanks Zoo Bird Department, especially Bob Seibels, Curator of Birds Emeritus, for their great passion and dedication. Without such professionalism and countless hours of dedication, the knowledge described in this text would never have been developed.

SOURCES FOR PRODUCTS MENTIONED

Kaytee exact (Original Hand-Feeding Formula and Kaytee exact Rainbow pellets), Kaytee Products Inc., 521 Clay St, Chilton, WI 53014, (800) Kaytee-1 or (920) 849-2321, www.kaytee.com.

Pedialyte Abbott Laboratories, Columbus, OH 43215, www.abbott.com.

Calcium Carbonate USP Precipitated Light, manufactured by PCCA, 9901 S Wilcrest, Houston TX 77099, (800) 331-2498, www.pccarx.com, Item# 30-1944-500.

Zupreem low iron softbill diet, Zupreem PO Box 9024, Mission, KS 66202, (800) 345-4767, www.zupreem.com.

Mazuri Zulife Soft-Bill Diet, (800) 227-8941, www.mazuri.com.

Nystatin, Bristol Myers Squibb, 345 Park Avenue, New York, NY 10154-0037, (212) 546-4000, www.bms.com.

REFERENCES

Howard, R. and Moore, A. 2003. A Complete Checklist of the Birds of the World. Princeton University Press, Princeton, New Jersey, pp 301–303.

33
Corvids

Elaine Friedman

INTRODUCTION

The information in this introduction is possibly the most important information included in this chapter. Corvids are highly intelligent birds with well developed social skills. They show anger, fear, jealousy, and the ability to deceive, which allows them to mask a physical problem. They are excellent observers and quick to notice any difference from the norm. They exhibit food preferences and have a wide range of personality traits. In order to successfully raise or rehabilitate corvid species, one must be a good observer and make judgment calls based on the history, body language, behavior, and physical condition of each individual bird. The caregiver must be able to adapt a set of instructions to each bird's particular needs. For example, too much food gavaged or force-fed to a weakened bird will be regurgitated and possibly aspirated.

These birds operate not only on instinct but also by the learned experiences they have had in their life. If they have never experienced red berries or a white mouse in their diet, putting this in their food bowl might cause them not to eat at all. And if as a neonate they never see natural foods in their diet, they might starve, once released, before locating food. These are birds that express thoughts and intentions in their vocalizations, feather position, and body language. Plan to research their natural history in more detail than presented here. Observe both wild and captive corvids and relate what you see and hear to the circumstances of the observation. And make a judgment call for the corvid in your care based not only on what you find described in a book but also on what you feel will work best. This chapter provides guidelines and insight to help you make educated decisions on how to proceed in raising an injured or orphaned corvid.

NATURAL HISTORY

The family Corvidae are members of the order Passeriformes, and include the largest of the songbirds, which are perching birds with three toes in front and one long toe behind. These birds are ruled less by instinct and more by their superior mental capabilities than other bird species. According to Sibley, there are 20 species of corvids grouped in 8 genera, including ravens, crows, magpies, jays, and Clark's Nutcracker, within the borders of the United States, with approximately 120 species worldwide. Protected by the federal government, corvids are included in the laws pertaining to migratory birds even though many members of the various corvid species do not migrate but may simply relocate to follow ample food supplies. It is illegal to keep a corvid as a pet.

These are social birds, often found in small to very large groups numbering thousands of birds. Some species, including the American crow, are cooperative breeders. The birds as a group are omnivorous, with some species being heavily dependent on certain food items including insects, nuts, and carrion. The focus of their diet fluctuates with the changing seasons and the natural foods available. Uneaten food and items of interest to the birds are cached. Caching techniques can be specialized, such as the spit caching of seeds on branches performed by the gray jay.

Flight for this group of birds is generally strong with rowing wingbeats. Due to their foraging skills, most of these birds spend periods of time at ground level with a member of the group posted as guard.

The nest for this family is a bulky cup of sticks in a tree or other convenient tall structure. At times some species will nest in a bush. Magpies add a roof when structurally possible and some ravens nest on ledges. Corvids have a reputation for being noisy and aggressive, but also of being quiet and secretive during nesting periods. An exception to this rule is the mobbing of predators like hawks and owls threatening the nest or fledglings.

Each species in the Corvidae family has specific behaviors relating to conspecifics and these behaviors may complicate release possibilities, especially if birds are not raised with siblings, similarly aged juveniles, or adults of the same species. Adult ravens, for example, may be intolerant of older juveniles, forcing the juveniles to form a group to defend food finds from the resident adults. Raven nestlings vocalize loudly back and forth to one another after feeding, which is not typical of the other species. Magpies are extremely aggressive to an inferior or poorly socialized member of the species.

There are excellent sources of information regarding the natural history of individual corvid species. It is imperative that an individual raising a particular species of corvid become familiar with the natural history of that species to prevent unintentional injury, taming, or imprinting of the bird being raised. Release criteria must be based on the needs of each species, especially the natural habitat and the expected interaction with wild conspecifics.

The natural diet of corvids consists of insects and other invertebrates, grains, seeds, fruits including berries, vegetables, nuts including acorns, small mammals, carrion, eggs and young birds, frogs, lizards, salamanders, worms, garbage, and just about any other natural food source found in the wild.

When raising corvids in captivity there are particular problems that appear that are related to the natural history of these birds. Crows and ravens are unusually large songbirds. Their size may cause human caretakers to ignore that they are still a juvenile and might not be self-feeding or that they might still be a nestling requiring a nest rather than a perch. Due to the social nature of the various corvid species, fledglings usually leave the nest well before becoming self-feeding, with the adults giving weeks or months of supportive care and training. The human caretaker of a juvenile corvid must supply more training than would be expected with other songbirds. Corvids are sensitive to changes in spatial relationships, an important component to a caching bird with a highly developed hippocampus portion of the brain. When in captivity, changes in housing may greatly affect corvids, which at times may cause them to stop eating. Corvid family nestlings appear more susceptible to overheating and dehydration than many other bird species, at times quickly becoming dehydrated after initial hydration even when housed in an incubator. Dehydration may cause the birds to become unresponsive to the stimuli that usually cause them to gape. If they are forcefully given food at this point, they lack the ability to successfully swallow or digest it. The bird may rapidly become critically ill unless the caretaker recognizes the cause of the problem and rehydrates the bird.

CRITERIA FOR INTERVENTION

Corvids may be brought into captivity for a variety of reasons. Hatchlings, nest and all, may be blown out of a tree during wind storms. Badly timed tree trimming or tree removal also accounts for many disruptions to nests. If nestlings are relocated to a neighboring tree or even put back into the same tree but not in an identical nest, the adults may not continue to support the birds. Older nestlings move about in the nest, stretching and flapping, possibly causing younger siblings or even themselves to fall out of the nest. Predators such as raccoons, owls, hawks, or even squirrels may injure a nestling or cause it to fall out of the nest.

During periods of low humidity and high temperatures, fledglings may become dehydrated and disoriented. If the area where the fledgling has landed appears unsafe for adult birds to support or assist the juvenile, the adults may vocalize to the younger bird but not give it supportive care. Because most fledglings must spend some time on the ground before they master flight, even a healthy fledgling may become frail from lack of food and hydration if parents are unwilling to risk their own safety to support the bird. Fledglings must not only learn to fly but also to eat on their own by following the example set by older birds and by trial-and-error pecking and exploring; hence they are vulnerable to injury by predators, including domestic pets.

Fledglings may be docile, especially if they are stunned or injured from a collision with a window or other object, and many times they are picked up by humans. A physical examination must be performed before any thought is given to reuniting a juvenile with its family, because a large percentage of corvids found by humans have injuries to the skeletal system or nervous system or are fatigued by lack of food and hydration. If a corvid is simply observed on the ground and adult birds are present, this may not be enough to ensure its safety. It is important to observe from a distance far enough away that adults are willing to approach the juvenile. If adults are observed repeatedly feeding the juvenile, no predators are present, and the juvenile appears alert and agile, it can probably be left undisturbed. But if adults are not actively feeding the juvenile or prodding it to a safe area or branch, the bird should be captured and evaluated. Returning the juvenile to the nest bears careful consideration. If other juvenile corvids are present in the nest and not quite ready to fledge, they might prematurely jump out of the nest when the sibling is returned. If the juveniles are not fully feathered and therefore more docile, returning a sibling to the nest is generally more successful for all of the birds. Some corvid nests, including those of ravens, are located on cliffs or in tall trees and would require an experienced climber or special equipment to reach the nest.

RECORD KEEPING

Corvids are covered under the Federal Migratory Bird Treaty and any time spent in captivity is, by law, regulated by the United States Fish and Wildlife Service. Injured or orphaned corvids should be cared for only by individuals or organizations licensed by both the state and the federal governments. An inexperienced caretaker raising a single bird is almost guaranteed to produce an imprinted or tame bird.

Basic information including species, age, location found, finder's contact information, reason for bringing the bird into captivity, behavior of the bird when found, medical problems found on initial exam, final disposition, and release location must be included in a record for each bird. A detailed medical record should include initial exam and updates, such as body weights, response to treatments, daily types and amounts of food consumed, behavioral notes, and results of laboratory tests.

Record the location the bird was found. Corvids are social birds, with family members congregated in a specific area. Returning a bird to a support network upon release will enhance its chance for survival. Detailed records about the habitat in the location the bird was found will allow a caregiver to pinpoint areas with habitat beneficial to a particular species of corvid. This will aid in the successful release of birds unable to be returned to their home territory for any reason.

Many organizations have multiple caregivers, which may result in inconsistent and inappropriate care. For this reason, feeding and housing instructions should be accessible to each caregiver including amounts to feed and feeding methods for each stage of the bird's growth or recovery.

Finally, corvids require the company of conspecifics to decrease stress and to develop social ties. They may carry illnesses or parasites that are infectious to other birds. Records should detail interactions or contact between birds in captivity to enable caregivers to keep social groups together through release and to track and locate transmission of contamination or illness.

INITIAL CARE AND STABILIZATION

A newly admitted corvid should be allowed to stabilize in a warm, quiet, and dark enclosure for at least 15 minutes before having an initial exam unless immediate care is indicated. The initial exam should consist of a systematic search for lesions, fractures, or other abnormalities. If indicated, further diagnostics may be conducted once the bird is stable. The bird should be weighed on a gram scale. This will aid in determining the quantity of fluids to offer initially. Hydration is of paramount importance. Without proper hydration, the bird cannot be fed or treated successfully. The safest method for rehydration is the administration of subcutaneous fluids. Give 2–3 percent of the body weight in fluids if the bird appears dehydrated. If hydration must be done orally, a corvid should be given initial fluids with a 1 ml syringe. For magpies and jays a narrow-tipped 1 ml syringe or a teat cannula (syringe extender) is useful. The bird must be warm before it can swallow and process fluids. A small portion, less than 0.1 ml, of warm oral solution (lactated Ringer's solution or equivalent), should be placed past the glottis down the bird's right side of the throat to ensure that it is capable of swallowing the liquid. Tissues become compressed and sticky when a bird is dehydrated, rendering it incapable of swallowing the liquid. In this case, subcutaneous fluids would be the optimal method for the initial rehydration. Once the bird exhibits the ability to gape and swallow, administer orally whatever portion of the calculated rehydration amount remains, divided over the next 2–3 hours.

For example: A 200 g corvid fledgling, 2% of its body weight in fluids would be: $200\,g \times 0.02 = 4\,ml$. This amount would then be divided and given to the bird orally over the next 2–3 hours. The size of the portion depends on the responsiveness of the bird. Weaker 200 g birds may be able to handle only 0.5 to 1 ml at a time.

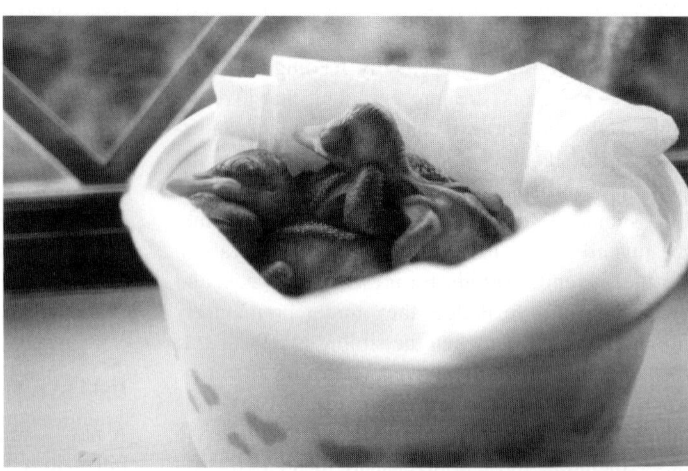

Figure 33.1. Western Scrub Jay chicks in a tissue-lined plastic container.

Administer only what the bird can manage at a given time regardless of the amounts quoted in the literature. The bird may have health problems preventing normal processing of fluids and could die if handled too aggressively. Once the bird begins to defecate, the focus may switch to the feeding regimen.

Housing during stabilization should be as stress-free as possible. Place hatchlings in an incubator if available, or use a heating pad set on the lowest heat setting, placed under the container the bird is housed in. Nestlings and hatchlings require a nest. Larger corvids such as crows and ravens might require a rolled towel placed in a donut shape as a nest to support their weight. Smaller birds may be placed in a plastic margarine-type container lined with multiple layers of toilet paper (see Figure 33.1). Use a plastic container that appears suitable in size for the species of hatchlings. The paper should be piled high enough to allow nestlings to defecate over the side of the nest; a hatchling should rest in an indentation in the toilet paper. The toilet paper should be crumpled enough to provide support for the birds to prevent splayed legs. If the heat supplied to a hypothermic bird in a nest is from a heating pad under the container, the layers of toilet paper will need to be increased as the bird warms to prevent overheating. Making a prewarmed nest available would be optimal. A sheet or two of toilet paper placed over the bird will also help keep warmth in the nest for hatchlings, especially if there is only a single bird.

Corvids tend to harbor pathogens that may be infectious to other birds. Do not combine a newly admitted bird with those already being hand-reared. A mouth and throat swab and accompanying microscopic exam for trichomoniasis, a fecal analysis for parasites or their eggs, and a thorough body exam for pox lesions and ectoparasites are recommended. Corvids are especially susceptible to West Nile Virus (WNV). Newly admitted corvids should be isolated if WNV is prevalent in the area; however, social needs of a new bird must be balanced with the stress of being isolated. If the single chick or fledgling appears healthy upon admission, it may be isolated for just for 2–3 days, even with the presence of WNV in the area. Then place the chick with only one or two others the first week and monitor closely.

COMMON MEDICAL PROBLEMS AND SPECIAL CARE PROBLEMS

Juveniles have a weaker immune system than adults. When introduced to an aviary, corvids at times develop bacterial infections or might have a rise in previously undetected parasites. If a bird appears quiet, is perched inappropriately—i.e., out in the sun when other birds are in the shade—is being picked on by the other birds, is perching much of the time with nictitating membranes or eyes shut, has a weak cry, is fluffed, or does not appear to be eating, remove the bird from the aviary and examine and weigh it. Bacterial infections may come from many sources in the aviary, especially when the weather has been hot. Consult a veterinarian regarding administering antibiotics. Observe for sprains, strains, or breaks that may develop as birds learn to fly. Periodic fecal analysis of samples in the aviary should prevent recurring problems with parasites.

Behavioral Issues

Activity at Dusk

Corvids naturally move to a roosting area at dusk, and this urge ignites in older juveniles with a frenzy. If the juveniles are still housed indoors at this point, place them in a room that may be darkened completely before dusk. If all else fails, cover the enclosure with a light blocking towel or cloth. Failure to do so may cause feather damage from the birds flying into the sides of the enclosure.

Aggression by Conspecifics

Be cautious when adding a new bird to a group of juveniles already in your care. Even removing a bird for an extended medical procedure and returning it to the group might lead to aggression from the group to the newcomer. If the newcomer is compromised or ignorant of social skills the bird might not be able to avoid aggressive overtures from members of the group. Injury or even death may result. When introducing a new bird, observe the interactions from a distance. It might be necessary to remove all of the resident birds from the housing, allowing the newcomer to acclimate. Then, one by one add the conspecifics. The new bird could also be housed with just one other resident until peace is declared. If the new bird has a health problem, it may need to fully recover before introduction to other birds. An imprinted bird might never achieve acceptance. The most aggressive of the corvids appear to be ravens and magpies when it comes to dealing with any new bird, especially those ignorant of accepted social rules.

Stress and Boredom

Wild birds in captivity will show signs of stress such as panic flight, open-mouthed breathing, repetitive movements, and feather picking. Corvids, with their high level of intelligence, need natural types of stimulation in captivity to lessen the possibility of negative behaviors. Introduce natural items such as rocks, pine cones, acorns, twigs, small branches with leaves, dried sunflowers, bark, and containers of soil to dig and cache in. Aviaries should have a substrate on the floor for foraging, digging, and caching. Add small trees or bushes in pots, impale fruit on branches, or hang suet baskets (Arcata Pet Supplies) with fruit, suet, mice, or other food inside. If they are indoors, allow the birds to see outdoors. Let in natural bird sounds. Avoid capturing the birds for occasional medication or examinations at the same time that they are being cleaned or fed. Otherwise, the birds will fear being caught every time the cleaning routine begins.

Feather Problems

Bald Head

This is normal in corvids if it occurs during the spring-summer-early fall molt period. Even the juveniles go through a body molt after flight feathers have established themselves. Magpies especially lose head feathers all at once. If a bird has experienced a traumatic health episode or has been in captivity for a period of time it may be more prone to a balding-head molt.

Feather Damage

If wing and tail feathers are broken on a juvenile, the feathers will not be replaced until a molt the following spring and summer. The same is true for an adult bird. Tail feathers may be successfully pulled under a veterinarian's care to stimulate early replacement of the feathers; however, this is usually not true of wing feathers. Corvid wing follicles tend to become damaged when the feathers are pulled. A better way to replenish damaged wing feathers is to house the bird in an aviary lined with a fine screen material (Pet Screen, Phifer Co.), fiberglass screening, shade cloth, or aviary netting. Provide steplike perching and do not have branches so close to perches that they brush against and break growing blood feathers. Supply a flutter climbing pole, which is a sturdy pole, such as a closet pole or straight tree branch covered with AstroTurf and long enough to rest against a horizontal perch at about a 45° angle to the ground. This allows a bird having difficulty with flight to sidestep up to a perch. It may flap its wings as it climbs up the pole, aiding the climb by the push of the flapping wings. Permitting a feather-damaged bird to get off the ground prevents further feather damage caused by failed attempts to jump from the ground to a perch.

Respiratory Distress

Corvids will demonstrate open-mouthed breathing when stressed or overheated; however, if this type of breathing is present when the bird is calm and at the proper temperature, it could be signs of a respiratory infection (bacterial or fungal) or signs of aspiration of food or liquids. Do not ignore the symptoms.

Dehydration

Corvids tend to become dehydrated easily in captive care. They become sluggish and may cease gaping. The solution to the problem is to rehydrate the bird, ensure that the food contains ample moisture, and ensure that the housing is not too warm.

Emaciation

A quickly determined sign of emaciation is a sharp keel. Evaluate total protein and packed cell volume to develop a course of action including the probability of survival, and whether a liquid diet or baby songbird food recipe diet (BSFR) should be provided. A corvid will regurgitate and possibly aspirate any food that its body cannot tolerate. Begin the feeding process more slowly than the feeding chart might suggest. As the bird gains strength, feeding amounts may be increased.

Eye Problems

Examine the eyes for discharge, swelling, or discoloration. Common causes of eye lesions may be injury, pox, bacterial infection, trichomoniasis, or mycoplasma. If the bird does not respond to visual stimuli correctly or exhibits a tracking-type of behavior with the head, suspect visual problems or impairment.

Foot Abnormalities

Abnormal Perching

Observe how the juvenile corvid perches or sits in the nest. If the bird repeatedly places the hallux forward together with the other toes, a wrap or cardboard shoe may be required to "train" the hallux into proper position. If left unattended, the hallux will continually fold under and prevent grasping of a perch. Care must be taken to allow for growth of the bird while a wrap or shoe is being used. A wrap applied too tightly may result in permanent damage to the foot.

Bumblefoot

Redness, hardening, swelling, or sores on the bottoms of the feet are signs of bumblefoot infections. Smooth perches or routinely standing on the aviary floor may lead to bumblefoot. If the condition is recognized early, a change of perching alternatives may solve the problem. Astroturf (Astroturf Solution) wrapped around a branch or pole provides an excellent perching surface. Advanced cases of bumblefoot will require antibiotics and veterinary care.

Head Injury

Many juvenile corvids fall from the nest or have unsuccessful initial flights, which may result in a head injury. A weak cry, labored breathing, eye problems, balance problems, or an abnormally quiet bird may be indications of a head injury. Keep the bird warm and quiet and seek veterinary assistance. Provide a rolled towel nest if support is needed to keep the bird upright and show caution in giving hydration and food, because the ability to swallow might be compromised.

Metabolic Bone Disease

Juvenile corvids often exhibit signs of metabolic bone disease. This is especially true if the bird was the runt of the clutch, was kept as a pet, or was raised by inexperienced parents or a member of the public. The BSFR diet will help in supplying necessary calcium to the bird, but extra supplementation of calcium may be necessary. Corvids seek out extra calcium in the wild, and have been seen peeling paint (which contains calcium) from houses during heavy snow periods when ground foraging is difficult. Captive corvids have been observed eating the shell of hard-boiled egg before any other food item offered. Supply a balanced diet. Offer corvids portions of hard-boiled egg with the shell on. Seek veterinary assistance concerning calcium supplements for birds showing signs of metabolic bone disease.

Infectious Diseases

Avian Pox

Examine the legs, feet, face, abdomen, vent, mouth, or any other exposed areas for raised areas or sores.

Pox is contagious to similar species by direct contact or an insect vector. Isolate all exposed birds for a minimum of 2 weeks. Birds exhibiting signs of the disease should be kept in a screened, insect-free area until lesions are healed. Disinfect all surfaces after use and discard contaminated cardboard crates or carriers. Poxvirus may be transmitted on clothing. Treatment involves supportive care to prevent secondary infections and promote healing. If pox lesions become grossly large or do not heal, the veterinarian should rule out bacterial or fungal infection or mite infestation.

West Nile Virus

As mentioned earlier, corvids are very sensitive to WNV, and the mortality of infected birds is high. The best treatment is prevention. If WNV is in your area, isolate newly admitted corvids for a few days in case they are carrying the virus but are not yet symptomatic. Placing new birds together in small groups exposes fewer birds if one bird develops symptoms and has WNV. Keep mosquitoes and other biting insects out of enclosures. Spray newly admitted birds for ectoparasites to make sure they are not carrying biting insects. Direct contact between birds may spread the illness. Check with your veterinarian for current treatment protocol if you suspect the corvid in your care has West Nile Virus.

Antibiotic Sensitivities

Trimethoprim sulfamethoxazole (Septra) may cause a corvid to regurgitate immediately or as much as an hour after dosing. If a bird is sensitive to this drug it may suffer from dehydration combined with lack of medication. Use this product only if necessary and watch the bird for problems.

Parasitic Diseases

External Parasites

Mites will appear as grayish patches on featherless areas, such as the legs and feet. A skin scraping and microscopic examination will help determine whether the bird has acquired burrowing mites that, if left unattended, may cause gross distortions that may look like grayish eruptions or protrusions with holes in the center. Treatment with Ivermectin and the application of an avian lice and mite spray will usually eradicate the parasites. Length of treatment depends on severity of the infestation.

Internal Parasites

Three of the more common parasites in corvids are capillaria, coccidia, and tapeworm. Feces should be tested soon after the bird is acquired, and prompt treatment is necessary to prevent infection of other birds. Praziquantel (Droncit) is effective for tapeworm, fenbendazole (Panacur) for capillaria, and sulfadimethoxine (Albon) for coccidia. When more than one parasite is present, do not administer Albon and Panacur simultaneously. Some corvids lose their appetite and become depressed after being dosed with this combination.

Trichomoniasis

Trichomoniasis infections are caused by protozoan parasites and may be present but visually undetectable. A wet mount of a mouth and throat swab should be examined under the microscope for the telltale "Pac Man"–like organisms. Carnidazole administered orally is routinely used to treat this condition. Check with your veterinarian for the correct dosage.

DIET RECIPES

Table 33.1 lists the ingredients for the BSFR.

Mash kibble with a fork after water has been absorbed. Puree egg and banana in a blender (see Tables 33.1, 33.2). Mix all the ingredients using a food processor. Freeze in small containers. Thaw only enough diet for 1 day. Warm the mixture by placing the container in warm water or on a warming plate set on low. If the air temperature is high, the

Table 33.1. Baby songbird food recipe (BSFR).

1 C (240 ml) Science Diet Canine Growth (Puppy) soaked in 1 C (240 ml) cold water
1 4 oz jar (112 g) baby banana or 4 oz (112 g) ripe banana
1 peeled hard-boiled egg
1 tsp (5 ml) bird vitamin (Superpreen, Arcata Pet Supply, or equivalent)
1 tsp (approximately 1800 mg) ground calcium carbonate

Table 33.2. Adult bird kibble mix.

4C Science Diet Canine Growth (Puppy) soaked in 2C water
1 tsp bird vitamin (Superpreen or equivalent)
1/2 hard-boiled egg
1/6C fruit, such as apples, pears
1/6C green vegetables, such as zucchini, cucumber
1/6C yellow or orange vegetable, such as carrots, squash

diet for a particular bird should be discarded midday and fresh diet supplied to finish the day.

Note: If the BSFR appears too stiff to feed via syringe, add a small amount of water the day of use and mix until the consistency is moist enough to easily syringe-feed but not too moist as to possibly cause aspiration of the food. Table 33.2 lists the ingredients for the adult bird kibble mix.

Ensure that the choice of fruits and vegetables will not spoil easily or be so watery as to make the kibble mushy. Pulse-chop eggs and fruit/vegetables in a food processor until coarsely chopped. Do not overprocess. Mix all ingredients. Store in refrigerator for up to 2 days.

DIET SUPPLEMENTS

Other items should be added to the kibble diet above to offer a variety of nutrients and textures. Do not overfeed any one of them as it may create an unbalanced diet. It is impossible to give absolutes on supplement additions. They are based on the caregiver observing the current status of the bird. A young bird just learning to eat will require mostly kibble plus a small amount of supplements to taste and move about. As the bird learns to manipulate food, more supplements may be given. Nuts must be cracked open at first and later may be supplied whole once the bird learns what to do with the nut. Add any of the following to the kibble mix:

- Chick (1 day old)
- Mouse, starting with pinkies or cut mice initially and working up to whole mice as the bird learns to grip and tear the food
- Hard-boiled egg, with shell on
- Unsalted nuts of all kinds, especially those found wild in the bird's native area
- Insects (including mealworms, waxworms, crickets, and those found naturally)
- Vegetable chunks
- Vegetable bits, i.e., frozen corn kernels, chopped string beans, broccoli bits, peas, fruit chunks, berries
- Fruit tidbits for pecking exploration stage—raisins, raisin-sized bits of strawberries, grapes, cantaloupe, and watermelon
- Cooked sweet potato as a good source for vitamin A
- Colored kibble bits, for example: Kit and Kaboodle cat food (Purina)
- Peanuts, unsalted, in the shell, cracked, and out of shell

When ravens become self-feeding, their diet is largely whole meats or carrion. Even in the final stages of hand-feeding they will reject the BSFR and gape only for cut-up meats like rats, chicks, or mice. Older juvenile crows also develop a taste for whole meats.

FEEDING PROCEDURES

All young birds must be warm and hydrated before introducing food. Once this is accomplished, if the young bird is actively gaping, begin syringe-feeding with the BSFR. If the young corvid is warm and hydrated but refuses to gape, it may be force-fed. During force-feeding or when feeding a corvid hatchling, support the head and extend the neck using gentle finger pressure. Place an appropriate-sized syringe (see Table 33.3) containing the BSFR down the right side of the bird's throat, positioning the tip past the glottis when force-feeding or when feeding a hatchling. For older, vigorous birds, the syringe may be placed in the back of the mouth and the bird will do the rest as the food is pushed in via the syringe. Use a 1 ml syringe with a stainless steel feeding tube or teat cannula syringe extender if necessary, for a tiny (25 g) or weak bird, and 0.5 ml or less of the BSFR for the initial portion for any corvid. Begin with small amounts of food and ensure that the bird does not expel the food or gag. Refer to Table 33.3 for approximate feeding amounts for the following categories: hatchlings (nakeds), nestlings (pinfeather birds and prefledglings), and fledglings.

EXPECTED WEIGHT GAIN

Corvids vary greatly in size when comparing species and even within a species. Charting the daily weight

Table 33.3. Feeding regimen.

Corvid	Age	Amount	Syringe	Frequency
Crow	Naked	1 ml or less	1 ml	Every 30–45 min
	Older naked	3–6 ml	1–3 ml	Every 30–45 min
	Pin (pinfeathers)	Up to 6 ml	1–3 ml	Every 30–60 min
	Prefledgling	6–12 ml	3 ml	Every 1–2 hr
	Fledgling	9 or more ml	3 ml	Every 1–3 hr
Scrub and Steller's Jays	Naked (1–6 days old)	0.1–1 ml or more	1 ml with teat cannula	Every 20 min from 7 a.m.–10 p.m.
	Naked (more than 6 days old)	Variable: 1–2 ml	1 ml; use teat cannula if not a strong gaper	Every 20–30 min from 7 a.m.– 9 p.m.
	Pins (with pinfeathers)	Variable: 1–3 ml	1 ml	Every 30–60 min from 8 a.m.–8 p.m.
	Prefledgling	Variable: 1–3 ml or more	1 or 3 ml For older prefledge (cut-off syringes)	Every 1–2 hr from 8 a.m.–8 p.m.
	Fledgling	Variable: 3 ml or more	3 ml (cut-off syringe)	Every 1–3 hr from 8 a.m.–7 p.m.
Magpies, Black and Yellow-Billed	Naked	0.1–2 ml or more if bird is still gaping	1 ml; use teat cannula for recently hatched or weak birds	Every 30 min from 7 a.m.–9 p.m.
	Pins (with pinfeathers)	Variable: 1–3 ml	1 ml	Every 30–60 min from 8 a.m.– 8 p.m.
	Prefledgling to fledgling	Variable: 1–6 ml	1 or 3 ml syringe (cut-off syringe; larger syringe for older, stronger birds	Every 45 min for younger birds up to every 120 min for older fledglings
Ravens	Naked to pin	Same as for crows, but increase amounts as bird gapes for more	For youngest raven, begin with 1 ml syringe and increase to 3 ml as soon as bird can tolerate it; use cut-off syringe	Every 30–60 min
	Prefledgling to fledgling	Ravens grow rapidly and vary greatly in size. An older bird may take as much as 20–30 ml. Allow bird to determine food amounts through gaping. Many ravens will refuse BSFR and need whole meats, such as cut-up mice	3 ml syringe or larger, (cut-off syringe); use forceps to feed cut-up meat	Every hr for prefledglings up to every 3 hr for oldest fledglings

Table 33.4. Developmental milestones in the American Crow (Emlen 1942).

Age/days	Weight/Grams	Integument	Eyes	Reaction to observer	Notes
1–3	15–30	Pink	Closed	Gaping	Brooding by parent; yolk sac persists
3–5	30–45	Smoky	Closed	Gaping	Brooding by parent; yolk sac persists
5–10	45–110	Black	Closed/ then slit	Gaping	Brooding by parent/tapers off; yolk sac persists
10–15	110–210	Growth of pins	Slit/then opening	Gaping	Brooding tapers off, then ends traces of yolk sac, then gone
15–18	210–255	Growth of feathers	Dull	Gaping	Voice changes to lower pitch
18–25	255–300	Growth of feathers	Clear gray-violet	Gaping, then crouching	Projection of middle primaries beyond sheaths is 2 in or less
25–30	approx. 300	Growth of feathers	Clear gray-blue	Crouching, then escape	Projection of middle primaries beyond sheaths is greater than 2 in

in grams for members of the common species in your area will be useful for future reference. The birds increase rapidly in size and weight, and then tend to level off as pinfeathers develop and change into feathers. Some birds bulk up in the aviary prior to release, significantly increasing their body weight (see Table 33.4).

An optimal method of weight evaluation of a corvid for an experienced rehabilitator is to palpate the amount of muscle on either side of the keel. A bird with small breast muscle mass is not ready to be released. If this evaluation is done after the bird has been in captivity for a number of weeks and the muscle mass is low, a reevaluation of the health status of the bird should be done, especially with respect to infection or parasites. If a diet has been used that varies from the ones listed in this chapter, a review of the nutrition supplied should also be done. As the weight of a bird begins to level off, usually around the prefledgling stage, pay attention to the hydration of the bird, because its food intake typically decreases. It may be necessary to supplement the syringed diet with oral fluids. First-year corvids tend to develop fat supplies to aid in getting them through their first winter. This has the potential of making them heavier than adult birds of similar dimensions in wingspan and body length.

HOUSING

Jays

Hatchlings should be placed in an incubator or in a heated, windowed cardboard pet carrier (Porta-pet); nestlings may go directly into a pet carrier. An optimal pet carrier is constructed of cardboard with a 7 × 9 in (18 × 23 cm) hole cut in one side and covered by a piece of flexible clear plastic taped in place with clear packaging tape (see Figure 33.2), creating a window. The pet carrier is lined on the bottom with a folded bath towel covered by a folded pillowcase.

A small towel rolled into a donut shape is provided in the carrier to be used as a nest or to hold in place a margarine container nest (lined with sheets of toilet paper) used for hatchlings. Hatchlings may require only a very light towel under the nest plus another towel wrapped around the nest to promote

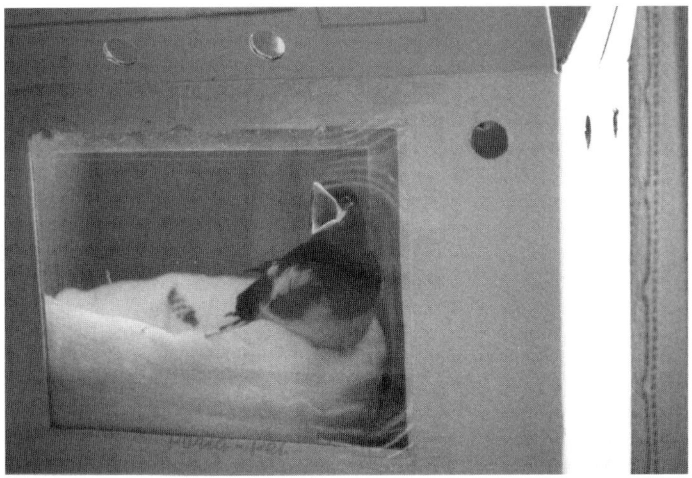

Figure 33.2. Juvenile magpie in a cardboard pet carrier fitted with a clear plastic window.

enough warmth from the heat source. Heat is supplied by placing a heating pad set on the lowest heat setting partially under the carrier for nestlings and fully under the carrier for hatchlings. Loss of heat may be adjusted by partially covering the top of the carrier with a pillowcase and by placing a layer of toilet paper over the nest. This carrier may be adapted for juvenile jays just leaving the nest by adding a sisal rope (natural fiber rope) perch. Two holes are made at perch level on the largest sides of the carrier. The sisal rope is strung through and held in place by knots tied on the outside of the carrier. Ensure that the rope placement leaves room for the bird to stand and also has ample room so the tail is not pushed against the carrier side. The window side of the carrier should be placed near a window to provide stress relief for the bird or birds inside.

Once the birds have demonstrated the ability to perch and sample food, they should be moved to a preflight cage. Line this cage with fiberglass screening to protect the feathers. A preflight cage is set up indoors, permitting birds to be hand-fed as they are learning to eat on their own. Perches in the cage should be arranged to allow the birds to hop back and forth easily. Food bowls should be placed away from areas where the birds defecate. Jays should be completely self-feeding before being placed in a larger enclosure or in an aviary. Even friendly juvenile jays become nervous about a radical housing change and may refuse to accept hand-fed food. The final step prior to release of a jay is for the bird to spend at least 2 weeks in an outdoor aviary.

Due to probing corvid beaks, most enclosures will sustain some damage, especially to lining materials. Pet Screen, (Phifer) is made to withstand dog and cat scratches, and it seems more resilient than other products. Cages and aviaries should have a variety of perches. Avoid using smooth branches. Corvid feet are prone to developing bumblefoot with the use of improper perching. Perches covered with a plastic turf material (AstroTurf, Solutia Inc.) are recommended for areas where the birds perch for extended periods. Perching alternatives include rough branches such as oak, live trees and plants, and sisal rope, which is a natural fiber rope that is rough enough to permit and support healthy bird feet.

Optimal incubator temperatures will vary among corvid hatchlings. Some songbird hatchlings are kept at temperatures as high as 90–95°F (32.2–35°C) and 40–50% humidity, but this is generally too hot for a corvid and could easily cause dehydration, especially if the incubator is not maintaining steady high humidity. Many rehabilitation centers keep a number of incubators warm with 5°F (2.8°C) differences between them. After placing a hatchling in an incubator, breathing and feeding patterns are observed. Open-mouthed breathing in a healthy hatchling indicates that the temperature is too warm. Decrease in gaping or inability to swallow indicates dehydration or that a bird is ill or cold. Even when the optimal temperature is attained, most corvid hatchlings need occasional replenishment of hydration, especially the recently acquired birds. The number of hatchlings placed together also makes a

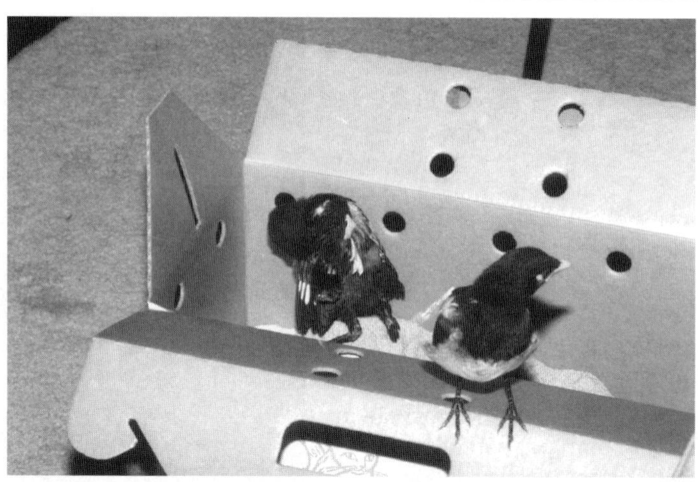

Figure 33.3. Juvenile magpies given the opportunity to stretch and flap their wings during pet carrier cleaning.

difference with corvids, because they have large bodies as compared to other songbirds. Single birds present a large unfeathered surface area from which to lose moisture; four to six birds grouped together supply a fairly resilient reservoir of warmth.

Larger Corvids (Ravens and Crows)

Larger corvid juveniles are usually started in a windowed pet carrier (see Figure 33.2) or a small kennel equipped with a rolled towel nest or plastic turf (Astroturf) perch, unless they are recently hatched. Follow the protocol under jays for recently hatched birds. If the bird's ability to eat or defecate normally is unclear, the bird should be kept in the carrier overnight for observation. Nestlings stay in the windowed carrier on a heat source until they begin to perch or become too large for the unit. They are then moved to a small kennel equipped first with a rolled towel nest, and then a perch. If the birds thrive in the small kennel, they are quickly moved to a larger kennel with a window view and one or two perches fitted with Astroturf that is cable-tied around a closet pole cut to fit the kennel width. The perch is wedged into the kennel using a washcloth or folded paper toweling at both ends. The birds should be given the opportunity to stretch and flap their wings during kennel-cleaning periods, either by placing them on top of the kennel (see Figure 33.3), on the floor (if they cannot yet fly), or in a mesh playpen covered with a blanket. The opportunity to build wing strength ensures a stronger bird upon placement in an aviary. The final housing before release is an outdoor aviary. If a small 6 × 6 × 6 ft (1.8 × 1.8 × 1.8 m) aviary is available, the birds may be placed outside while they are still gaping. The small aviary allows hand-feeding of the still-gaping birds. Once the birds become self-feeding and comfortably go down to the ground to eat rather than just from hanging bowls, they are moved to the large aviary.

SOCIAL GROUPINGS

Form small groups of juveniles upon admission and allow the birds to remain with this social group throughout the rehabilitation period. Release the birds as a group. Corvid social bonds are strong, and disrupting the bonds will cause stress. Do not mix or switch the birds as new birds are admitted.

AVIARY

Check with your state Fish and Game agency for their specifications for aviary size for corvids. Another good source is the *Minimum Standards*, published by the National Wildlife Rehabilitation Association, www.nwrawildlife.org. A 10 × 10 × 7 ft (3 × 3 × 2 m) aviary would suffice for magpies and jays and 20 × 10 × 7 ft (6 × 3 × 2 m) is enough for the larger corvids, such as ravens and crows. Line the aviary with insect screening to prevent feather damage and to protect from mosquito-borne illness. Pet Screen (Phifer) is stronger than regular insect screening and appears to sustain less damage from corvids. Most damage occurs to the aviary sides where the ends of perches contact the netting. These areas may be further lined with plastic hardware cloth to deter probing beaks. A variety of perching must be supplied both for prevention of bumblefoot and to familiarize the birds with perching possibilities in the wild. The highest perch should be placed in a protected area of the aviary and it is recommended that this perch be covered with plastic turf material (Astroturf). This is where the birds will spend much of their time. Sisal rope, rough natural branches, and live plants are good alternatives. Most corvids are hesitant to go to the ground to eat or drink when first placed in an aviary. This behavior may last for a number of days. To prevent dehydration and starvation, hang bowls containing water and basic foods near the most frequently used perch for the first few days of aviary usage. Favorite foods may be placed at ground level to inspire exploration. The bowls used to hold food and water at ground level should be sturdy nontip crocks. Always have climbing poles, fitted with plastic turf material reaching from the ground up to a perch in the aviary, to allow nonflighted birds to climb to a perch where they will feel safe. The perch should not be so high that they might fall and be injured. This aids in stress relief and encourages healthy feather growth. Nonflighted birds left on the ground often injure themselves trying to gain height. If even simple changes are made to the aviary after adding birds, such as putting in a larger water bowl, the birds may stop eating for a period of time. Corvids are highly spatially oriented and notice the slightest change in environment. The aviary must be partially covered for protection from the elements and have a substrate on the floor to inspire digging and caching. Bark and 0.75–1.5 in (2 × 3.8 cm) smooth light pebbles (Lodi rock) are good choices.

WEANING

In the wild, corvids may spend many months learning from their parents and other relatives. The birds fledge well before they are self-feeding and may be supported and protected out of the nest by an extended family group. When raising a corvid, time and effort must be spent to prepare the bird for what it will face upon release to the wild. It must be able to locate food, water, and shelter and be aware of what to fear. It will not have the benefit of the family support group, so to improve survival, the bird must be educated before release. Because of their high sensitivity to spatial relationships, corvids fear unknown areas and might be too afraid to seek food in a new area. Juvenile corvids benefit greatly by being housed in an outdoor environment replicating as much as possible what the release area will be like. The best positive factor would be to house the bird with a surrogate or other adult corvid of the same species so the young bird can learn from the more experienced bird.

Based on the these facts, weaning should involve being placed in enclosures, which allow the bird to experience live plants; tree branches; substrates such as dirt, bark, and rocks to dig and cache in; and logs to pound on and use for cracking nuts. Additionally, the bird should be able to hear other wild bird sounds, especially those of the species involved, so that the bird can learn which vocalizations are connected with what dangers located outside of the enclosure. Present the natural foods that will be in season when the bird is released for recognition purposes. Expose the bird to seed feeders, suet baskets, fruit, and nuts hung on branches of bushes' nuts wedged in pine cones' food wedged in the cracks of logs; and anything else you can devise to educate the birds on finding food. In some areas, crows frequent fast food restaurants and picnic grounds, so they are taught to tear apart a paper bag.

The weaning process also involves allowing the bird to test natural food items while learning to eat on its own. As soon as a bird begins to leave the nest it should be given food items to explore. When the bird begins to hold some food in its mouth rather than swallow during syringe-feeding, it means that it is eating some food on its own but probably not enough to sustain itself. When gaping becomes intermittent, make feed intervals longer, maintaining at least four feedings a day. As the bird becomes more proficient at eating, reduce the number of feedings per day to three, then two, then one, and finally cease feed support while keeping weight records on the bird. Most caregivers give fresh food in the morning and allow the bird to eat and explore the fresh food, and then offer support later in the day until the bird is no longer gaping and is maintaining its weight. Evidence that the bird is eating is also present in profuse defecation and normal activity level. Changes made in a corvid's enclosure usually result in a period of time in which the bird will refuse to eat. In the weaning period, offer support if the enclosure must be changed, and continue the support until it is evident that the bird has resumed eating on its own. This process may be aided by supplying food and water in hanging cups at perch level in a kennel and especially in an aviary. During the weaning period, avoid replenishing only one type of food offered in the enclosure. Fledglings need to explore, taste, and move about natural food items as they learn to take in enough food to support themselves. Sprinkling a few wiggly worms on fruits, kibble, and other food items will encourage exploration. Bright colors like corn kernels also inspire probing beaks. Colored items such as egg yolks, persimmon, watermelon tidbits, and blood-red mouse parts will often elicit at least a taste. Allow the bird to practice its eating prowess, to learn to crack nuts, and to pull apart a whole mouse before placing it in a large enclosure where progress is not easily monitored. Before a bird is moved outside, it must be acclimated to more adverse conditions than that of a temperature-controlled environment. A bird should be gradually exposed to more extreme temperatures during the weaning process.

PREPARATION FOR WILD RELEASE

Preparation for wild release of the bird should begin upon entry of the bird into your care. Never treat a wild bird as a pet. Introduce it to a natural environment and natural foods to ensure that, upon release, the bird recognizes the things that will keep it alive. Corvids are social birds and should never be raised alone. A bird devoid of the social rules of its species will be shunned or possibly injured by birds that would ordinarily socialize with the bird. Find another caregiver with a bird similar in age to the one in your possession or arrange to pair the bird with an injured adult or permanently injured captive adult. During the time you are waiting to combine birds, supply the singlet in your care with a mirror at eye level, a species-specific stuffed toy, or an actual mount to view up close. If the stuffed toy is the size of the actual bird, place it in the nest with the bird so the "companion" can be leaned on and pushed against. Face an indoor enclosure up against a window so that the bird views the outdoors rather than human activity. Interact with the bird only when necessary and then not in a way you would with a pet.

Once in the aviary, the birds will demonstrate distrust of humans if they have been successfully reared. A wild-raised fledgling is usually already fearful of humans and therefore does not require as much concern over taming or imprinting.

RELEASE

To be considered for release, a corvid should be parasite- free, well fleshed, difficult to catch in the aviary, and fully feathered with the feathers having a water-repellent quality called *weathered.* The fledgling should be adapted to varying temperatures and able to fly easily to the top of a tree, eat on its own, identify and locate natural foods, successfully interact with others of its species, and be fearful of people and predators before being considered a candidate for release. A minimum of 3 weeks in an outdoor aviary with other birds of the same species is necessary to acclimate a corvid and maximize its survivability in the wild. Realize that for the first week the bird might not come down to the aviary floor and that the bird must be comfortable foraging on the ground in order to survive.

Release a corvid in an area where there are others of its own kind. Optimally return any bird to its family territory. If this is not possible, find an area where multiple groups gather so that the new bird will have a better chance of acceptance. Release groups of corvids raised together in the same location so that they continue to interact with and support one another. It is especially important with ravens to release a juvenile in an area with other juveniles if the original parents cannot be found. Juveniles support one another and lead each other to food, and adults might chase an unknown juvenile.

Because these birds are diurnal, release them early in the day in good weather.

SOURCES FOR PRODUCTS MENTIONED

AstroTurf Solutia Inc, PO Box 66760, St. Louis, MO 63166-6760, www.astroturfmats.com.

Kit and Kaboodle cat food, Purina Mills, Nestlé Purina PetCare Company, Checkerboard Square, St. Louis, MO 63164, (314) 982-1000, www.purina.com.

Pet Screen, Phifer Inc., P O Box 1700, Tuscaloosa, AL 35403-1700, (205) 345-2120, www.phifer.com.

Portapet-Cardboard Pet Carrier 24″ × 12″ × 18″, Item # 60000: UPCO, 3705 Pear St, St. Joseph, MO 64503, (800) 254-8726, www.UPCO.com.

Super Preen, Item ##835–837: Arcata Pet Supplies, (877) 237-9488, www.arcatapet.com.

Suet Baskets, Item #1472: Arcata Pet Supplies, (877) 237-9488, www.arcatapet.com.

Sisal Rope (natural fiber rope): LeHigh, 2834 Schoeneck Road, Macungie, PA 18062, (610) 966-9702, www.Lehighgroup.com.

Trimethoprim-sulfamethoxazole (Septra), King Pharmaceuticals, Bristol, TN 37620, (888) 840-5370, www.kingpharm.com

Teat Cannula (Cannula Item # J): www.squirrelstore.com.

REFERENCES

Angell, T. 1978. Ravens, Crows, Magpies, and Jays. University of Washington Press, Seattle, Washington.

Caffrey, C. 2003. Determining impacts of West Nile Virus on crows and other birds. In American Birds, Summary of the 103rd Christmas Bird Count. Audubon, pp. 12–13.

Ehrlich, P.R., Dobkin, D.S., and Wheye, D. 1988. The Birder's Handbook. Simon and Schuster Inc., New York, pp. 406–421.

Elston, C.F. 1991. Ravensong. Northland Publishing Co., Flagstaff, Arizona.

Emlen, J.T., Jr. October, 1942. Notes on nesting colony of Western Crows. In Bird Banding, 13, pp. 143–154.

———. 1936. Age determination in the American Crow. In The Condor, XXXVIII, May–June: 99–102.

Friedman, E. 2004. Magpie rehabilitation. In Wildlife Rehabilitation, Vol. 22. National Wildlife Rehabilitation Association, St. Cloud, Minnesota.

Friedman, E. and Petersen, S. 2001. Care for the Western Scrub Jay and Steller's Jay. In Wildlife Rehabilitation, Vol. 19. National Wildlife Rehabilitation Association, St. Cloud, Minnesota.

Goodwin, D. 1976. Crows of the World. Cornell University Press, New York, pp. 173–183.

Heinrich, B. 1999. Mind of the Raven. HarperCollins Publishers, Inc., New York.

Kilham, L. 1989. The American Crow and the Common Raven. A&M University Press, College Station, Texas.

Madge, S. and Burn, H. 1994. Crows and Jays: A Guide to the Crows, Jays and Magpies of the World. Houghton Mifflin Company, New York.

NWRA. www.nwrawildlife.org.

Savage, C. 1997. Bird Brains—The Intelligence of Crows, Ravens, Magpies, and Jays. Sierra Club, San Francisco.

Save Those Eggshells. 1998. Birder's World. Kalmbach Publishing Co., Waukesha, Wisconsin.

Sibley, D.A. 2001. The Sibley Guide to Birds. Alfred A. Knopf. New York, pp. 350–361.

Terres, J.K. 1991. The Audubon Society Encyclopedia of North American Birds. Wings Books, Avenal, New Jersey, pp. 124–144.

34
Passerines: Hand-Feeding Diets

Rebecca Duerr

INTRODUCTION

In the wild, nearly all passerine chicks in North America are fed insects in order to provide adequate levels of protein to fuel rapid growth rates. Even species that as adults are specialists on other foods, such as seeds, almost always feed their chicks insects. Ideally, chicks in captivity should be fed exactly the same foods the parents would have fed them in the wild; however, duplicating this is an extremely challenging task. Human caregivers may have dozens or even hundreds of chicks in care at one time, may have a limited selection of commercially available insects from which to choose, or may have financial constraints limiting expenditures on live foods. Consequently, there is a significant need to have hand-feeding diet recipes available that enable caretakers to provide chicks with an excellent plane of nutrition while taking cost, effort, and accessibility into account.

Investing in high-quality diets is a wise choice under any circumstances. Well-nourished chicks are less prone to disease and grow faster than chicks fed lower-quality diets. In a rehabilitation context, this may lead to fewer mouths to feed at any given time, which is especially important when raising large numbers of birds simultaneously.

Many articles have been written in recent years describing the nutritional needs of juvenile passerines and how to meet those needs in captivity (MacLeod and Perlman 2001, 2003; Winn 2002; Finke and Winn 2004a, b). In addition to other educational opportunities, the International Wildlife Rehabilitation Council (IWRC) offers an advanced course called *Wildlife Feeding and Nutrition*, which provides training on diets for captive wildlife. See Appendix 1, "Important Contacts," for IWRC contact information, or their website at www.iwrc-online.org for upcoming training dates and locations. See Appendix 2, "Energy Requirements for Growing Birds," for a table of caloric requirements for growing passerines based on body size.

Many foods fed to young passerines by the uninformed are wholly inadequate and should never be used: bread and milk, condensed milk, hamburger, and uncooked rice to name a few. Feeding these items may result in the death of the bird. See Chapter 1, "General Care," for short-term diet suggestions. Hand feeding diets based on dog food are not adequate for growing passerines, nor are commercial diets intended for baby parrots. An exception to this may be Kaytee Exact Hand Feeding Formula, which some rehabilitators report as effective when fed to House Finches. Other passerines fed parrot diets may survive and appear of healthy weight, but plumage is likely to be of poor quality. Parrots have significantly lower protein requirements than passerines, and the protein supplied is primarily of plant origin rather than the high-quality animal-based (e.g., insect) protein needed by passerines. Dog food–based diets also typically produce fledglings with inferior feather quality. Caregivers should beware becoming so familiar with the appearance of low-quality plumage that it appears normal. Plumage on birds raised for wild release must be indistinguishable from wild chicks of the same age.

To avoid development of metabolic bone disease in chicks, any hand-feeding formula must have the calcium and phosphorus balanced in a 2 : 1 ratio by weight, with calcium comprising approximately 2% of the diet as calculated by dry weight. Corvids, Northern Mockingbirds, and American Robins are at especially high risk of developing metabolic bone disease. Calcium carbonate is the most commonly

Table 34.1. MacDiet© 2006 by Astrid MacLeod and Janine Perlman.*

Amount	Ingredient
2/3 C (160 ml)	Water
1/2 C (120 ml or 65 g)	Super-premium feline growth dry kibble; soak refrigerated in above water until fully softened; do not discard any unabsorbed water
2	Hard-boiled egg whites, sieved through a fine mesh strainer
3 Tbsp (45 ml)	Canned super-premium feline growth food, drained of liquid
2 Tbsp (30 ml)	Freeze-dried insects, soaked/reconstituted in a minimum of water; drain excess water
1/2 Tbsp (8 ml)	"Knox Blox" powdered gelatin
1800 mg	Elemental calcium from 4.5 g powdered calcium carbonate
50 mg	Vitamin C (ascorbic acid)
1 small pinch (volume in 2 sesame seeds)	Powdered B-complex vitamins
4 drops (0.3 ml)	Fish (body, not liver) oil
1 small drop (0.08 ml)	Vitamin E oil
1 slightly rounded Tbsp (20 ml)	Low or nonfat plain yogurt

*Reprinted courtesy of Janine Perlman.

used supplemental form of calcium. Powdered calcium carbonate products vary quite widely in density, from as low as 700 mg per teaspoon to over 1600 mg per teaspoon. Consequently, caregivers must weigh calcium powder on an accurate scale measuring to milligrams, such as a balance beam scale, until they are familiar with a given product's measure of milligrams calcium per unit volume (e.g., per teaspoon). Weights and measures should be rechecked every time a new shipment is received or a new brand is used. Calcium carbonate is 40% elemental calcium by weight, hence 1 g (1000 mg) of calcium carbonate powder supplies 400 mg of elemental calcium.

Caregivers must make every effort to not get food on feathers or in eyes. Sloppy feeding techniques lead to feather damage, possible permanent feather follicle damage, skin and eye infections, and a host of other problems. Any food spilled on feathers must be promptly removed with a moist cotton swab or equivalent, and food must be immediately flushed from eyes with ophthalmic saline solution.

The recipes in Tables 34.1–34.3 are excellent options, although all are works in progress and are continually being updated as new knowledge becomes available. All are intended to be used with live insects as a significant portion of the diet. Do not delete ingredients or the nutrients may be out of balance. A summary of typical San Diego Zoo passerine feeding protocols is presented last, where chicks are fed almost exclusively animal protein until a gradual transition to adult diet when nearing weaning age.

MACDIET

Be sure to weigh or measure amounts; do not estimate or leave out ingredients. For each 6 ml of MacDiet fed, also feed 10 large mealworms, 5 waxworms, and 3 large crickets. The MacDiet recipe supplies the amount of calcium needed for this proportion of dietary insects. Provide as many drops of water as the bird wants after each feeding. All ingredients except vitamins and yogurt can be blended, frozen as cubes, and stored for up to 1 month. Thaw a day's portion and add a proportional amount of vitamins and yogurt.

For birds 1–3 days posthatch, feed only mealworm guts, beheaded waxworms, and cricket abdo-

Table 34.2. Formula for Nestling Songbirds (FoNS©) 2006, by Mark Finke and Diane Winn.*

Amount	Ingredient
135 g (1 C)	ZuPreem Premium Ferret Diet, presoaked in approximately 1.5 C water
71 g (1 jar)	Beech-Nut Chicken & Chicken Broth Baby Food
12 g (2 Tbsp)	Dried powdered egg white
5 g (0.5 tsp)	Active-culture plain yogurt
3 g	Calcium carbonate (provides 1200 mg calcium)
1 g (0.25 tsp)	Avi-Era (Lafeber) avian multiple vitamins

*Reprinted courtesy of the International Wildlife Rehabilitation Council.

mens, in approximately the proportions above, in a mash. Add a tiny amount of yogurt into the mash. Add digestive enzymes as follows: use a tiny (poppy-seed–sized) amount of pancreatin (e.g., Pancrea-zyme) powder per feeding, mix thoroughly into the insect gut mash, and incubate at room temperature for 15 minutes before feeding. Providing fecal microflora for gut colonization is essential. Twice a day, give the bird a tiny speck of fresh feces from a healthy adult conspecific. If this is added to food, discard remainders and thoroughly wash all implements. Be sure to feed 100 mg/day of elemental calcium as powdered calcium carbonate for every 3–4 g insects fed (approximately 20 mixed insects). Provide copious amounts of additional water or hypotonic fluids; more uninjured hatchlings are lost due to dehydration than for any other reason.

FORMULA FOR NESTLING SONGBIRDS

Table 34.2 presents the Formula for Nestling Songbirds (FoNS©). Blend in food processor until smooth. Add water if needed to achieve desired consistency for feeding. Soaking time is reduced if ferret kibble is pulverized in a food processor prior to adding water. Calculated composition as fed: 73% water, 1.27 kcal/g; by dry weight: 50% protein, 23% fat, 17% carbohydrate, 2.0% calcium, 1.0% phosphorus (see Finke and Winn 2004b for additional information).

Table 34.3. Basic nestling diet.

Amount	Ingredient
1 C (240 ml)	Purina ProPlan Kitten Chicken and Rice dry kibble
1.25–1.5 C (300–360 ml)	Water
2 Tbsp (30 ml)	Powdered egg white
1/2 tsp (2.5 ml)	Avi-Era (Lafeber) avian vitamins
1850 mg	Calcium carbonate powder (provides 750 mg calcium)

BASIC NESTLING DIET

Table 34.3 details a basic nestling diet. Soak kibble for 20–30 minutes. Add the rest of the ingredients and blend until smooth. This diet is not as high quality as the previously described diets. However, it is relatively inexpensive, easy to make, and may be a good choice for some circumstances. This diet has been used with success in a large urban shelter raising several thousand chicks a year.

SAN DIEGO ZOO TYPICAL PASSERINE PROTOCOL

Hatchlings of passerine species such as Bird-of-Paradise or Metallic Starlings start life fed 33% bee larvae with 40% chopped pinkie mice and 27% crickets. There are minor variations in proportions of food items fed for each species. Bee larvae are particularly fed at the first and last meals of the day due to their high moisture content. Additional bee larvae are fed to chicks that tend to be dehydrated. Chicks are fed nine times a day, every 1.5 hours. Calcium carbonate is supplemented at 1% of the weight of the food fed the previous day. Chicks are also supplemented with Apatate (liquid vitamin B complex for children) at 1 ml per 50 g food fed. Chicks are fed 30–35% of body weight per day at hatch, rising to 55–60% of body weight by day 5.

At 5 days of age, feeding of bee larvae is discontinued. Chicks are fed 50–55% chopped pinkie mice, 35% 3-week-old crickets and 10% papaya. At 7–9 days, papaya is raised to 20% of the diet, and feedings are decreased to seven times daily, every 2 hours. At 10 days, Metallic Starlings receive 5% of the diet as soaked soft-bill pellets, plus 45% fuzzy mice, 30% crickets, and 20% papaya. Birds-of-Paradise have 5% mealworms added to the mix of 35% chopped fuzzy mice, 25% mealworm halves, 20% crickets, and 20% papaya. From days 11–20, the diet is gradually shifted from the high-protein juvenile diet to the adult diet mix. The amount fed per day reaches a maximum of about 65% of body weight between days 6–10, and declines thereafter as birds begin to be offered adult diet.

White-crowned Shrike hatchlings are fed 25% each bee larvae, pinkies, crickets, and waxworms. After day 5, the bee larvae are no longer fed and are replaced by carnivore meat. At day 10, chicks are fed 25% each pinkies, adult crickets, molted mealworms, and carnivore meat. At day 17, shrikes are fed 35% fuzzies, 35% carnivore meat, 10% soaked Iams cat chow, 10% mealworms, and 10% crickets. Daily food intake starts at 25% of body weight and rapidly climbs to 50–75% by day 10. Feedings are every 1.5 hours nine times daily from days 0–5, every 2 hours seven times daily from days 6–8, and every 3 hours five times daily until weaning begins in earnest at day 25. Calcium and B vitamins are supplemented in the same manner as the other species.

ALL DIETS

Warm only enough diet to be used within 2–3 hours. Refrigerate excess food and use refrigerated diets within 48 hours. Do not feed chilled or hot food; rather, feed diet warm or at room temperature. Do not heat diets in microwave ovens to avoid problems with super hot areas of food potentially causing burns. When warming cold diet, place a dish of diet in a larger pan of hot water until no longer chilled. Change food and feeding implements several times a day. Each container of chicks should have its own dish of food and own feeding implements to reduce risk of disease transmission between groups of chicks. All feeding tools should be cleaned and disinfected before and after use.

ACKNOWLEDGMENTS

Many thanks to Janine Perlman, Astrid MacLeod, Diane Winn, Mark Finke, International Wildlife Rehabilitation Council, and Pat Witman for providing diet information; Nancy Eilertsen and Linda Hufford for helpful discussions; and Penny Elliston and Jennifer Gursu for logistical assistance. Thanks to Guthrum Purdin for editorial assistance.

SOURCES FOR PRODUCTS MENTIONED

Avi-Era avian vitamins: Lafeber Company, 24981 North East Road, Cornell, IL 61319, (800) 842-6445, www.lafeber.com.

Beech-Nut Chicken & Chicken Broth Baby Food: Gerber Products Co. Fremont, MI 49413, www.gerber.com.

Calcium carbonate powder: Life Extension Foundation, P.O. Box 229120, Hollywood, FL 33022, (800) 544-4440, www.lef.org.

Iams cat food: The Iams Company, Dayton OH 45414, (800) 675–3849.

Powdered egg white: John Oleksy Inc., PO Box 34137, Chicago, IL 60634, (888) 677-3447, www.eggstore.com.

ProPlan Total Care Kitten Chicken and Rice Formula: Purina ProPlan products, www.proplan.com.

ZuPreem Premium Ferret Diet: Zupreem, PO Box 9024, Mission, KS 66202, 10504 W. 79th St, Shawnee, KS 66214 (800) 345-4767, www.zupreem.com.

REFERENCES

Finke, M. and Winn, D. 2004a. Insects and related arthropods: A nutritional primer for rehabilitators. Journal of Wildlife Rehabilitation 27(3–4): 14–27.

———. 2004b. Formula for Nestling Songbirds (FoNS)©: Updates for 2006. Journal of Wildlife Rehabilitation 27(3–4): 28.

MacLeod, A. and Perlman, J. 2001. Adventures in avian nutrition: Dietary considerations for the hatchling/nestling passerine. Journal of Wildlife Rehabilitation 24(1): 10–15.

———. 2003. Food for thought: Songbird nestling diets, 2004. Journal of Wildlife Rehabilitation 26(3): 26–27.

Winn, D. 2002. Formula for nestling songbirds: Down payment on fitness and survival. Journal of Wildlife Rehabilitation 25(3): 13–18.

35
Passerines: House Finches, Goldfinches, and House Sparrows

Rebecca Duerr and Guthrum Purdin

NATURAL HISTORY

House Finches and goldfinches are classified in family Fringillidae, subfamily Carduelinae. Other members of family Fringillidae include chaffinches, bramblings, and Hawaiian Honeycreepers. The cardueline finches also include grosbeaks, siskins, canaries, crossbills, and redpolls among others. The taxonomy of these species is somewhat controversial and may become revised with time. Adults of these species typically show pronounced sexual dimorphism, with males often possessed of striking plumage. There are approximately 150 species of fringillid finches worldwide, with 17 species occurring in North America (Elphick et al. 2001).

House Finches commonly nest in human habitation areas, including in hanging planters, under eaves, or on trellises. In temperate areas, pairs may produce up to three broods of four to five chicks per season. Young are fed regurgitated seeds; they are unusual among North American passerines in that they do not feed their young insects. There are three species of goldfinches in North America: Lesser, American, and Lawrence's Goldfinches. These species lay four to six eggs per clutch and may have two broods per season. Young are fed regurgitated milky seed pulp and some insects (Ehrlich et al. 1988).

The European House Sparrow is an introduced and well-established species in North America, and is not especially closely related to native North American sparrows. There are also introduced Eurasian Tree Sparrows breeding in a small area of central North America, but this species is not as ubiquitous as the House Sparrow. These two species are classed in Family Passeridae, the Old World sparrows. House sparrows often nest in urban areas: shopping malls, nestboxes intended for other species, eaves, drain spouts, Spanish tile roofs, and other enclosed spaces. As cavity nesters these birds may outcompete native species for nest sites, particularly Eastern Bluebirds and Cliff Swallows. House Sparrows have up to three broods of four to six chicks per season. Chicks are fed primarily insects (Ehrlich et al. 1988); however, chicks hatched at shopping malls may be fed random human food debris as well.

Finch versus Sparrow

House Finches and House Sparrows are among the most common chicks presented for rehabilitation in North America, with goldfinches presented less often. Chicks of these species are often confused with other species and with each other. All hatch small chicks (<1–2 g) with distinctly red-colored mouths and pink skin (see color image of gaping House Finch nestlings on cover). These species all display the typical anisodactyl passerine toe arrangement with three toes forward and one back.

House Finch chicks have four rows of whitish down on their heads: two rows on the crown and a small row above each eye. Goldfinch chicks have one row of grayish down over each eye, and another row crossing the back of the head to form a triangle of down. The down on House Finches and goldfinches persists as the body feathers come in, and may give the chicks the appearance of having cobwebs on their heads. House Sparrow chicks do not have any down at all, but rather hatch completely naked. By the time their eyes begin to open at 3–5

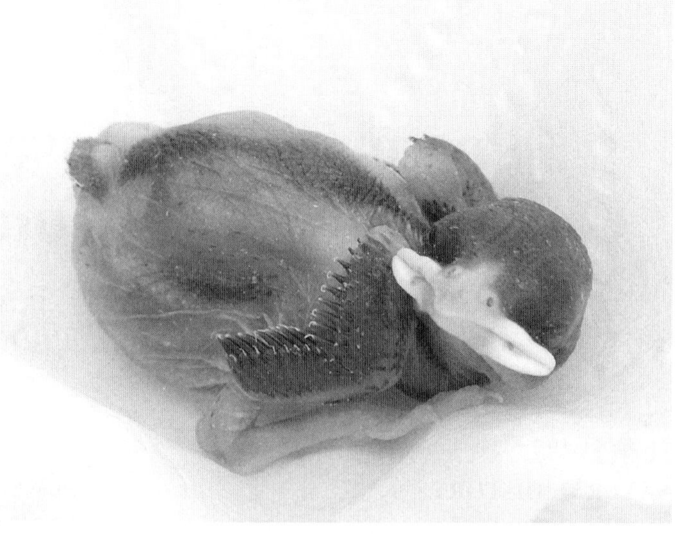

Figure 35.1. House Sparrow nestling with body and flight feathers just starting to come in. Note complete lack of downy feathers (photo courtesy of Jackie Wollner).

days of age, they typically have feather tracts beginning to emerge with a "5 o'clock shadow" appearance (see Figure 35.1). Well-nourished House Sparrow chicks may near adult weight before developing significant feathering. House Sparrows are the largest in this group, with House Finches being slightly smaller. Goldfinches are approximately half the size and weight of the others at any given age as determined by feather development. Adult weights are as follows: House Sparrow 28 g, House Finch 21 g, American Goldfinch 13 g, Lawrence's Goldfinch 11.5 g, Lesser Goldfinch 9.5 g (Sibley 2000). Young American Goldfinches can be differentiated from other goldfinches by the presence of distinctly black feathering on the wings with peach wing bars apparent as soon as feathers emerge. With experience, caregivers may also recognize each species' distinctive vocalizations.

CRITERIA FOR INTERVENTION

These species are common victims of cat attack. Additionally, chicks may be found on the ground covered in mites. Chicks may be presented for care when drain spouts are cleaned, or when house painting or construction is occurring. House Sparrow hatchlings frequently land on concrete when falling from urban nests and consequently may present with intraabdominal bleeding or leg fractures. House Finch fledglings are commonly "kidnapped" by well-meaning people who erroneously believe them to be abandoned. See Chapter 1, "General Care," for more information on whether a chick requires rescue.

RECORD KEEPING AND INITIAL CARE AND STABILIZATION

Small plastic leg bands may be used to differentiate individuals from each other (Red Bird Products). Individual identity is important for monitoring progress, body weights, or tracking effectiveness of treatment. See Chapter 1 for more information.

COMMON MEDICAL PROBLEMS AND SOLUTIONS

Lacerations from predators should be cleaned, debrided, and closed primarily whenever possible, to speed healing and reduce development of stress bars on growing feathers. All debris should be removed from wounds, and the feathers carefully plucked within 3–5 mm of the margin, with the exception of flight feathers. Take care to avoid tearing skin by gently plucking in the direction of feather growth or toward the wound edge, if close to margins. For very young chicks or for wounds that do not have much tension, surgical glue such as Nexaband (Abbott) may provide adequate closure. Semipermeable self-adhesive dressings such as

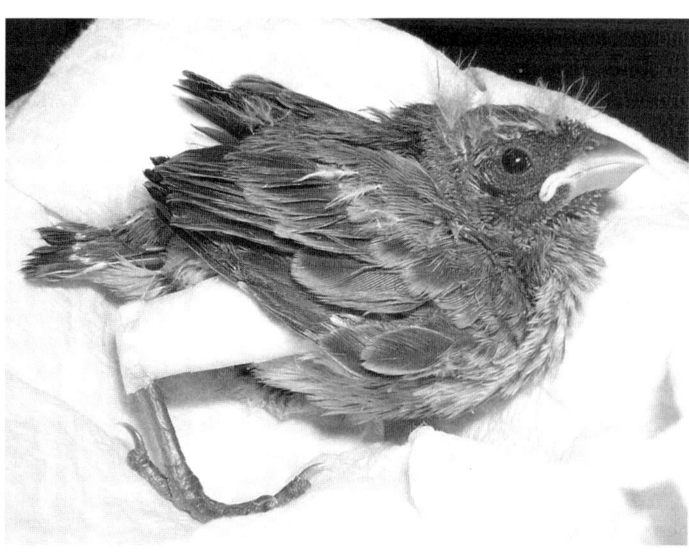

Figure 35.2. House Finch nestling with fractured tibiotarsus in minimally restrictive splint.

Biodres (DVM Pharmaceuticals) or Tegaderm (3 M) may be used for wounds that are unable to be sutured or glued. The authors' preference is to suture, glue, or dress all open wounds, especially in crowded wild bird nursery situations. Whenever possible, facilitate the fastest possible wound healing in order to lead to rapid progress through rehabilitation and an expeditious release. The longer the bird must stay in captivity, the more likely it is to develop secondary problems.

Subcutaneous emphysema (air under the skin) is a common result of a cat attack or severe impact, where one or more air sacs have been ruptured and leak air into subcutaneous spaces. This often resolves without treatment, but it may be helpful to remove the pressure if it is interfering with mobility or if it is causing the bird to become depressed. If necessary, puncture the bubble with a sterile needle, avoiding any visible skin blood vessels. Many cases will reinflate quickly and may require repeat punctures several times over the course of a few days. This problem may manifest 24–48 hours after presentation.

All chicks with wounds, including subcutaneous emphysema, should be placed on a course of broad-spectrum antibiotics that is likely to cover *Pasteurella multocida*, such as amoxicillin with clavulanic acid (Clavamox, Pfizer), at 125 mg/kg orally twice daily or cephalexin at 100 mg/kg orally twice daily until the problem resolves (Carpenter 2005). Be sure antibiotics are not discontinued until the wound has completely healed. Some wildlife veterinarians continue antibiotics for several days after external wounds have healed to reduce the likelihood of complications, especially in cases of body cavity punctures.

Midshaft tibiotarsus fractures are quite common in these chicks and often heal well with little impact on time in captivity. The authors use a minimally restrictive splint reminiscent of a miniature hockey shin guard (see Figure 35.2) to splint these fractures. Even tiny nestling goldfinches may be splinted with a neatly constructed lightweight splint. Splints for this fracture must hold the broken bone at the correct length to prevent the loose ends from overriding each other, and must provide rotational stability to keep the foot facing forward. As long as these requirements are met, it is not necessary to fully restrain the hock or knee joints, or bind the leg to the body. The goal should be for the bird to be able to use its leg as normally as possible while the fracture heals. Binding a rapidly growing leg to the body is not ideal. Fractures heal extremely quickly in these chicks. Remove splints in 1 week; if any motion is detected at the fracture site, reapply the splint for 1 more week, with size adjusted for growth if necessary. The younger the chick and the smaller the species, the faster fractures heal. Wing fractures are much less common in this age group than in adults.

Intestinal parasites are uncommon in House Finches and goldfinches, but House Sparrows occa-

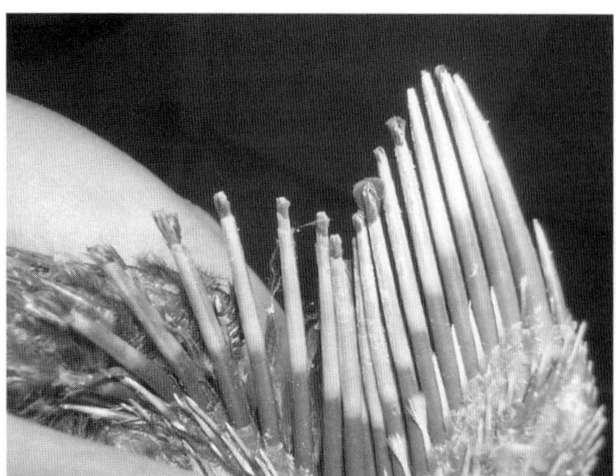

Figure 35.3. House Sparrow wing with feather sheaths that need to be preened off.

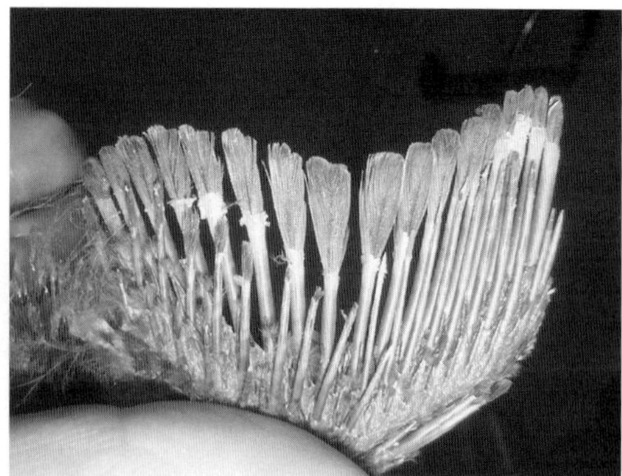

Figure 35.4. House Sparrow wing after preening. Note whitish areas were removed, but blood feather zones were unharmed.

sionally have coccidia. Diagnosis is by fecal float or smear. Treatment is with toltrazuril (Baycox, Bayer) at 7–25 mg/kg once daily for 2 days. Gastrointestinal yeast infections are not uncommon. Diagnosis is by fecal cytology or wet mount of a crop swab. Treatment is with Nystatin (Mycolog, Bristol-Myers Squibb) at 300,000 IU/kg twice daily for 7–14 days. Trichomoniasis occurs in these chicks, especially when raised in crowded nurseries. Many rehabilitation centers treat incoming animals for this disease prophylactically with carnidazole (Spartrix, Janssen) at 25 mg/kg orally once (Carpenter 2005). The authors have found it efficacious to repeat the dose once per week when this disease is a recurring problem in shelters. House Finches typically display signs as nestlings and fledglings and may show vomiting, slow or absent crop emptying time, or other nonspecific signs of illness. Close attention must be paid to disinfection of feeding implements and hygiene of caging. Each container of chicks should have its own food container to reduce potential spread of pathogenic organisms.

Poor Feather Condition in Sparrows

House Sparrows often require manual preening to remove the feather sheaths from their flight feathers (see Figure 35.3). If this is not done, birds often develop stress marks at the spot where the sheath constricted the feather. To remove feather sheaths, gently scrape a thumbnail along the white, nonblood feather portion of the feather to break the sheath (see Figure 35.4). Do not attempt this higher on the growing feather or damage to the blood feather zone may result. House Finches and goldfinches do not generally require this assistance.

Sparrows sometimes present as runts, with feather development suggesting age far older than body size would indicate. These birds typically do not do well, and although they may be frisky on arrival they often decline and die within a few days. Feather condition is usually poor as well. Normal-size sparrows may present with abnormally white feathers, or feathers in terrible condition. These birds are often unable to grow normal feathers, neither with plucking nor with long-term care to wait for a normal molt. Birds with inadequate body feather coverage may do poorly once outside or even die abruptly in the aviary. Euthanasia should be considered for House Sparrows with extremely poor feather condition. Because possession of House Sparrows is not regulated in many areas of the United States, permanent captivity may be a viable option in some circumstances. Check with local wildlife agencies if uncertain of applicable regulations.

Sick Finches

House Finches sometimes develop a disease syndrome colloquially known to rehabilitators as "Sudden Finch Death Syndrome," which may make them very frustrating birds to raise. It occurs as House Finches approach weaning age, when a significant portion of them may start to decline and eventually sicken and die. The authors' opinion on this issue is as follows:

- The onset of problems is not sudden if adequate attention is paid. Chicks that are in trouble have slowed crop clearance time, appear fluffed, may exhibit vomiting, or develop dirty feathers secondary to vomiting. These signs are seen 24 hours or more before deaths occur.
- Placing birds exhibiting signs of poor thrift on a cocktail of antibiotic, antiprotozoal, and antifungal medications turns many cases around quickly, which suggests an infectious organism may be the problem despite often negative diagnostic tests.
- Susceptibility to disease may be due to reduced immune function, which may be secondary to nutritional issues and stress. Premature weaning likely contributes to the problem. Overfeeding is also a common problem because finches will continue gaping when already overfull. Stretched-out crops have poor motility. A poorly motile, overly large crop provides an excellent site for growth of pathogenic organisms.
- For many wildlife veterinarians including the author (RD), overgrowth of Clostridium is the primary suspect agent. Problems appear reduced when House Finches are raised with a daily dose of metronidazole (Flagyl, Pfizer). This medication covers many anaerobic intestinal bacteria such as Clostridium and is effective against flagellates as well.

Recommendations for Caregivers Having Problems with Sick Finches

Keep feathers, nests, caging, and feeding implements scrupulously clean. Provide a calm, quiet environment. Do not keep finches next to noisy species such as starlings, or species that carry trichomonas such as doves or pigeons. Feed small, frequent meals of no more than 5% body weight every 30–45 minutes for 12–14 hours a day. Do not attempt to wean birds until tail feathers are fully grown out, body feathers are held sleek to the body instead of erect like a fledgling, birds are not frantically begging, and birds are at or above normal adult weight (18–21 g). Treat all affected and at risk chicks with metronidazole (Flagyl, Pfizer) at 50 mg/kg once daily until weaned. Separate sickly chicks from healthy chicks. Subcutaneous fluids may be needed for chicks having delayed crop emptying. Consult an avian veterinarian for diagnostic tests and further treatment.

HAND-FEEDING DIETS

These species do quite well on the diets listed in Chapter 34, "Passerines: Hand-Feeding Diets." Additionally, many rehabilitators use Kaytee Exact Hand Feeding Formula on these species with good results; this is an exception to the usual rule of not feeding parrot hand-feeding formulas to passerines. House Sparrows, however, will have higher-quality plumage when raised on higher protein diets.

Food Presentation

Once birds are leaving the nest and starting to explore, a diverse mix of small seeds should be offered. "Canary Mix" or "Finch mix" or similar undyed mixes work well, especially if other seeds such as niger (thistle) are mixed in for variety. Goldfinches are particularly attracted to thistle seeds and millet spray. Fresh plant material such as broccoli florets, parsley sprigs, minced greens, and halved grapes are popular first foods. House Sparrows may also eat insects. Other possible foods include fennel, crushed nuts, currants, minced apple or cherries, crumbled hard-boiled egg, and ground kitten kibble. Present food as an array of easily visible items. Shallow lids make excellent seed dishes, although scatter some seed on the floor as well. Broccoli florets and halved sideways grapes may be impaled on a bamboo skewer as "shish kabobs" and placed within easy reach of perches. Another presentation option is to drill a hole in one side of the long arm of a wooden clothespin big enough to snugly fit a short bamboo skewer segment. Fill the skewer with fresh fruits and vegetable chunks, wedge one end in the clothespin, and then clamp the clothespin to the perch with the skewer sticking up. Millet spray dangled next to perches may act as a needed enticement for reluctant eaters. Shallow water dishes should also be offered as soon as the birds are exploring their environment. Once birds are being weaned, keep food dishes large and wide to maximize visual stimulus. Wall-mounted food dishes may be useful in some circumstances, but may end up serving as litter boxes instead when birds perch on them while facing toward the center of the basket.

FEEDING PROCEDURES

House Finches and goldfinches of all ages eat best when fed in small bites (0.05–0.2 ml per bite depending on age) delivered to the back of the mouth. Nestlings that are frightened may be stimulated to gape by gently tapping a clean syringe tip on the side of the beak. It is helpful in encouraging gaping to imitate the species' begging noise in a soft whistle. Older chicks that are too frightened to gape may gape if beak tapping occurs while gently held in the feeder's hand and while the whistling begging sound is made. Be patient. Within a few feedings, healthy chicks will begin to understand that we are trying to feed them not eat them.

A 1 ml syringe with an attached cannula tip (Jorgensen) works well for all ages of House Finches and goldfinches, and hatchling House Sparrows (see Figure 1.6). Once House Sparrows have grown strong enough to pull on the cannula tip at around 10 g, there is significant risk that the bird will pull the cannula tip off the syringe and swallow it. Use a 1 ml syringe without the extra tip for older sparrows. Once a feeding syringe has been filled, all extraneous food should be wiped from the outside of the syringe and tip before feeding to reduce spillage.

When feeding a nest full of chicks it is useful to give one bite to each bird and move around in a circle until all chicks have had enough. This allows each bird to fully swallow their last bite before receiving more. House Sparrows are quite competitive for food. It is necessary to make sure each chick is receiving its share. The smallest, weakest House Finch in a clutch may end up on the bottom of the nest, necessitating the counting of heads when feeding.

Some rehabilitators use other feeding implements, including feeding picks (see Figure 1.6) and clean paintbrushes, to deliver food. In these authors' experience, the paintbrush technique tends to result in chicks that have been "painted" with food. In the hands of a dedicated caregiver, that is likely not the case, because some experienced personnel prefer this method. Feeding picks may be problematic due to the propensity of finches for jumping around a lot when begging, potentially brushing against a loaded pick and becoming dirty. Neither of these methods allows quantification of the amount fed.

Overfeeding may cause problems in these species, as they will continue begging for food until well after they are full. Consequently, caregivers must control the amount of food fed and cannot rely on the bird stopping gaping when it is full. Goldfinches are very prone to infections from having their plumage dirtied by excessive meal size or sloppy feeding techniques.

Hatchlings and Nestlings

Young chicks should be fed every 20–30 minutes for 14 hours a day. House Finch and goldfinch crops are easily visible on young chicks and should never be filled larger than 2/3 the size of the bird's head. This amount is approximately 5% of body weight (1 ml per 20 g body weight), but amounts to be fed depend on the diet chosen. Crops should empty between feedings. Hatchlings may weave their head while gaping. A cotton swab may be needed to steady the head during feedings, or gentle, steadying fingers. Sharp vision is required to feed tiny chicks, because it is easy to miss the mouth and get birds dirty.

Hatchlings have a higher requirement for water than older chicks. Their diet should either be thinned to a runny but not watery consistency, or amounts of more solid foods should be kept small and a corresponding amount of water fed with the meal. Pay close attention to droppings. If droppings stop being produced with every meal or if the chick stops gaping, palpate the chick's abdomen; it should always feel soft. Hatchlings that are becoming dehydrated may lack enough fluid to move food through the gut and it may feel firm to the touch. Give these birds small amounts of oral fluids, or subcutaneous fluids if not swallowing well, until food currently in the body has passed. Once the abdomen is soft again and stools are being passed, start feeding diet again with higher moisture content.

Fledglings

Fledglings should be fed every 45 minutes for 12–14 hours a day. House Finches that stay in the nest until quite mature are the easiest to wean, and they tend to have relatively high body weights. Allow birds to stay in the nest as long as they want. As soon as birds are perching and moving about the cage, they should be offered solid foods. These species start nibbling on food items well in advance of being able to effectively crack open seeds, so caregivers may be fooled into thinking birds are self-feeding prematurely. Hand-feeding should continue until birds are no longer frantically begging. Continue using the 1 ml syringe with cannula tip for goldfinches and House Finches until weaning. Do not use cannula tips for House Sparrow fledglings.

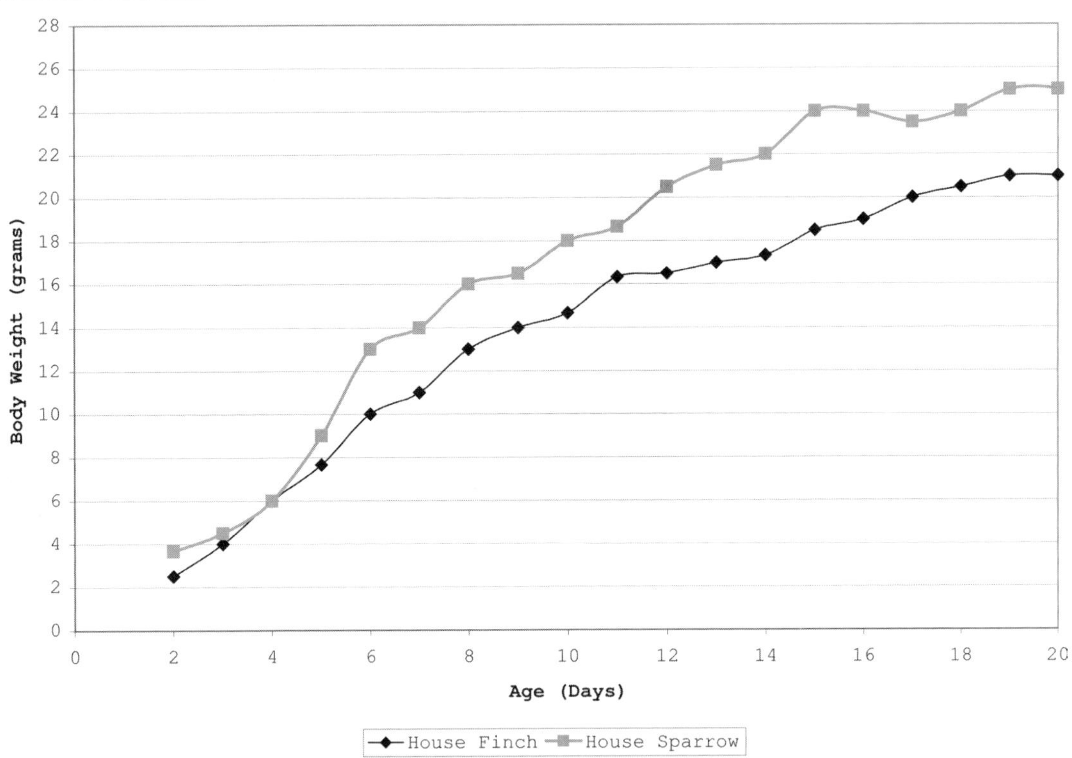

Figure 35.5. Typical growth of House Finch and House Sparrow chicks.

EXPECTED WEIGHT GAIN

See Figure 35.5 for a chart of typical growth of House Finch and House Sparrow chicks.

HOUSING

Hatchlings

Hatchlings should be kept in appropriately sized nest replacements inside an incubator such as an Animal Intensive Care Unit (Lyon Technologies). House Sparrows enjoy the security of having the nest covered with a tissue between feedings or using a cavelike structure as a nest (see Figure 37.3). Temperatures should be kept at 90–95°F (32–35°C) with 40–50% humidity. Other options for high heat housing are discussed in Chapter 1.

Never keep chicks on flat surfaces because of the possible development of splayed legs. Nests must have texture on the inside that will allow growing feet and legs something to grip, such as coiled or crumpled tissue. Keep hatchlings scrupulously clean by removing fecal material or spilled food immediately, changing tissue as needed.

Nestlings and Fledglings

When chicks are fully feathered nestlings, they may be moved out of the incubator. Place the nest in a large basket on a heating pad set on "low" (see Figure 35.6). Large laundry baskets with window screening covering all holes make excellent housing, as do reptariums (see Chapter 37, "Passerines: Swallows, Bushtits, and Wrens"). Use large pieces of window screening secured with clothespins as a ceiling on baskets. Older House Sparrows are excellent escape artists and tend to hide under furniture once out and about, so be sure to adequately secure all caging lest caregivers have to waste time chasing birds around the facility.

Baskets should have normal daylight-level illumination, preferably with a full-spectrum lighting fixture. Fledglings will be more difficult to wean if lighting levels are too dim. Birds require 9–10 hours

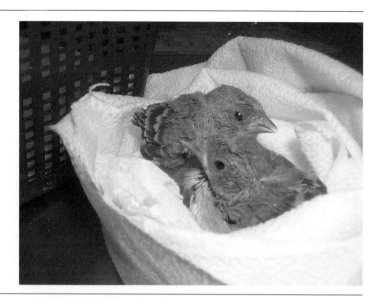

Figure 35.6. Lesser Goldfinch nestlings in berry basket nest.

of sleep nightly and will continue begging until the lights are turned out for the evening. Cleaning and other activities that require light for human activity should take this need for darkness into account. If lights are left on while tasks are finished, birds will continue to be active and may go to bed hungry.

As birds begin to leave the nest and explore their environment, add perching materials such as wild collected sticks and trimmings from natural food items, including dandelion heads or green tips of small branches of unsprayed lilac, honeysuckle, or forsythia with buds. Do not overfill baskets with natural vegetation, because birds will need easy access to food when weaning begins. Once birds no longer return to the nest, discontinue the supplemental heat. Keep perches placed close to the ground, because these species tend to perch on the highest spot available. Perches near the floor put fledglings in close proximity to food dishes.

House Sparrows may spend a lot of time hiding, as is to be expected from a cavity-nesting species. This can complicate ensuring that every chick gets enough to eat, because one chick may continually poke its head out to eat while others simply hide. It may occasionally be necessary to remove hiding places and add them again when birds are well on their way to eating on their own.

WEANING

It is critical to not try weaning small seed-eating birds too soon. It can be very tempting to reduce the number of daily feedings as soon as they are observed manipulating solid food, especially when raising large numbers of birds simultaneously. These birds are fed by their parents well after they have fledged from the nest. In the wild, chicks follow their parents from place to place learning how to forage. It is a common sight to see House Finch fledglings that appear very mature perching outdoors begging and being fed by an adult. This is a crucial period when fledglings experiment with finding food and perfecting their food-handling skills while their beaks continue to mature. By waiting until birds are a little older, caregivers will produce healthier birds in less time. Birds that are weaned too early may become sickly and remain in care for a longer period.

Weaning House Finches is a relatively easy procedure, but it involves scrupulous attention to detail to be successful. Once fledglings reach about 16 g, they start becoming interested in seed (see Figure 35.7). Many caregivers use this as a cue to cut back on formula feedings, thinking the birds are becoming self-sufficient; however, they are still too uncoordinated in handling seed and their beaks are too soft to properly shell seed. Adults may pick up, shell, and swallow a seed in less than a second. Fledglings may carry the same seed around for 20 minutes, practicing manipulation. They may, in fact, simply lift and drop seed after seed. The amount of seed they consume is inadequate for health and the final stages of development.

Syringe feeding must continue at 45-minute intervals. If a 16 g bird has copious seed in the crop, the

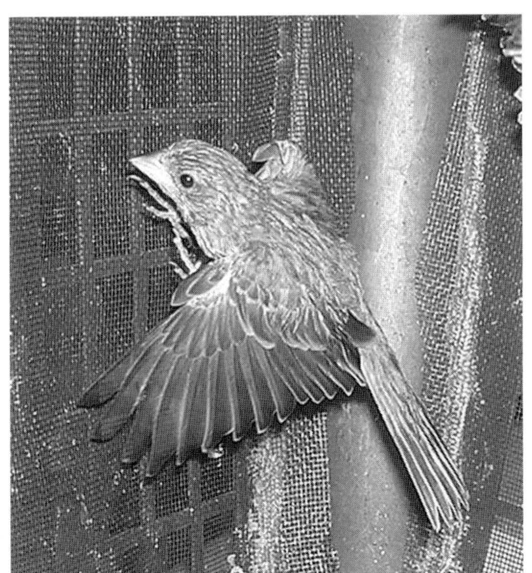

Figure 35.7. Fledgling House Finch at weaning age.

ration size of 1 ml can be lowered, but with caution. Birds at this age that are not begging should be suspected of having a health problem and should be examined. Never try to wean a frantically begging bird or one that is weak, vomiting, depressed, or generally sickly.

Well-nourished fledglings will happily investigate offered food. To facilitate fledglings' experiments in self-feeding, provide a fresh skewer of broccoli and grapes twice daily. It is also acceptable to offer chopped broccoli florets and grapes in a small, low dish on the floor of the basket. Use a separate dish or jar lid from the seed dish for easy disposal when wetter food items become chewed over. Make sure the produce is fresh and change often. These items are soft, sweet, and highly palatable to finches. House Finches eat green plant buds and green seeds in the wild; broccoli florets approximate these soft green buds. It will often be the first thing they eat on their own. They can become very excited when getting greens intermittently during the day. A small sprig of millet is well received by young birds. It is best to use only a small sprig because millet is not especially nutritious. However, as long as a high percentage of the diet is still a balanced, prepared formula, a controlled amount of palatable but nutritionally deficient foods is acceptable. The key is to get them eating and to make it something pleasant for them to do.

The decision to start weaning House Finches is based on observation of the whole bird. The tail must be fully grown out and the notch in the distal tip noticeable. Birds unready for weaning will have a fluffy, immature appearance to the head feathers. When old enough to wean, the head will look smooth and sleek. Be aware that when begging, they will erect those feathers and may look younger. Observe birds at rest when not being fed. The wispy, white natal down may be entirely absent by this point, but a few plumes can persist for quite awhile. The beaks start to look somewhat heavier, with gape flanges nearly gone. If a bird bites the caregiver's finger, it may have noticeable pressure. Some birds in the basket may be showing less of the wild enthusiasm for the syringe seen in nestlings. Birds being weaned should be sleek and starting to have the silhouette of adults.

Key at this point is weight. Finches can be best weaned at 18–21 g. On the morning of day 1, weigh all birds in the basket to be weaned. If all birds are at least 18 g increase the feeding interval to every 1 hour. Provide a very large dish of seed and scatter seed on the floor. This should be a diverse mix of regular finch seed, thistle, and can include canary mix for diversity. Provide a skewer of fruits and vegetables. Continue hourly feedings the rest of the day. Weigh birds again the next morning. If all birds are behaving normally and accepting the syringe, there's no problem. If one or more birds are gaping frantically and look like they are starving, reevaluate those birds. If they are maintaining their weight above 18 g leave them on the new schedule. If one's weight is below 18 g, consider moving that bird to a basket of younger birds. If they are all losing weight, return to the previous 45-minute schedule. Do not force-feed birds that are not taking food from the syringe unless they are losing weight.

The morning of day 3–4, weigh all birds. If weights are still 18 g or above, increase the feeding interval to once every 2 hours. Some birds may be fully self-feeding, but chances are most are still begging. Give up to 1 ml of formula during feedings. Ample seed and water must always be available. Beware of other personnel sneaking extra feedings to weaning birds; this may confound conclusions of how birds are doing while hand-feedings are cut back. Birds that act desperate for food at any point should be critically evaluated. It may be a signal of illness. Sometimes groups develop a personality and may appear especially dependent or independent. Some groups may all beg wildly. Others may refuse all syringe food on their first day. Look at the birds during each feeding and cleaning to get a sense for their condition. If there is any uncertainty, leave them at 1 hour.

On day 5–6, check weights and follow the above observational recommendations. If all weights are still above 18 g, decrease formula feedings to every 3 hours. Many or all fledglings may be uninterested in the syringe. If birds can maintain weight for 1 day on this small amount of supplemental feeding, they must be eating significant amounts on their own because 1 ml every 3 hours is insufficient to maintain body weight. If any birds are still actively taking syringe food, it is fine to wait until day 7 to change the feeding schedule. Even if still begging, they can be safely cut off thereafter as long as they appear healthy and vigorous. Weigh them 24 hours after ending the last syringe feeding. If weight is maintained, they are self-feeders and can be considered for prerelease aviary time.

Some rehabilitators complete the later steps of weaning while the birds are in outdoor quarters, to more closely replicate what would occur with wild parents. This is an excellent option but may be impractical in some circumstances, such as when birds are being raised in large numbers or with large numbers of volunteer caregivers. It is more feasible for professional staff to oversee weaning when birds are indoors and can be individually managed as necessary.

It's best to record weights during weaning to monitor individual variation. Daily weighing is a good idea if time permits and can be done while cleaning the basket. Just put the weanlings in a small plastic holding cage and weigh after zeroing the scale. Some finches are small. The author (GP) has found about 5% of House Finches wean at 17 g. Ultimate judgment on weaning status is made on overall appearance, especially head (sleek) and tail (long, notched), and demeanor (vigorous, active, no frantic begging). If unable to weigh birds daily, monitor the keel musculature closely. If sharp, the bird is thin. Young, growing birds, though, even in good weight, don't have the plump, firm pectoral muscles of wild adults. These will develop once they reach the aviary and can fly regularly.

In summary, on day 1 increase the feeding interval from 45 minutes to 1 hour. On day 3, offer feedings every 2 hours. Baskets that are doing well can go to 3-hour feeds on day 5 and by day 7 are likely to be fully self-feeding.

House Sparrows can be weaned on the same basic schedule with a few species-specific considerations. A sparrow of 20–27 g with tail feathers grown in to at least 1–1.5 in (2–3 cm) long is likely ready for weaning. Sparrows ready to wean will have resorbed their bright yellow gape flanges. Their beaks will be becoming grey-beige and hard. Their bites will become painful, and their bodies are fully feathered. They act restless in the basket and start to become an escape risk. Sparrows tend to progress very quickly to fully self-feeding once the daily number of syringe feedings is reduced. Work from the basic weight check and increasing feed interval plan for finches; however, it may be found that all birds are refusing formula after a day or two. Do not force-feed, and just monitor weights. If they're staying over 21 g and appear bright and alert, they should be fine. After a few days, evaluate for transfer to the aviary.

House sparrows that are raised singly may be difficult to wean because they may overfocus on the caregiver. Use a visual barrier of light-colored cloth that allows normal illumination but blocks view of human activity. Cheesecloth is a good choice for visual barriers. Singly raised House Sparrows may be aggressive if introduced to other birds at the aviary stage; hence, ensure that all birds have at least one conspecific companion in order to gain social skills.

Goldfinches notoriously gape long after their crops are full. Once they start eating seed, monitor how full their crops are before syringe feeding to avoid overfilling the crop. The formula ration needs to be carefully monitored. When offering solid food, mix in a liberal amount of thistle. Wean Lesser Goldfinches at 9–10 g, but, again, evaluate feathering and demeanor to determine maturity. Lesser Goldfinches are dangerously thin if they drop back down to 7 g. American Goldfinches generally run 2 g or so larger. Regional differences should be expected in any bird species. The weaning plan may need adapting to local variations in body size.

HINTS FOR CARE IN LARGE FACILITIES

If rotating volunteer caregivers are feeding chicks, training in feeding techniques is very important before allowing new persons to feed chicks. It only takes one feeder with poor technique to mess an entire room of chicks.

These species do well in a shelter environment, but need consistent care and daily attention from management staff. Birds that become fluffed, stop producing droppings, or refuse food when not being weaned must be promptly evaluated. Hatchlings may require micromanagement-level attention several times daily, because troubleshooting problems in hatchling passerines is beyond the skill level of most general care volunteers.

PREPARATION FOR WILD RELEASE

Aviaries for these species are recommended to be at least 4 × 8 × 8 ft high (1.2 × 2.4 × 2.4 m) for four to six birds (Miller 2000). Aviaries should be constructed with 0.5 × 0.5 in (1 × 1 cm) hardware cloth or wire mesh outer walls, and the interior should be fully lined with fiberglass window screen to prevent injury and damage to feathers. To provide protection from digging predators, the floor should have hardware cloth embedded below the substrate. At least one third of the ceiling, sides, and back of the aviary should be of solid material to provide shade and privacy. A variety of perching opportunities should be available, such as branches, shrubs, and sisal rope. The central area of the aviary should be left open to provide room for active flight exercise. As much natural food as possible should be provided, with seed mixes offered as well. Multiple elevated feeding dishes should be used to present food. Birds should spend 7–10 days in the aviary before release. They must be strong flyers, waterproof, and able to forage on a wide variety of food items.

RELEASE

Goldfinches should be released into a flock if possible. Releasing House Finches back into the area each bird was found may be optimal, but since birds from different areas are often raised together, the authors prefer to release birds as a group into good habitat with adults of the species nearby.

Release of nonnative House Sparrows is controversial. If birds are to be released, choose locations where there are already well-established populations. Do not release into naive habitat or into parkland where they are known to be outcompeting native birds.

Because these species are diurnal, release in the morning to allow birds to orient themselves before dark. Choose the release day with at least 3 days of nonextreme weather forecasted.

ACKNOWLEDGMENTS

Many thanks to Lessie Davis and Martha Kudlacik. Thanks to Debbie Daniels, Sarah Brockway, and Jackie Wollner for their enthusiasm and dedication to the birds, and a special thank you to the thousands of finches and sparrows that have wound up in our hands over the years, for teaching us about their needs.

SOURCES FOR PRODUCTS MENTIONED

BioDres: DVM Pharmaceuticals, Subsidiary of IVAX Corporation, 4400 Biscayne Blvd, Miami FL 33137, (305) 575-6000.

Carnidazole (Spartrix): Janssen Animal Health, available in the U.S.A. through Global Pigeon Supply 2301 Rowland Ave, Savannah, GA 31404, (800) 562-2295, www.globalpigeon.com.

Kaytee products: 521 Clay St, P.O. Box 230, Chilton, WI 53014, (800) KAYTEE-1.

Leg Bands: Red Bird Products, P.O. Box 376, Mt. Aukum, CA 95656, (530) 620-7440, www.redbirdproducts.com.

Metronidazole: Pfizer Inc., 235 East 42nd St, New York, NY 10017, (212) 733-2323.

Nexaband: Abbott Animal Health, North Chicago, IL 60064, (888) 299-7416.

Nystatin: Bristol Myers Squibb, 345 Park Ave, New York, NY 10154-0037, (212) 546-4000, www.bms.com.

Reptarium screen enclosures: LLLReptile and Supply Company Inc., 609 Mission Ave, Oceanside, CA 92054, (760) 439-8492, www.lllreptile.com.

Teat Infusion Cannula J-12 (Jorgensen Laboratories Inc., Loveland CO) and O-Ring syringes available from www.squirrelstore.com.

Tegaderm: 3 M Corporate Headquarters, 3 M Center, St. Paul MN 55144-1000, (888) 364-3577.

Toltrazuril (Baycox): Bayer Animal Health, available in the U.S.A. through Global Pigeon Supply, 2301 Rowland Ave, Savannah, GA 31404, (800) 562-2295, www.globalpigeon.com.

REFERENCES

Carpenter, J.W., ed. 2005. Exotic Animal Formulary, 3rd Edition. Elsevier Saunders, Philadelphia, pp. 135–344.

Ehrlich, P.R., Dobkin, D.S., and Wheye, D. 1988. The Birder's Handbook: A Field Guide to the Natural History of North American Birds. Simon and Schuster Inc., New York, 785 pp.

Elphick, C., Dunning J.B., Jr., and Sibley, D.A. 2001. The Sibley Guide to Bird Life and Behavior. Alfred A. Knopf Inc., New York, 588 pp.

Hill, G.E. 1993. House finch (*Carpodacus mexicanus*). In The Birds of North America, No. 46 (Poole, A. and Gill, F., eds. Philadelphia: The Academy of Natural Sciences; Washington, D.C.: The American Ornithologists' Union.

Miller, E.A., ed. 2000. Minimum Standards for Wildlife Rehabilitation, 3rd Edition. National Wildlife Rehabilitation Association, St. Cloud, Minnesota, 77 pp.

Rule, M. Songbird Diet Index. Coconut Creek Publishing Co, Coconut Creek, Florida 161 pp.

Sibley, D.A. 2000. The Sibley Guide to Birds. Alfred A. Knopf Inc., New York, 544 pp.

36
Passerines: American Robins, Mockingbirds, Thrashers, Waxwings, and Bluebirds

Janet Howard

NATURAL HISTORY

The "thrush relatives" are a group of six families of passerines including the Turdidae (bluebirds, thrushes, and robins), the Timaliidae (wrentits), the Mimidae (mockingbirds and thrashers), the Sturnidae (starlings), the Motacillidae (wagtails & pipits) and the Bombycillidae (waxwings). These families are closely related taxonomically through DNA studies and share similar diets. However there is substantial variation in appearance, nesting, migration, and habitat.

Fruit and insects are the bulk of the diet of the thrush relatives, with a seasonal focus on insects during breeding and fruits during summer through winter. Nests are typically open cup–shaped, typically built in a tree or shrub but sometimes in a manmade or natural cavity (bluebirds). The typical clutch size is four to five eggs, incubated by the female for 10–17 days, with two to three broods per year. Hatchlings are altricial and sparsely covered with down.

All the birds in these families have the typical passerine anisodactyl toe arrangement, with three toes pointing forward and one toe pointing backward (see Figures 36.1, 36.2). Their bills are distinguished by their slender but not sharply pointed shape, adapted for eating soft foods like insects and berries. Many of these species have characteristic foraging behaviors, such as waxwings passing berries from bird to bird down a long line of individuals, or a classic American Robin standing in the grass with head cocked hunting earthworms.

CRITERIA FOR INTERVENTION

The thrush relatives are among the most common species of passerine brought into captivity, because fledglings are frequent victims of well-intentioned kidnapping. Many of these birds commonly leave the nest 1–5 days before they are adept at flying. American Robins in particular commonly fledge while flight feathers are still in sheaths, leading well-meaning people to think they have fallen out of the nest or been abandoned, sometimes amid the protests of their parents. This preflight fledgling period also makes them a common victim of cat and dog attacks, as well as car accidents. Any bird that has been in a cat's mouth should be brought into care for treatment, but most uninjured fledglings can be successfully returned to their parents.

Bluebirds are another common entrant to rehabilitation due to the close monitoring of bluebird nestboxes by birding enthusiasts. Healthy chicks may be brought in if a parent is known to have been killed or injured, and it should be noted that healthy bluebird babies may be successfully fostered by other bluebirds that have young of the same age. It may be beneficial for rehabilitators to maintain contact with a network of people monitoring bluebird boxes so that any single, healthy chick can be fostered rather than coming into a captive environment.

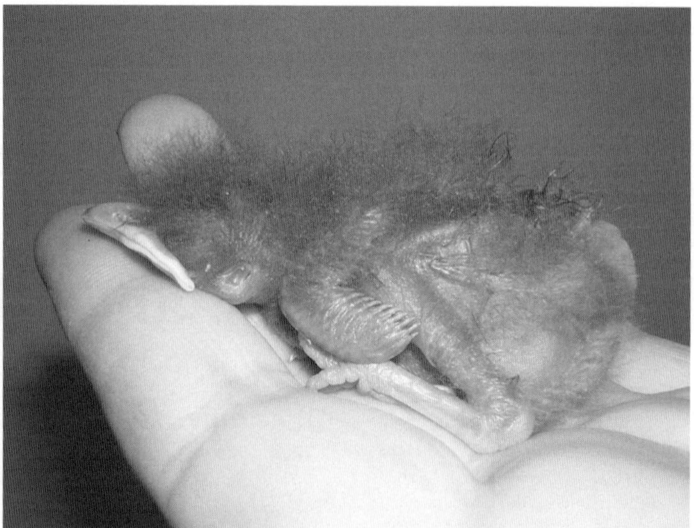

Figure 36.1. Northern Mockingbird hatchling. Note thick gray down over head and back and thin gape flange margins, which are offwhite not yellow. Inside of mouth is yellow. Lower beak does not protrude beyond upper (photo courtesy of Rebecca Duerr).

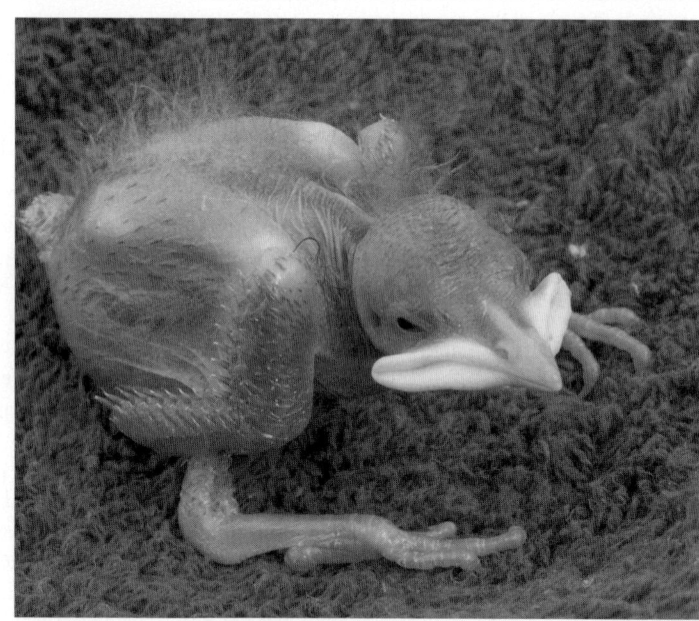

Figure 36.2. European Starling young nestling with eyes just opening. Note enlarged lower beak with thick gape flange margins. Mouth is bright yellow. Down is sparse and gray on head, shading to whitish on rump (photo courtesy of Jackie Wollner).

When fostering bluebirds, the total number of nestlings should not exceed a number normally found in bluebird nests in the area (usually 5–6).

RECORD KEEPING

Many of these birds form flocks or family groups, so it is often helpful to know their exact rescue location so they may be returned there when they are released. In addition, detailed records for each bird will help gauge each individual bird's health and growth, so daily updates of information, including body weights, diet, wellness, and health, are helpful to monitor progress toward release.

INITIAL CARE AND STABILIZATION

Passerines are very susceptible to complications caused by stress, so care should be taken upon examination to minimize stress. New intakes should be

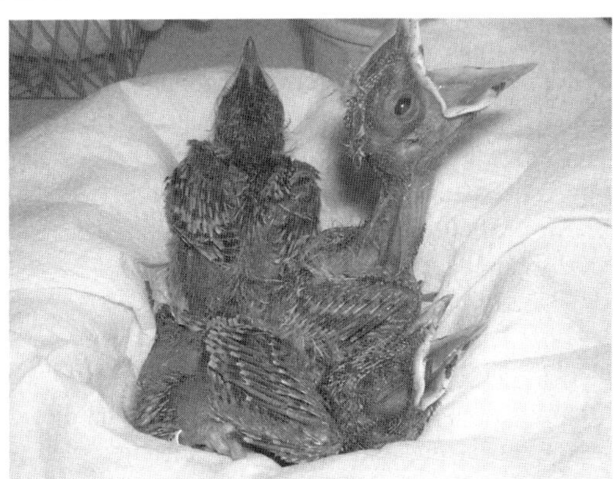

Figure 36.3. Newly admitted nestling American Robins in replacement nest (photo courtesy of Rebecca Duerr).

placed in an incubator (such as a Brinsea Octagon TLC4) or warm room at 90–95°F (32–35°) if unfeathered, 85°F (30°C) if at least partially feathered, and allowed to warm in a dark, quiet place to minimize stress. It is important that chicks be kept at a steady temperature, even during the exam, and no feeding should be attempted until the animal's body temperature has stabilized.

Once the animal is warm, hydration should begin, using an isotonic rehydration solution such as warmed lactated Ringer's solution. Most hatchlings and fledglings will produce droppings with each feeding, but with dehydrated birds, often several attempts 15–20 minutes apart are necessary before droppings are produced. After droppings are produced, feeding can begin (see Figure 36.3).

COMMON MEDICAL PROBLEMS AND SOLUTIONS

Thrush relatives often present with lacerations and broken bones from animal attacks, subcutaneous emphysema or ruptured air sacs, dehydration, or complications from being fed a poor or inadequate diet by well-meaning rescuers. Antibiotics are frequently given to cat attack victims; however, it should be noted that trimethoprim/sulfamethoxazole may cause vomiting in many of the thrush relatives, so amoxicillin, cephalexin, enrofloxacin, or ciprofloxacin are often preferable with these species.

Caregivers should take care to search any cat or dog attack victims for two injuries, caused by upper and lower teeth. Commonly there is one major laceration, with an accompanying bruise, broken bone, or smaller laceration opposite the primary injury. Lacerations should be cleansed and closed primarily whenever possible with sutures or surgical glue. However, surgical glue alone is not strong enough to hold thigh lacerations in older jumpy fledglings, especially in fledgling American Robins. Hygroscopic dressings may be used when lacerations are not closeable or necrotic tissue is present. Silver sulfadiazine cream may also be of use with some wounds, because it helps keep the wound moist while providing antibiotic and antifungal protection. This cream is water soluble, so it is much preferred to any sort of oil-based antibiotic ointment. See Chapter 1, "General Care," for more information on wound treatment in young birds.

Some veterinarians prefer to allow subcutaneous emphysema to resolve on its own, and this may be preferable if it is not causing the bird much discomfort. Others prefer to deflate affected areas with a large gauge sterile needle.

Robins are often fed earthworms by their parents or their human rescuers before arriving, and therefore are subject to gapeworm (*Syngamus trachea*) infections. Earthworms are an intermediate host to the parasite, the eggs of which are ingested, and larvae later migrate to the trachea. Many robins arrive in care making a characteristic "snick" or soft coughing sound, as they cough up the parasite's eggs and swallow them. Other symptoms are difficulty swallowing or in advanced cases, difficulty breathing. Treatment is a single dose of ivermectin or fenbendazole. Fenbendazole has been associated with feather abnormalities when given while feathers are actively growing, but many rehabilitation centers use this drug for deworming juvenile passerines without problem.

Routine fecal flotation and smears are advisable for most of the thrush relatives. American Robins and mockingbirds frequently present with other parasitic infections such as coccidia, tapeworms, or capillaria. Some American Robins will present with many of these at once. Many rehabilitation centers have protocols in place to routinely deparasitize American Robins on arrival because heavy parasite loads are so common. Trichomoniasis is also seen, especially in mockingbirds, and may be diagnosed by throat swab. In addition to being affected by many of the previously mentioned parasites, European Starlings in North America are also often infected with Giardia. Consult your avian veterinarian for antiparasitic drug dosage information. Drugs commonly used to treat parasites in these species include carnidazole, ronidazole, metronidazole, praziquantel, fenbendazole, toltrazuril, and ivermectin.

Cedar Waxwings have the unique problem of arriving in care after becoming drunk on fermented berries. Waxwings are known to frequently gorge themselves on fruit, and late season fermented berries can intoxicate them, making them prey to animals, people, and cars. This problem is usually seen after breeding season is over, but should be kept in mind as a possibility for birds presenting as fledglings. In addition, if the fruit has been treated with pesticides, death can occur. As with cases of intoxication in people, time will improve the birds' condition, but if poisoning is suspected a treatment of activated charcoal may be necessary.

Mockingbirds and robins are prone to metabolic bone disease. If they have been inadequately fed by rescuers for an extended period of time, they may have broken or malformed bones, or may have difficulty standing. Frequently a well-meaning rescuer has not fed the bird enough calcium and will think the birds are developing properly; but on their first flight, the birds break bones attempting to land. Sometimes the smallest bird in a clutch will show signs of this disease if the parents were unable to provide adequate nutrition for all chicks. Affected birds should be supplemented with calcium glubionate orally at 150 mg/kg once or twice per day (Carpenter 2005) and placed on a balanced diet. Lightweight supportive splints may be required if pathologic fractures have occurred. Padded perches and cage bottoms may also increase the comfort of affected birds. Euthanasia should be considered for severely affected birds with joint abnormalities or poor prognosis.

The thrush family (thrashers, thrushes, and mockingbirds in particular) is also prone to avian pox. Many birds arrive in rehabilitation with pox lesions covering the nonfeathered portions of their body, such as eyes, mouth, and feet. Unfortunately, avian pox is a frequently deadly virus, and only supportive care may be offered. Because pox can be transmitted through insect bites or direct contact, birds should be quarantined from other birds, and all feeding utensils, dishes, and caging should be disinfected before use with other birds. Handlers should also wear gloves when handling affected birds to avoid being a mechanical vector of virus. Lesions in the mouth may cause difficulty eating, and the birds may need to be tube fed until the lesions improve. If the lesions cover the throat and food cannot be swallowed or a tube cannot be passed, the bird should be euthanized. If lesions impair the animal's vision, it should be placed in a small container so that it does not have trouble finding food and water. If quarantine facilities are not available, it is preferable to euthanize affected birds rather than put healthy birds at risk.

DIET RECIPES

The thrush relatives respond well to a varied diet of live insects, fruit, and a hand-feeding diet such as FoNS or Mac Diet (see Chapter 34, "Passerines: Hand-Feeding Diets). Because of their varied diet, it is critical that they get the correct proportions of calcium to phosphorus (2:1 by weight), enough calcium to ensure proper bone development, and enough high-quality animal protein to ensure proper feather development. A very successful ratio of foods for fledglings is 1/3 hand-feeding diet, 1/3 live insects, and 1/3 other foods such as fruits, berries, raisins, oranges or melons, hard boiled egg, peanut butter crumble, corn, and suet. Start nestlings on a hand-feeding diet plus freshly killed insects (mealworms, waxworms, crickets) and then graduate slowly, one food item at a time starting with soft fruit pieces, to the fledgling/adult diet to avoid any abrupt changes in their digestion.

In addition, robins should have a limited number of earthworms, preferably in loam, to provide foraging practice. Loam becomes an essential part of the diet of robins; however, the number of earthworms should be limited to avoid gapeworm infections. An attractive first food for these birds is a mixture of peanut butter crumble with dried adult flies (or a mixture of dried adult, pupae, and larvae) such as Bird Bug Cuisine from Arbico Organics. The author finds that this mixture is frequently a first choice of thrushes and robins beginning to self feed.

Peanut Butter Crumble

- 2C Hills Science Diet feline maintenance dry food
- 2C toasted wheat germ
- 2 Tbsp AviEra avian vitamins (Lafeber)
- 1200 mg calcium from 3 g calcium carbonate powder
- 1/2C "old fashioned" peanut butter (no salt, sugar, or other additives)

Table 36.1. Percent of plant foods in diet.

Species	Spring	Summer	Autumn	Winter
Mockingbird	17%	35%	67%	59%
Catbird	20%	60%	81%	76%
Brown Thrasher	28%	46%	71%	78%
American Robin	21%	60%	81%	64%
Wood Thrush	5%	35%	77%	N/A
Hermit Thrush	7%	15%	47%	60%
Eastern Bluebird	7%	17%	38%	39%
Starling	7%	41%	39%	68%
Cedar Waxwing	74%	80%	90%	97%

Pulverize the dry cat food in a food processor or coffee grinder and mix dry ingredients thoroughly. Add the peanut butter and mix well until it becomes loose, crumbly, and nonoily. Store mixture in a tightly sealed container in the refrigerator.

A variety of foods will help keep these birds interested and help them develop their skills with foraging and finding a variety of fruits and insects (see Table 36.1). Captive foods can include chopped grapes, berries (wild and cultivated), cherries, raisins, minced apple or pear, sections of orange, mealworms, waxworms, crickets, moths, crumbled hardboiled egg yolk, dried flies, peanut butter crumble, nutmeats, sunflower seeds, cracked or fresh corn, and suet bits.

FEEDING PROCEDURES

Many of the thrush relatives are prone to overeating, so it is critical to be sure they have swallowed their food between each mouthful, and they should not be overfed. Because the passerine stomach can hold approximately 5% of body weight, the food amount should be calculated and the appropriate amount be fed at each meal. When the birds are overfed, vomiting or poorly formed droppings may occur. If the droppings look like undigested food, the amount of each feeding should be reduced. It should be noted, however, that the droppings of fruit-eating birds are often the same color as the berries they are eating, and the stool color is not a cause for concern as long as the droppings look well formed and otherwise normal.

The thrush relatives are stimulated by movement in the nest, especially before their eyes are open. If they are difficult gapers, the caregiver can jostle the nest to simulate the feeling of the parent landing on the nest.

Hatchlings

Hatchlings should be fed 5% of their body weight (1 ml of food for a 20 g bird) every 20–30 minutes for 12–14 hours a day. One ml syringes are excellent feeding implements. The thrush relatives, particularly starlings and waxwings, are very enthusiastic eaters, and they may gape again before they have swallowed the previous mouthful. Care should be taken to ensure that food is placed in the back of the throat on the right side to encourage swallowing and to feed small amounts at a time so they do not choke on any food still in their mouth.

Nestlings and Fledglings

Fully and partially feathered birds should be fed every 45–60 minutes for 12–14 hours a day. One ml syringes are usually a good size, although as they grow the larger birds, such as starlings and robins, may require a 3 ml syringe.

Fledglings that come into captivity after fledging frequently have difficulty adapting to their new diet and caregiver. The birds are attracted to movement and they can be drawn to a syringe by moving it around and softly tapping their beak. Feeding live insects on the first day may also acclimate them to their new environment, because they will be drawn to the movement, particularly with live crickets.

Cedar Waxwings in the wild feed chicks primarily insects for the first 2 days, and then they increase

Table 36.2. Maturity data for eight species of thrush-relatives.

Species	Breeding Season	Hatch Weight	Days to Fledge	Weight at Fledging	Self-Sufficient (Post-fledge)	Adult Weight
Eastern Bluebird	Mid-April to July	2.4 g	18–20	28–29 g	2–3 weeks	31 g
Wood Thrush	Mid-May to Early August	4.2 g	12–14	35 g	2–3 weeks	47
American Robin	Mid-April to Mid-August	5.5 g	13–15	48–50	4 weeks	77 g
Catbird	May to August	3 g	10–11	26–28 g	2–3 weeks	37 g
Mockingbird	Mid-April to July	3.5 g	11–13	32 g	2–4 weeks	49 g
Brown Thrasher	Mid-April to July	5–6 g	10–11	40 g	2 weeks	69 g
Starling	Mid-April to July	5.5–7 g	20–23	50 g	1.5–2 weeks	82 g
Cedar Waxwing	June to Mid-October	3 g	14–18	30 g	2 weeks	32 g

the percentage of fruits so that nestlings near the fledging age are fed approximately 85% fruits. The challenge is for the caregiver to ensure that the nestlings and fledglings are getting enough fruit as to approximate a wild diet, but enough protein and calcium to support growing bones and feathers. The adult birds' protein requirements are less than half of those of the American Robin or wood thrush, and unlike other fruit-eating members of the thrush family, Cedar Waxwings have intestinal sucrase, allowing them to efficiently digest sucrose from sugary fruits.

These birds are very curious and active, and it is not uncommon for them to be less interested in food on the day they fledge. They become interested in exploring the area outside their nests, so they may refuse some feedings or gape less in general. Usually, their appetites will return to normal after a day or so, and caregivers should be careful to ensure that they get enough food on the days after fledging.

Robins can be stimulated to self feed by providing a shallow dish filled with soil and earthworms. They will be drawn to the movement in the soil, and often their first self-feeding attempts are on the earthworms.

Live insects are a critical aid in encouraging self-feeding, particularly crickets and moths, which move quickly and develop the birds' feeding skills. As their skills develop, fruit can be hidden among the leaves or other cage materials, fresh foliage can be added to the enclosures, and food can be scattered at the bottom of the cage to encourage natural foraging behaviors. If possible, provide branches with berries attached. Mockingbirds will often exhibit wing flashing at live insects.

Many of the thrush relatives are cooperative breeders, with older siblings or other flock members helping to feed and raise the young. These birds develop best in captivity when housed with others of their same species, and frequently older robins will encourage their younger cagemates to forage and eat on their own, or may even assist with feeding the younger fledglings.

EXPECTED WEIGHT GAIN

Most of the thrush relatives are small (2–4 g) at hatching and then steadily gain weight until the days prior to fledging, when they are generally 60–70% of their adult weight (see Table 36.2). It is common for these birds to lose weight in the day prior to or after fledging and then continue to grow at a rapid pace until they reach their adult size 2–4 weeks later.

HOUSING

Hatchlings should be kept at 95°F (32.2–35°C). Nests can be created using toilet paper or paper towels formed inside a berry basket or small bowl (depending on the size of the chick). It is important that the birds be able to sit with their legs underneath them, and that they have enough support on their sides so that their legs do not splay out to the sides to ensure proper limb development.

After each feeding, each bird should defecate, usually moving their hindquarters to the edge of the

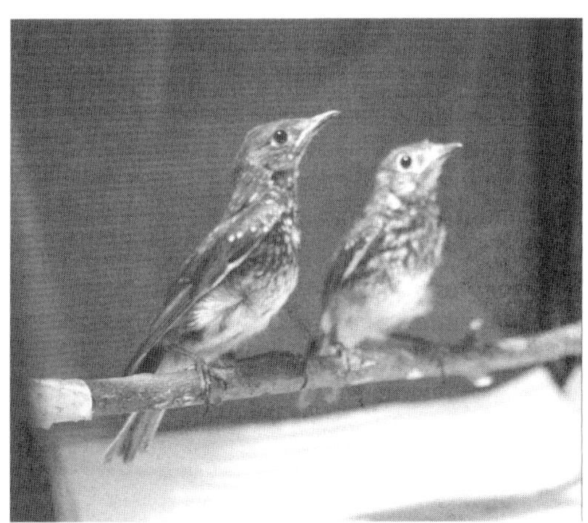

Figure 36.4. Eastern Bluebird fledglings perching in Reptarium.

nest and dropping a fecal sac over the side. The caregiver can catch the fecal sac as the parent would and remove it from the nest site to avoid soiling, or change the nest materials after each feeding so that the birds do not become soiled. Birds with diarrhea typically do not have an encapsulated fecal sac.

Once the birds fledge, they can be kept in a larger container. The best containers for these birds will not have large openings that would allow live insects to escape, and will have soft sides that will allow the fledglings to explore with their beaks without injuring themselves, such as a Reptarium (38 gal or larger; Dallas Manufacturing Company, Inc.) or a large laundry basket with window screen lining (see Figure 36.4). Wire cages are to be avoided unless they are lined with window screening, since they will allow live insects to escape and may cause feather damage.

Caging should be cleaned several times a day. These birds tend to be messy, because they will explore all areas of their enclosure as they develop their foraging skills. They are also adept at tipping over food and water dishes, so stable dishes are recommended.

Perching materials should be provided as soon as the birds fledge, and the materials should be adjusted and changed as they grow. Bluebirds should also be provided with a sheltered area or a small box, and they will often huddle together at night as they would in the wild.

Human toddler playpens make excellent indoor fledgling housing with the addition of a clipped-on window screen ceiling and a full spectrum light on top. Swinging natural stick perches give birds still being hand fed practice balancing and jumping onto moving targets.

Supply normal daylight–level illumination to caging, with a normal day/night–light/dark cycle. Weaning may be delayed if birds are not kept in adequately illuminated environments. These species need at least 8–10 hours of sleep at night at all ages.

WEANING

As the birds grow accustomed to their postnest environment, natural materials should be added to allow them to experience a more natural environment and encourage foraging behavior. Large branches, small logs or pieces of bark, and full branches with leaves can provide both shelter and a stimulating environment (see Figure 36.5). As the birds begin to self-feed, their skills can be developed by hiding food in the bark, under leaves, or on branches.

Robins, thrashers, and other thrushes are stimulated when caregivers put earthworms or mealworms in soil, or mix mealworms with crumbled suet cake, dried flies, and small pieces of nutmeats in one shallow bowl so that the birds can dig through the food to find what they want.

Once these birds have begun to self feed, the weaning process can begin. Weighing the birds on a regular basis becomes critical, because it is the best indicator of how well the bird is eating. Each bird should gain weight throughout the day, and then will lose weight while they sleep each night, but their weight should remain stable or continue to increase during the entire weaning period. Feedings can be reduced slowly over a period of days, and when the birds are regularly eating on their own, they can be weighed in the morning and then later in the day to ensure that their food intake is sufficient to cut back and then discontinue. If the bird loses weight during the day, feedings should be added back in until the bird can naturally increase its weight during the day through food it eats on its own. Most of the thrush relatives will naturally begin to refuse feedings as they become adept at feeding themselves, so the caregiver should watch their activity for clues as to when handfeedings can be stopped (see Figure 36.6).

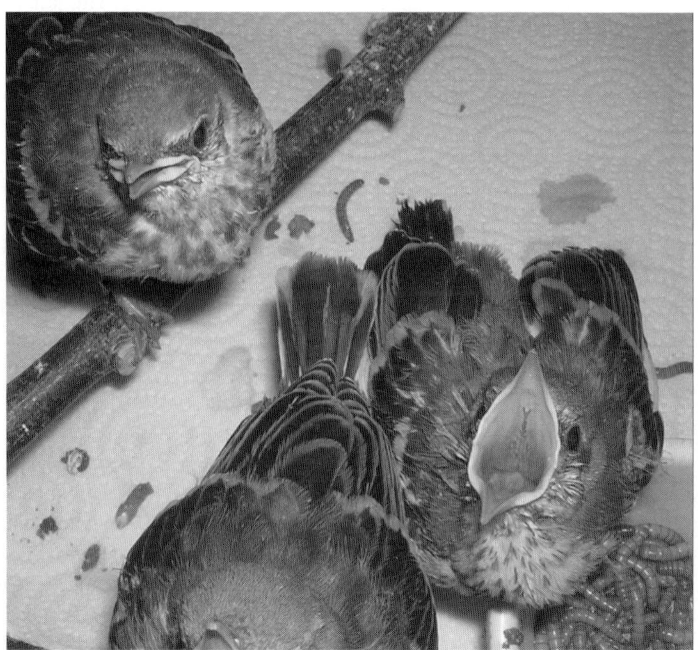

Figure 36.5. Fledgling mockingbirds gaping for hand feeding (photo courtesy of Rebecca Duerr).

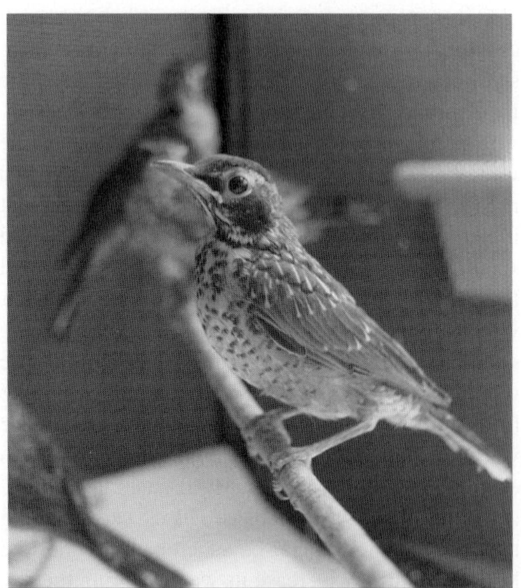

Figure 36.6. Fledgling American Robin.

PREPARATION FOR WILD RELEASE

Due to the dependence on foraging, the enclosures should become increasingly large and more fully featured as the birds develop. Thrushes, robins, starlings, and thrashers particularly enjoy bathing, and they should be given a bathing water source in addition to their drinking water at least once a day. Birds that do not automatically bathe can be stimulated to preen by misting them once or twice a day with water.

The birds should be acclimated to the outdoors gradually by moving them near an open window or bringing their enclosure outdoors for increasing periods of time, and finally moving it to an outdoor aviary. The aviary should be at least 4 × 8 × 8 ft (1.2 × 2.4 × 2.4 m) for most groups, and 8 × 8 × 16 ft (2.4 × 2.4 × 4.9 m) for larger bodied species or groups of birds. Most of the thrush relatives will easily tolerate being in mixed species groups in a large aviary; however, the total number of birds should not exceed approximately 8–10. The enclosure should contain as many natural features as possible, such as trees, bushes, and foliage, along with leaves or grassy areas and water for bathing and drinking. If possible, distribute or hide foods throughout the enclosure so the fledglings can practice foraging in a large space before release. Be sure any parasitic infections have been adequately treated before moving birds to the aviary to avoid contaminating the aviary with parasite eggs.

RELEASE

Birds should spend a minimum of 7–10 days acclimating to the outdoors in an aviary before release. They should be able to fly well, find adequate shelter in the environment, shed water when misted, and successfully forage for insects and other food.

The birds can be released either in their home environment, or can be soft released near the rehabilitation facility, with food and shelter provided after release until they decide to move on. Cedar Waxwings are communal birds and must be released into an active flock.

Release dates should be selected to avoid weather extremes in the day or two following release, allowing birds to find shelter and develop a home territory before rain or storms may inhibit their movement.

ACKNOWLEDGMENTS

Thanks to Casey Levitt, who taught me everything in this chapter and more. Thanks also to Astrid MacLeod and Janine Perlman, for answering hundreds of questions over the years.

SOURCES FOR PRODUCTS MENTIONED

Brinsea Octagon TLC4: Brinsea Products Inc., 704 N. Dixie, Ave, Titusville FL 32796, (888) 667-7009.

Bird Bug Cuisine: Arbico Organics, P.O. Box 8910, Tucson, AZ 85738-0910, (800) 827-2847.

Reptarium®: Dallas Manufacturing Company Inc., 4215 McEwen Road, Dallas, TX 75244, (800) 256-8669.

REFERENCES

Carpenter, J.W., ed. 2005. Exotic Animal Formulary, 3rd Edition. Elsevier Saunders, Philadelphia, pp 135–344.

Cavitt, J.F. and Haas, C.A. 2000. Brown Thrasher (*Toxostoma rufum*). In The Birds of North America, No. 557 (Poole, A. and Gill, F., eds.) The Birds of North America, Inc., Philadelphia.

Cimprich, D.A. and Moore, F.R. 1995. Gray Catbird (*Dumetella carolinensis*). In The Birds of North America, No. 167 (Poole, A. and Gill, F., eds.) Philadelphia: The Academy of Natural Sciences; Washington, D.C.: The American Ornithologists' Union.

Derrickson, L.C. and Breitwisch, R. 1992. Northern Mockingbird. In The Birds of North America, No. 7 (Poole, A., Stettenheim, P., and Gill, F., eds.) Philadelphia: The Academy of Natural Sciences; Washington D.C.: The American Ornithologists' Union.

Eilertsen, N. and MacLeod, A. 2001. A Flying Chance: A Manual for Rehabilitating North American Passerines, and a Survival Guide for the North American Passerine Rehabilitator. East Valley Wildlife, Phoenix, Arizona.

Elphick, C., Dunning, J.B., Jr., and Sibley, D.A., eds. 2001. The Sibley Guide to Bird Life & Behavior. Alfred A. Knopf, New York, 588 pp.

Gowaty, P.A. and Plissner, J.H. 1998. Eastern Bluebird (*Sialia sialis*). In The Birds of North America, No. 381 (Poole, A. and Gill, F., eds.) The Birds of North America, Inc., Philadelphia.

Martin, A.C., Zim, H.S., and Nelson, A.L. 1951. American Wildlife & Plants: A Guide To Wildlife Food Habits. New York, McGrawHill, 500 pp.

Sallabanks, R. and James, F.C. 1999. American Robin (*Turdus migratorious*). In The Birds of North America, No. 462 (Poole, A. and Gill, F., eds.) The Birds of North America, Inc., Philadelphia.

Sibley, D.A. 2000. The Sibley Guide to Birds. Alfred A. Knopf, New York, 544 pp.

Stokes, D. 1979. Stokes Nature Guides: A Guide to Bird Behavior, Vols. I and II. Little, Brown & Co., Boston.

Witmer, M.C., Mountjoy, D.J., and Elliot, L. 1997. Cedar Waxwing (*Bombycilla cedrorum*). In The Birds of North America, No. 309 (Poole, A. and Gill, F., eds.) Philadelphia: The Academy of Natural Sciences; Washington, D.C.: The American Ornithologists' Union.

37
Passerines: Swallows, Bushtits, and Wrens

Veronica Bowers

NATURAL HISTORY

Swallows

There are approximately 90 species of swallows found worldwide, except in Antarctica, and the greatest number of species is found in Africa. Eight of the 90 species occur in North America. All North American swallows are migratory, spending the breeding season in the U.S. and migrating as far as South America during the winter.

Swallows have long pointed wings, short bills, short legs, small delicate feet, and an anisodactyl toe arrangement with three toes forward and one toe back. Swallows are more aerial than other passerines and are graceful while in flight, much like swifts. All swallows are aerial insectivores, frequenting open areas for foraging, often near bodies of water. Swallows feed almost exclusively on flying insects. Tree Swallows are the only North American swallows known to occasionally consume certain types of berries during the winter.

Some species, such as Tree and Violet-green Swallows, nest in dispersed territories. Others, such as Barn Swallows, nest in aggregated groups. Cliff and Bank Swallows nest in colonies. Nest sites range from burrows to holes in trees, banks, and cliffs, to nest-boxes or cup or gourdshaped nests made of mud.

All species hatch altricial, naked, blind, and helpless young. Incubation ranges from 13–18 days. Both parents care for the young in all swallow species. Young swallows fledge the nest at approximately 3 weeks of age.

Bushtits

Bushtits are one of the smallest North American passerines. Their range extends throughout western North America. Adults are approximately 4 in (10 cm) in length and weigh only 6 g. Their bodies are gray with light brown on the head, long slender tails, dark pointed bill, and dark long legs. They are strictly insectivorous. At one time, Bushtits were grouped by ornithologists with the chickadees and titmice in the family Paridae. Recent research has shown that they are most closely related to the old-world group known as long-tailed tits.

Bushtits are highly social birds. During the non-breeding season, large flocks of up to 40 or more birds can be seen foraging together. The flocks are usually comprised of several family groups. While foraging, they remain in constant contact with each other, using light, high-pitched call notes. They roost communally in dense cover and huddle closely together for warmth. They are very active foragers, spending the majority of daylight hours searching for food. As foliage gleaners, Bushtits pick insects and spiders from leaf and twig surfaces hanging upside down to reach prey items on the underside of leaves. Bushtits are often seen foraging in mixed species groups, such as with chickadees, kinglets, and titmice.

During the breeding season, birds pair off and become somewhat territorial. They construct a fully enclosed pendulous nest suspended from a group of small twigs in a tree. The foundation of the nest is bound together with spider webs, and then a variety of plant materials such as moss and small leaves is used to camouflage the exterior. The interior is lined with feathers and animal hair; dryer lint is also a common nest material. Average clutch size is five to seven, with one to two broods per season. Most Bushtits typically complete their breeding cycle by late June. The male and female build the nest, incubate the eggs, and brood and feed the young. Some pairs have helpers. Helpers are usually unmated male Bushtits or adults whose own nest has failed. In exchange for helping raise their young, helpers are allowed to roost in the nest at night.

Wrens

There are 76 species of wrens worldwide, 7 of which occur in North America. Wrens are small brown birds that are very active and vocal. They dwell in scrubby habitat and dense undergrowth, from marshes and forests to deserts. They are strictly insectivorous and use their slender pointy bills to glean their food from the ground, plant surfaces, and cracks and crevices of rocks and trees. Some wrens, like the Carolina and Bewick's, are known to consume tiny amounts of berries and seeds during the winter. Some species of wrens in North America are migratory; others are not.

Wrens are well known for their complex and loud song and can develop large repertoires of song. Young wrens learn their paternal song between 30 and 60 days of age. Wrens use their song to defend territory and attract a mate. Wrens are extremely territorial during the breeding season, and nonmigratory species defend their territory all year.

All wrens nest in some form of enclosed space, including rock crevices, tree hollows, nestboxes and even abandoned automobiles. Both the male and female participate in nest building and raising the young. Clutch sizes range from 3–10 eggs. Young fledge the nest at 10–23 days of age depending on the species. The distinctive uppointed tail posture of wrens can be discerned on nestlings as soon as the tail feathers begin to emerge, aiding in identification.

CRITERIA FOR INTERVENTION

Swallows

The mud nests of barn and cliff swallows are frequently knocked down by humans. Nests can also legitimately fall from structures on their own if an old nest was reused or there is a prolonged spell of wet weather.

If a barn swallow nest has fallen, the nest remains mostly intact, and the young in the nest are uninjured, a nest replacement should be considered. To replace the nest, construct a cup-shaped basket out of 0.25 in (0.5 cm) chicken wire and affix the basket in the exact location of the original nest. Make sure the basket is free of sharp edges or protruding pieces of wire that could cause injury to parent birds arriving at the nest or young in the nest. Insert the original nest with the chicks in the wire basket. Observe the nest from a distance until there is confirmation that the parents are tending to their young.

Nest replacement for cliff swallows is often not practical due to the physical structure of their fully enclosed gourd-shaped mud nests and the nature of their colonial nesting habits. When a human knocks a cliff swallow nest down, they usually remove a significant portion of or the entire colony, which may lead to dozens or a hundred or more nestlings requiring care simultaneously. Fostering of a few orphaned nestlings into nests of other families is possible, but must be done with extreme care. To evaluate potential foster families for an orphaned cliff swallow (or barn swallow), consider the following: age of young in the nest, number of chicks in the nest already, and health of the orphaned swallow. The ages of the foster family and orphan must be the same, the number of chicks in the nest should not exceed four, and the orphaned swallow must be in good health without injuries, illness, or parasites. The nest must also be accessible by a human. Due to the structural nature of cliff swallow nests, it can be very difficult to make these observations, especially if the young in the potential foster nest are less than 10 days old. Never stick hands into cliff swallow nests because there is a high risk of damaging nests. Fostering an orphaned barn swallow into another barn swallow family is less challenging because their nests and young are visually accessible, making them easy to evaluate.

Tree and Violet-green Swallows are cavity nesters. They will nest in tree hollows as well as nestboxes. If an active nest is destroyed by tree removal, healthy vocal nestlings can easily be re-nested in a nestbox mounted on a pole in the same location where the tree was. Remove the nest and nestlings from the cavity of the tree and place in the nestbox. Observe the nestbox from a distance and watch for the parents to respond to the food cries of the young. Do not leave the young alone in the nestbox until parents have been observed entering the nestbox and feeding the young.

Fledgling swallows are often brought into rehabilitation centers for care after they have collided with a structure or car or have had an unfortunate encounter with a domestic cat. Sometimes they are victims of kidnapping. Swallows are flight capable when they first fledge the nest. During the first day out of the nest they may not be strong enough to sustain flight for extended periods of time, so it is common to find youngsters resting on the ground or other precarious locations looking very vulnerable. Fledgling swallows found on the ground are not always ill or injured and can often be left alone for the parents to care for. If parents are observed actively tending to a fledgling, human intervention is not necessary. If parents are not observed for several hours, intervention may be required. A thorough examination should always be conducted before reuniting the youngster with its parents.

Bushtits

Bushtit nests are extremely well camouflaged and are commonly cut down during springtime tree trimming. If the nest is undamaged and the nestlings are uninjured, the nest should be reattached to the tree. If the nest is still attached to the branch that was cut, the entire branch should be reattached using wire to secure it to another branch in the tree. The nest should be placed no more than 1 ft (30 cm) from its original location and should not be accessible or visible to predators. Do not attempt to put the nest in another tree. The nest should be observed for at least 1 hour from a distance of 30 ft (9 m) or more to be certain the parents find the nest and continue to care for the young.

Domestic cats, jays, and squirrels are common predators of Bushtit nests. If a nest has been disturbed or destroyed by a jay or squirrel and there are surviving nestlings, attempts should not be made to re-nest the youngsters because the predators will return and predate the nest again. If a domestic cat has attacked a nest of Bushtits, all survivors should be brought to a wildlife rehabilitator for care because cats carry bacteria in their mouths and claws that can be lethal to birds.

Wrens

Wrens may choose inappropriate nest sites. Nest relocation is rarely successful because wrens are shy species and very wary of change in their surroundings. Chicks are also often admitted after being caught by cats.

RECORD KEEPING

See Chapter 1, "General Care."

INITIAL CARE AND STABILIZATION

The majority of young swallows presented for care will have some degree of dehydration or emaciation, or both. Gaping active hatchling, nestling, and fledgling swallows can easily be rehydrated orally with a rehydration fluid appropriate for the condition of the bird. More severely dehydrated birds may require fluids to be administered subcutaneously. It is not uncommon to keep a dehydrated swallow on fluid therapy for several days after intake. The oral rehydration solution listed in the IWRC Wildlife Feeding and Nutrition manual (IWRC 2003) works exceptionally well as part of initial care when working with emaciated swallows. Fully feathered but emaciated birds should be kept in an incubator set at 85–87°F (29–30°C) to allow incoming nutrition to be utilized for rebuilding body tissues rather than generation of heat.

Bushtits and wrens are very prone to stress in captivity. Consequently, oral administration of fluids is much preferred over subcutaneous injection in order to minimize handling. See Chapter 1 for more information on initial stabilization.

COMMON MEDICAL PROBLEMS AND SOLUTIONS

Cat-caught birds should immediately begin a course of an antibiotic such as Clavamox (see Chapter 1). Small wounds should be cleaned with warm water or dilute betadine. Bushtits and wrens are very small birds, which may make it difficult to palpate fractures or locate puncture wounds. Using a damp cotton swab can be helpful to brush back feathers when looking for puncture wounds. A tiny amount of silvadene cream, or other water-soluble ointment can be applied if necessary.

Fractured wings must be carefully evaluated. Swallows are migratory aerial insectivores and therefore must have 100% recovery from a wing fracture. Fractured legs are less common, but have a better prognosis for recovery due to swallows' feeding behavior and perching preferences. Bushtits and wrens must also have full recovery of flight agility to qualify for release. Bushtits are intensive foragers, spending the day in constant search of food with their flockmates. They must be able to keep up with the flock at all times and require full use of their legs and feet to dangle from tips of branches while gleaning insects from the underside of leaves.

Damaged feathers may be a common condition presented in Cliff Swallows. There are several causes for damaged feathers. Deer mice are known to predate Cliff Swallow nests. The mice enter the nest and chew on the developing feathers of the nestlings. When the bird is ready to fledge the nest they are often unable to fly due to missing or poorly developed feathers that are the result of being chewed upon by the mice. When humans remove active nests, it may result in injuries or feather damage, particularly when high-pressure washing is used to knock the nests down. Poor feather condition may also be the result of improper housing while in captivity. Broken and damaged feathers should be pulled to allow healthy new feathers to grow in before it is time for the birds to migrate. Pulling feathers can be very painful for the bird and should be done only under the supervision of an avian veterinarian.

Ectoparasites, such as mites and lice, are common among these species and are easily treated with a pyrethrin spray such as Ultracare Mite and Lice Bird Spray (8 in 1). Mist the spray onto a cloth first, and then loosely wrap the bird in the cloth. Do not enclose the head in the cloth and never spray directly onto the bird. Change the bedding and caging frequently until parasites are no longer present. Quarantine infested birds until all parasites are gone. An oral dose of diluted ivermectin at 200 μg/kg once (Carpenter 2005) may be necessary for severe infestation. Other ectoparasites such as botfly or blowfly are unusual, but do occur and should be treated with ivermectin and possible antibiotic. Remove larvae and eggs from the bird's body and feathers.

These species rarely present with internal parasites, but it is always good practice to conduct a fecal smear or float. In 2006, the author experienced an outbreak of oral trichomoniasis among several dozen young swallows and found that a course of Ronidazole was an effective treatment; Carnidazole was ineffective on that occasion.

Stress in captivity can be detrimental to any wild bird, but Bushtits and wrens are especially susceptible to stress. When hand-raising these species, they are best cared for under the supervision of one caregiver and must be provided a quiet and calm environment.

DIET

These species should only be hand-raised on a diet that is specifically designed for young insectivores, such as MacDiet supplemented with a variety of live insects (see Chapter 34, "Passerines: Hand-Feeding Diets," for recipe). The hand-feeding formula should not be thin or watery. When using MacDiet, it should be prepared to resemble a thick puddinglike consistency. Never use commercial parrot hand-feeding formulas or homemade formulas that are high in sugar or contain soy or dairy products such as cottage cheese. Depending on the age of the bird, live insects can include mealworms, waxworms, crickets, fly larvae, houseflies, and fruit flies. Live cultivated insects such as mealworms and crickets should be fed a diet that is high in calcium and protein. When purchasing cultivated insects, small (not to exceed 0.5 in/1.25 cm in length) mealworms and crickets should be ordered. Medium and large-sized insects are difficult for swallows to digest and to manipulate with their bills. They are inappropriate for birds the size of swallows. Commercially available freeze-dried flies are a good addition to the diet of self-feeding swallows when sprinkled over a dish of live mealworms.

FEEDING PROCEDURES

Swallows

Swallows do not possess a true crop and therefore must be fed small amounts of food at frequent intervals. Overfeeding can cause the food to back up into the throat, aspirate the bird, dirty the feathering, or even rupture the proventriculus. To achieve optimum growth and healthy weight, young swallows must be kept on hand-feeding schedules 14–16 hours each day every 20–30 minutes until they are completely self-feeding. Perfect feather condition is essential to their survival upon release, so extreme care must be used to keep their feathers free of food and fecal matter at all times.

Observe the droppings at each feeding. Loose runny feces can be the result of overfeeding. A lack of droppings can be a sign of dehydration. Droppings with an orange color can be a sign of underfeeding or bacterial infection. If whole undigested insects are present, use smaller pieces of insect and tenderize insect bodies first by squishing with forceps before feeding them to the birds. Healthy droppings should be well formed, moist, and contained in a fecal mucous envelope.

It is advisable to establish a food call when hand-feeding swallows; a short soft double whistle is usually effective. This is helpful in stimulating a gape response and can be used later during the

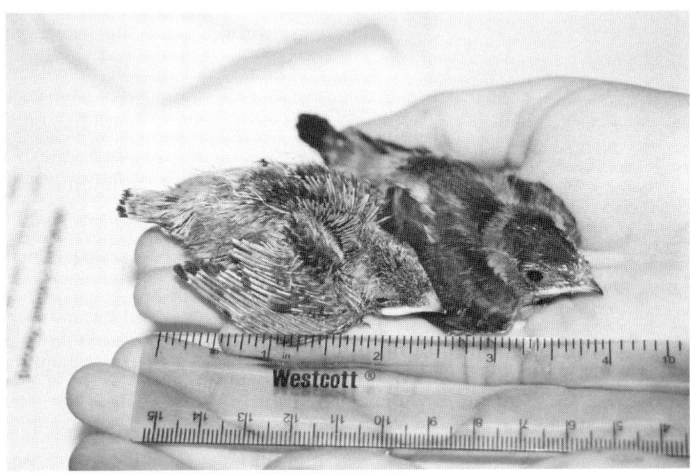

Figure 37.1. Nine- and twelve-day-old Cliff Swallows. Note dramatic change in feather development.

weaning process once the birds are in the aviary for prerelease conditioning.

Healthy young birds will readily gape when they are hungry. If a nestling or hatchling swallow is not gaping, it may be dehydrated, cold, or have another physical condition that needs to be addressed. It is common for older nestling and fledgling swallows to be fearful of humans and reluctant to gape when they are first brought into care. If they are in good health, they should be housed with another swallow of similar age that is gaping well. This will teach the reluctant gaper the new means of receiving food. If a nestmate is unavailable, a mirror placed next to the nest can helpful in stimulating a gape response. This should be used as a temporary solution. Swallows should never be raised singly. If necessary, call another rehabilitation center to locate swallow nestmate of similar age.

Hatchlings

Hatchlings should be fed small amounts of the MacDiet using a 1 ml syringe with a cannula tip (Jorgensen) attached to the end and tiny pieces of white mealworms (mealworms that have recently shed their exoskeleton) or small fly larvae with heads pinched using a pair of bluntend forceps. Feedings should be small and frequent, every 20 minutes for at least 14 hours a day; 16 hours a day is optimum.

Nestlings

Nestling swallows will continue to be fed the same diet every 20 minutes, 14–16 hours a day (see Figure 37.1). Each feeding should include 1/3 insects and 2/3 MacDiet. Insects fed to nestlings should be prekilled. Insects with tough exoskeletons, such as mealworms and crickets, require tenderizing by squeezing the body with forceps and removing the legs.

Fledglings

Fledgling swallows need to be fed every 20 minutes, 14–16 hours a day, until they are self-feeding. At fledging age (approximately 21–23 days old), the swallows will begin to refuse syringe feedings and gape only for insects offered on forceps. Insects can be dipped in the MacDiet formula to ensure the birds are still receiving sufficient vitamins and minerals. It is essential that feeder insects are fed a nutritious diet in order to provide proper nutrition. Insects with tough exoskeletons, such as mealworms and crickets, may still require tenderizing by squeezing the body with forceps and/or removing legs.

Bushtits and Wrens

Young Bushtits and wrens require small frequent feedings every 15 to 20 minutes for 14 hours a day to ensure healthy weight gain and development. Hatchling and nestling Bushtits may take only two bites of food per feeding. It is imperative that they are not overfed. Overfeeding can result in diarrhea and other digestive problems and possibly death. Hatchlings days 1 to 3 should be fed MacDiet with alterations for hatchlings developed by Janine Perlman (see Chapter 34, MacDiet section). Hatch-

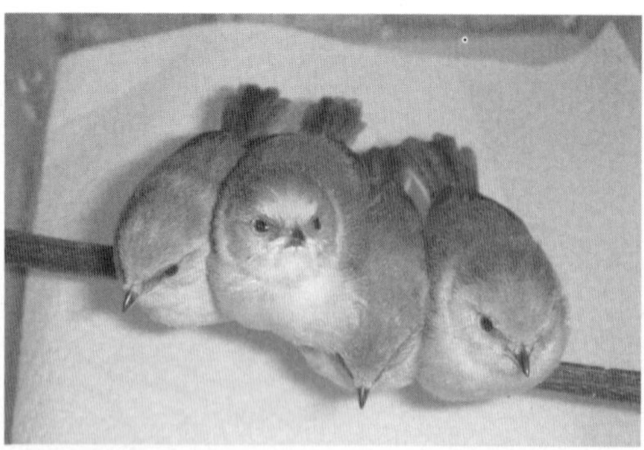

Figure 37.2. Bushtits like to huddle when perching.

lings 3 days and older and nestlings should be fed the MacDiet and killed insects, such as fly larvae and very small white mealworms. Heads of mealworms should be pinched and bodies of the mealworms should be tenderized by pinching with forceps. Use a cannula tip attached to a 1 ml syringe to administer formula and forceps to feed the insects.

Keep the nest and nestlings clean. Bushtits and wrens are very small birds, and even the tiniest amount of food or feces left on the bird can damage feathers, or if near the face, it can cause infection. While in the nest, Bushtits raise their rear ends almost over their heads to defecate toward the center of the nest (see Figure 37.2). This is normal behavior and usually perfectly timed during their scheduled feeding. Fecal sacs can easily be removed from the nest with forceps at this time.

Fledgling wrens are especially fearful when they are brought into captivity. Be patient and use extreme care if forcefeeding is necessary. Offer only insects initially, which are more recognizable as a source of food than a syringe. A wiggling worm held at the tip of forceps is likely to pique the interest of a shy but hungry fledgling wren.

As the birds get older continue feeding small amounts of the MacDiet and insects on a frequent feeding schedule every 20 to 30 minutes for 14 hours per day. Two thirds of daily feedings should be comprised of insects. As birds continue to pick up more food on their own, gradually reduce the frequency of their feedings. Bushtits and wrens can be slow to wean. Careful observation of self-feeding is critical. Although birds may be observed picking up insects and killing them on their own, they may not be ingesting enough food to sustain themselves. As soon as the birds are no longer begging for food and have been self-feeding proficiently for at least 3 days, they can be moved to an aviary for prerelease conditioning.

EXPECTED WEIGHT GAIN

Hatchling swallow weights range from 5–8 g for birds 3–5 days old depending on the species. Nestling swallow weights vary widely, depending on the species. The greatest rate of growth and development occurs between days 5 and 10 for all species, with average weight gain of 2 g per day. Fledgling swallows will typically exceed adult weights by 2–3 g. It is important to chart weights over time to determine optimal body weights for species in each region.

HOUSING

Swallows

Hatchlings

Hatchling swallows should be kept in an incubator set at 90–95°F (32–35°C) with 50% humidity. An artificial nest can be created using a round plastic container lined with a washcloth and then filled in the center with crumpled tissue to form the shape of a natural nest. Proper texture of the lining and shape of the nest provide important support for the developing young bird. Choose a size of container that will comfortably accommodate the number of nestlings to inhabit the nest. Never house more that five swallows in a nest because overcrowding and soiling each other with fecal matter may become an issue.

Hatchlings and nestlings of cavity-nesting species such as Tree, Cliff, and Rough winged Swallows, should have their nests placed in an artificial nest cavity. This can be done by creating a cave using a thick terry cloth hand towel folded in half and placed over the nest (see Figures 37.3, 37.4). The opening of the towel cave should be large enough to allow nestling cliff swallows to defecate out the entrance of the nest. There should also be space left around the edge of the nest for other nestling swallow species to defecate over the side of the nest. It is essential to keep enclosures and nests clean. Towels and tissues must be changed as soon as they become soiled with fecal matter or food.

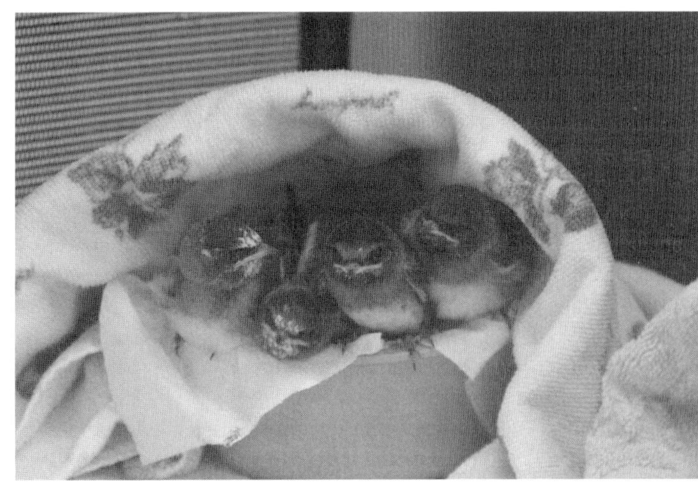

Figure 37.3. Cliff Swallows close to fledging. Using a covered domestyle nest increases the comfort and security of many species.

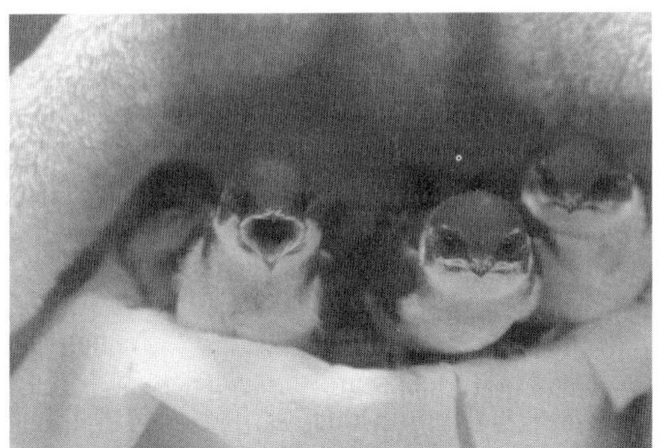

Figure 37.4. Prefledging Violet-green Swallows in dome nest.

Nestlings

Nestlings can be housed in the same manner as hatchlings. As they grow and begin to develop feathers, the temperature of the incubator can be dropped by 1 degree each day. By day 10, healthy birds are able to thermoregulate and the temperature may be lowered to 80°F (27°C).

By 18 days of age, swallows will begin perching on the edge or entrance of their nests. At this point, the nest and towel cave should be moved to a larger enclosure with soft sides, such as a 38 gal mesh reptarium (see Figure 37.5). The end of the enclosure with the nest should be place on a heating pad set on the lowest setting.

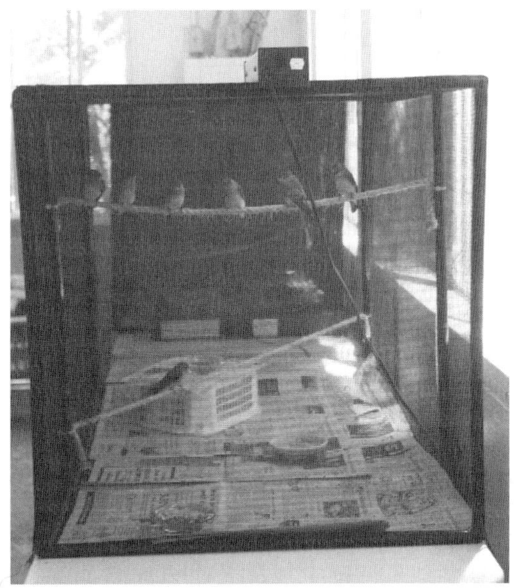

Figure 37.5. Large reptarium for housing swallows indoors. Note sisal rope perches, elevated glass food dishes reachable from perch, low, flat water dish, full spectrum lighting fixture on top.

Fledglings

Swallows will fledge the nest between day 20 and 23, depending on the species. At this time, natural perches such as branches and logs should be provided in the enclosure. The nest should remain in the enclosure until the birds are no longer returning to sleep in it. Some swallows will continue to take naps during the day and sleep at night in the nest up to 1 week after fledging.

Indoor enclosures for fledgling swallows should contain lowsided clear dishes of mealworms and a wide shallow dish of water for drinking and bathing. Hanging dishes used for pet birds can be filled with mealworms and attached to the wall of the enclosure placed at perch level. As the activity of the swallows increases, the size of the enclosure should be increased. If swallows are to be housed indoors until they are self-feeding, they should be kept in an enclosure that is at least 4 × 3 × 3 ft (1.2 × 0.9 × 0.9 m). No more than 10 swallows should be housed in an enclosure of this size. Softsided mesh reptariums are ideal indoor enclosures, but a wire cage fully lined with fiberglass window screen to protect feather condition also works well.

Bushtits and Wrens

Hatchlings and Nestlings

Create an artificial nest using a plastic container or berry basket lined with paper towel. Fill the center of the nest with tightly crumpled tissue to provide enough texture so that the nestlings have something to grip with their feet. A cover made from a folded face cloth should be folded over the top of the nest to create a dome. Enclosing the nest in this manner will create an environment in which the nestlings feel more secure and will minimize stress. Placing the nest in a small nestbox within the incubator is also a comfortable option for some wren species. The nestbox must have an opening mechanism for ease of hand-feeding the birds. Wren nestlings must be kept in an incubator set at 90°F (32°C) with at least 50% humidity, Bushtits should be kept slightly hotter at 95°F (35°C). As feathers develop and unfurl, the temperature can gradually be reduced by 1°F (0.5°C) each day until room temperature.

Never raise or release a single Bushtit. Chickadees are compatible nestmates for Bushtits, but Bushtits will still require the company of at least one other Bushtit during prerelease conditioning in the aviary and upon release.

Fledglings

Wrens and Bushtits hatch sequentially and therefore fledge the nest in the same manner. Nests must remain in the enclosure until fledglings are no longer returning to the nest to roost at night. When fledglings begin to leave the nest, move them from the incubator into a small enclosure such as a small basket lined with fiberglass window screen, or nylon netting and a lid made of similar material. During the first week of fledging the nest, the size of the basket should be increased every 2 to 3 days. This gradual process will minimize stress and reduce unnecessary expenditure of energy. Check the weight, overall condition, and general behavior of each bird before it graduates to the next enclosure. Baskets should be furnished with natural foliage, hanging dishes of very small mealworms set at perch level, and perches that are an appropriate diameter for small feet. Wrens are shy, so provide a hollow log or large piece of bark propped against the side of the basket to create a comfortable place to hide.

After they have been in the various baskets for 1 week, the birds can be moved to a fledge cage with plenty of room to fly back and forth. The cage should be approximately 3 × 2.5 × 2.5 ft (90 × 75 × 75 cm) with a small entrance. Once flight-capable, wrens and Bushtits are quick to escape their enclosure if given the opportunity. A small square of window screen secured at the top of the entrance with safety pins or clothespins between the cage and the door of the cage to cover the entrance will prevent unwanted escapes when the cage door is opened for feeding and cleaning. Furnish the cage with perches at different heights and natural branches complete with leaves to encourage foraging. Hang dishes of small mealworms and fly larvae at varying heights in the cage. For wrens, place dishes of small mealworms on the floor of the cage hidden behind logs and pieces of bark. Scatter leaf litter and grass on the bottom of the cage and include a shallow dish of water and shallow dish of clean dirt. Wrens enjoy dust baths.

In the fledgling cage, most wren species will roost at night in cavity of some sort. Young wrens enjoy roosting in enclosed domestic finch nests. The size of the nest will depend on the number of wrens in the enclosure. Place crumpled tissue in the nest and change the bedding regularly. They will often retreat to the nest during the day for short naps.

Young wrens must be exposed to the song of their species. There is current research that shows song development in many species of young passerines is critical to their survival. Recordings of bird songs are readily available on the Internet as well as on CDs. Research the available materials for the species in question. Make a recording of the song and play it for the birds intermittently throughout the day.

When combining Bushtit families into a cage, be observant and watch for squabbles. A dominant bird in the flock may attack other members.

PRERELEASE CONDITIONING

Swallows

It is the author's preference to move fledgling swallows to an aviary as soon as they are fully flight-capable and no longer returning to the nest to sleep at night. Hand-feeding will need to continue at regular intervals until the swallows are completely selffeeding. When hand-feeding swallows in an aviary, birds should be encouraged to take their food on the wing. This can be done easily by holding an insect in the forceps up in the air several feet away from the birds while they are perched. Giving a food call to the birds and bobbing the forceps up and down a few inches will attract the swallow's attention. When the bird approaches the forceps to snap up the food, it is important to remember to release the food so the bird may take it. They should be encouraged to do this at least once at the beginning of each feeding. This technique encourages natural foraging skills as well as flight conditioning. The remainder of each feeding can be administered while the birds are perched and should be continued until the birds are no longer begging for food. Behavior and weight of the birds must be closely monitored using this hand-rearing technique and should not be done with more than 10 birds in an aviary. It may become difficult to feed and monitor the condition of individual birds if there are too many birds in the aviary.

Aviaries should be a minimum of 16 × 8 × 8 ft high (4.9 × 2.4 × 2.4 m high); larger is obviously better, allowing the birds more room for banking and turning while in full flight. Aviaries should be of wood frame construction with an exterior of protective wire, such as hardware cloth to keep the birds safe from predators, and the interior should be fully lined with fiberglass window screen to prevent injury and damage to feathers. One third of the aviary should be fully enclosed on the sides, back, and top with plywood to provide shade, privacy, and a safe place to roost and flee from the sight of predators. The substrate of the aviary can be composed of one or combination of the following: sod, concrete, earth, gravel, wood.

The aviary should be furnished with a variety of perches. A line of sisal rope should be provided at each end of the aviary in addition to natural branches with leaves and a shallow shelf lined with artificial turf. Keep all perching areas at the ends of the aviary and do not obstruct the flight path. A roost box should be placed high in a corner at the covered end of the aviary.

Provide dishes of mealworms at different levels in the aviary, but do not place dishes on the ground. Dishes can be placed on small shelves affixed to the walls of the aviaries, large shallow dishes can be placed in hanging plant holders and suspended from the ceiling of the aviary and they can also be placed on platform-style birdfeeding trays placed in the middle of the aviary. Wide shallow dishes of water should be provided for bathing and drinking.

An abundance of flying insects must be provided in the aviary to encourage natural foraging. Dishes of mealworms are not sufficient when hand-raising an aerial feeding insectivorous species. Flying insects can be provided by introducing wild-caught moths and flies into the aviary and by stocking the aviary with commercially purchased live fly pupae that will hatch into flying houseflies. Compost buckets of rotting fruit can be established to attract and cultivate fruit flies. As a precaution, compost buckets should be covered with aviary wire.

Bushtits and Wrens

An 8 × 8 × 8 ft (2.4 × 2.4 × 2.4 m) aviary lined with fiberglass window screen to prevent feather damage and injury works well for 2–3 wrens (see Figure 37.6); a 12 × 8 × 8 ft (3.6 × 2.4 × 2.4 m) enclosure works well for 3–6 wrens or Bushtits. One third of the aviary should include a covered roof and solid walls to protect against weather and provide a secure place to roost and flee from visual range of predators. The outside of the aviary should be lined with hardware cloth for protection against predators. The aviary should be enriched with ample vegetation to simulate an appropriate habitat for wrens and Bushtits. Suspend freshly cut leafy branches from the roof to create a forest canopy and introduce wild insects. Potted living shrubs and trees as well as logs with rough bark are also excellent enrichments to add in the enclosure. Vegetation should be dense at each end of the aviary for foraging and roosting, but the middle should be left open to leave ample room for flight without obstructions. Using metal binder clips, fasten small hanging domestic bird dishes of small mealworms to

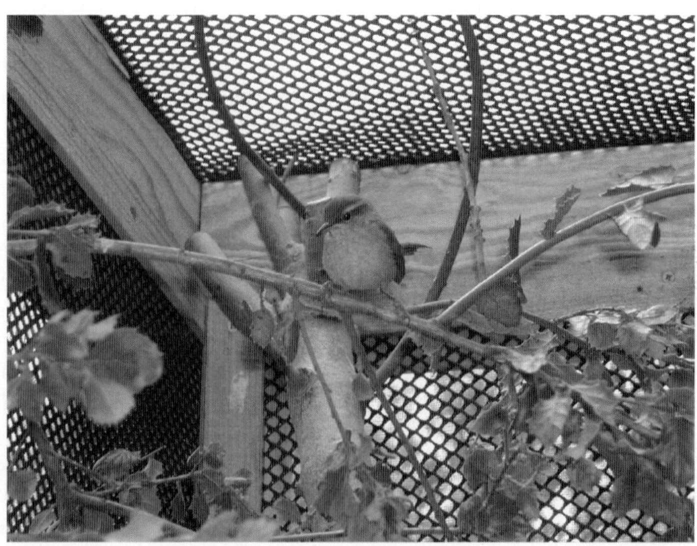

Figure 37.6. Bewick's Wren in outdoor aviary. Wrens are shy and require ample hiding places.

branches. Change branches frequently to introduce fresh wild bugs. Water dishes for bathing and drinking should be provided as well as a shallow pan of fresh clean dirt for dust baths on the floor of the aviary.

Brush piles are essential because wrens spend a great deal of time foraging low to the ground. Create brush piles using cut branches from trees or sections of artificial Christmas trees. Dishes of worms and fly larvae should be hidden in the piles of brush. Additional insects can be provided by purchasing small crickets and commercially cultivated tiny stingless wasps that can be hatched in the aviary or by creating a compost bucket of rotting fruit to attract fruit flies. When using a compost bucket, cover the bucket with small gauge aviary wire to prevent accidents and then cover the bucket with brush. The insects will climb out of the bucket onto the leaves of the brush providing a natural environment for foraging.

Self-feeding Bushtits should spend at least 1 full week in the aviary for prerelease conditioning. Self-feeding wrens should spend 10–14 days in the aviary for prerelease conditioning. A roost box and nest-boxes should be secured high in the enclosure for roosting at night.

RELEASE

Swallows

Once the swallows have been self-feeding in the aviary for 10–14 days, they should be evaluated for release back to the wild. Swallows are long-distance migrants and have stringent requirements for survival in the wild. A swallow ready for release should be able to sustain continuous flight for at least 5 minutes with ease, demonstrate the ability to catch flying insects on the wing, be a healthy weight for the species, show an appropriate fear response to predators, have impeccable feather condition, and be waterproof.

Swallows should be released back to their natal territory if their colony or family is still present. If their family has dispersed, select another release site with suitable habitat for the species where other swallows are present. Release day should take place on a clear forecast of at least 3 days of good weather. Before setting the swallows free from their transport carrier, check for predators. If there are swallows calmly feeding and flying about in the sky above, that is a good indication that the area is free of predators. Swallows should be released in the early morning to allow for exploration and adjustment to the new environment before it is time to find a roost for the night.

Bushtits and Wrens

Bushtits and wrens should be aerobically fit, waterproof, have excellent feather condition, be totally self-feeding and able to forage successfully. Bushtits must be released in a group in the appropriate habitat where there are other Bushtits present. Never raise or release a single Bushtit. Wrens should be released back to their natal territory. However, if that is not possible, select a location with appropriate habitat for the species. Release should occur in the morning upon forecast of 3 days of clear weather.

OVERWINTERING SWALLOWS

Overwintering may be a consideration when a young swallow is not ready for release in time for the fall migration. Well-managed, longterm care will be required to maintain good health throughout the winter. Proper lighting by natural sunlight and artificial UV light must be provided, as well as meticulously maintained hygienic conditions and a balanced diet. Nails and bill will require grooming approximately every 30 days. Weight should be monitored. Feathers should be carefully examined and checked frequently for ectoparasites and cleanliness. Feet should be checked regularly because swallows are prone to bumblefoot (pododermatitis) if they are sedentary. They must also be housed with another swallow. Swallows kept singly become depressed and their general health will deteriorate.

ACKNOWLEDGMENTS

Thanks to my husband Lance Groody for his assistance and support. Special thanks to Melanie Piazza and Brenda Goeden of WildCare in Marin County, California, and Mary Pierce, Marcia Johnson, and Doris Duncan of Sonoma County Wildlife Rescue. And of course, my sincere gratitude to the amazing passerines whose beauty and song grace this earth each day.

SOURCES FOR PRODUCTS MENTIONED

Ultracare Mite and Lice Bird Spray: 8 in 1 Pet Products, Hauppauge, NY, (800) 645-5154.

Mesh reptariums, logs and bark: LLLReptile and Supply Company Inc., 609 Mission Ave, Oceanside, CA 92054, (760) 439-8492, www.lllreptile.com.

Mealworms, waxworms and crickets: Rainbow Mealworms, 126 E. Spruce St, Compton, CA 90220, (800) 777-9676. https://www.rainbowmealworms.net/home.asp.

Live insects, fly pupae, fly larvae and dried bugs: Biconet, 5116 Williamsburg Road, Brentwood, TN 37027, (800) 441-BUGS, www.biconet.com.

REFERENCES AND FURTHER READING

Bent, A.C. 1942. Life Histories of North American Flycatchers, Larks, Swallows and their Allies. United States Government Printing Office, Washington D.C.

Elphick, C., Dunning, J.B. and Sibley, D.A., eds. 2001. The Sibley Guide to Bird Life and Behavior. Alfred A. Knopf, Inc., New York, 588 pp.

Graham, K. 1999. Captive Care of Swallows. Wildlife Rehabilitation Bulletin 17(3).

International Wildlife Rehabilitation Council. 2003. Wildlife Nutrition and Feeding. IWRC, Oakland, California, 73 pp.

MacLeod, A. and Perlman, J. 2001. Adventures in avian nutrition: Dietary considerations for the hatchling and nestling passerine. Journal of Wildlife Rehabilitation 24(1): 10–15.

Rule, M. 1993. Songbird Diet Index. Coconut Creek Publishing Co., 161 pp.

Winn, D., Dunham, S. and Mikulski, S. 2003. Food for insects and insects as food: Viable strategies for achieving adequate calcium. Journal of Wildlife Rehabilitation, 26(1): 4–13.

38
Passerines: Exotic Finches

Sally Huntington

NATURAL HISTORY

The term "finch" has been used as a vague reference to any bird with a beak suitable for cracking seed. These popular cage and aviary birds are from Order Passeriformes, family Estrildidae. They are small, generally 9–23 cm (3.5–9 in) in length and weigh 7.5–35 g. They are active, quiet, brightly colored birds easily cared for as pets.

Over the past several decades, most of these finches have been wild-caught and imported into the United States and Europe in huge numbers from their native Africa, South America, Southeast Asia, Pacific Islands, and Australia. The seemingly unrestricted importation of unlimited quantities of these small finches made them inexpensive beauties taken for granted as one of the staples of the pet trade. The growing scarcity of some finch species during the late 20th century, including some to the brink of extinction such as the Red Siskin, (*Carduelis cucullata*), has caused an increased appreciation of these finches' true value in aviculture, the pet trade, and their impact on agriculture and agricultural pests. Renewed worldwide attention to conservation has led to several finch species being listed under CITES conventions, and this has led to restrictions on the number of imported birds. This restriction has both increased the dollar value of individual birds, and has increased captive-breeding numbers to become approximately 50% of U.S. finches sold. For example, during the 1980's, the common St. Helena Waxbill Finch (*Estrilda astrild*) sold in retail pet stores for $29.50 a pair. By early 2006, the pet store price was $250.00 per pair, an eightfold increase.

In the U.S. all Australian finches are captive-bred, and only 50% of African birds are captive-bred. With the exception of the Society Finch (*Lonchura domestica*), it is thought that even fewer Asian finches are captive-bred, but exact figures are not available.

CRITERIA FOR INTERVENTION

Finches rely on swiftness of flight to avoid predators in the wild. This beneficial instinct for quick flight in response to perceived danger saves lives, but it also may result in abandonment of chicks. Solitary chicks may be abandoned when their presence appears insufficient to stimulate first-time parents into nurturing behavior. Sometimes a chick is abandoned by confused parents due to changes around their nest site, such as when chicks accidentally fall out of nests, when parents flee in night-fright panic caused by predators, or when parents do not return due to flight accidents.

RECORD KEEPING

Keeping thorough records is the best way to keep track of the overall health of each chick. Weigh the chick on a gram scale at least twice a day at the same time to provide a weight record for comparison to existing charts or for developing new milestones for the rarer finch where information may be scarce or nonexistent. At a minimum, records should include the species, approximate date of hatch, why chicks are being hand-raised, location found if taken from the wild, medical observations, weight gain (or loss), maturation behaviors (begging, wing practice, preening and beak practice), banding date and band identification, diet changes, and the final disposition of the bird.

INITIAL CARE AND STABILIZATION

Hand-rearing finch chicks is a time-consuming and often exasperating experience, but hand-reared chicks typically have a better than 50% chance of survival. Without intervention and hand-rearing, an abandoned or cold chick cannot hope to survive.

The first thing a chick in distress needs is warmth. Usually a newly discovered abandoned chick will feel cold to the human palm. The optimal air temperature for young chicks is approximately 90–95°F (32.2–35°C). Warming of a newly discovered chick can begin immediately by clasping the chick in one's warm palm during transport or while readying a warming device, and periodically blowing warm breath into your cupped hand. Any commercial pet-type heating pad, reptile rock or the newer iron-powered instant heat-pack such as a Uniheat Small Pets Shipping Warmer (American Pioneer) can be used if monitored closely to maintain proper temperature. Temperature may be monitored by use of an integrated thermometer within a nest or by use of a Raytek Minitemp laser thermometer (Raytek International), which can be used from outside the nest.

Use a small ceramic bowl to replicate the nest size (see Figure 38.1). Two to three facial tissues can be used as pads inside the bowl on top of the heat source. The tissues are easy to change after each feeding. Do not feed the chick until it is warm. It cannot digest food taken into a cold crop. New hatchlings do not have to be fed for 20–24 hours after hatching. Chicks with their eyes still closed or not feathered are best kept in a dark container (with a lid) to mimic a covered nest environment. Opening the lid permits light to enter the container, which becomes a cue to being fed. This container will hold the heat source and the ceramic dish, and allows easy access for feeding.

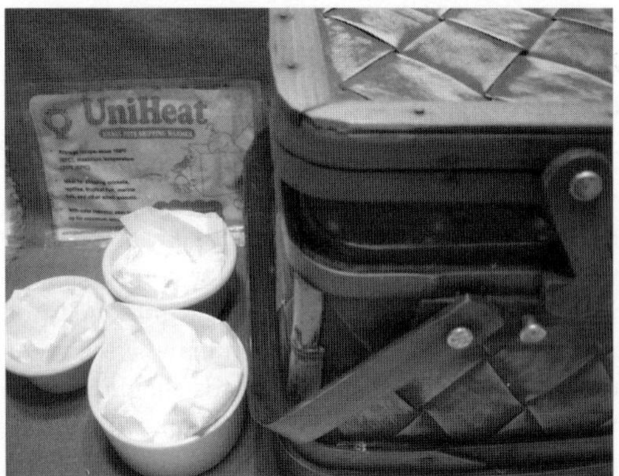

Figure 38.1. Three sizes of ceramic nest replacement bowls, with tissue bedding, Uniheat Small Pets Shipping Warmer, and large covered basket.

Once warm, the first couple of feedings are to hydrate the chick and insure normal body functions. Initially, feed an isotonic rehydration fluid such as Pedialyte at 80°F (31°C). This serves to flush through any parent-provided food or seed, which may otherwise go sour in the chick's system. When the translucent crop appears empty and the chick passes a stool, the "system" is working. At this point a hand-feeding diet may be introduced. Once fed food, the chick should pass droppings that have form after each feeding. See Chapter 1, "General Care," for more information on initial care of chicks.

HAND-FEEDING DIETS

Commercial hand-rearing formulas such as Kaytee Exact work well for finches. Follow instructions on the package: watery for young chicks, "soupy" to "thick" for older chicks. Food can be kept warm for ongoing use by placing a small-enough container of the food in a mug or large cup of warm water, which rests on a commercially available electric cup-warmer. Rinse the feeding utensil after each use. Do not mix large amounts of formula because it will dry out, become clumpy, and sour within 3–4 hours. Be aware of food quality by smell; do not feed sour formula.

FEEDING PROCEDURES

Good feeding implements include glass or plastic eye droppers or 1 ml O-ring syringe for most finches (see Figure 38.2). However, a small pipette works best with very tiny newly hatched waxbills. These instruments provide a free-flowing feeling to the fingers of the feeder and are sensitive to resistance in the crop, a sign that the chick is not receptive to the food. If food is forced against resistance through the dropper, the risk of aspiration is very high and may prove fatal.

First, encourage begging behavior by gently tapping the side of the beak with the clean tip of the filled eye dropper. The chicks will learn to accept and actually suck on the end of the dropper. While

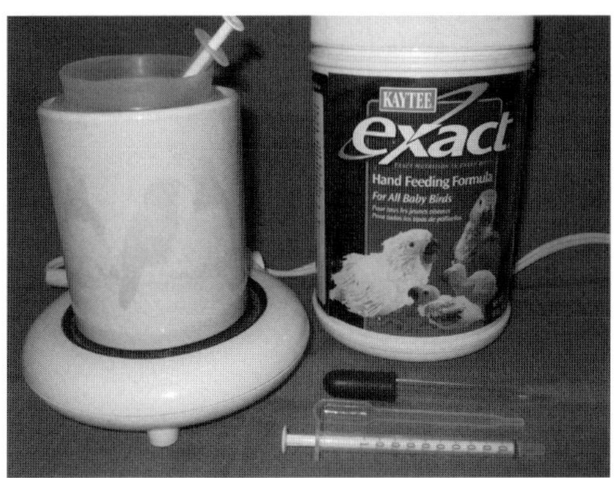

Figure 38.2. Cup warmer for keeping diet warm, Kaytee Exact Hand Feeding Formula, eye dropper, small pipette, 1 ml O-ring syringe.

the chick begs with mouth open, carefully touch the inside of the mouth with the dropper tip, releasing a drop or two into the chick until the chick seems to accept and actually suck on the dropper while swallowing. Keep the quantity fed in one meal small until certain how much the bird can comfortably eat. Do not allow the chick's mouth to become overfull with food. The chick cannot breathe when its mouth is full, and the bird may aspirate if it is not swallowing well. Check the vent after each feeding. Make sure the vent is clean because the chick will normally pass a stool immediately after feeding. This stool should have some form, similar to, but not as thick as, toothpaste coming from a tube.

Monitor crop size. Generally, Estrildid finch crops fill equally on each side of the neck, and fringillidae finches (native North American spp.) fill only on the right side. A good rule of thumb is the following: the total crop capacity, whether on each side of neck or on one side of the neck, should be about half the size of the chick's head when the crop is full of food. Aim to feed the amount of food the chick can move out of the crop every 2 hours for the most success. The Estrildid chicks are eager beggars and will gape and tend to overeat. Overeating causes food to remain in the crop too long, and it tends to sour. Do not overfeed beyond this 1/2 size-of-head rule.

At night, keep the chick warm and in the dark, allowing the chick to sleep 9–10 hours. Cover the chick with a crumpled tissue to mimic parental nocturnal brooding behavior.

Hand-rearing is more successful when there is more than one chick in a nest. Another chick should be introduced to the nest of single chicks, and it does not have to be of the same species. Society or Bengalese (*Lonchura domestica*) or Zebra Finches (*Poephila guttata*) of about the same age (or size) are good warm friends and their eager begging often stimulates the other chick to gape.

COMMON MEDICAL PROBLEMS

Weight loss, lethargy, a lack of begging, gas bubbles in the crop, crop stasis, or mustard-yellow–colored stools without shape indicates that the chick may have contracted an illness, is responding to an incorrect diet or missed feeding schedule, or has become chilled. Another major problem of hand-reared finches is poorly formed stool adhering to the vent and vent feathers thereby blocking the vent. Clean the vent as necessary with warm water.

Be alert to crop spasms caused by bacteria or fungus. The crop may be seen expanding and contracting slowly in a sort of rolling motion, often turning red in color. To treat this condition, flush the crop with small amounts of hydration fluids until the contents pass, and then administer a commercially available antibiotic or probiotic. Follow the directions of the manufacturer.

See Chapter 1, "General Care," for more detailed medical information and Chapter 35, "Passerines: Finches, Goldfinches, and House Sparrows," for information on similar species.

EXPECTED WEIGHT GAIN

Case Study: Blue Capped Cordon-bleu Waxbill (*Uraeginthus cyanocephalus*) Reared with an Orange-breasted Zebra Finch (*Peophila guttata*)

A Blue Capped Cordon-bleu Waxbill was found on the floor of the aviary. The estimated age was 4–5 days old because the eyes were not quite open yet. The chick was not cold to the touch and began begging when touched. The weight was monitored closely (twice a day) the first 48 hours to make sure the chick was gaining weight (see Figure 38.3). The amount of 0.4 ml was fed approximately eight times during the day with a 1 ml O-ring syringe. The amount fed was raised to 0.5 ml eight times per day at 8 days of age. At 10 days of age, the bird began pecking at food items. At 14 days of age, the chick was thriving and picking at seeds and egg food. The

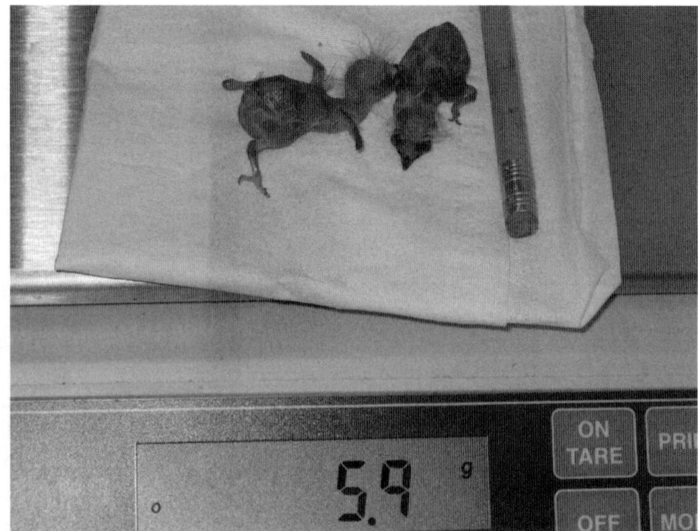

Figure 38.3. Two Blue Capped Cordon-bleu Waxbill chicks on scale.

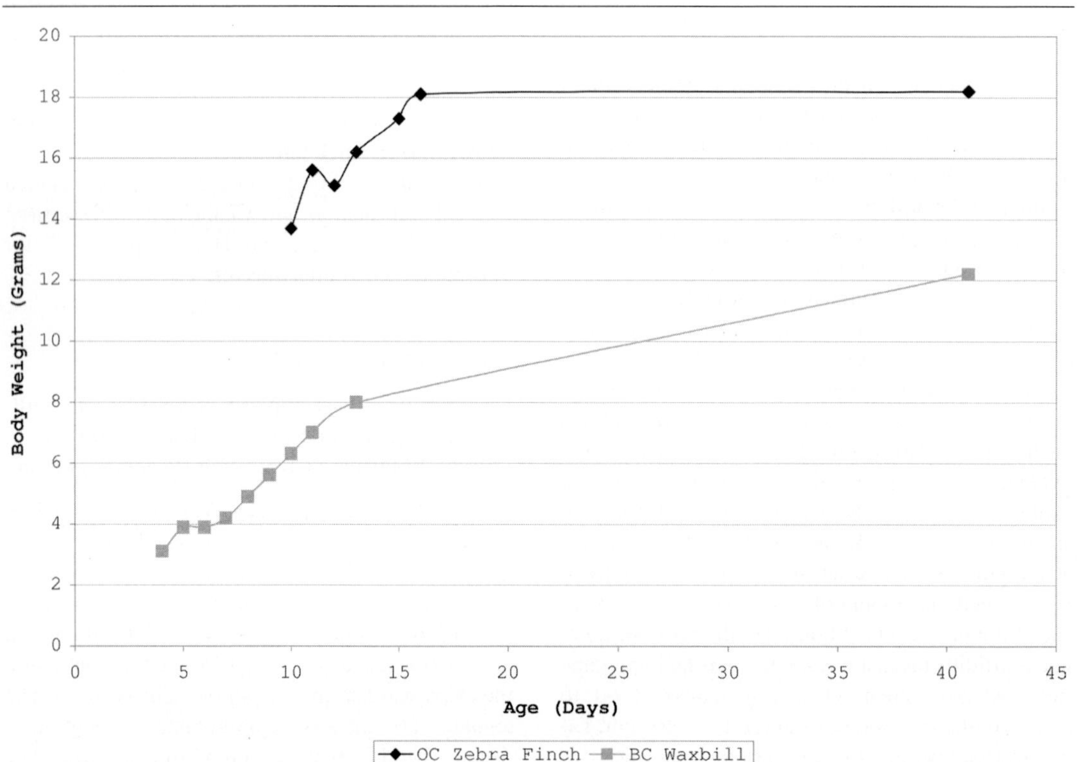

Figure 38.4. Weight gain of two chicks: a Blue Capped Cordon-bleu Waxbill and an Orange-breasted Zebra Finch.

last weight is the adult bird. An Orange-breasted Zebra Finch chick was brought in to be a "warm friend" for the Blue Capped Cordon-bleu. The zebra finch was about 10 days old. This chick was fed with an eye dropper 1.5–2.0 ml eight times daily until 16 days of age. This chick began pecking behavior at 15 days of age. See Figure 38.4 for a weight gain chart from these two chicks.

HOUSING

Young chicks do quite well in a small basket with a lid so that the caretaker can easily access the birds for cleaning and frequent feedings. Once the chicks are fully feathered and want to perch they should be moved to a cage at least 12 × 12 × 12 in (30 × 30 × 30 cm) with perches, water holders, and easy access for continued feeding and cleaning. Weaning begins when the finch occasionally refuses to be hand-fed. Begin to cautiously skip feedings. Continue to offer food until the finch weans itself. Continue to offer food from the eight times a day originally followed, to seven, six, five, and four times a day until it is totally refused for 2 days. As the chicks become more feathered and mobile and are well into wing practice and short flights, the caretaker must be creative in the choice of containers, which permit not only perching and continued easy access for feeding and cleaning, but do not let the birds escape. A flap of window screening can be placed over cage doors to prevent escape while a hand is inserted through the door for feedings.

WEANING

In the wild, these species fledge between 19 and 28 days and are usually weaned by 33–44 days of age. Hand-reared finches take longer to wean but will eventually do so. Just before the chicks fledge they begin preening and vigorously flapping their wings while holding onto a perch. Fledging occurs within 2–3 days of the chicks' first wing practice. Once they fledge, hand-reared finches seldom return to the ceramic nest site. Fledging behavior is also accompanied by curiosity, head-cocking and peering, exploration with their beaks, improving flight coordination, tearing strips of tissue or other paper items, tugging on nestmate's feathers, and other active behaviors. At this point, the chick's daily weight gain slows considerably as it approaches or reaches adult weight.

INTRODUCTION TO CAPTIVE FLOCK

Chicks must spend time with their species to learn the social skills needed to interact with other birds. This is safely accomplished by placing their weaning cage near a mature bird aviary for a few days so that the juvenile can observe adult behaviors. The fledgling will learn by observation of the adults and slowly wean itself from hand-feeding, shifting to eating the adult diet. When possible, place the fledglings with friendly adult birds of their species, or with Society Finches (*Lonchura domestica*) that will model adult social behaviors and skills such as how to drink, hull seeds, bathe, and gather nesting materials. Frequent handling by the caretaker will produce a "pet bird" that is habituated to humans.

ACKNOWLEDGMENTS

My thanks and appreciation to my husband and editor, Vince Huntington; my late father, Dr. Jimmy Cutler, DVM; and the many national and international "bird talking aviculturists," including Roy Beckham, Robert Black, Kateri Davis, Julie Duimstra, Mary Hibner, Frank Jones, Russell Kingston, Mareen Shanahan, Hal Vokaty, and others.

SOURCES FOR PRODUCTS MENTIONED

Kaytee Exact: Kaytee products, 521 Clay St, PO Box 230, Chilton, WI 53014, (800) KAYTEE-1.

O-ring syringes: available from Chris's Squirrels and More, LLC, P.O. Box 365, Somers CT 06071, (860) 749-1129, http://www.thesquirrelstore.com.

Raytek Minitemp laser thermometer: Raytek International, (800) 227-8074.

Uniheat Small Pets Shipping Warmer: American Pioneer International, PO Box 402, Orinda, CA 94563.

REFERENCES AND FURTHER READING

Black, R. 1999. Problems with Finches. Black Publishing, Lafayette, California, pp 77–78.

Clement, P., Harris, A., and Davis, J. 1993. Finches and Sparrows. Princeton University Press, Princeton, New Jersey, pp 11–18.

Goodwin, D. 1982. Estrilidid Finches of the World. Cornell University Press, New York, pp 23–29.

Huntington, S. 2002. Breeding the White-eared Bulbul. AFA Watchbird 24(1): 16–20.

———. 2003. Meet the companion finch. Bird Talk Magazine 21(6): 60–69.

———. 2005. The Red-headed finch. Just Finches and Softbills Magazine 5: 3–6, 29.

Kingston, R. 1998. Keeping and Breeding Finches. Indrus Productions Queensland Australia, pp 60–61.

Restall, R. 1997. Munias and Mannikins. Yale University Press, New Haven and London, pp 20–21.

Appendix I
Important Contacts

UNITED STATES MIGRATORY BIRD PERMIT OFFICES

The information in this appendix is based on information provided by the National Wildlife Rehabilitator's Association.

The following list includes only the U.S. Fish and Wildlife Service Migratory Bird Permit Offices

Region 1
Tami Tate-Hall
Migratory Bird Permit Office
911 NE 11th Ave
Portland, OR 97232-4181
503-872-2715
503-231-2019 (fax)
tami_tatehall@fws.gov

Region 2
Kamile McKeever, Permits Administrator
U.S. Fish and Wildlife Service
Migratory Bird Office
P.O. Box 709
Albuquerque, NM 87103-0709
505-248-7882
505-248-7885 (fax)
kamile_mckeever@fws.gov
http://www.fws.gov/permits/mbpermits/birdbasics.html

Region 3
Andrea Kirk
Migratory Bird Permit Office
1 Federal Dr
Fort Snelling, MN 55111
612-713-5449 (direct office)
612-713-5436 (general line)
andrea_kirk@fws.gov

Region 4
Carmen P. Simonton
Wildlife Compliance Specialist
U.S. Fish and Wildlife Service
Migratory Bird Permit Office
404-679-7049
404-679-4180 (fax)
Carmen_Simonton@fws.gov

Region 5
Peggy Labonte
U.S. Fish and Wildlife Service
Migratory Bird Permit Office
300 Westgate Center Dr
Hadley, MA 01035-0779
413-253-8643
http://www.fws.gov/migratorybirds
http://www.fws.gov/northeast/migratorybirds
http://www.fws.gov/permits/mbpermits/birdbasics.html

Region 6
Janell Suazo
U.S. Fish & Wildlife Service
Migratory Bird Permit Office
P.O. Box 25486
Denver Federal Center 60154
Denver, CO 80225-0486
303-236-8171 ext 630

Region 7
U.S. Fish and Wildlife Service
Migratory Bird Permit Office (MS-201)
1011 E. Tudor Rd
Anchorage, AK 99503
907-786-3693
http://www.fws.gov/permits/mbpermits/birdbasics.html

STATE AND U.S. TERRITORY WILDLIFE PERMIT OFFICES (LISTINGS ARE ALPHABETICAL BY STATE OR U.S. TERRITORY ABBREVIATION)

Karen Blejwas, Wildlife Biologist
Permits Section
Dept of Fish & Game
P.O. Box 115526
Juneau, AK 99811-5526
907-465-4148

Craig Hill, Assistant Chief
Law Enforcement Section
Div of Wildlife/Freshwater Fisheries
P.O. 301456
Montgomery, AL 36130-1456
334-242-3467

Karen Rowe, Non-game Migratory Bird Program Leader
AR Game & Fish Commission
31 Halowell Lane
Humphrey, AR 72073
870-873-4302
krowe@agfc.state.ar.us

Sandy Cate, Coordinator
Adobe Mountain Wildlife Center
AZ Game and Fish Dept
2221 W Greenway Rd
Phoenix, AZ 85023
623-582-9806

Nicole Carion
CA Dept of Fish & Game
Wildlife Programs Branch
1812 9th St
Sacramento, CA 95814-2090
916-445-3694
ncarion@dfg.ca.gov

Kathy Konishi
CDOW/Special Licensing
6060 Broadway
Denver, CO 80216
303-291-7143
Kathy.konishi@state.co.us

Laurie Fortin, Wildlife Technician
Dept of Environmental Protection
Wildlife Division
79 Elm St
Hartford, CT 06069
860-424-3011
860-424-4078 (fax)
laurie.fortin@po.state.ct.us

Kenneth M. Reynolds
Program Manager II
DE Division of Fish and Wildlife
4876 Hay Point Landing Rd
Smyrna, DE 19977
302-653-2883
302-653-3431 (fax)
302-222-5604 (cell)
Kenneth.Reynolds@state.de.us

Wildlife Permit Officer
FL Fish & Wildlife Cons Comm
620 S Meridian St
Tallahassee, FL 32399-1600
850-488-6253

Special Permit Unit
Wildlife Resources Division
GA Dept of Natural Resources
2065 US Hwy 278 SE
Social Circle GA 30025-4714
770-761-3044
706-557-3060 (fax)

Norma I. Bustos
Wildlife Program Specialist
HI Dept of Land & Natural Resources
Division of Forestry and Wildlife
1151 Punchbowl St, Rm 325
Honolulu, HI 96813
808-587-0163
808-587-0160 (fax)
norma.i.bustos@hawaii.gov

Daryl Howell
IADNR
Wallace State Office Bldg
502 E 9th St
Des Moines, IA 50319-0034
515-281-8524
daryl.howell@dnr.state.ia.us

Non-game Wildlife Program Manager
Dept of Fish & Game
Box 25
Boise, ID 83707-0025
208-334-2920

Brian Clark
Dept of Natural Resources
1 Natural Resources Way
Springfield, IL 62702-1271
217-782-6431
bclark@dnrmail.state.il.us

Linnea Petercheff
Operations Staff Specialist
Division of Fish and Wildlife
402 W Washington St, Rm W273
Indianapolis, IN 46204
317-233-6527
317-232-8150 (fax)
lpetercheff@dnr.i.gov

Wildlife Permit Officer
KS Dept of Wildlife & Parks
512 SE 25th Ave
Pratt, KS 67124-8174
620-672-5911

Wildlife Permit Coordinator
KY Dept of Fish & Wildlife Resources
#1 Sportsmans Lane
Frankfort, KY 40601
502-564-7109

Non-Game Wildlife Biologist
LA Dept of Wildlife and Fisheries
2000 Quail Dr
P.O. Box 98000
Baton Rouge, LA 70898-9000
225-763-3557
225-765-2452 (fax)

Dr. Tom French, Assistant Director
Heritage & Endangered Species
MA Wildlife Field Headquarters
North Drive
Westboro, MA 01581
508-792-7270 ext 163

Mary Goldie
DNR
580 Taylor Ave
Tawes State Office Bldg E-1
Annapolis, MD 21401
410-260-8540
http://www.dnr.state.md.us/wildlife/rehabpermit.asp

Susan Zayac
Dept of Inland Fish & Wildlife
284 State St Station #41
Augusta, ME 04333-0041
207-287-5240
susan.zayac@maine.gov

Wildlife Rehabilitation Permit Coordinator
MI Dept of Natural Resources
Law Enforcement Division
P.O. Box 30031
Lansing, MI 48909
517-373-1230

Nancy Huonder, Wildlife Rehab Program Coordinator
DNR Nongame Wildlife Program
500 Lafayette Rd, Box 25
St. Paul, MN 55155-4025
651-259-5108
nancy.huonder@drn.state.mn.us

Lynn Totten
Dept of Conservation
P.O. Box 180
Jefferson City, MO 65102-0180
573-522-4115 ext 3322

Richard G. Rummel
Dept of Wildlife, Fish & Parks
MS Museum of Nat Science
2148 Riverside Dr
Jackson, MS 39202-1353
601-354-7303 ext 109
richardr@mmns.state.ms.us

Wildlife Permit Coordinator
MT Fish, Wildlife & Parks
23 S Rodney
Helena, MT 59601

Tammy Minchew
Special Permits Coordinator
NC Wildlife Resources Commission
1724 Mail Service Center
Raleigh, NC 27699-1724
919-707-0060
919-707-0067 (fax)

Sandra Hagen
Non-game Biologist
ND Game & Fish Dept
100 N Bismarck Expressway
Bismarck, ND 58501-5095
701-328-5382
shagen@state.nd.us

Wildlife Permit Officer
Game & Parks Commission
105 W 2nd St Suite 201
Valentine, NE 69201

Sgt. Bruce Bonenfant
NH Fish and Game Dept
11 Hazen Dr
Concord, NH 03301
603-271-3127

Amy Wells
NJ Division of Fish & Wildlife
P.O. Box 400
Trenton, NJ 08625-0400
609-292-2965
amy.wells@dep.state.nj.us

Rhonda Holderman
Special Uses Permit Manager
NM Dept of Game and Fish
P.O. Box 25112
Santa Fe, NM 87504
505-476-8064
505-476-8166 (fax)
rhonda.holderman@state.nm.us

Julie Meadows, Program Officer 1
License Office-special licenses NV
Dept of Wildlife
4600 Kietzke Lane D-135
Reno, NV 89502
775-688-1512

Patrick P Martin
NYS Dept Env Conservation
625 Broadway
Albany, NY 12233-4752
518-402-8985
pxmartin@gw.dec.state.ny.us

Caroline Caldwell, Program Administrator
Wildlife Management & Research
Division of Wildlife
2045 Morse Rd, Bldg G
Columbus, OH 43229-6693
614-265-6330
carolin.caldwell@dnr.state.oh.us

Jim Edwards
Law Enforcement Division
OK Dept of Wildlife Conservation
P.O. Box 53465
Oklahoma City, OK 73152-3465
405-521-3719

Carol Turner
Wildlife Biologist
OR Dept Fish & Wildlife
3406 Cherry Ave NE
Salem, OR 97303
503-947-6318
503-974-6330 (fax)
joel.a.hurtado@state.or.us
www.dfw.state.or.us

Wildlife Permit Officer
PA Game Commission
2001 Elmerton Ave
Harrisburg, PA 17110-9797
717-783-8164

Lori Gibson
Wildlife Permit Officer
Division of Fish & Wildlife
277 Great Neck Rd
West Kingston, RI 02892
401-789-0281
lori.gibson@dem.ri.gov

Wildlife Permit Coordinator
Sandhills Research & Educ Center
P.O. Box 23205
Columbia, SC 29224-3205
803-419-9645

Wildlife Permit Officer
Game, Fish & Parts Dept
Division of Wildlife
412 W Missouri, Suite 4
Pierre, SD 57501
605-773-4191

Walter Cook
Captive Wildlife Coordinator
TWRA/Law Enforcement Division
P.O. Box 40747
Ellington Ag Center
Nashville, TN 37204
615-781-6647

Texas Parks and Wildlife
Nongame Permits Specialist
4200 Smith School Rd
Austin, TX 78744-3291
800-792-1112

DNR Division of Wildlife Resources
1594 W N Temple, Suite 2110
P.O. Box 146301
Salt Lake City, UT 84114-6301
801-538-4701

Diane Waller
VA Dept of Game & Inland Fisheries
P.O. Box 11104
Richmond, VA 23230-1104
804-367-9588

Judy Pierce
Division of Fish & Wildlife
6291 Estate Nazareth 101
St. Thomas, VI 00802-1104
340-775-6762

Law Enforcement Assistant
Agency of Natural Resources
Fish & Wildlife Dept
103 S Main, Ste 10
South Waterbury, VT 05671-0501
802-241-3727

Peggy Crain
Dept of Fish & Wildlife
600 Capitol Way N
Olympia, WA 98501-1091
360-902-2513
crainpsc@dfw.wa.gov

Wildlife Rehabilitation Liaison
DNR
Box 1721, WM/6
Madison, WI 53707-7921
608-267-6751
http://dnr.wi.gov/or/land/wildlife
Jennifer.haverty@dnr.state.wi.us

Wildlife Permit Officer
Division of Natural Resources
Wildlife Resources
1900 Kanawha Blvd
Bldg 3, Rm 816
Charleston, WV 25305
304-558-2771

WL Law Enforcement Coordinator
Game & Fish Dept
3030 Energy Lane
Casper, WY 82604
307-473-3400

CANADA PROVINCIAL AGENCIES (LISTINGS ARE ALPHABETICAL BY PROVINCE)

Ron Bjorge, Acting Executive Director
Wildlife Management Branch
Fish and Wildlife Division
Sustainable Resource Development
2nd Floor
9920-108 St
Edmonton, AB T5K 2M4
CANADA

Yvonne Foxall
Permit & Authorization Service Bureau
P.O. Box 9372 STN PROV GOVT
Victoria, BC
V8W 9M3
CANADA
http://www.env.gov.bc.ca/pasb

Dr. James R. Duncan, Manager
Biodiversity Conservation Section
Wildlife and Ecosystem Protection Branch
Manitoba Conservation
Box 24, 200 Saulteaux Crescent
Winnipeg, MB R3J 3W3
CANADA
204-945-7465 work
204-945-3077 (fax)
jduncan@gov.mb.ca
www.manitoba.ca/conservation/wildlife
http://web2.gov.mb.ca/conservation/cdc/

Gerard MacLellen
Environmental Monitoring and Compliance
P.O. Box 697
5151 Terminal Rd, 5th Floor
Halifax, NS B3J 2T8
CANADA
902-424-2547

Delbert Miller
Senior Fish & Wildlife Specialist, Aylmer District
Ministry of Natural Resources
615 John St N
Aylmer ON N5H 2S8
CANADA
519-773-4709
519-773-9014 (fax)
delbert.miller@ontario.ca

John Sullivan
Canadian Wildlife Service
465 Gideon Dr
P.O. Box 490 Lambeth Station
London, ON N6P 1R1
CANADA
519-472-5750

Tamara Gomer
Wildlife in Captivity Specialist
Policy and Program Development
Ontario Ministry of Natural Resources
300 Water St, 5th Floor N
Peterborough, ON K9J 8M5
CANADA
705-755-1999
tamara.gomer@mnr.gov.on.ca

Ministère des Ressources naturelles et de la Faune
Direction des territoires fauniques et de la réglementation
Édifice Bois-Fontaine—2e étage
880, chemin Sainte-Foy
Québec, PQ G1S 4X4
CANADA
418-627-8691
418-646-5179 (fax)

Ms Penny Lalonde
Saskatchewan Environment
Resource Stewardship Branch
2nd Floor
3211 Albert St
Regina, SK SKS 5W6
306-787-6218

U.S. STATE REHABILITATION ASSOCIATIONS (LISTINGS ARE ALPHABETICAL BY STATE ABBREVIATION)

California Council for Wildlife Rehabilitators (CCWR)
P.O. Box 434
Santa Rosa, CA 95402
415-541-5090
info@ccwr.org
www.ccwr.org

Colorado Council for Wildlife Rehabilitation (CCWR)
c/o Sigrid Ueblacker
R.R. 2 Box 659
Broomfield, CO 80020
303-665-5670

Connecticut Wildlife Rehabilitators Association, Inc. (CWRA)
P.O. Box 3556
Amity Station
New Haven, CT 06525
203-389-4411
info@cwrawildlife.org
www.cwrawildlife.org

Delaware Wildlife Rehabilitators Association (DWRA)
Robin Coventry, President
276 Cambridge Rd
Camden, DE 19934
302-698-1047
coventrybird@verizon.net

Florida Wildlife Rehabilitation Association (FWRA)
P.O. Box 1449
Anna Maria, FL 34216
941-778-6324
www.fwra.org

Iowa Wildlife Rehabilitators Association (IWRA)
Beth Brown, Treasurer
Box 217
Osceola, IA 50213
651-342-2783

Illinois Wildlife Rehabilitators Association (IWRA)
P.O. Box 28
Tremont, IL 61568
309-925-5321
309-922-3204
wildan@dpc.net

Louisiana Wildlife Rehabilitators Association (LAWRA)
P.O. Box 90201
Lafayette, LA 70509
www.lawraonline.com

Wildlife Rehabilitators' Association of Massachusetts, Inc. (WRAM)
62 Common St
Groton, MA 01450
978-448-2912

Maryland Wildlife Rehabilitators Association (MWRA)
c/o Roxy Brandenburg
6616 A Debold Rd
Sabillasville, MD 21780
410-255-4737
www.mwra.org

ReMaine Wild
P.O. Box 113
Newcastle, ME 04553

Minnesota Wildlife Assistance Cooperative (MWAC)
P.O. Box 130545
Roseville, MN 55113
info@mnwildlife.org
www.mnwildlife.com

Wildlife Rehabilitators of North Carolina (WRNC)
2542 Weymoth Rd
Winston-Salem, NC 27103

Wildlife Rehabilitators Association of New Hampshire (WRANH)
Ann McDermott, President
P.O. Box 1274
Lincoln, NH 03251
603-536-2592
admin@wranh.org

New Jersey Association of Wildlife Rehabilitators (NJAWR)
c/o Dave Purdy
24 Mountain Church Rd
Hopewell, NJ 08525

New York State Wildlife Rehabilitation Council (NYSWRC)
Kelly Martin, President
Box 246
Oswego, NY 13827
www.nyswrc.org
607-687-1584
brancher@clarityconnect.com

Ohio Wildlife Rehabilitators Association (OWRA)
c/o Betty Ross
175 RT 343
Yellow Springs, OH 45387-1895
937-767-7648
baross@antioch-college.edu
www.owra.org

Pennsylvania Association of Wildlife Rehabilitators (PAWR)
4991 Shimerville Rd
Emmaus, PA 18049-4955
570-739-4393
redcreekwildlife@comcast.net
www.pawr.com

Texas Wildlife Rehabilitators Association
P.O. Box 114
Cat Spring, TX 78933
Txhuff@aol.com

Wildlife Rehabilitation Association of Virginia (WRAV)
Robin Eastham, President
Portaferry Farm
Batesville, VA 22924
540-456-8324
540-456-8788 (fax)
robinjane@cstone.net

Wild In Vermont
Nancy J. Carey, President
P.O. Box 163
Underhill Center, VT 05490
802-899-1027

Washington Wildlife Rehabilitation Association (WWRA)
Shelley McGuire, President
14299 Rosario Rd
Anacortes, WA 98221
360-421-0914
shelley.mcguire@att.net

Wisconsin Wildlife Rehabilitators Association (WWRA)
South 3091 Oak Knoll Rd
Fall Creek, WI 54742
262-662-2224
wwra_org@yahoo.com

CANADA PROVINCIAL REHABILITATION ASSOCIATIONS (LISTINGS ARE ALPHABETICAL BY PROVINCE)

Bill Tomlinson, President
Alberta Wildlife Rehabilitators Association (AWRA)
P.O. Box 79113
70-1020 Sherwood Dr
Sherwood Park, AB T8A 2QA
CANADA
a_w_r_a@hotmail.com

Liz Thunstrom, Vice President
Wildlife Rehabilitators' Network of British Columbia (WRNBC)
1388 Cambridge Dr
Coquitlam, BC V3J 2P7
CANADA
604-939-9571
www.wrn.bc.ca

OWREN (Ontario Wildlife Rehabilitation and Education Network)
40—1110 Finch Ave W, Ste 1071
Toronto, ON M3J 3M2
CANADA
905-735-6885 (fax)
info@owren-online.org
www.owren-online.org

ZOO AND AVICULTURE RESOURCES

American Federation of Aviculture (AFA)
www.afabirds.org

American Zoo and Aquarium Association
www.aza.org

Avicultural Society of America (ASA)
Membership Secretary
P.O. Box 5516, Riverside, CA 92517-5516.
www.asabirds.org

National Finch & Softbill Society (NFSS)
Membership
7421 Whistlestop Dr
Austin, TX 78749
www.nfss.org

Organization of Professional Aviculturists, Inc. (OPA)
OPA Membership
P.O. Box 927
Littleton, NC 27850-0927
www.proaviculture.com

Appendix II Energy Requirements for Growing Birds

GENERAL INFORMATION

See Tables A2.1 and A2.2 for energy requirements of growing birds. Sick and injured young birds have extremely high energy requirements but may have a reduced capacity to metabolize food. In such cases, growth may be delayed while healing occurs. Caregivers should provide the chick with as much ample high-quality diet as it is able to digest. Energy needs change daily in rapidly growing chicks.

CALCULATIONS

- Passerine Bird Basal Metabolic Rate (BMR) = body weight in $kgs^{0.75} \times 129$
- Non-passerine Bird Basal Metabolic Rate (BMR) = body weight in $kgs^{0.75} \times 78$
- Maintenance Energy Requirement (MER) in kcal/day = BMR × 1.5
- Adjustment for Growth = MER × 1.5–3.0
- Adjustment for Sepsis = MER × 1.2–1.5
- Adjustment for Mild Injury = MER × 1.0–1.2
- Adjustment for Severe Injury = MER × 1.1–2.0

Source: Carpenter J.W., ed. 2005. Exotic Animal Formulary, Third Edition. Elsevier Saunders, St. Louis, p 559.

Table A2.1. Energy requirements of passerine chicks.

Body Weight (grams)	Basal Metabolic Rate (BMR)	Maintenance Energy Requirement (MER) in kcal/Day	Kilocalories per Day for Growth when Healthy
2	1.2	1.8	2.7–5.5
4	2.1	3.1	4.6–9.2
6	2.8	4.2	6.3–12.5
10	4.1	6.1	9.2–18.4
12	4.7	7.0	10.5–21.0
14	5.3	7.9	11.8–23.6
16	5.8	8.7	13.1–26.1
18	6.3	9.5	14.3–28.5
20	6.9	10.3	15.4–30.9
25	8.1	12.2	18.2–36.5
30	9.3	13.9	20.9–41.8
35	10.4	15.7	23.5–47.0
40	11.5	17.3	26.0–51.9
45	12.6	18.9	28.4–56.7
50	13.6	20.5	30.7–61.4
60	15.6	23.5	35.2–70.4
70	17.6	26.3	39.5–79.0
80	19.4	29.1	43.7–87.3
90	21.2	31.8	47.7–95.4
100	22.9	34.4	51.6–103.2
120	26.3	39.5	59.2–118.4
140	29.5	44.3	66.4–132.9
160	32.6	49.0	73.4–146.9

Table A2.2. Energy requirements of non-passerine chicks.

Body Weight (grams)	Basal Metabolic Rate (BMR)	Maintenance Energy Requirement (MER) in kcal/Day	Kilocalories per Day for Growth when Healthy
30	6.3	9.4	14–29
40	7.8	11.7	18–35
50	9.2	13.8	21–41
60	10.5	15.8	24–48
70	11.8	17.8	27–53
80	13.1	19.6	29–59
90	14.3	21.4	32–64
100	15.5	23.2	35–70
120	17.7	26.6	40–80
140	19.9	29.9	45–90
160	22.0	33.0	50–99
180	24.0	36.1	54–108
200	26.0	39.0	59–117
225	28.4	42.6	64–128
250	30.8	46.1	69–138
275	33.0	49.6	74–149
300	35.3	52.9	79–159
350	39.6	59.4	89–178
400	43.8	65.6	99–197
450	47.8	71.7	107–215
500	51.7	77.6	116–233
600	59.3	89.0	133–267
700	66.6	99.9	150–300
800	73.6	110.4	166–331
900	80.4	120.6	181–362
1000	87.0	130.5	196–392
1250	102.8	154.3	231–463
1500	117.9	176.9	265–531
1750	132.4	198.6	298–596
2000	146.3	219.5	329–658
2500	173.0	259.5	389–778
3000	198.3	297.5	446–892

Appendix III
Resources for Products Mentioned

DIETS AND DIETARY SUPPLEMENTS

Cyclop-eeze, Argent Chemical Laboratory, 8702 152nd Ave. N.E., Redmond, WA 98052, (800) 426-6258, www.argent-labs.com.

Dried egg products: John Oleksy Inc., P.O. Box 34137, Chicago, IL 60634, (888) 677–3447, www.eggstore.com.

Dried egg yolk and eggs: Honeyville Grain Inc., 11600 Dayton Drive, Rancho Cucamonga, CA 91730, (888) 810-3212 ext. 107, www.honeyvillegrain.com.

Gerber Products Co. Fremont, MI 49413, www.gerber.com.

Hagen: 50 Hampden Rd, Mansfield, MA 02048, (800) 225-2700, www.hagen.com.

Harrison's Bird Diets: 7108 Crossroads Blvd, Suite 325, Brentwood, TN 37027, (800) 346-0269, www.harrisonsbirdfoods.com.

Kaytee Exact Hand Feeding Formula and Kaytee exact Rainbow pellets: Kaytee Products Inc., 521 Clay St., Chilton, WI 53014, (800) Kaytee-1 or (920) 849-2321, www.kaytee.com.

Kit and Kaboodle cat food: Purina Mills, Nestlé Purina PetCare Company, Checkerboard Square, St. Louis, MO 63164, (314) 982-1000, www.purina.com.

Lafeber Company, 24981 North East Rd, Cornell, IL 61319, (800) 842-6445, www.lafeber.com.

Layena: Purina Mills, 555 Maryville University Drive, St. Louis, MO 63141, (800) 227-8941, www.purinamills.com.

Lory life Pre-Mix Nectar Diet: Avico, Cuttlebone Plus, 810 North Twin Oaks Valley Rd, #131, San Marcos, CA 92069, (760) 591-4951 or (800) 747-9878, www.cuttleboneplus.com.

Mazuri Flamingo Complete, ZuLiFe Soft-Bill Diet, and Maintenance Primate Biscuit (low protein): Mazuri, P.O. Box 66812, St. Louis, MO 63166, (800) 227-8941, www.mazuri.com.

Nekton products: www.nekton.de.

Nutri-cal: Vetoquinol USA/Evsco Pharmaceuticals, 101 Lincoln Ave., Buena, NJ 08310, (800) 267-5707.

Pretty Bird International, Inc., P.O. Box 177, Stacy, MN 55079, (800) 356-5020, www.prettypets.com.

Purina Mills Poultry Diets: 2005. SunFresh Recipe Products Index Page. St. Louis, MO, www.rabbitnutrition.com/flock/index.html.

Rainbow Landing, P.O. Box 462845, Escondido, CA 92046-2845, (800) 229-1946, lorynectar@earthlink.net.

Rodents (frozen): LLLReptile and Supply Company Inc., 609 Mission Ave, Oceanside, CA 92054, (760) 439-8492, www.lllreptile.com.

Roudybush: Box 908, Templeton, CA 93465-0908, (800) 326-1726, www.roudybush.com.

STAT high calorie liquid diet: PRN Pharmacal, Inc., Pensacola, FL 32504, www.prnpharmacal.com.

SuperRich Yeast (not "brewers yeast"): Twin Laboratories, 50 Motor Parkway, Suite 210, Hauppauge, NY 11788.

Vital HN (hydrolyzed protein enteric diet powder): Ross Products, (800) 258-7677, a division of Abbott Laboratories, Abbott Park, IL. Vital HN may be obtained in single packages from Chris's Squirrels and More (860) 749-1129, (877) 717-7748.

Zupreem Low Iron Softbill Diet: Zupreem, P.O. Box 9024, Mission, KS 66202, 10504 W. 79th St. Shawnee, KS 66214 (800) 345-4767, www.zupreem.com.

Invertebrate Food

Arbico Organics: P.O. Box 8910, Tucson, AZ 85738-0910, (800) 827-2847.

Biconet, 5116 Williamsburg Rd, Brentwood, TN 37027, (800) 441-BUGS, www.biconet.com.

Fluker Farms, 1333 Plantation Ave, Port Allen, LA 70767-4087, (800) 735-8537, www.flukerfarms.com.

Rainbow Mealworms, 126 E. Spruce St, Compton, CA 90220, (800) 777-9676. https://www.rainbowmealworms.net/home.asp.

DISINFECTANTS

Betadine: Purdue Pharma L.P., Stamford, CT, (800) 877-5666, (203) 588-8000, www.pharma.com.

Nolvasan: Fort Dodge, Wyeth, 5 Giralda Farms, Madison, NJ 07940, (800) 533-8536, www.wyeth.com.

EGG MONITORING DEVICES AND CANDLING DEVICES

Egg Buddy (Egg monitoring device): Avian Biotech International, 1336 Timberlane Rd, Tallahassee, FL 32312-1766, (850) 386-1145, (800) 514-9672, www.avianbiotech.com/buddy.htm.

Egg Candlers: Lyon Technologies, Inc., 1690 Brandywine Ave, Chula Vista, CA 91911, (888)596-6872, www.lyonelectric.com.

FEEDING NEEDLES, TUBES, SYRINGES, AND NIPPLES

ACES Animal Care Equipment and Services, Inc., 4920-F Fox St, Denver, CO 80216, (303) 296-9287 (worldwide), (800) 338-2237 (North America), (303) 298-8894 (fax), www.animal-care.com.

Catac nipples: Catac Products Limited, Catac House, 1 Newnham St, Bedford Mk40 3jr England, +44 (0) 1234 360116 (tel), +44 (0) 1234 346406 (fax), www.catac.co.uk. Also available from Chris's Squirrels and More, LLC, P.O. Box 365, Somers CT 06071, (860) 749-1129, www.squirrelsandmore.com.

Feeding Tube and Urethral Catheter available from Tyco Healthcare/Kendall, (800) 962-9888, www.kendallhq.com. Sizes 8 through 18 French.

Syringes with catheter tip available from Tyco Healthcare/Kendall, (800) 962-9888, www.kendallhq.com. Monoject, 60 ml.

Teat Cannula (Jorgensen Laboratories Inc.) and O-Ring syringes, www.squirrelsandmore.com.

FURNISHING AND HOUSING ITEMS

Astroturf, Solutia Inc, P.O. Box 66760, St. Louis, MO 63166-6760, (800) 723 8873, www.astroturfmats.com.

Netting: Nylon Net Company, 845 N Main St, Memphis, TN 38107, (800) 238-7529.

Netting: Christensen Net Works, 5510 A Nielsen Ave, Ferndale, WA 98248, (800) 459-2147.

Pet Carriers: Petmate, P.O. Box 1246, Arlington, TX 76004-1246, (877) 738-6283, www.petmate.com/Catalog.plx.

Pet Screen, Phifer Inc., P.O. Box 1700, Tuscaloosa, AL 35403-1700, (205) 345-2120, www.phifer.com.

Portapet-Cardboard Pet Carrier 24″ × 12″ × 18″: UPCO, 3705 Pear St, St. Joseph, MO 64503, (800) 254-8726, www.UPCO.com, Item #60000.

Reptarium screen enclosures: LLLReptile and Supply Company Inc., 609 Mission Ave, Oceanside, CA 92054, (760) 439-8492, www.lllreptile.com.

Reptarium screen enclosures: Dallas Manufacturing Company Inc., 4215 McEwen Rd, Dallas, TX 75244, (800) 256-8669.

Rubber pans and tubs: Fortex Fortiflex (800) 468-4460, www.fortexfortiflex.com/rubberpans.html.

Sisal Rope (natural fiber rope): LeHigh, 2834 Schoeneck Rd, Macungie, PA 18062, (610) 966-9702, www.Lehighgroup.com.

Suet Baskets: Arcata Pet Supplies, www.arcatapet.com, (877) 237-9488, item #1472.

INCUBATORS, HATCHERS, BROODERS, AND HEATING PADS

Incubators, Brooders, and Contact Incubation Systems (Contaq X3): Lyon Technologies, Inc., 1690 Brandywine Ave, Chula Vista, CA 91911, (888) 596-6872, www.lyonelectric.com.

Brinsea Octagon TLC-4: Brinsea Products Inc., 704 N. Dixie Ave, Titusville, FL 32796, (888) 667-7009.

Heating pads available from Gaymar Industries, Inc., (716) 662-2551, (716) 662-8636 (international), www.gaymar.com.

Portable Brooder, Dean's Animal Supply, P.O. Box 701172, St. Cloud, FL 34770, (407) 891-8030, www.thebrooder.com.

ThermoCare Portable ICS Units: ThermoCare Inc., P.O. Box 6069, Incline Village, NV 89450, (800) 262-4020, www.thermocare.com.

REHYDRATION SOLUTIONS

Pedialyte: Abbott Laboratories, 100 Abbott Park Rd, Abbott Park, IL 60064-3500, (847) 937-6100, www.abbott.com.

Ross Consumer Products Division, Abbott Laboratories, 625 Cleveland Ave, Columbus, OH 43215, (800) 227-5767, http://www.pedialyte.com.

RECORD-KEEPING AND IDENTIFICATION AIDS

Leg bands: National Band and Tag Company, 721 York St, Newport, KY 41072-0430, (800) 261-TAGS (8247).

Leg bands: Red Bird Products P.O. Box 376, Mt. Aukum, CA 95656, (530) 620-7440, www.redbirdproducts.com.

Computer Program: Minitab Inc., Quality Plaza, 1829 Pine Hall Rd, State College, PA 16801-3008, (814) 238-3280, www.minitab.com.

SCALES

American Weigh Scales Inc., 1836 Ashley River Rd, Suite 320, Charleston, SC 29407, (866) 643-3444.

Lyon Technologies, Inc., 1690 Brandywine Ave, Chula Vista, CA 91911, (888) 596-6872, www.lyonelectric.com.

Pelouze Scales, Rubbermaid Commercial Products, 3124 Valley Ave, Winchester, VA 22601, (800) 950-9787, (888) 761-8574, www.pelouze.com.

VETERINARY SUPPLIES

Antibiotics and Antifungal drugs and Vaccines

Carnidazole (Spartrix): Janssen Animal Health, available in the U.S.A. through Global Pigeon Supply, 2301 Rowland Ave, Savannah, GA 31404, (800) 562-2295, www.globalpigeon.com. or Jedds, 1165 North Red Gum, Anaheim, CA 92806, (800) 659-5928, www.jedds.com.

Lasix: Aventis (Sanofi-Aventis): 300 Somerset Corporate Blvd, Bridgewater, NJ 08807-2854, (800) 981-2491, (800) 207-8049, http://products.sanofi-aventis.us/lasix/lasix.html.

Nystatin: Bristol Myers Squibb, 345 Park Ave, New York, NY 10154-0037, (212) 546-4000, www.bms.com.

Roche Pharmaceuticals, Hoffman-La Roche, Inc., 340 Kingsland St, Nutley, NJ 07110, (973) 235-5000, www.rocheusa.com/products/rocephin/pi.pdf.

Toltrazuril (Baycox): Bayer Animal Health, available in the U.S.A. through Global Pigeon Supply, 2301 Rowland Ave, Savannah, GA 31404, (800) 562-2295, www.globalpigeon.com.

Trimethoprim-sulfamethoxazole (Septra): King Pharmaceuticals, Bristol, TN 37620, (888) 840-5370, www.kingpharm.com.

West Nile Virus Vaccine: Fort Dodge Animal Health, West Nile Vaccine Product Manager, P.O. Box 25945, Overland Park, KS 66225-5945, (800) 477-1365 (U.S.A.), (800) 267-1777 (Canada), www.equinewestnile.com/index.htm.

Bandaging, Splint, and Wound Products

BioDres: DVM Pharmaceuticals, Subsidiary of IVAX Corporation, 4400 Biscayne Blvd, Miami, FL 33137, (305) 575-6000.

Op-site Flexifix dressing: Smith & Nephew, Inc., 11775 Starkey Rd, P.O. Box 1970, Largo, FL 33779-1970, (800) 876-1261, www.opsitepostop.com/

SAM Splint: SAM Medical Products, 7100 SW Hampton St, Ste 217, Portland, OR 97223, (800) 818-4726.

Tegaderm and Vetrap: 3M, 3M Center, St. Paul, MN 55144-1000, (888) 364-3577.

Vetrap (3M) available from Jeffers, (800) 533-3377, www.jefferspet.com. Sizes: 2″ wide × 5 yards and 4″ wide × 5 yards.

Parasite Control

Kelthane miticide: Dow AgroSciences LLC, 9330 Zionsville Rd, Indianapolis, IN 46268, (317) 337-3000.

Sevin Dust: GardenTech, P.O. Box 24830, Lexington, KY 40524-4830, (800) 969-7200.

Ultracare Mite and Lice Bird Spray: 8 in 1 Pet Products, Hauppauge, New York, (800) 645-5154.

VITAMIN AND MINERAL SUPPLEMENTS

Avi-Con: Lloyd, Inc., P.O. Box 130 Shenandoah, IA 51601, (800) 831-0004.

Avi-Era Avian Vitamins: Lafeber Company, Cornell IL 61319, (800) 842-6445, www.lafeber.com.

Avimin: Lambert-Kay, Cranbury, NJ 08512 (available in many pet stores).

Calcium Carbonate Powder (1 kg bottles): Life Extension Foundation, P.O. Box 229120, Hollywood, FL 33022, (800) 544-4440, www.lef.org.

Calcium Carbonate USP Precipitated Light: manufactured by PCCA, 9901 S. Wilcrest, Houston, TX 77099, (800) 331-2498, www.pccarx.com, Item# 30-1944-500.

Mazuri Auklet Vitamin Mix (5M25-3M): Mazuri, 1050 Progress Drive, Richmond, IN 47374, (800) 227-8941, www.mazuri.com, Product information at: www.mazuri.com/PDF/52M5.pdf.

Mazuri Vita-Zu Bird Tablet (5M25): Mazuri, 1050 Progress Drive, Richmond, IN 47374, (800) 227-8941, www.mazuri.com, Product information at www.mazuri.com/Home.asp?Products=2&Opening=2.

Quikon Multivitamin: Orchid Tree Exotics, 2388 County Rd EF, Swanton, OH 43558, (866) 412-5275, www.sunseed.com.

SeaTabs: Pacific Research Laboratories, El Cajon, CA.

Superpreen: Aracata Pet Supplies, (800) 822-9085, www.arcatapet.com, item #'s 835-837.

Vionate powder: Rich Health Inc., Irvine, CA.

Index